Bottom Line's
HEALTH
BREAKTHROUGHS 2016

**Bottom Line
Books**
www.MyBottomLine.com

10 9 8 7 6 5 4 3 2 1

ISBN 0-88723-733-9

Health**Day**

Selected articles in this book were written by reporters for HealthDay, an award-winning international
daily consumer health news service, headquartered in Norwalk, Connecticut.

Bottom Line Books® publishes the advice of expert authorities in many fields.
These opinions may at times conflict as there are often different approaches to solving problems.
The use of this material is no substitute for health, legal, accounting or other professional services.
Consult competent professionals for answers to your specific questions.

Telephone numbers, addresses, prices, offers and websites listed in this book are accurate
at the time of publication, but they are subject to frequent change.

Bottom Line Books® is a registered trademark of Boardroom® Inc.
281 Tresser Boulevard, Stamford, Connecticut 06901

www.MyBottomLine.com

Bottom Line Books® is an imprint of Boardroom® Inc., publisher of print periodicals,
e-letters and books. We are dedicated to bringing you the best information from the most
knowledgeable sources in the world. Our goal is to help you gain greater wealth,
better health, more wisdom, extra time and increased happiness.

Printed in the United States of America

Contents

3 • BRAIN HEALTH

4 • CANCER

5 • CONSUMER HEALTH ALERTS

6 • DIABETES

7 • DIET, NUTRITION AND FITNESS

Contents

Contents

19 • WOMEN'S HEALTH

Preface

We are proud to bring you the all-new *Bottom Line's Health Breakthroughs 2016*. This collection represents a year's worth of the latest health news and scientific discoveries in a broad spectrum of fields.

When you choose a Bottom Line book, you are turning to a stellar group of experts in a wide range of specialties—medical doctors, alternative practitioners, renowned nutrition experts, research scientists and consumer-health advocates, to name a few.

We go to great lengths to interview the foremost health experts. Whether it's cancer prevention, breakthrough arthritis treatments or cutting-edge nutritional advice, our editors talk to the true innovators in health care.

How do we find all these top-notch professionals? Over the past 40 years, we have built a network of leading physicians in both alternative and conventional medicine. They are affiliated with the world's premier medical institutions. We follow the medical research, and with the help of our partner HealthDay, an award-winning service that reports on evidence-based health news, we bring the latest information to our readers. We also regularly talk with our advisers in teaching hospitals, private practices and government health agencies.

Bottom Line's Health Breakthroughs 2016 is a result of our ongoing research and contact with these experts, and is a distillation of their latest findings and advice. We hope that you will enjoy the presentation and glean helpful information about the health topics that concern you and your family.

As a reader of a Bottom Line book, please be assured that you are receiving reliable and well-researched information from a trusted source. But, please use prudence in health matters. Always speak to your physician before taking vitamins, supplements or over-the-counter medication... changing your diet...or beginning an exercise program. If you experience side effects from any regimen, contact your doctor immediately.

The Editors, Bottom Line Books, Stamford, Connecticut.

Allergies, Asthma and Respiratory Conditions

How Cooking Oil with the Right Vitamin E Can Help You Breathe

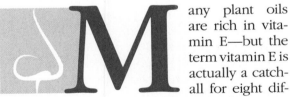

Many plant oils are rich in vitamin E—but the term vitamin E is actually a catchall for eight different chemical compounds, each with its own antioxidant profile. And the problem is that we may be getting way too much of one certain type of vitamin E that's not good for us.

WHAT'S IN YOUR OIL?

We know from animal experiments that a type of vitamin E called D-alpha tocopherol and another type called D-gamma tocopherol have completely opposite effects on lung function…one good, the other bad. Never mind animals…what about the effects in people? A team of researchers from the Feinberg School of Medicine at Northwestern University in Chicago and other universities compared blood levels of vitamin E against the results of lung-function tests (which measure how much air a person can exhale in one big breath) of more than 4,500 people. *And the researchers confirmed that these two different vitamin Es—D-alpha tocopherol and D-gamma tocopherol—have the different effects…*

•**D-gamma tocopherol was associated with worse lung function for everyone,** and the higher the level, the worse the lung function.

•**D-alpha tocopherol was associated with better lung function for everyone. The study also showed that increases in D-alpha tocopherol could counteract the effects of D-gamma tocopherol.**

What's behind this? It seems that D-alpha tocopherol inhibits allergic inflammation—that is, inflammation that is set off by allergies—while D-gamma tocopherol promotes allergic

Joan M. Cook-Mills, PhD, professor of medicine, department of allergy/immunology, Feinberg School of Medicine, Northwestern University, Chicago. Her study was published in *Respiratory Research*.

inflammation. Sometimes your body wants and needs temporary inflammation, for example, to help isolate causes of tissue injury, such as bacteria and toxins. But a steady diet (literally!) of a substance that enhances inflammation—even if it is a vitamin—is going to hurt you. Another recent study found that too much D-gamma tocopherol in the body can aggravate osteoarthritis—so its effects aren't limited to the lungs but, in all likelihood, extend anywhere that inflammation can develop.

BREATHING EASIER

You are what you eat, they say, and it's becoming clearer that Europeans, for example, may breathe easier than Americans in part because they have two to six times less D-gamma tocopherol in their bodies than American adults do—and the main reason is that Europeans use more olive oil or safflower oil, which are low in D-gamma tocopherol and high in D-alpha tocopherol. Americans, on the other hand, consume more soy, corn and canola oils, which are very high in D-gamma tocopherol.

So, even if you never get asthma or another disease that compromises your ability to breathe, the evidence suggests that you can help your lungs be healthier and stronger and naturally breathe better by making some very simple food choices.

HOW TO GO
FOR MORE D-ALPHA

Cooking oils that are richer in D-alpha than D-gamma tocopherol include olive, sunflower and safflower, which can replace soy, corn and canola oils. Sunflower seeds, hazelnuts, almonds and wheat germ are also rich in D-alpha tocopherol. What about vitamin E supplements? Some contain only D-alpha tocopherol, some only D-gamma tocopherol, and some a mixture of the two types. If you want to take a supplement, consult with a doctor specifically trained in nutrition (a naturopathic doctor or a chiropractic doctor)—or a nutrition specialist (registered dietician).

Allergy Drops: Pain-Free Help for Allergy Sufferers

Michael L. Lewin, MD, faculty member, Weill-Cornell Medical College, New York City, and allergist in private practice, Wilton, Connecticut, and New York City. *Lewin Allergy.com*

If you've been getting allergy shots to control your allergy symptoms—or if you've avoided shots because of the pain and hassle but hate living with the runny nose, itchy eyes and wheezing—you'll be happy to know about an alternative that has long been used in Europe and is finally gaining popularity in the US. It's called sublingual (under the tongue) immunotherapy, aka allergy drops.

In addition to being a pain-free, do-it-at-home treatment, allergy drops have other advantages over shots. *Here's how they work and why they're worth considering...*

HOW DROPS DO THE JOB

Immunotherapy works by desensitizing the body to a particular allergen (allergy-producing substance) that it perceives as a threat, whether that allergen is ragweed or dog dander or something else. Subcutaneous immunotherapy (allergy shots) is one form of immunotherapy... sublingual immunotherapy is another.

Allergy drops are customized for each patient based on the results of allergy testing. The liquid extract that's used contains a very small amount of one particular allergen or of multiple allergens. Gradually, in incremental amounts, the allergen dosage is increased, enabling the body to build up tolerance. Over time, as the treatment calms the immune system's reaction to the allergen, symptoms are reduced or prevented altogether.

Which allergies can be eased: Allergy drops can replace shots for a wide range of allergens, including those related to cats...dogs...dust mites...cockroaches...molds...grasses...ragweed...trees...and others. In addition, drops can treat some allergies that shots can't treat, including those to poison ivy...formalin (a preservative used in many fragrances, cleaning products, textiles and adhesives)...and even some foods, including peanuts and milk.

Note: Bee sting allergies can be treated only by injection, not with drops.

Allergy drop evidence: Many dozens of studies conducted in Europe have demonstrated allergy drops' benefits, and now researchers in the US are finding similar positive results...

• In a review of 63 studies involving 5,131 patients, researchers from The Johns Hopkins University School of Medicine found moderate-to-strong evidence for significant improvement of asthma symptoms, runny/stuffy nose and eye inflammation among patients using sublingual immunotherapy for a wide range of allergies.

• A study published in *The Journal of Allergy and Clinical Immunology* found allergy drops effective in reducing symptoms and the need for allergy medication in patients allergic to ragweed, one of the most common allergens.

• A study that dealt with peanut allergy was particularly promising, given that accidental peanut ingestion can be fatal for people who are highly allergic. Published in *The Journal of Allergy and Clinical Immunology*, it reported that 70% of participants who received allergy drops for 44 weeks were able to tolerate at least 10 times as much peanut powder without developing symptoms as they could before treatment began.

In the US, the FDA approves specific antigens (substances that stimulate the production of antibodies)—and these antigens are the active ingredients in extracts used for allergy shots. It is legal for doctors to prescribe these same antigens "off-label" in the sublingual formulations used for allergy drops.

DROPS VERSUS SHOTS

The main question for many allergy sufferers is this—Do drops work as well as shots? Unfortunately, we don't yet have a clear answer to this due to a shortage of high-quality, head-to-head comparison studies. Among the limited studies that do exist, some find shots to be somewhat more effective...others rate the two therapies about the same. The World Health Organization endorses sublingual immunotherapy—and in my own practice, where I administer both shots and drops, I have found both methods effective.

Allergy drops do have some distinct advantages over injections...

• **Convenience.** You can administer the drops to yourself at home instead of having to go to the doctor's office.

Caveat: You do have to remember to take the drops every day—whereas shots generally are given only every one to four weeks.

• **Comfort.** Unlike shots, which hurt and may leave red, tender lumps that linger for a day or more, drops involve no discomfort and taste pleasant.

• **Speedy relief.** Drops start to work much faster than shots do. Injection immunotherapy generally requires about a year of treatment before significant improvement in symptoms is experienced, where as most of our drops patients see significant improvement within several months of beginning treatment.

• **Seasonal option.** For seasonal allergies—trees, grasses and ragweed—there is a preseasonal drops protocol that allows patients to experience relief with just a six-week course of sublingual immunotherapy each year. Patients start taking daily drops in late February or early March for tree allergies...in April for grass allergies...and in July for ragweed allergies. This preseasonal therapy is administered prior to the emergence of the seasonal pollens and is discontinued once those pollens emerge. In contrast, shots are taken all year, even for seasonal allergies.

Important: For nonseasonal environmental allergies—dust, molds, animal dander, etc.—drops, like shots, generally are taken year-round.

• **Long-lasting effects.** With both shots and drops, treatment typically continues for three to five years, after which many patients are able to discontinue treatment. For some patients, the relief is permanent...for others, symptoms return years later, at which point treatment can resume. For a small minority of patients, continuous treatment is needed to keep symptoms under control. The possibility does exist for allergies to return fairly quickly after discontinuing treatment, but this appears to occur less frequently with allergy drops than with shots.

• **Safety.** Allergy injections can trigger a rare but potentially life-threatening allergic reaction known as anaphylaxis. This is why a patient receiving allergy shots typically needs to wait in the doctor's office for 30 minutes after an injection, to make sure that no adverse reaction occurs. In contrast, current studies indicate that there have been no reports of anaphylactic reactions to allergy drops. That's why patients can safely take the drops on their own at home. Side effects of allergy drops generally are limited to occasional, temporary and mild throat irritation, itchy tongue and/or swollen lips.

Very important: Neither allergy drops nor shots are appropriate treatments for acute allergy attacks, and they cannot be substituted for a rescue inhaler, EpiPen or other emergency treatment.

• **What about cost?** Insurance policies in the US generally do not cover allergy drops, nor does Medicare. If your insurance covers shots but not drops, it may be cheaper for you to get shots, depending on your copay. However, if you are paying out of pocket, drops provide a significant cost savings because they require far fewer doctor visits. Patients receiving drops generally need only about four visits per year, while patients getting shots typically need from 13 to 52 visits per year. As for the cost of the extract itself, the antigens for drop formulations cost significantly less than for shots.

Are you intrigued by the idea of escaping allergy shots and giving allergy drops a try? You can find allergists in your area by checking the directory of the American Academy of Allergy, Asthma and Immunology at its website, *aaaai. org*. To learn whether a particular physician uses sublingual immunotherapy, you'll need to contact his/her office…but the trend is that an increasing number of allergists in the US are offering allergy drops to patients who are happy to put their painful shots behind them.

Natural Hay Fever Self-Defense

Jamison Starbuck, ND, naturopathic physician in family practice and a guest lecturer at the University of Montana, both in Missoula. She is past president of the American Association of Naturopathic Physicians and a contributing editor to *The Alternative Advisor: The Complete Guide to Natural Therapies and Alternative Treatments.*

If you're suffering from hay fever, most doctors will send you straight to the drugstore to pick up one of the dozens of medicines that are designed to treat allergy symptoms. But what if you could prevent your hay fever before it ever takes hold?

Well, that's where my natural spring allergy prevention protocol comes in. If you start following the regimen below sometime in March or early April, you've got a much better chance of being stronger and more resilient when the pollen really starts flying in many parts of the US. All of these remedies can be continued throughout allergy season, though you may be able to reduce your dose if you're not having symptoms.

My natural hay fever–fighting defense regimen…*

• **Flavonoids.** These compounds, which are found in fruits (especially citrus and berries) and vegetables, help strengthen your nasal membranes. To prevent allergies, it's crucial to keep irritating particles, such as pollen, from entering your bloodstream through the membranes of your upper-respiratory tract. Quercetin and hesperidin are my favorite flavonoids for allergy prevention.

Typical hay fever–fighting dose: 300 mg of a product that combines quercetin and hesperidin, four times a day.

• **Stinging nettle.** Like flavonoids, nettle helps by strengthening your defenses against the attack of allergens. Unless you are allergic to the plant itself (it grows in the wild in many parts of the US and is in the Urticaceae family),

---

*The remedies here are safe to take with conventional allergy medicine if needed, but check first with your doctor if you take other medications, such as blood thinners—these supplements could interact. If symptoms persist, see your doctor for advice.

Better Care for Allergies

Stress doesn't cause allergy attacks, but it can make them worse, a recent study reports.

Details: Among 179 allergy patients, those who had higher stress levels (as measured by daily online diaries) had more frequent flare-ups.

Why: Stress can disrupt the endocrine and immune systems, which could contribute to allergy episodes.

To reduce stress: Try positive thinking… eat right…get plenty of sleep…exercise regularly—and see a therapist, if necessary.

William Malarkey, MD, associate director, Institute for Behavioral Medicine Research, The Ohio State University, Columbus.

nettle is safe. Commonly known as one of "nature's best antihistamines," it also contains lots of flavonoids, is rich in minerals and fights inflammation. You can purchase this herb in capsules, tincture and as a dried herbal tea.

Typical hay fever–fighting dose: Two capsules or 60 drops of tincture in two ounces of water, three times a day, away from meals to increase absorption. If you prefer tea, use two teaspoons of dried nettle leaf per 10 ounces of water and steep, covered, for five minutes. Drink 24 ounces a day.

•**Pantothenic acid (vitamin B-5).** This vitamin plays a key role in the synthesis of the adrenal steroid hormones that fight inflammation and allergic reactivity.

Typical hay fever–fighting dose: 100 mg per day, taken in the morning with food when adrenal activity is highest.

•**Omega oils.** You might already be taking omega-3 fatty acids—it's widely known that they are good for the heart and brain and may even help prevent certain types of cancer. But few people realize that these healthful fats are also necessary to maintain healthy respiratory membranes. Omega oils help strengthen your immune system's resistance to perceived threats, including pollen.

Typical hay fever–fighting dose: At least 1,700 mg of fish, flax or borage oil daily. For best absorption, take this supplement with a meal.

Is It Really Sinusitis?

Murray Grossan, MD, an otolaryngologist and head-and-neck surgeon with the Tower Ear, Nose and Throat Clinic at Cedars-Sinai Medical Center in Los Angeles. He is author of *Free Yourself from Sinus and Allergy Problems Permanently.* GrossanInstitute.com

Don't assume that it's merely a bad cold when you're stuffed up and feeling lousy for more than the usual seven to 10 days. It could be something worse—and much harder to get rid of. It could be sinusitis.

Sinusitis is a condition where the nasal passages become inflamed and swollen. It's usually caused by a cold, but it could be triggered by allergies or a bacterial or fungal infection.

Here's how to tell if you have sinusitis and what to do about it if you do…

STEP 1: MAKE THE DIAGNOSIS

Long-lasting congestion, accompanied by tenderness around the eyes, forehead and/or cheeks, is the hallmark of sinusitis. Mucus will probably be yellow or greenish rather than clear.

Sinusitis can persist for weeks, months or even years. Colds never last that long. Another hint is when you get sick. If your symptoms are predictable—they occur only in the spring or summer, for example, or when you eat certain foods—you might have sinusitis triggered by allergies.

Most people with sinusitis have slow-moving cilia, microscopic filaments in the respiratory tract that propel mucus out through the nose or down the back of the throat. After an allergy or a cold, the cilia slow down. Also, some people with certain conditions such as cystic fibrosis have chronic slow-moving cilia. Impaired mucus transport is what causes congestion, which can become a breeding ground for infection.

STEP 2: IRRIGATE THE NASAL CAVITIES

Irrigation is the best treatment for congestion-related problems, including sinusitis, colds and allergies. It thins and flushes away mucus and helps the sinuses drain. It also washes out allergens and infection-causing bacteria.

Mix about one teaspoon of salt and one-half teaspoon of baking soda in two cups of warm sterile water. Pour it into a squeeze bottle or another type of nasal-irrigation device. (Or you could try a system I invented called the Hydro Pulse Sinus System, available online—it applies the low, steady pressure needed to create suction and pull out mucus.)

Keeping the head centered, put the solution into one nostril. Keep it flowing until the solution begins to flow out the other nostril. Gently blow your nose, then repeat on the other side.

Caution: If you're using a squeeze bottle, try to maintain steady pressure. A University of Pennsylvania study found that infected mucus can backflow into squeeze bottles and cause a reinfection.

STEP 3: SHRINK THE SWELLING

Much of the discomfort of sinusitis comes from swollen mucous membranes. To reduce swelling, apply moist heat to the sinus area. Soak a washcloth in warm-to-hot water, and drape it over the nose and cheeks. When it cools, resoak and reapply it several times a day.

Another way to reduce swelling and congestion is to lift the tip of your nose. It sounds (and looks) silly, but it works because a downward-dipping nose (common in older adults) can block the nasal openings. At night, loop a piece of one-half-inch-wide medical-grade tape under the end of the nose…pull the ends slightly upward…and stick them between the eyes. It will keep the nasal passages open while you sleep.

Also helpful: My Clear-ease natural fruit enzyme tablets. Follow the label directions. Fruit-based enzymes such as bromelain and papain reduce sinus swelling.

STEP 4: CLEAN YOUR HOME

Pollens, molds and dust mites, along with plain old dust, can cause sinusitis.

You don't have to give your home the "white-glove treatment." But do wash bedding weekly in hot water to kill dust mites and their eggs. Also consider dust mite–proof mattress and pillow covers. Vacuum carpets once a week, preferably with a vacuum equipped with a HEPA filter. It's also a good idea to keep dogs and cats out of the bedroom to minimize nighttime exposure to dust and dander from their coats.

Nasal Swab to the Rescue!

Doctors routinely prescribe antibiotics for sinusitis even though only about 10% of patients actually need them. A new swab test (in development) identifies bacterial sinusitis in just five minutes.

The Ohio State University Center for Clinical and Translational Science.

STEP 5: MORE VITAMIN C

Vitamin C can reduce the intensity and duration of coldlike symptoms, including congestion. It's a mild antihistamine that reduces mucus production and sinus swelling. When sinusitis flares, increase your dietary intake of vitamin C by eating plenty of salads, leafy green vegetables, citrus, etc.

Caution: Some fresh fruits such as strawberries contain high levels of natural histamines, but canned or cooked do not. If you notice an increase in congestion and/or head pain after eating certain foods, avoid them until you're feeling better.

STEP 6: USE A DECONGESTANT

I don't recommend decongestants before trying drug-free treatments. But if you've had sinusitis for a few weeks or longer, your body's defenses are probably exhausted. Using a decongestant spray once or twice will provide relief and give your natural defenses a chance to catch up.

Any decongestant spray, tablet or liquid can help, but I like Patanase Nasal Spray. It's a prescription spray that quickly clears congestion and doesn't contain a corticosteroid. Menthol inhalers such as Vicks and Benzedrex also can provide relief.

STEP 7: DE-STRESS

Doctors have known for a long time that emotional stress can dampen immunity and increase the risk for infection. It also tends to increase the incidence (and discomfort) of colds, allergies and sinusitis.

Stress creates a cycle known as anxiety reinforcement. The more stress you experience, the more likely you are to get sick—and the more you'll notice the discomfort.

My advice: Practice biofeedback. It's easy—and effective. Once or twice a day, sit in front of a mirror. Slowly inhale for a count of four, then exhale for a count of six. As you exhale, consciously relax the muscles in the face, jaw and shoulders. It's physiologically impossible to feel anxiety when your muscles are relaxed.

People who practice this technique soon learn that they can reduce stress-related symptoms at any time, not just when they're in front of the mirror.

WHEN TO SEE YOUR DOCTOR

By taking the steps in this article, you might be able to avoid a trip to the doctor's office, which could save you $100 or so. However, if you still have sinusitis symptoms after several weeks, do see your doctor. He/she may recommend other treatments including an antibiotic (usually *amoxicillin*) if you have a bacterial infection.

SWEET SELF-TEST

Open a package of saccharin, and put a few of the granules inside your nostrils. See how long it takes before you taste sweetness. If you taste the saccharin in about five minutes, you probably don't have sinusitis. If it takes 20 to 30 minutes, sinusitis is likely.

Vitamin D Helps Relieve Chronic Hives

Jill Poole, MD, associate professor of internal medicine at University of Nebraska Medical Center, Omaha, and principal investigator of a study published in *Annals of Allergy, Asthma & Immunology*.

Many patients with this distressing condition take a standardized combination of three allergy drugs—*cetirizine* (Zyrtec), *montelukast* (Singulair) and *ranitidine* (Zantac).

Recent finding: People who also took 4,000 international units (IU) of vitamin D-3 daily for 12 weeks had significantly less severe symptoms than patients who took only 600 IU daily.

Researchers Focus on Eczema-Food Allergy Link

King's College London, news release.

The skin disease eczema may be an important factor in the development of food allergies in infants, a recent British study suggests.

The breakdown in the skin barrier that occurs in eczema could play a key role in triggering food sensitivity in babies, the researchers from King's College London and the University of Dundee said.

"This is a very exciting study, providing further evidence that an impaired skin barrier and eczema could play a key role in triggering food sensitivity in babies, which could ultimately lead to the development of food allergies," said Carsten Flohr, MD, PhD, clinician scientist, senior lecturer, dermatologist, King's College London.

The researchers said the discovery suggests that food allergies may develop via immune cells in the skin rather than in the gut and that the findings indicate that eczema may be a potential target for preventing food allergies in children.

A link between eczema and food allergies has been known for some time, but this study—published in a July 2013 issue of the *Journal of Investigative Dermatology*—adds to growing evidence of the skin barrier's role in the process, according to the researchers.

STUDY DETAILS

The study included more than 600 infants who were three months old and exclusively breast-fed from birth. They were tested for eczema and checked to see if they were sensitized to the six most common allergenic foods.

Egg white was the most common allergen, followed by cow's milk and peanuts. The more severe the eczema, the stronger the link to food sensitivity, independent of genetic factors.

It's believed that the breakdown of the skin barrier in infants with eczema leaves active immune cells found in skin exposed to environmental allergens—in this case food proteins—which then triggers an allergic immune response, the researchers explained.

They also noted that food sensitivity does not always lead to food allergy and they're conducting a follow-up of the infants in this study.

IMPLICATIONS

"This work takes what we thought we knew about eczema and food allergy and flips it on its head. We thought that food allergies are triggered from the inside out, but our work shows that in some children it could be from the outside in, via the skin," Dr. Flohr explained. "The skin barrier plays a crucial role in protecting us from allergens in our environment, and we can see here that when that barrier is compromised, especially in eczema, it seems to leave the skin's immune cells exposed to these allergens."

This finding opens up the possibility that by repairing the skin barrier and preventing eczema, it might be possible to reduce the risk of food allergies, Dr. Flohr added.

info The American Academy of Dermatology has more about eczema at *http://www.skincarephysicians.com/eczemanet/FAQ.html*.

Exposing Babies to Peanuts May Help Curb Allergy Risk

Gideon Lack, MD, department of pediatric allergy, King's College London, England.

Rebecca Gruchalla, MD, PhD, departments of internal medicine and pediatrics, University of Texas Southwestern Medical Center, Dallas.

American Academy of Allergy, Asthma & Immunology annual meeting, Houston.

New England Journal of Medicine, online.

Giving peanut products to infants at high risk for peanut allergy may reduce the risk of developing the allergy by 80%, a startling recent study suggests.

For years, the conventional wisdom was to avoid giving peanuts to infants who were at risk for developing an allergy to them. And although that recommendation was retracted in 2008, many parents continued to avoid giving peanut products to their infants, said lead researcher Gideon Lack, MD, from the department of pediatric allergy at King's College London in England.

Dry-Roasted Allergies?

Peanut allergies are common in the US, but not in Asian countries, where raw or boiled peanuts are the norm.

Possible reason: High-heat roasting produces proteins that can trigger an allergic response.

The Journal of Allergy and Clinical Immunology

"However, eating peanut [products] in the first year of life protects against the development of peanut allergy in a high-risk group of children," he said. "This is the exact opposite of what was recommended."

Babies who have a high risk of developing a peanut allergy are those who have severe eczema and/or have an allergic reaction to eggs, Dr. Lack said.

STUDY DETAILS

In the study, Dr. Lack's team selected 640 infants, aged four months to 11 months, who were at high risk of developing peanut allergy.

The babies were randomly selected either to eat at least 6 grams of peanuts in food served three or more times a week, or to avoid peanut products until they were five.

Dr. Lack said that even some children who could not tolerate peanuts developed some immunity. Overall, at age five, the prevalence of peanut allergy in all children who ate peanut products was just over 3%, compared with slightly more than 17% among those who avoided foods or snacks with peanuts in them, the researchers found.

"This is a greater than 80% reduction in the prevalence of peanut allergy," Dr. Lack said.

Moreover, introducing peanut products early was safe and well tolerated, the researchers added. Infants were not given whole peanuts because of the risk of choking, they noted.

The recent study was published online in the *New England Journal of Medicine*, to coincide with a planned presentation of the findings at the American Academy of Allergy, Asthma & Immunology annual meeting in Houston.

EXPERT COMMENT AND CAUTION

Rebecca Gruchalla, MD, from the departments of internal medicine and pediatrics at the University of Texas Southwestern Medical Center at Dallas and coauthor of an accompanying journal editorial, said, "This study clearly shows that early introduction of peanut [products] leads to a decrease in peanut allergy."

Dr. Gruchalla cautioned, however, that giving peanut products to high-risk infants needs to be done in consultation with a pediatrician and an allergy specialist.

Peanut allergy and other allergies have been increasing around the world, she said. Why this is so, however, isn't clear. "That's the million dollar question. Is it lifestyle changes? Is it food changes? Is it genetic? We don't know," she added.

RECOMMENDATIONS

Dr. Lack recommended that infants at risk for peanut allergy have a skin test for peanut at four months of age. If the skin test shows no reaction, they should be given peanut products regularly until the age of five.

However, if the skin test shows a reaction to peanuts, the authors recommend giving the infant a trial of peanut-containing food in the doctor's office. If there is no reaction during the observed trial of peanut products, then the infant should continue eating them. If the infant reacts to the food containing peanuts, immediate treatment by the physician may be needed to quell the allergic symptoms brought on by the peanut product.

info For more information about peanut allergies, visit the American College of Allergy, Asthma & Immunology at *http://acaai. org/allergies/types/food-allergies/types-food-allergy/peanut-allergy.*

FDA Cautions Against "Undeclared" Food Allergens

U.S. Food and Drug Administration, news release.

Some food labels may not reliably list all possible food allergens, according to the U.S. Food and Drug Administration.

The agency added that these "undeclared allergens" are the leading cause of FDA-requested food recalls.

Under federal law, foods marketed in the US are required to identify all major food allergens—such as milk, eggs, fish, crustacean shellfish, tree nuts, wheat, peanuts and soybeans—on product labels. This mandate is to prevent life-threatening allergic reactions, according to the FDA.

The FDA can seize any foods that do not contain this allergen information on their labels. Most food manufacturers, however, will recall their products voluntarily.

To prevent these recalls, the FDA said it is investigating why some possible allergens are omitted from food labels. The FDA is also working with the food industry to improve testing for the presence of possible allergens.

HOW CONSUMERS CAN HELP

Consumers can help by reporting any allergic reactions to food to their local FDA consumer complaint coordinator, said Steven Gendel, FDA food allergen coordinator.

In sorting through recall data, the FDA said it has already identified noticeable trends, such as…

Between September 2009 and September 2012, roughly one-third of all foods reported as serious health risks involved allergens that were not included on food labels. Most often,

Thank You, Fido!

Dogs may help protect babies against allergies and asthma. When mice were exposed to dust from households with dogs that were allowed outdoors, the mice's gut microbes changed significantly and they had reduced allergic responses to well-known allergy triggers.

Theory: Children in homes with dogs that are allowed outside develop intestinal bacteria that provide better immunity against many allergens.

Animal study by researchers at University of California, San Francisco, published in *Proceedings of the National Academy of Sciences*.

the foods involved were bakery products, snack foods, candy, dairy products, and dressings or sauces.

The allergens involved most frequently in recalls were milk, wheat and soy.

Several recalls involved candy made with dark chocolate that contained undeclared milk. The FDA said these chocolate-coated snack bars had labels that indicated the products were "dairy-free" or "vegan." "This represented a significant risk for milk-allergic consumers," said Gendel.

Labeling errors most often occur due to the use of the wrong label, the FDA found. This can happen when similar products are sold in similar packages, but contain different ingredients, including allergens.

Based on these findings, the FDA said the number of food allergen recalls can be reduced by increasing awareness about food allergens and improving the way food packages, labels and ingredients are handled.

The FDA advised consumers to learn about recalled products on the agency's website, the Food Allergy Research and Education (FARE) website and from food manufacturers.

info The U.S. Department of Health and Human Services provides more information on how to protect yourself from food allergies at *http://www.foodsafety.gov.*

Many People Misuse Devices for Asthma, Allergic Reaction

Aasia Ghazi, MD, Allergy and Asthma Specialists of Dallas, and adjunct assistant professor, University of Texas Medical Branch, Galveston, Texas.
Jennifer Appleyard, MD, chief of allergy and immunology, St. John Providence Health System, Detroit.
Annals of Allergy, Asthma and Immunology, online

Few people know how to properly use the medical devices that contain lifesaving medications for severe allergic reactions and asthma attacks, a recent study shows.

A life-threatening allergic reaction is known as anaphylaxis. The incidence of anaphylaxis is rising, according to background information in

the study. A shot of epinephrine—a stimulating hormone—into a muscle can stop anaphylaxis, according to the study authors.

Asthma inhalers can be used to deliver medicine to stop an asthma attack, or they can deliver preventive medications that help stop asthma attacks from occurring. They can be used alone or along with an additional device called a spacer. Spacers are chambers that temporarily hold the medication, which can be especially helpful when giving medication to children, according to the American Lung Association.

Misuse of asthma inhalers or spacers can lead to too little medicine being used. That means symptoms might not be treated properly. It can also lead to overuse of medication, according to background information in the study.

Just 16% of the patients in the study knew the correct way to use an epinephrine injector for someone with a life-threatening allergy. And only 7% knew how to use an asthma inhaler as directed.

"This isn't a new concern. We always worry about our patients, especially those with food allergies," said one of the study's authors, Aasia Ghazi, MD, from the Allergy and Asthma Specialists of Dallas.

"We had a patient call in the middle of a reaction, and she didn't remember how to use the epinephrine injector. That's why we looked to see what's going on, and what are the barriers that keep patients from using these devices properly?" Dr. Ghazi explained.

STUDY DETAILS

Dr. Ghazi and her colleagues recruited 102 patients prescribed epinephrine and 44 prescribed asthma inhalers or spacers for the study. Eleven percent of those prescribed epinephrine had used the device before. Eighty percent of those with asthma reported having used an inhaler—also called a metered-dose inhaler, or MDI—or a spacer before, the researchers said.

The study volunteers demonstrated how to use a device to the researchers.

Of the 84% who misused the epinephrine, more than half missed three or more steps involved in the correct use of the device. The most common error was not leaving the shot in for 10 seconds.

"We instruct patients to leave the unit in place for 10 seconds to make sure 100% of the medication is injected," Dr. Ghazi said.

Of the 93% who misused asthma inhalers or spacers, 63% missed three or more steps. The most common mistake was not exhaling before depressing the canister to inhale the medication, according to the study.

Time appeared to be a significant factor in patients' memories. For those prescribed epinephrine injectors within a year, 10% had perfect use. If they had the device for one to five years, just 5% had perfect use. If someone had been given the device five years prior, perfect use dropped to just 1%, the study found.

PRACTICE MAKES PERFECT

Jennifer Appleyard, MD, who was not involved with the study, said that epinephrine injectors come in kits that have training devices. She also suggested practicing with expired devices by injecting a piece of fruit, such as an orange. "It's important to feel comfortable with the injector. Everyone needs to practice," Dr. Appleyard said.

"This study really drives home the need to reinforce the use of these devices every time a patient comes in," said Dr. Appleyard, who is chief of allergy and immunology at St. John Providence Health System in Detroit. "And, it's not enough to just give instructions. People need to show me how they use the device," she added.

Some devices have instructions written on them, and others will talk you through the steps, according to Dr. Ghazi.

Both experts said if your doctor hasn't shown you how to use your medical devices, you need to speak up. "Talk to your caregiver, and make sure you're getting instructions whenever you visit. Make sure you're getting it right, and clarify any doubts you have," Dr. Ghazi said.

"A life can be saved with an epinephrine injection. It's a big deal," said Dr. Ghazi.

The study was published online in the *Annals of Allergy, Asthma and Immunology*.

info Read more about how to use an epinephrine injector from the U.S. National Library of Medicine at *www.nlm.nih.gov* (search "epinephrine injection").

CART: A Better Way to Catch Your Breath If You Have Asthma

Study titled "Controlling asthma by training of Capnometry-Assisted Hypoventilation (CATCH) vs slow breathing: a randomized controlled trial," by researchers in the department of psychology and the Anxiety and Depression Research Center at Southern Methodist University, Dallas, published in *Chest*.

Asthma. The very mention of the word can make you feel like you have a boa constrictor wrapped around your chest. If you have asthma, chances are that when you feel that squeezing, suffocating feeling of an attack, you take deep breaths—gasping for air—but this is actually wrong. Or maybe you have heard that taking deep, slow and paced breaths is the right way to go. But the latest research shows that there really is a much better way to catch your breath.

WHEN LESS IS MORE

In an attempt to catch their breaths, asthmatics gulp air and breathe too rapidly during an attack. It's a natural reaction, but this can cause a decrease in the body's level of carbon dioxide (CO_2), resulting in hyperventilation and its characteristic symptoms of dizziness, breathlessness and pins and needles. The lungs become hyperreactive, stuffy and dry, making the asthma attack far worse and scarier than it needs to be.

Now consider this: Shallow breathing does the opposite…it increases CO_2 levels. Knowing this and knowing that shallow breathing helps people with panic disorder (who also tend to hyperventilate), researchers from Southern Methodist University in Dallas decided to test the effectiveness of a shallow-breathing technique, successfully used in people with panic disorder, in adults with asthma.

They randomly assigned 120 asthma sufferers to receive either a standard breathing therapy called slow-breathing and awareness training (SLOW) or a therapy called capnometry-assisted respiratory training (CART). SLOW teaches asthmatics to take slow, full breaths through awareness and control of their respiratory rate (the number of breaths they take per minute). CART also trains its users to control their respiratory rate but encourages shallow breathing and control of CO_2 levels through use of a device called a capnometer. The capnometer provides feedback about CO_2 levels so that a person can practice how to breathe to prevent CO_2 from dipping too low.

The study participants practiced their therapies for four weeks on their own and with respiratory therapists and used their asthma medications as needed. The researchers monitored asthma attacks, need for medication and various aspects of respiratory function during this time and for six months' follow-up—and patients kept journals of the impact of SLOW or CART therapy on their asthma.

The results? Whereas both techniques resulted in an 81% improvement in lung function, the CART group was in better shape six months down the road than the other group. Their airways had become more widened and their CO_2 levels were more normalized than those of patients practicing SLOW, and that difference remained consistent throughout further follow-up. Patients practicing CART also coped better when under the stress of an acute asthma attack because they felt more in control of their symptoms and what exactly was happening in their bodies during attacks.

LEARNING TO BREATHE

If you have (or know someone who has) asthma and are unfamiliar with breath retraining therapies, such as SLOW and CART, it's a good idea to ask your doctor for a referral to a respiratory therapist—especially someone who knows about CART. These therapies are not a substitute for asthma medication, but they clearly work as add-ons and can help you improve lung function so that you can possibly rely less on medication. As for which therapy is better for long-term improvement, this study, at least, points to CART.

Keep a Common Cold Out of Your Lungs— Especially if You Have Asthma

Richard Firshein, DO, director and founder, The Firshein Center for Integrative Medicine, New York City.

If you're prone to bronchitis or pneumonia or have asthma, you may freak out any time someone near you coughs or sneezes, as viral droplets waft through the air, landing on pens, doorknobs, your clothes—or in your eyes or nose. You may pull out all the stops to prevent getting sick, but what if, despite your best efforts, you get snagged by a head cold? *Here's how to keep that cold from taking over your lungs...*

KEEP A COLD OUT OF YOUR CHEST

There are two ways that a head cold can burrow into your lungs, according to Richard Firshein, DO, director of the Firshein Center for Integrative Medicine in New York City. One is just that the same virus causing the head cold moves from the nose and throat to the lungs. The other is that another infection—usually bacterial—takes advantage of the weakened immune system. No matter what, you can avoid this one-two punch.

As soon as you feel the first symptoms of a cold coming on, Dr. Firshein recommends taking vitamin C and zinc. "This regimen is not a cure-all, but it will help shorten the duration of the problem, and, for many people, it will keep the immune system healthy enough to get through the head cold without it turning into a chest cold," he said.

Dr. Firshein recommends at least 500 milligrams (mg) per day of vitamin C, taken in a split dose (250 mg twice per day) for three to five days. Don't take more than 1,500 mg daily or else you will risk side effects, such as painful

---

No-Stink Asthma Trigger

According to a recent study, when asthma patients believed that an odor—even if it was neutral and contained no irritants—would worsen asthma symptoms, their symptoms did increase.

Journal of Psychosomatic Research

kidney stones and soft stools or full-blown diarrhea. As for zinc, whether in lozenge or tablet form, Dr. Firshein recommends a dosage of 10 mg to 25 mg twice a day until symptoms clear. Be aware, though, that zinc lozenges and tablets can cause upset stomach or a metallic taste.

"Most people will do fine with vitamin C and zinc," Dr. Firshein said, "but some people, such as the elderly and those with certain health conditions such as asthma or heart disease, may need to add other supplements to fortify their immune systems." *Dr. Firshein's go-to supplements for people who need an extra boost include...*

Echinacea. This herb, from the daisy family, has antioxidant and antiviral properties and fortifies the immune system against bacterial attack. In all, it can reduce the length and severity of colds. Dr. Firshein prefers a liquid extract dispensed by dropper and recommends formulations marketed by Herbs Pharm and Gaia.

Cordyceps. Cordyceps is a potent immune-strengthening nutrient derived from a fungus that grows inside caterpillars that live high in the Himalayan mountains. It's expensive...and natural cordyceps supplements can be hard to find. Dr. Firshein recommends these brands—Host Defense and Jarrow Formulas. He suggests a starting dosage of two 500-mg capsules once per day.

EXTRA DEFENSE FOR ASTHMATICS

If you have asthma, you especially want to guard against chest colds. The combination of swelling and mucus production from a chest cold makes breathing even more difficult. It can also bring on dangerous—and deadly—constriction of the airways (bronchospasms).

"People with asthma have to be more vigilant," said Dr. Firshein. "They should use all of the vitamins and supplements mentioned above and fortify their immune systems with N-acetylcysteine (NAC) and magnesium."

NAC is an antioxidant that can dissolve and loosen mucus, so it will help clear the airways. Dr. Firshein recommends a dosage of 250 mg twice a day. Magnesium is a natural bronchodilator, so it will also help open up the airways. Again, Dr. Firshein recommends 250 mg twice a day.

As a final word to the wise, Dr. Firshein urges that you see a doctor if your symptoms worsen instead of improve. Also see your doctor if an asthma attack occurs during a cold, if a bad cough doesn't go away after other cold symptoms resolve or if your temperature climbs over 99.4°F.

Relieve COPD Flare-Ups with Vitamin D

Study titled "Vitamin D3 supplementation in patients with chronic obstructive pulmonary disease (ViDiCO): a multicenter, double-blind, randomized controlled trial," from Centre for Primary Care and Public Health, Blizard Institute, Barts and London School of Medicine and Dentistry, Queen Mary University of London, published in *The Lancet Respiratory Medicine*.

Chronic obstructive pulmonary disease (COPD) is a crippling combination of chronic bronchitis and emphysema. If you have it, you're worn out by a constant cough, phlegm, shortness of breath and chest tightness. The symptoms can be managed (though never cured) by breathing exercises and physical therapy, bronchodilator and corticosteroid drugs and—worst-case scenario—being hooked up to an oxygen tank. And every so often, symptoms will flare up to an extreme.

Breakthrough news: If you or a loved one is a COPD sufferer, taking supplements of a certain essential nutrient can significantly reduce your risk of flare-ups.

D TO THE RESCUE

Researchers from Queen Mary University of London expanded on a small study that looked at vitamin D deficiency and supplementation in people with COPD and confirmed the earlier findings—vitamin D supplements reduced risk of flare-ups.

The current study recruited 240 patients with COPD from across Britain and conducted a full-fledged placebo-controlled study.

The researchers first tested these patients' current vitamin D levels to keep track of who was low, normal or high. Then, about half the participants were treated with a 3-milligram dose (120,000 IU) of vitamin D, taken in the form of oral drops given every two months for a year. (This is a very large megadose of the vitamin that is, basically, only used in research studies and in people with severely low vitamin D levels. The average person should never take this amount of the vitamin on his or her own.) The other participants were given a placebo.

The results: Supplementation reduced the risk of COPD flares by 43% in patients who had borderline-to-low vitamin D levels to begin with (blood levels of less than 50 nanomoles per liter [nmol/L]) but did not do much for patients who already had normal or high levels of the vitamin (blood levels of 50 nmol/L or greater). But most people with COPD do have low levels of vitamin D or outright vitamin D deficiencies. In this study, 87% had insufficient-to-deficient levels.

The researchers are not yet sure exactly how vitamin D helps stop COPD flare-ups, but they think it might have to do with the vitamin's protective antimicrobial and anti-inflammatory properties. COPD flares often are caused by either infections or irritation of the respiratory system (from exposure to cigarette smoke or other pollutants, for example). Vitamin D likely helps the immune system fend off these onslaughts.

BEWARE TOO MUCH D

Although no serious side effects were attributed to vitamin D in the study, more D was not better. In fact, patients who already had vitamin D blood levels of 100 nmol/L or greater were slightly more susceptible to flares. So, even though the large majority of people with COPD are low in D and could use a supplement, don't just start taking it on your own. Instead, speak to your doctor about having a blood test to know exactly what your vitamin D level is before starting a supplement.

Having too much vitamin D in your system is dangerous. It can cause itchy skin, calcium build-up in the arteries, daytime sleepiness, headaches,

Cigars Are Not a Safe Smoke

Cigar smoking, which many smokers believe is safer than cigarettes, has more than doubled in the US since the year 2000. But a large-scale analysis found that cigar smokers had higher levels of several toxic substances in their blood and urine than nonsmokers, with levels of at least one potential cancer-causing agent comparable to that found in cigarette smokers.

Jiping Chen, MD, PhD, MPH, epidemiologist, FDA Center for Tobacco Products, Silver Spring, Maryland.

heart rhythm abnormalities, muscle pain, stomach issues, kidney stones, and high blood pressure.

If your vitamin D level is very low, your doctor may prescribe a very large dose of D that you take, for example, once a week or once a month—as the patients in this study did. But this is definitely not a regimen that anyone should do on his or her own without close medical supervision for the reasons explained above.

More than likely, your levels are just a bit low, and your doctor will recommend a high-quality daily supplement in a dosage that is right for you. The recommended daily allowance of vitamin D for people who are one to 70 years of age is 600 IU, and it's 800 IU for people 71 and older...but up to 4,000 IU per day has been considered safe by the US National Academy of Sciences Institute of Medicine.

One-Sided Breathing OK?

Murray Grossan, MD, Los Angeles–based otolaryngologist in private practice and author of *Stressed? Anxiety? Your Cure Is in the Mirror. GrossanInstitute.com*

Is it a problem if you breathe through only one side of your nose?

It could be, depending on the cause. A growth in the nasal cavity or a deviated septum (a displacement of the thin wall between the nostrils) can affect breathing and trigger nosebleeds, sinus infections and headaches.

Sleep also can be affected. A nasal obstruction can cause snoring and other disorders, such as sleep apnea, a condition in which abnormal pauses in breathing reduce oxygen flow to the brain.

Try this: Stand in front of a mirror, and raise the tip of your nose. Can you breathe through both nostrils? If you can, use a three-inch-long strip of medical tape (from under the nose to between your eyes) to keep your nose slightly raised during sleep. If not, see an ear, nose and throat doctor.

How to Cure Snoring with a Song

Murray Grossan, MD, otolaryngologist and head-and-neck surgeon with the Tower Ear, Nose & Throat Clinic at Cedars-Sinai Medical Center in Los Angeles. He is author of *Free Yourself from Sinus and Allergy Problems Permanently. GrossanInstitute.com*

If your spouse complains about your early-morning habit of singing *O Sole Mio* in the shower, just explain that it's better than an all-night concert of wall-shaking snores.

Nearly half of all adults snore occasionally, and about 25% do it all the time when they're sleeping.

What happens: Air passages in the back of the throat tend to sag when you sleep. The movement of air through the narrowed openings triggers vibrations that are heard as snoring.

Anyone can snore, but it tends to be worst in elderly or overweight men.

Singing exercises strengthen and tighten tissues in the throat and soft palate (the area at the back of the roof of the mouth), just as weight lifting tightens flabby arms. British researchers found that people who practiced singing exercises daily for three months slept better and had a reduction in the frequency, severity and loudness of snoring.

THE STOP-SNORING WORKOUT

Follow these steps, which include tongue exercises, singing and humming. They can help reduce snoring and obstructive sleep apnea, interruptions in nighttime breathing caused by blocked airways. Do these exercises even if you snore only occasionally because occasional snoring can develop into sleep apnea over time.

•**Press the tongue firmly (and repeatedly) against the hard palate (the roof of the mouth behind the front teeth).** Then press as much of the tongue as possible against the middle of the roof of the mouth…and then against the back. Keep pressing and moving your tongue for about three minutes.

•**Press the tip of your tongue firmly behind the front teeth** while simultaneously pressing the back of the tongue against the floor of the mouth. This is difficult to do, but just trying to do it is helpful.

•**While holding the tongue against the hard palate,** sing each of the vowel sounds—"Aaaa"…"Eeee"…"Iiii"…"Oooo"…and "Uuuu"—for three minutes at a time. While singing the vowel sounds, vary the pitch from high to low. Changes in pitch cause variations in vibration that exercise the tissues more completely. Just plain singing (that song in the shower!) helps, too.

•**Hum.** You can do this for a few minutes throughout the day—for example, when you're driving or working around the house.

•**Whenever you swallow, try to keep the tongue pressed against the roof of the mouth.** You'll feel tension at the back of your throat.

FORCEFUL BLOWING

This is another technique that reduces snoring and sleep apnea.

A few times a day, blow up balloons. Breathe in deeply through your nose, then blow out hard to fill the balloons.

If you're musically inclined—or would enjoy giving it a try—play a wind instrument, such as a trumpet, kazoo or didgeridoo (an Australian wind instrument). A study published in *British Medical Journal* found that people who played the didgeridoo for 15 to 30 minutes daily snored less and also had improvements in sleep apnea and daytime sleepiness.

Important: Be aware that these steps will take at least a few months to work, but the results can be dramatic. I advise patients who struggle with snoring and sleep apnea to do the exercises before considering surgery or other treatments. You can stop doing the exercises when there's no more snoring.

The Buzz About Positional Therapy for Sleep Apnea

Lawrence J. Epstein, MD, program director of the Sleep Medicine Fellowship Program and associate physician, division of sleep and circadian disorders, departments of medicine and neurology at Brigham & Women's Hospital, and instructor in medicine at Harvard Medical School, all in Boston.

It happened again—a night's sleep was wrecked by the gasping for air, snoring and snorting caused by obstructive sleep apnea (OSA). The symptoms strike whenever you roll over onto your back, and even though you know a CPAP machine would fix the problem, you just can't get yourself to use one. You might even have a machine gathering dust in a corner of your bedroom.

No worries. If lying on your back really is what sets off your OSA, there is, in fact, a new way to avoid symptoms and get some shut-eye.

Half of people with OSA generally have symptoms only when they are sleeping on their backs. This is called positional OSA. Until recently, CPAP was the main and doctor-preferred treatment for positional OSA even though simply not sleeping on your back prevents symptoms, too. Studies have shown that, although not quite as effective as CPAP, positional therapy—which offers a variety of techniques to keep a sleeper off his or her back—is adequate to control OSA symptoms in people who won't or can't use a CPAP machine.

Until now, positional therapy has been pretty basic, involving use of low-tech objects such as tennis balls, body pillows or foam belts that discourage or prevent a person from rolling onto his back during sleep. Now, a new approach, called vibro-tactile positional therapy, uses vibration to prevent a person from sleeping on his back. And the device, called Night Shift, does not restrict movement like the older options do.

NO LOST SLEEP

Night Shift is a relatively thin neck collar with a sensor that vibrates when you roll onto your back. The intensity of the vibration increases until you change your sleep position.

Surprisingly, this vibrating gadget will not disrupt sleep and keep you up as much as your OSA will, says Lawrence J. Epstein, MD, an expert in sleep medicine and positional therapy from Harvard Medical School and past president of the American Academy of Sleep Medicine. Although you might be briefly roused to roll over, you usually won't completely awaken, he said. You simply will shift position and fall right back into deeper sleep.

The device also electronically monitors how often you roll onto your back, how long you stay in that position before shifting and how much you snore or have breathing problems during sleep, explained Dr. Epstein. "This information can be downloaded onto a computer and sent to your doctor to determine how effective the device is for you," he said.

According to a small published study sponsored by Advanced Brain Monitoring, Inc. (the makers of Night Shift) and conducted by the inventors of the device, Night Shift reduced sleep apnea by more than half in 83% of the study participants who used the device nightly for four weeks. This had a greatly improved effect on snoring, daytime depression and sleepiness and, most importantly, getting enough oxygen during sleep. At some point though, a larger, independent study will need to confirm Night Shift's effectiveness and also compare it to CPAP. But the bottom line is that using any technique that will help prevent OSA is better than nothing.

HOW TO GET THE DEVICE

Night Shift is available by prescription only, so if you want to try it, speak with your doctor. Dr. Epstein advised that it may be worth your while to see a board-certified sleep specialist rather than your primary care physician to get a prescription for the device. Unlike a primary care doctor, a sleep specialist (a physician with training and board certification in sleep medicine) can ensure that positional therapy is right for you. Such a doctor will also best use the product's technology to closely monitor your response to treatment.

Although Night Shift is not yet widely covered by insurance, at $349, it's about one-third of the price of a CPAP machine.

Don't Let Central Sleep Apnea Silently Suffocate You

Robert S. Rosenberg, DO, board-certified sleep doctor with sleep labs in Prescott Valley and Flagstaff, Arizona. He is author of *Sleep Soundly Every Night, Feel Fantastic Every Day: A Doctor's Guide to Solving Your Sleep Problems. AnswersForSleep.com*

You probably know that sleep apnea is a disorder that interrupts sleep with repeated stops and starts in breathing. You may think it's something that only snorers or overweight people have to worry about. If so, think again. There is a type of sleep apnea that happens silently without any snoring or other noises. It could be happening to you even if you think you sleep well—and a bed partner might not even notice.

This type of sleep apnea, called central sleep apnea (CSA), is getting more attention among doctors as they learn about how much sneakier

Check Your Tongue

According to a recent study, obese men and women with sleep apnea had significantly larger tongues with more fat than those who didn't have the sleep condition.

Problem: A larger tongue (which also can be present in people of normal weight) can block the airway during sleep, causing breathing to briefly stop.

What to do: Ask your doctor to check your tongue size to help determine your risk for sleep apnea.

Richard J. Schwab, MD, professor of medicine, Hospital of the University of Pennsylvania, Philadelphia.

and more dangerous it is than the commonly known obstructive sleep apnea (OSA). To really take charge of the situation, sleep specialists have recently banded together to create a web portal called Sleep Apnea Doctors for consumers and physicians alike, where folks can become informed about all types of sleep apnea, find specialists in their area who treat it and even get online consultations and guidance about insurance coverage.

But if CSA can't be seen or heard, how do you know whether you have it so you can seek medical help?

SUFFOCATING IN SILENCE

Although OSA generally occurs in overweight people who usually snore because of it, CSA can develop whether you are slender or chubby. Unlike the mini-suffocations of OSA that are characterized by grunts, gasps and snores, those of CSA are, as mentioned, virtually silent. Because signs and symptoms of CSA are easily missed, serious and even permanent health problems are more likely to occur than they are for people with OSA. These health problems can include diabetes, atrial fibrillation (irregular heartbeat), high blood pressure, sexual dysfunction and emotional disorders. CSA can even lead to a decrease in the brain's gray matter, resulting in poorer planning skills, working memory, attention span, problem solving and verbal reasoning.

Over time, the hippocampus, the part of the brain that controls memory, can become irreversibly damaged, and this may be why some people with sleep apnea are misdiagnosed with early Alzheimer's disease.

Whereas OSA is triggered by something blocking the airway, such as fat deposits or simply anatomy, CSA can happen when the central nervous system, which contains the brain's respiratory control center, fails to send a signal to the respiratory system to breathe.

HOW TO KNOW IF YOU HAVE CENTRAL SLEEP APNEA

Although CSA can be hard to detect, certain symptoms can offer clues that it may be happening. *Red flags include…*

17

Sleep Device Bonus

When a person with sleep apnea begins treatment with a continuous positive airway pressure (CPAP) device, which forces air into the lungs during sleep, the person's resistance to insulin (a hallmark of diabetes) improves dramatically.

If you have sleep apnea: Treatment with a CPAP device may not only improve your sleep but also help lower diabetes risk.

Imran H. Iftikhar, MD, assistant professor of internal medicine, University of South Carolina, Columbia.

•**Abrupt awakenings accompanied by shortness of breath,** including shortness of breath that's relieved by sitting up.

•**Difficulty staying asleep** (insomnia, that is) or excessive daytime sleepiness (hypersomnia).

•**"Brain fog,"** characterized by difficulty concentrating and poor memory.

•**Morning headaches.**

•**Daytime tiredness, lack of energy, moodiness and/or irritability**—symptoms that can build into anxiety, depression or another mood disorder.

Also, although CSA is a lot more of a challenge for a bed partner to detect than OSA, it can be done. A partner who listens carefully may hear a few rapid breaths followed by no breath at all for 15 seconds or longer—that's a telltale sign. A person with CSA may also lightly snore.

GETTING A DIAGNOSIS

If CSA, or any sleep disorder, is suspected, its presence must be confirmed by a sleep study. This may require an overnight stay at a sleep center, which may be in a hospital or free-standing clinic. Your respiration, brain waves and maybe even muscle movements will be recorded while you sleep, and you may be videotaped as well. Make sure that the sleep center you visit is accredited by the American Academy of Sleep Medicine (AASM). These facilities are staffed only by AASM board-certified sleep doctors. You can find an accredited

sleep lab or a sleep apnea doctor in your area, as well as get more information on sleep disorders, at the AASM website.

FIXING IT

Fortunately, CSA is treatable, but the treatment is individualized and depends on the particular cause. Sometimes the remedy is as simple as getting supplemental oxygen at night, which consists of sleeping with a mask over your nose or your nose and mouth that is connected to a canister of oxygen. In other cases, working with a cardiologist to improve heart function is the key, or else it might be getting off opiate pain medications.

Although continuous positive airway pressure (CPAP) machines, which mechanically push air through the windpipe, are often prescribed for people with OSA, another device is better and recommended for people with CSA. It is called an adaptive servo-ventilator (ASV). This device, which, like OSA machines, requires wearing a mask, analyzes normal breathing patterns and stores the data in a computer. If you stop breathing, the device automatically delivers pressurized air, sometimes with extra oxygen, until normal breathing resumes. ASV is approved by most insurers and Medicare, and that's great news. So if you at all suspect that you or a bed partner might be having interrupted breathing while asleep, don't suffocate in silence. Use the resources now available to find the right doctor and get evaluated for a referral to a sleep disorder clinic so you can work toward a solution.

Healthy Diet Linked to Lower Risk of Lung Disease

Raphaelle Varraso, PhD, researcher, epidemiological and public health approaches, unit of aging and chronic diseases, National Institute of Health and Medical Research, Villejuif, France.
BMJ, online

A healthy diet low in red meat and rich in whole grains might reduce the risk of developing the crippling chronic lung disease known as COPD, recent research suggests.

Researchers tracked more than 120,000 men and women and found healthy eaters were one-third less likely to develop COPD compared with big consumers of red meat, refined grains, sugary drinks and alcohol.

COPD, or chronic obstructive pulmonary disease, is an umbrella term for several chronic lung diseases, including emphysema and bronchitis, that lead to blocked air passages and restricted oxygen flow. Routine breathing can be difficult for someone with COPD—the third leading cause of death in America, according to the American Lung Association.

"The predominant risk factor for COPD in the developed world is cigarette smoking," said study lead author Raphaelle Varraso, PhD, a researcher with the unit of aging and chronic diseases at the National Institute of Health and Medical Research in Villejuif, France. "But up to one-third of COPD patients have never smoked, suggesting that other factors are involved. This novel finding supports the importance of diet in COPD [development]."

The finding builds on a wide body of prior research suggesting that a healthy diet lowers the risk for heart disease and cancer. And good eating habits seem to lower COPD risk for both smokers and nonsmokers alike, the researchers found.

Be Patient with Coughs

Most coughs last an average of 18 days. And because most coughs are caused by viruses, they are not relieved by antibiotics. But patients often believe that a cough should last no more than a week and ask their doctors for antibiotics. Even many doctors estimate that a cough is expected to last only seven to nine days.

Study of 493 people by researchers at University of Georgia College of Public Health, Athens, published in *Annals of Family Medicine*.

STUDY DETAILS

To explore the impact of diet on COPD risk, the investigators focused on the health and eating habits of more than 73,000 women who participated in the U.S. Nurses' Health Study between 1984 and 2000. They also looked at the nutrition profiles of over 47,000 men enrolled in the Health Professionals Follow-Up Study between 1986 and 1998.

Most of the participants were white, and all worked as health professionals.

By the end of each study's time frame, 723 women and 167 men developed COPD. The subsequent analysis indicated that COPD risk was far lower among those whose diets were light on red meat, sweetened drinks and alcohol, and rich in vegetables, complex carbohydrates such as green vegetables and whole grains, and polyunsaturated fats and nuts.

Polyunsaturated fats include soybean, safflower, corn and canola oils, and fish such as salmon, trout and herring.

The finding that a healthy diet was independently related to lower COPD risk appeared to hold up even after accounting for other factors, including smoking history, age, race, exercise habits and being overweight.

Nevertheless, Dr. Varraso cautioned against concluding that diet has a direct impact on COPD risk, given that the study participants were medical professionals with a presumably greater focus on health and healthy behavior than the general public. However, the findings underscore the need for more research into how eating patterns affect lung health, Dr. Varraso suggested.

"Although COPD prevention efforts should continue to focus on smoking cessation, our results encourage clinicians to consider the potential role of the combined effect of foods in a healthy diet in promoting lung health," said Dr. Varraso.

info Visit the U.S. National Institutes of Health at *www.nhlbi.nih.gov* for more information about COPD.

Sweet Drink Beats Lingering Cough

Neda Raeessi, MD, researcher, Baqiyatallah University of Medical Sciences, Tehran, Iran.

According to a recent study, a warm honey-coffee drink relieves persistent coughing better than corticosteroids or cough syrups.

To make: Mix one-half teaspoon of instant coffee granules with two-and-a-half teaspoons of honey. Stir into seven ounces of warm water. Drink three servings a day. Honey is a well-known remedy for cough, and caffeine dilates bronchi and stimulates breathing. If your cough hasn't eased after a few weeks of using this remedy, see your doctor.

Nearly Half of Older Adults With Asthma, COPD Still Smoke

Patricia Folan, RN, DNP, director, Center for Tobacco Control, North Shore-LIJ Health System, Great Neck, New York.
NCHS Data Brief, National Center for Health Statistics. U.S. Centers for Disease Control and Prevention.

Close to half of U.S. adults over 40 who have trouble breathing due to asthma or COPD still continue to smoke, federal health officials recently reported.

"With assistance, quitting may still be challenging but it is possible," said Patricia Folan, director of the Center for Tobacco Control at North Shore-LIJ Health System in Great Neck, New York.

These recent CDC statistics come a day after the release of another agency report, which found that 15% of Americans between 40 and 79 years of age suffer from some form of lung obstruction—typically asthma or chronic obstructive pulmonary disease (COPD).

STUDY DETAILS

In the new study, CDC researchers led by Ryne Paulose-Ram, PhD, looked at data from the U.S. National Health and Nutrition Survey for the years 2007-2012.

They found that during that time, about 46% of adults aged 40 to 79 who had a lung-obstructing illness currently smoked. That number rose to 55% when the researchers looked only at cases involving "moderate or worse" disease.

Smoking rates were similar between the sexes, and rose as levels of education fell, the CDC said.

The agency noted that rates of smoking for people with lung obstruction were more than double that of people without such illnesses—about 20%.

WHY SICK PEOPLE STILL SMOKE

Why do people whose illnesses are brought on or exacerbated by smoking continue with the deadly habit? Folan said the issues are often complex and tough to change.

"Approximately 40% of those with COPD experience high levels of depression and anxiety, making it more difficult to comply with treatment and quitting smoking," she said.

"What works best to help patients with COPD quit smoking is treatment for their depression," Folan said.

Also effective, she added, is "information about and availability of the most effective ways to quit, including FDA-approved cessation medications, empathetic counseling, motivational interviewing, and ongoing support from professionals, family and friends."

The alternative—to continue smoking—exacerbates COPD symptoms and raises the odds for death, Folan said. Also, "since it is difficult to eat with shortness of breath, poor nutrition and unintended weight loss are also often consequences associated with COPD," she said.

"For patients with COPD, the single best thing they can do for their lungs is quit smoking," Folan said.

 For more about COPD, visit http://*www.nhlbi.nih.gov/health/health-topics/topics/copd*

Blood Pressure and Cholesterol

Don't Let Them Drug You for Mild High Blood Pressure

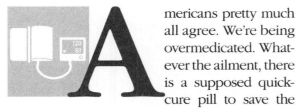**A**mericans pretty much all agree. We're being overmedicated. Whatever the ailment, there is a supposed quick-cure pill to save the day. Although we are very fortunate to have access to certain lifesaving drugs, we must resist the pharmaceutical-industry onslaught with its risks and side effects!

Latest case in point: Blood pressure control. The latest research shows clearly that many physicians are way too quick to break out their prescription pads when simple lifestyle changes may do the trick to control high blood pressure without the risk of side effects. You might very well be taking unneeded blood pressure medication. *Here's how to know...*

ONE SIZE DOESN'T FIT ALL

Of all the people the world over who have high blood pressure, more than 60% have a mild form of it. Although evidence doesn't show that treating mild high blood pressure with drugs changes the risk of a first heart attack or stroke (except for people with diabetes or chronic kidney disease), most patients with mild high blood pressure are treated with medication anyway. Some health organizations want to change the guidelines, but most are resisting. This got Stephen A. Martin, MD, an assistant professor from the University of Massachusetts Medical School, along with a team of American and Canadian doctors, to argue in a recent article in the medical journal *The BMJ* that things have got to change.

For one, they point out, guidelines to treat everyone with mild high blood pressure with drugs are not based on evidence but "expert opinion." Evidence, on the other hand, tells us that deciding who should be treated with drugs

Stephen A. Martin, MD, assistant professor, University of Massachusetts Medical School, Barre, Massachusetts. His article appeared in *The BMJ*.

is a little more complicated and should depend not on a number on a blood pressure monitor, but on age, sex and specific risk factors such as diabetes or kidney disease.

In other words, one size does not fit all—despite what the drug companies or even some lackadaisical doctors might want!

According to the American Heart Association, you have mild high blood pressure (also called hypertension) once your blood pressure hits 140/90. The first number represents systolic blood pressure—the maximum pressure when your heart muscle is contracting. The second number represents diastolic pressure—the lowest pressure when your heart is relaxed. Before we go further, here's a quick reference on blood pressure readings…

Desired range: Systolic 90–119 / diastolic 60–79.

Prehypertension: Systolic 120-139 / diastolic 80-89.

Mild hypertension: Systolic 140–159 / diastolic 90–99.

Hypertension: Systolic 160 and higher / diastolic 100 and higher.

The definition of mild hypertension was decided back in 1977 (based on expert opinion, not clinical evidence). Doctors didn't prescribe drugs for it then, but now they virtually all do, so that 94% of people age 65 and older who have any type of hypertension are on a drug, according to Dr. Martin. But an analysis conducted by a team of researchers and published as a Cochrane Review showed that antihypertensive drugs do not reduce risk of heart attack or stroke any better than placebo in people with mild hypertension. The analysis from *The BMJ* also noted that studies that show the benefit of antihypertensive drugs in people with severe hypertension are deceptively used to justify use of these drugs in people with milder forms of it.

Why? Follow the money. The estimated cost of treating mild hypertension in the United States is $32.1 billion per year!

A BETTER APPROACH

Dr. Martin and his colleagues pointed out that medicating people with mild hypertension is often an incentive for them (and their doctors)

Check BP at Home

Monitoring blood pressure at home instead of only in the doctor's office is more effective for diagnosing and treating hypertension.

Bonus: A recent study found that patients using home blood pressure–monitoring kits saved insurance companies up to $1,364 over 10 years, which could translate into lower premiums. Home blood pressure monitoring is also helpful for those at risk for hypertension.

Alejandro Arrieta, PhD, assistant professor of health policy and management, Florida International University, Miami.

not to make necessary lifestyle changes. Why bother when you can just take a pill? Rather than overdiagnosing hypertension and overprescribing antihypertensive drugs, Dr. Martin says, much more effort needs to be put into encouraging healthy lifestyle changes, while reserving drug treatment for people who really need it—those who are known to be truly at risk for heart disease, such as people with diabetes, chronic kidney disease, metabolic syndrome and blood pressure that is 160/100 or higher.

Besides that, Dr. Martin and his coauthors point out that blood pressure readings by doctors are often inaccurate. Doctors often do not consider, for example, whether a patient has just smoked a cigarette (taken nicotine) or plied him- or herself with caffeine, which can affect blood pressure readings. And then there's "white-coat syndrome," in which anxiety over being examined temporarily increases blood pressure exactly at a time when an accurate reading is needed—while at the doctor's office! Considering that 20% of people with any level of high blood pressure also have white-coat syndrome, there are almost certainly legions of people out there who have been misdiagnosed with mild hypertension and told to take drugs.

WHAT YOU CAN DO

To better ensure that you get an accurate blood pressure reading, do it yourself at home. Yes, home blood pressure monitoring is preferred, according to Dr. Martin, because it removes white-coat syndrome from the picture and also allows a person to take multiple readings instead of just one. Multiple readings give a better sense of what is really happening.

Blood pressure–monitoring devices are widely available. The AHA recommends cuff-style monitors that fit over the upper arm because they are more accurate than wrist and finger monitors. *The AHA gives this guidance for blood pressure monitoring…*

•**Take two.** Measure your blood pressure twice per day at the same times each day, such as morning and evening. And each time you measure it, take two or three readings one minute apart. (Some home monitors will automatically perform three readings in a row and average the results—all you have to do is sit patiently for a few minutes.)

•**Relax.** Don't drink caffeinated beverages or exercise (or smoke) within the 30 minutes before measuring your blood pressure.

•**Keep a log.** Accurately document the date and time of each of your blood pressure readings, and keep that log for presentation to your doctor. (Some monitors have built-in memory to store readings or apps to download the reading to a website for later access.)

If you are told by your doctor that you have mild hypertension and should go on medication, question why and whether lifestyle changes would be the better alternative. Read on for more information on how blood pressure regulation is not a one-size-fits-all discipline.

How Low to Go for Blood Pressure Control

Study titled "Pharmacotherapy for Hypertension in Older Adults: A Systematic Review" by department of pharmacy practice, Oregon State University College of Pharmacy, published in *Drugs & Aging*.

Many of you in your 60s or older who have been fit and health-conscious may be worried—or aggravated—about what your doctor is telling you about your blood pressure. It's up a little. In fact, it has been creeping upward to the point where now the doctor wants to put you on meds, even though research says that most people with mild high blood pressure don't need medication.

Or maybe you're already on a blood pressure–lowering drug because your pressure really was quite high—and it has stayed somewhat high even with medication. Your doctor is still scaring you with factoids about heart attack and stroke and wants to increase your medication dose.

Before you become a victim of your doctor's prescription pad, here's important news that puts a new light on blood pressure control in older people. The treatment, and the blood pressure goals, that make sense for people who are middle age and younger are not necessarily right for more mature folks. As people age, their blood pressure naturally tends to increase, and older bodies metabolize drugs differently than younger ones. Given these facts, it does not make sense to treat high blood pressure in older people based on information gathered from younger people. It might even be harmful.

A recent study showed that, if you are on an antihypertensive drug, you'll probably be just fine without upping your medication dosage or switching to a stronger drug as long as your treatment keeps your systolic blood pressure (the first number on your blood pressure readings) at about 150 mmHg (in the range of mild high blood pressure). So, take a deep breath, relax and read on.

MORE MEDS DON'T EQUAL MORE BENEFIT

To learn more about cardiovascular disease and medication-related risks in hypertensive people age 65 and older, a team of researchers from the Oregon State University College of Pharmacy analyzed a group of well-designed published studies on the topic. The studies compared different types of antihypertensive drugs against either each other or placebo and/or looked at the benefits and risks of using drugs to achieve different blood pressure targets as recommended by different sets of guidelines and/or evaluated the risks and benefits of antihypertensive drugs.

The results: Whereas antihypertensive drugs were more beneficial than no treatment for older people in terms of lowered incidence of heart attack and stroke, strict control of systolic blood pressure (getting it down to 140 mmHg or lower) was no better than mild control (getting it to 150 mmHg). As for diastolic blood pressure, most of the studies reviewed didn't emphasize or report the findings.

As for the risks and benefits of antihypertensive drugs, some studies showed no age-related side effects and some showed that, compared with younger people, older people were more likely to experience dizziness and weakness, possibly due to orthostatic hypotension (a condition in which blood pressure suddenly drops when you stand up), and bradycardia (slowed heart rate), which itself causes faintness, weakness, shortness of breath, chest pains and mental confusion.

WHAT DOES THIS MEAN FOR YOU?

The study authors note that more research is needed to determine the best methods for managing high blood pressure in older people. So the take-home from this study is that, if you're a mature adult and need medication to control high blood pressure, discuss these recent findings with your physician and ask if your current treatment goals are the right ones for you.

Better Blood Pressure Testing

Swapnil Hiremath, MD, MPH, assistant professor of medicine, University of Ottawa, Canada.

When researchers compared readings from home blood pressure monitors with those from validated mercury monitors in the doctor's office, up to 15% of home monitor readings were inaccurate. And in about 8% of the cases, the readings were off by more than 10 points—a significant difference that could change a doctor's treatment advice.

If you have a home monitor: Take it to your doctor's office every year or two to validate its accuracy.

6 Dangerous Myths About Your Blood Pressure

Mark C. Houston, MD, associate clinical professor of medicine at Vanderbilt University School of Medicine in Nashville and author of What Your Doctor May Not Tell You About Hypertension *and* What Your Doctor May Not Tell You About Heart Disease.

About one of every three adults in the US has high blood pressure (hypertension). But only about half of these people have it under control. This unfortunate statistic is due, in part, to some common misconceptions about hypertension.

Six myths—and the facts…

MYTH #1: In-office blood pressure tests are the gold standard. The automated devices in most doctors' offices are convenient, but they're not as precise as the manual (mercury) blood pressure kits. It's common for automated office blood pressure machines to give readings that are off by several points. The old-fashioned monitors tend to give more precise measurements, since doctors use a stethoscope to listen to the sound of blood flowing.

To get an accurate blood pressure reading, the patient should have rested in a seated position for at least five minutes, and his/her arm should be supported on a table or held by the person giving the test.

Blood Pressure Alert

One in 12 adults age 65 and older who began taking thiazide diuretics for high blood pressure had adverse effects, such as low levels of sodium and/or potassium and decreased kidney function.

Upshot: Older adults need to be monitored with a metabolic blood test within a month of starting thiazide diuretics. In some cases, a potassium supplement may be prescribed.

Anil N. Makam, MD, assistant professor of medicine, The University of Texas Southwestern Medical Center, Dallas.

Important: Both types of monitors can give a skewed reading due to "white-coat hypertension," higher readings that result from anxious feelings during a doctor's visit.

Fact: You can get accurate blood pressure readings at home as long as you use an automatic, cuff-style monitor that properly fits over your upper arm (not over your wrist or finger) and follow the instructions. The device should be approved by the Association for the Advancement of Medical Instrumentation (AAMI). This ensures that the device has undergone extensive studies to validate its accuracy. To tell if a monitor has AAMI approval, check the label on the device's package.

MYTH #2: It's fine to check your blood pressure now and then. Checking your blood pressure every few days or just once a week is fine for maintaining good blood pressure readings but not for achieving good control in the beginning.

New approach: 24-hour ambulatory blood pressure monitoring (ABPM). It's done routinely in the UK but is still a novelty in the US. That's likely to change because studies show that it's the most effective way to measure blood pressure (see page 26).

With ABPM, patients wear a device (usually around the waist) that controls a blood pressure cuff that measures brachial pressure (inside the arm at the elbow crease). ABPM, which takes readings every 15 to 60 minutes over a 24-hour period, allows your doctor to choose medications and doses more precisely. The test costs $100 to $350, but it is usually covered by insurance with proper diagnostic coding (such as labile, or "episodic," hypertension or resistant hypertension).

My advice: Have the test once when diagnosed with hypertension, and repeat it once or twice a year to see how treatment is working.

MYTH #3: It's OK to take blood pressure medication at your convenience. Blood pressure normally drops 10% to 20% during sleep. But about 25% of blood pressure patients (known as nondippers) don't experience this nighttime drop. Their blood pressure is always elevated, and they need to time their medications accordingly.

If a 24-hour test shows that you're a nondipper, your doctor will probably advise you to take medications at night. Taking medications at night—say,

---

Easy Exercise Fixes Blood Pressure

People taking medication for high blood pressure lowered their systolic (top number) blood pressure by five points by squeezing a handgrip exerciser three times a week for eight weeks. Participants squeezed the exerciser a total of four times at each session. Researchers speculate that using a handgrip exerciser may produce small changes in pathways that affect the autonomic nervous system, which controls heart rate, blood pressure and blood vessel function.

Study by researchers at McMaster University, Hamilton, Ontario, published in *Scandanavian Journal of Medicine & Science in Sports.*

---

at about 9 pm—can reduce the risk for cardiovascular events (such as a heart attack) by 61% compared with taking them in the morning. Nighttime medications can also help lower the surge in blood pressure that occurs in the morning.

MYTH #4: Sodium isn't a big deal for everyone. Much of what we hear or read about blood pressure these days includes references to "salt sensitivity." For people who are salt-sensitive, even small amounts of sodium can cause a rapid rise in blood pressure. But don't assume that you're safe just because your blood pressure doesn't seem to rise when you consume sodium.

Fact: Excessive salt causes vascular damage even in people without hypertension…and it increases the risk that you'll eventually develop high blood pressure.

The recommended daily limit for sodium is 1,500 mg for adults age 51 and over. People who are salt-sensitive should get even less. People who cut back on salt usually see a drop in systolic (top number) blood pressure of six to seven points and a drop in diastolic (bottom number) pressure of three to four points.

Also: Don't assume that sea salt is safe. It has only slightly less sodium chloride than table salt.

MYTH #5: You need drugs to control blood pressure. If your blood pressure is 140/90 or higher, your doctor will probably prescribe one or more medications.

But certain nutritional supplements can help boost the effectiveness of those drugs. One study found that 62% of patients who used the DASH 2 diet, exercised, lost weight and took specific supplements for six months were able to reduce or stop their use of blood pressure medications.* *Supplements to discuss with your doctor…*

•**Coenzyme Q10 (CoQ10)** reduces blood pressure by an average of 15/10 points. About half of people who take it can eventually discontinue blood pressure medications.

Typical dose: 120 mg to 225 mg daily.

•**Taurine,** an amino acid, can lower blood pressure by 9/4.1 points.

Typical dose: 2 g to 3 g daily. Larger doses may be needed in some cases.

•**Lycopene** is an antioxidant in tomatoes, grapefruit and other fruits. It reduces blood pressure, blood fats and inflammatory markers such as C-reactive protein. Consider taking this supplement if you don't eat a lot of lycopene-rich foods.

Typical dose: 10 mg to 20 mg daily.

MYTH #6: Food won't help your blood pressure. Foods rich in potassium can reduce blood pressure. Try to get at least two-and-a-half times more potassium than sodium in your diet—the ratio that blocks sodium's negative effects.

Good high-potassium foods: A medium-sized potato with skin has 926 mg of potassium, and a medium-sized banana has 422 mg.

*For more information on the Dash 2 diet, go to *HypertensionInstitute.com* and search under "nutritional services."

Wearable Monitors May Help Spot Hypertension

Margaret Piper, PhD, MPH, senior investigator, Kaiser Permanente Center for Health Research, Portland, Oregon.

Elliott Antman, MD, associate dean of clinical and translational research, Harvard Medical School, and president, American Heart Association.

Kim Allan Williams, MD, chief of cardiology, Rush University Medical Center and president-elect of the American College of Cardiology.

People suspected of having high blood pressure may soon be asked to wear what's known as an "ambulatory" blood pressure monitor for a day or so to confirm the diagnosis, according to draft recommendations issued by the U.S. Preventive Services Task Force.

Ambulatory blood pressure monitoring involves a blood pressure cuff worn constantly around the upper arm, and an attached monitoring device. The cuff automatically inflates at regular intervals, providing a more complete picture of how blood pressure fluctuates. The data is stored in the device and later downloaded, explained Margaret Piper, PhD, MPH, a senior investigator at the Kaiser Permanente Center for Health Research.

Patients are also asked to keep a diary of their activity during the day, and doctors use data from the monitor and the diary to weigh whether a person truly has high blood pressure.

The data gathered by wearing a monitor throughout a person's daily routine was up to 40% better at predicting future heart attacks, strokes and heart disease than individual blood pressure checks done in a doctor's office, said Dr. Piper. Dr. Piper is also the lead author of the evidence review.

"We found that the ambulatory blood pressure monitoring did a better job of predicting future events, and it's more accurate at predicting the population of patients who would benefit from treatment," she said.

The review was published online in a December 2014 issue of the *Annals of Internal Medicine.*

A second study in the same issue of the journal found that people with even mild high blood pressure benefit from taking blood pressure-lowering medicine.

Both studies are important, given that deaths from high blood pressure increased almost 40% between 2001 and 2011, said Elliott Antman, MD, an associate dean of clinical and translational research at Harvard Medical School and president of the American Heart Association.

"About a third of adults in the United States have high blood pressure," said Dr. Antman, who was not involved with the study. "We need to get on top of this now."

If the task force recommendation becomes final, health insurers would be required to pay for ambulatory blood pressure testing. Under the Affordable Care Act, preventive procedures approved by the task force must be covered.

WHO BENEFITS FROM A BODY MONITOR

Patients who experience "white coat syndrome" stand to benefit most from the change, Dr. Antman said. Such patients become "very nervous and their blood pressure becomes unusually elevated in the presence of a medical environment," which can lead to a false diagnosis of high blood pressure.

White coat syndrome may affect as many as 30% of people with suspected high blood pressure, Dr. Piper said.

Other people who might benefit include people who had a single bad test and people close to the threshold of high blood pressure, she said.

"That way, you don't treat the people who wouldn't benefit from treatment and might actually be harmed by it," Dr. Piper said. "It's going to refine the initial screen performed in a doctor's office, and give you more accurate results."

Another group of patients that might benefit are those who react the opposite way. These people may have lower pressure at the doctor's office than at home, said Kim Allan Williams, MD, chief of cardiology at Rush University Medical Center and president-elect of the American College of Cardiology.

"Some people's blood pressure is naturally higher at home," Dr. Williams said. "They take their medicine when they know they're coming to the doctor, or they have a lot of social stress at home."

Ambulatory monitors have been around for some time now, Dr. Antman said, adding that new versions are easier to use than ever. Some cuffs now wirelessly connect to a patient's smartphone, so they don't have to carry a clunky monitor around.

Restaurants Are Cooking Smart

Chain restaurants are reducing the salt in their food. Large chains reduced sodium in food by 1.5% annually, on average, from 2009 to 2013. Subway reduced sodium by 30% across its whole menu. Burger King cut sodium by 27%.

Center for Science in the Public Interest, Washington, DC.

NOT THE SAME AS SELF-MONITORING

Dr. Piper stressed that ambulatory blood pressure monitoring is not the same as self-monitoring performed at home by patients. In self-monitoring, patients choose when they will perform their blood pressure check, using a device they've purchased themselves.

"We had data for self-monitoring that seemed to follow the same pattern as ambulatory monitoring, but there were far fewer studies, so we didn't feel we had enough data to draw conclusions," she said.

Getting a correct diagnosis of high blood pressure is clearly important. The second blood pressure study found that people with early high blood pressure who took medication lowered their risk of stroke by almost 30%. They also cut risk of heart-related death by 25%, and their risk of heart failure by 20%, according to the study.

Drs. Antman and Williams said the results of the medication study are encouraging, but that patients should first adopt lifestyle changes before taking medication. Such changes might include exercising more, losing weight, and eating a healthier diet that cuts back on cholesterol, simple carbohydrates and sodium.

"I take this as more evidence to support the concept that lower is better, especially if you can get there with means other than drugs and using as little drugs as necessary," Dr. Williams said.

info For more on lowering blood pressure, visit the American Heart Association at *www.heart.org.*

Fish Oil's Omega-3s Lower Blood Pressure

Study titled "Long-Chain Omega-3 Fatty Acids Eicosapentaenoic Acid and Docosahexaenoic Acid and Blood Pressure: A Meta-Analysis of Randomized Controlled Trials," published in *American Journal of Hypertension.*

Eat less salt, get more exercise, drink less alcohol. Yeah, yeah, yeah. You've heard this advice a hundred times, but you don't always do it…even though you know it could help lower your blood pressure. Or maybe you do do it quite conscientiously...but it's not enough to get your blood pressure down where it ought to be.

Well, listen to this. There's a drug-free way to reduce blood pressure that can work as well as or even better than these lifestyle modifications, according to a huge recent study. It's easy to do, and it's inexpensive—and it can make a significant enough difference that some people wind up not even needing the medication they would otherwise have to take.

The key: Fish and fish oil.

THE 70-STUDY MEGA-INVESTIGATION

High blood pressure (hypertension) is a huge problem in this country. Nearly one-third of Americans have the dangerous condition already...fewer than half of them have it under control...and 20% of them don't even know they've got it. Another 30% have prehypertension, meaning blood pressure that's higher than normal but not yet in the hypertension range. All are at increased risk for heart attack and stroke. Medications can help lower blood pressure, but they have risks, too—so safe, natural alternatives are of keen interest.

Numerous studies have looked at whether the omega-3 fatty acids eicosapentaenoic acid (EPA) and docosahexaenoic acid (DHA), found primarily in fish oil, can help reduce blood pressure. But the study designs have been all over the map and results have been inconsistent. To remedy that, researchers conducted a meta-analysis, combining the results of 70 high-quality randomized, placebo-controlled clinical trials—the gold standard in studies—that examined the effects of EPA/DHA on blood pressure in adults.

The average length of the studies was 69 days. The average dose of EPA/DHA was 3.8 grams (g) per day...and sources included different types of seafood, omega-3-fortified foods and various omega-3 supplements, such as fish oil, algae oil and purified ethyl esters. The placebos were mostly vegetable oils, especially olive oil.

What the researchers found: People who consumed EPA/DHA had lower average numbers for both systolic blood pressure (the top number of a blood pressure reading, which indicates the force during the heart's contraction) and diastolic blood pressure (the bottom number, which indicates the force in between the contractions). *For instance, compared with placebo users...*

•**Overall, participants who consumed EPA/DHA** had a 1.52-point lower systolic reading...and a 0.99-point lower diastolic reading.

•**Among people who had documented high blood pressure** and who were not taking medication to reduce it, results were most impressive—EPA/DHA consumers had a 4.51-point lower systolic reading...and a 3.05-point lower diastolic reading.

Comparison: The improvement in the systolic number with EPA/DHA is on par with or even beats the average systolic blood pressure reductions seen with lifestyle modifications—3.6 points for reducing sodium intake...4.6 points for increasing physical activity...and 3.8 points for reducing alcohol consumption.

•**People with normal blood pressure benefited, too**—EPA/DHA consumers had a 1.25-point lower systolic reading...and a 0.62-point lower diastolic reading.

•**When evaluating only those studies in which participants took fish oil supplements,** the EPA/DHA consumers had a 1.75-point lower systolic reading...and 1.11-point lower diastolic reading.

Check This Before Starting a Statin

Before starting a statin, have a coronary artery calcium (CAC) test. The CAC test more accurately predicts cardiovascular risk than factors such as cholesterol, blood pressure, current smoking and diabetes. In 35% of people considered high risk according to those factors, a CAC test showed that risk was relatively low and could be managed by lifestyle modifications instead of medication. The test is widely available...takes about three minutes...and costs $75 to $100, which may be covered by insurance.

Khurram Nasir, MD, MPH, a cardiovascular disease specialist and director of wellness and prevention research at Baptist Health South Florida, Miami Beach. He is senior author of a study published in *European Heart Journal*.

•**As for dosage,** the most benefit overall was seen with daily doses of 2.0 to 4.0 g of EPA/DHA per day.

GAINING PERSPECTIVE

The blood pressure reductions seen in this meta-analysis may not seem huge to you—but they are clinically meaningful.

Consider this: In adults, systolic blood pressure normally rises by 0.6 points each year—so the 1.25-point reduction seen among participants who did not have high blood pressure would be enough to delay a person's progression from pre-hypertension to hypertension by two years. And the 4.51-point reduction seen among unmedicated hypertension patients could be enough to allow such a person to avoid having to start taking blood pressure drugs. EPA and DHA probably help blood pressure by improving the function of the endothelium (inner lining of the blood vessels), thus reducing vascular resistance.

Disclosure: This study was funded by Global Organization for EPA and DHA Omega-3s (GOED), an association of manufacturers, marketers and supporters of omega-3 fatty acids. However, GOED had no role in the study design or management of the data collected…and because this study was a meta-analysis, the data came from other published studies that were not funded by GOED.

Getting your omega-3s: Fish oil supplements are a convenient way to boost EPA/DHA intake—but the pills can increase bleeding risk, so it is important to get your doctor's OK and discuss dosage before taking them, especially if you are on blood-thinning medication or are anticipating any surgery. Eating fatty fish such as salmon, mackerel and sardines also is a great way to get your omega-3s.

Probiotics Help Reduce Blood Pressure

Janet Bond Brill, PhD, RD, LDN, a nutrition, health and fitness expert in Valley Forge, Pennsylvania, and author of *Blood Pressure Down.*

A recent Australian study found that people who regularly ate dairy products containing live probiotic bacteria had a modest but significant reduction in blood pressure. They lowered systolic (top) pressure by 3.56 millimeters of mercury and diastolic (bottom) pressure by 2.38 millimeters.

Best: Aim for one serving of yogurt with live probiotic cultures every day.

5 Foods That Fight High Blood Pressure

Janet Bond Brill, PhD, RD, a nationally recognized nutrition, health and fitness expert who specializes in cardiovascular disease prevention. She has authored several books on the topic, including *Blood Pressure DOWN, Prevent a Second Heart Attack* and *Cholesterol DOWN.* DrJanet.com

Is your blood pressure on the high side? Your doctor might write a prescription when it creeps above 140/90—but you may be able to forgo medication. Lifestyle changes still are considered the best starting treatment for mild hypertension. These include not smoking, regular exercise and a healthy diet. In addition to eating less salt, you want to include potent pressure-lowering foods, including…

RAISINS

Raisins are basically dehydrated grapes, but they provide a much more concentrated dose of nutrients and fiber. They are high in potassium, with 220 milligrams (mg) in a small box (1.5 ounces). Potassium helps counteract the blood pressure–raising effects of salt. The more potassium we consume, the more sodium our bodies excrete. Researchers also speculate that the fiber and antioxidants in raisins change the biochemistry of blood vessels, making them more pliable—important for healthy blood pressure. Opt for dark raisins over light-colored ones because dark raisins have more catechins, a powerful type of antioxidant that can increase blood flow.

Researchers at Louisville Metabolic and Atherosclerosis Research Center compared people who snacked on raisins with those who ate other packaged snacks. Those in the raisin group had drops in systolic pressure (the top number) ranging from 4.8 points (after four weeks) to 10.2 points (after 12 weeks). Blood pressure barely budged in the no-raisin group. Some people worry about the sugar in raisins, but it is natural sugar (not added sugar) and will not adversely affect your health (though people with diabetes need to be cautious with portion sizes).

My advice: Aim to consume a few ounces of raisins every day. Prunes are an alternative.

BEETS

Beets, too, are high in potassium, with about 519 mg per cup. They're delicious, easy to cook (see the tasty recipe on the next page) and very effective for lowering blood pressure.

A study at The London Medical School found that people who drank about eight ounces of beet juice averaged a 10-point drop in blood pressure during the next 24 hours. The blood pressure–lowering effect was most pronounced at three to six hours past drinking but remained lower for the entire 24 hours. Eating whole beets might be even better because you will get extra fiber.

Along with fiber and potassium, beets also are high in nitrate. The nitrate is converted first to nitrite in the blood, then to nitric oxide. Nitric oxide is a gas that relaxes blood vessel walls and lowers blood pressure.

My advice: Eat beets several times a week. Look for beets that are dark red. They contain more protective phytochemicals than the gold or white beets. Cooked spinach and kale are alternatives.

DAIRY

In research involving nearly 45,000 people, researchers found that those who consumed low-fat "fluid" dairy foods, such as yogurt and low-fat milk, were 16% less likely to develop high blood pressure. Higher-fat forms of dairy, such as cheese and ice cream, had no blood

pressure benefits. The study was published in *Journal of Human Hypertension.*

In another study, published in *The New England Journal of Medicine*, researchers found that people who included low-fat or fat-free dairy in a diet high in fruits and vegetables had double the blood pressure–lowering benefits of those who just ate the fruits and veggies.

Low-fat dairy is high in calcium, another blood pressure–lowering mineral that should be included in your diet. When you don't have enough calcium in your diet, a "calcium leak" occurs in your kidneys. This means that the kidneys excrete more calcium in the urine, disturbing the balance of mineral metabolism involved in blood pressure regulation.

My advice: Aim for at least one serving of low-fat or nonfat milk or yogurt every day. If you don't care for cow's milk or can't drink it, switch to fortified soy milk. It has just as much calcium and protein and also contains phytoestrogens, compounds that are good for the heart.

FLAXSEED

Flaxseed contains alpha-linolenic acid (ALA), an omega-3 fatty acid that helps prevent heart and vascular disease. Flaxseed also contains magnesium. A shortage of magnesium in our diet throws off the balance of sodium, potassium and calcium, which causes the blood vessels to constrict.

Flaxseed also is high in flavonoids, the same antioxidants that have boosted the popularity of dark chocolate, kale and red wine. Flavonoids are bioactive chemicals that reduce inflammation throughout the body, including in the arteries. Arterial inflammation is thought to be the "trigger" that leads to high blood pressure, blood clots and heart attacks.

In a large-scale observational study linking dietary magnesium intake with better heart health and longevity, nearly 59,000 healthy Japanese people were followed for 15 years. The scientists found that the people with the highest dietary intake of magnesium had a 50% reduced risk for death from heart disease (heart attack and stroke). According to the researchers, magnesium's heart-healthy benefit is linked to its ability to improve blood pressure, suppress irregular heartbeats and inhibit inflammation.

My advice: Add one or two tablespoons of ground flaxseed to breakfast cereals. You also can sprinkle flaxseed on yogurt or whip it into a breakfast smoothie. Or try chia seeds.

WALNUTS

Yale researchers found that people who ate two ounces of walnuts a day had improved blood flow and drops in blood pressure (a 3.5-point drop in systolic blood pressure and a 2.8-point drop in diastolic blood pressure). The mechanisms through which walnuts elicit a blood pressure–lowering response are believed to involve their high content of monounsaturated fatty acids, omega-3 ALA, magnesium and fiber, and their low levels of sodium and saturated fatty acids.

Dr. Janet's Roasted Red Beets with Lemon Vinaigrette

Beets are a delicious side dish when roasted, peeled and topped with a lemony vinaigrette and fresh parsley. This recipe is from my book *Prevent a Second Heart Attack*.

6 medium-sized beets, washed and trimmed of greens and roots
2 Tablespoons extra-virgin olive oil
2 teaspoons fresh lemon juice
1 garlic clove, peeled and minced
1 teaspoon Dijon mustard
¼ teaspoon kosher salt
¼ teaspoon freshly ground black pepper
¼ cup chopped fresh flat-leaf Italian parsley

Preheat the oven to 400°F. Spray a baking dish with nonstick cooking spray. Place the beets in the dish, and cover tightly with foil. Bake the beets for about one hour or until they are tender when pierced with a fork or thin knife. Remove from the oven, and allow to cool to the touch.

Meanwhile, in a small bowl, whisk together the olive oil, lemon juice, garlic, mustard, salt and pepper for the dressing. When the beets are cool enough to handle, peel and slice the beets, arranging the slices on a platter. Drizzle with vinaigrette, and garnish with parsley.

Serves six.

Bonus: Despite the reputation of nuts as a "fat snack," the people who ate them didn't gain weight.

The magnesium in walnuts is particularly important. It limits the amount of calcium that enters muscle cells inside artery walls. Ingesting the right amount of calcium (not too much and not too little) on a daily basis is essential for optimal blood pressure regulation. Magnesium regulates calcium's movement across the membranes of the smooth muscle cells, deep within the artery walls.

If your body doesn't have enough magnesium, too much calcium will enter the smooth muscle cells, which causes the arterial muscles to tighten, putting a squeeze on the arteries and raising blood pressure. Magnesium works like the popular calcium channel blockers, drugs that block entry of calcium into arterial walls, lowering blood pressure.

My advice: Eat two ounces of walnuts every day. Or choose other nuts such as almonds and pecans.

High Cholesterol Increases Risk for Breast Cancer

Rahul Potluri, MD, honorary clinical lecturer in cardiology, Aston Medical School, Aston University, Birmingham, England. He is lead author of the *ACALM* study presented at the Frontiers in CardioVascular Biology 2014 Conference in Barcelona.

A recent British study found that women diagnosed with high cholesterol, defined by counts higher than 200 mg/dL, were 64% more likely to develop breast cancer than women without high cholesterol. Researchers reviewed the medical records of 664,159 female patients between 2000 and 2013. The researchers decided to do the study after a recent mouse study linked aggressive breast cancer to a chemical created by the body's processing of cholesterol. Further research is needed to confirm the findings. In the meantime, there is strong evidence that exercising regularly and maintaining a healthy weight can help lower the risk of developing breast cancer after menopause. The British study also suggests that taking statins (prescription drugs to reduce high cholesterol) could help prevent breast cancer, but a clinical trial of the use of statins for breast cancer would need to be conducted before statins could be prescribed for that.

Eat This to Lower Your Cholesterol

Penny Kris-Etherton, PhD, RD, distinguished professor of nutrition, The Pennsylvania State University, University Park.

Adults who ate a small avocado every day for five weeks instead of a sugary dessert or beverage had significantly lower cholesterol than those who didn't eat one.

Explanation: Avocados contain monounsaturated fat, fiber, phytosterols and other nutrients believed to lower the amount of cholesterol in the blood.

Tip: Add avocado to salads, sandwiches or lean protein, such as chicken or fish dishes, and eat guacamole with fresh veggies—not high-sodium chips.

Low-Dose Statins Work Best for Some Heart Patients

Kimberly Gudzune, MD, MPH, assistant professor, medicine, Johns Hopkins University School of Medicine, Baltimore.

Carl Lavie, MD, professor, medicine, and medical director, cardiac rehabilitation and preventive cardiology, John Ochsner Heart and Vascular Institute, New Orleans, and Ochsner Clinical School, University of Queensland School of Medicine, Brisbane, Australia.

Annals of Internal Medicine, online

A recent analysis suggests that people at high risk for heart disease who can't take high-dose statin drugs to lower their cholesterol might benefit from a treatment combination that includes taking a low-dose statin.

The American College of Cardiology and the American Heart Association cholesterol guidelines recommend moderate- or high-intensity statin therapy for people whose medical conditions or cholesterol levels put them at risk for heart disease—the leading cause of death for both men and women in the United States.

With this recent research, scientists at Johns Hopkins reviewed published studies to compare the benefits and harms of a lower-intensity statin when combined with one of several other cholesterol-lowering treatments in adults at high risk for heart disease.

Study author Kimberly Gudzune, MD, MPH, said combining a low-dose statin with either a so-called bile acid sequestrant or Zetia (*ezetimibe*)—both of which are medications that also work to lower cholesterol levels—lowered "bad" (LDL) cholesterol. Taking a high-dose statin by itself also lowered LDL levels.

But some patients don't respond to high doses of statins and some suffer from side effects, including muscle pain, she explained.

"At least in the short term, this strategy seems to be as effective as the high-dose statin alone, although there were two major caveats: We don't know much about side effects and we don't know about long-term effectiveness," said Dr. Gudzune, an assistant professor of medicine at Johns Hopkins.

She also said the researchers were not able to draw conclusions about mortality or heart problems such as heart attacks.

There was not enough evidence regarding LDL cholesterol reduction when it came to using a low-dose statin with fibrates, niacin or omega-3 fatty acids, Dr. Gudzune said. Fibrates can lower levels of blood fats known as triglycerides and can sometimes raise levels of "good" (HDL) cholesterol.

The review was published online in the journal *Annals of Internal Medicine.*

THE PROBLEM WITH HIGH-DOSE STATINS

"It doesn't happen infrequently that patients come in and say, 'I'm having muscle pains on this statin,'" Dr. Gudzune said. "So we wanted

Walk Away Heart Disease

Taking a five-minute walk every hour counters the negative effects of sitting at a desk or on a couch for long hours. Extended sitting is bad for blood pressure and cholesterol and contributes to obesity. Researchers believe the increase in muscle activity aids blood flow, which improves arterial function and could even prolong life span.

Study by researchers at Indiana University School of Public Health, Bloomington, published in Medicine & Science in Sports & Exercise.

to review the literature and help shed a little bit of light on it for those patients."

Dr. Gudzune said they aren't yet sure of the long-term benefits of combining low-dose statins and other medications.

"Unfortunately, we weren't really able to examine the risk for [heart] events like heart attacks or strokes," she said. "We aren't sure if it translates into decreased [heart] risk."

EXPERT RESPONSE

"This is a nice paper," commented Chip Lavie, MD, medical director of cardiac rehabilitation and preventive cardiology at the John Ochsner Heart and Vascular Institute in New Orleans. "But I suspect that many clinicians . . . already know that a lower-dose statin combined with a second lipid agent—most know this best with ezetimibe—produced at least similar but probably slightly better [results]...compared with lower-dose statins alone."

Based on the most recent guidelines, Dr. Lavie said, doctors should try to get patients to tolerate the proven therapies before resorting to other less proven "but potentially very effective treatment approaches."

The American Heart Association has more on cholesterol at *heart.org*.

Cancer-Cholesterol Mix

Emma Allott, PhD, is a former researcher at Duke University School of Medicine, Durham, North Carolina, and lead author of a study in *Cancer Epidemiology, Biomarkers & Prevention.*

Cholesterol is linked to prostate cancer recurrence. According to a recent finding, patients with high blood levels of triglyceride fats—above 150 mg/dL—had a 35% increased risk for recurrence following prostate cancer surgery. Elevated total cholesterol—above 200 mg/dL—also was associated with increased risk (9% for every 10-mg/dL rise).

But: Higher levels of HDL ("good") cholesterol were linked to reduced risk (39% decrease for each 10-mg/dL improvement) in men with low HDL. Cholesterol and triglyceride levels can be improved through lifestyle changes and/or statin drugs.

Niacin and Statins Don't Mix

Robert H. Eckel, MD, professor of medicine...professor of physiology and biophysics...and Charles A. Boettcher II Chair in Atherosclerosis at University of Colorado Anschutz Medical Campus, Aurora. He also is past president of the American Heart Association.

Niacin has few benefits for people taking statins and significant risks. Niacin is prescribed with statins to lower LDL (bad cholesterol) and triglycerides and to raise HDL (good cholesterol). But statins by themselves are just as good at preventing heart attack and stroke. Niacin increases patients' risk for gastrointestinal, musculoskeletal, infectious, bleeding-related and diabetes-related side effects—and even death, according to a recent study of more than 25,000 people.

Brain Health

Alzheimer's Symptoms Reversed

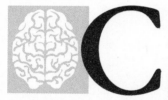

Can Alzheimer's symptoms be reversed? A breakthrough treatment suggests that they can. In a study recently published in the journal *Aging*, Dale Bredesen, MD, director of the Alzheimer's Disease Program at UCLA's David Geffen School of Medicine, presented an all-natural, multicomponent treatment program that reversed memory loss in four people with Alzheimer's and in five people with either subjective cognitive impairment or mild cognitive impairment (the stages of memory loss that typically precede Alzheimer's). *Here he describes the breakthrough…*

NEW THINKING

The current, widely accepted theory of Alzheimer's says that the protein beta-amyloid forms plaques outside neurons in the brain… somehow triggering the production of abnormal tau tangles inside neurons…thereby interfering with synapses, the information-laden connections between neurons that create memory and other mental activity.

New thinking: Normal mental function depends on a balance between synaptoblastic (synapse-making) and synaptoclastic (synapse-destroying) activity. If there is more synaptoclastic activity, memory loss may ensue. If there is chronic synaptoclastic activity, our research suggests that Alzheimer's occurs.

My colleagues and I have identified 36 unique synapse-affecting factors (including beta-amyloid). Addressing only one or two of these factors—with a drug, for example—will not reverse Alzheimer's. But addressing many factors—10, 20 or more—can effectively reverse the symptoms.

Here are several key factors in what we call the MEND (Metabolic Enhancement for Neuro

Dale Bredesen, MD, the Augustus Rose Professor of Neurology and director of the Mary S. Easton Center for Alzheimer's Disease Research, the Alzheimer's Disease Program and Neurodegenerative Disease Research in the David Geffen School of Medicine, UCLA.

Degeneration) program—factors anyone can use to prevent, slow, stop or potentially even reverse memory loss…

RESTORING MEMORY

Synapse-making and synapse-destroying factors function in a "loop" that develops momentum, like a snowball rolling downhill. In the synapse-destroying momentum of Alzheimer's, you gradually lose memories, ultimately even basic ones such as the faces of loved ones. But because the synapse-making factors in the MEND program are so effective, they can reverse the momentum of Alzheimer's. The more of them that you incorporate into your daily life, the more momentum there is to protect and restore memory.

•**Optimize diet.** Eliminate simple carbohydrates such as anything made from white flour and/or refined sugar. Don't eat processed foods with either "trans fats" or "partially hydrogenated vegetable oil" on the label. If you're sensitive to gluten, minimize your consumption of gluten-containing foods, such as wheat and rye (there are simple tests to determine whether you are indeed gluten-sensitive). Emphasize fruits and vegetables. Eat nonfarmed fish for neuron-protecting omega-3 fatty acids.

Why it works: This dietary approach reduces inflammation and high levels of insulin (the hormone that regulates blood sugar), both of which are synapse-destroying.

Important: Dietary changes have more impact than any other factor in preventing or reversing memory loss.

Helpful: Four books that have diets consistent with MEND are *Eat to Live* by Joel Furhman, MD…*The Blood Sugar Solution* by Mark Hyman, MD…*The Spectrum* by Dean Ornish, MD…and *Grain Brain* by David Perlmutter, MD.

•**Have a nightly "fast."** Don't eat three hours before bedtime. Ideally, 12 hours should pass between the last time you eat at night and when you eat breakfast.

Example: Dinner ending at 8:00 pm and breakfast starting at 8:00 am.

Why it works: This eating pattern enhances autophagy (the body's ability to "clean up" dysfunctional cells, such as beta-amyloid) and ketosis (the generation of ketones, molecules that can help protect neurons). It also reduces insulin.

•**Reduce stress.** Pick a relaxing, enjoyable activity—walking in the woods, yoga, meditation, playing the piano, etc.—and do it once a day or every other day for at least 20 to 30 minutes.

Why it works: Stress destroys neurons in the hippocampus, the part of the brain that helps create short- and long-term memory. Stress also boosts cortisol, a synapse-damaging hormone. And stress increases corticotropin-releasing factor (CRF), a hormone linked to Alzheimer's.

•**Optimize sleep.** Sleep seven to eight hours every night.

Why it works: Anatomical changes during sleep flush the brain of toxic, synapse-damaging compounds. If you have trouble sleeping, we have found that 0.5 mg of melatonin at bedtime is the best dose for restorative sleep.

•**Exercise regularly.** I recommend 30 to 60 minutes per day, four to six days per week. Combining aerobic exercise (such as brisk walking) with weight-training is ideal.

Why it works: Among its many benefits, exercise produces brain-derived neurotrophic factor (BDNF), a powerfully synaptoblastic compound.

•**Stimulate your brain.** Brain-training exercises and games stimulate and improve your ability to remember, pay attention, process information quickly and creatively navigate daily life.

Why it works: Just as using muscle builds muscle, using synapses builds synapses. (Scientists call this ability of the brain to change and grow plasticity.)

Helpful: Brain HQ (*BrainHQ.com*) and Lumosity (*Lumosity.com*) are good, science-based online programs for stimulating your brain.

•**Take folate, vitamin B-6 and vitamin B-12.** These three nutrients can reduce blood levels of the amino acid homocysteine, which is linked to an increase in tau, increased age-related shrinkage of the hippocampus and double the risk for Alzheimer's disease.

Sniffing Peanut Butter Can Diagnose Alzheimer's

One of the first areas of the brain to be affected by Alzheimer's is the one that controls the sense of smell. People with Alzheimer's couldn't smell a teaspoon of peanut butter until it was five centimeters (about two inches) away. People without Alzheimer's could smell it when it was 17 centimeters (about seven inches) away, on average.

Study by researchers at McKnight Brain Institute Center for Smell and Taste, University of Florida, Gainesville, published in *Journal of the Neurological Sciences*.

However: To work, these supplements must undergo a biochemical process called methylation—and many older people don't "methylate" well, rendering the supplements nearly useless. To avoid the problem, take a form of the supplements that already is methylated (or activated)—folate as L-methylfolate, B-6 as pyridoxal-5-phosphate and B-12 as methylcobalamin.

• **Take other targeted supplements.** Along with the three B vitamins, there are many other supplements that target synaptoblastic and synaptoclastic factors. Check with your doctor about the right dosages. The supplements include vitamin D-3 (low levels double the risk for Alzheimer's)...vitamin K-2...vitamin E (as mixed tocopherols and tocotrienols)...the minerals selenium, magnesium and zinc (zinc, for example, lowers copper, which is linked to Alzheimer's)...DHA and EPA (anti-inflammatory omega-3 fatty acids)...coenzyme Q10, N-acetyl-cysteine, alpha-lipoic acid (they nourish mitochondria, energy-generating structures within cells)...and probiotics (they improve the microbiome, helping to strengthen the lining of the gut, reducing body-wide inflammation).

Also, certain herbs can be helpful. These include curcumin (1 gram per day), ashwagandha (500 mg once or twice per day) and bacopa monnieri (200 mg to 300 mg per day). These have multiple effects, such as reducing inflammation and amyloid-beta peptide and enhancing neurotransmission.

4 Supplements That Can Impair Your Brain

Cynthia Kuhn, PhD, professor of pharmacology, cancer biology, psychiatry and behavioral sciences at Duke University School of Medicine in Durham, North Carolina. Dr. Kuhn is also coauthor, with Scott Swartzwelder, PhD, and Wilkie Wilson, PhD, of *Buzzed: The Straight Facts About the Most Used and Abused Drugs from Alcohol to Ecstasy*.

I t's hardly news that supplements—just like drugs—can have physical side effects.

Recent development: Researchers are now learning more and more about unwanted mental changes that can occur when taking popular supplements (such as herbs and hormones).

These supplements can be a hidden cause of depression, anxiety, mania and other mental changes because patients—and their doctors—often don't realize how these products can affect the brain.

Supplements that may cause unwanted mental changes...

MELATONIN

Melatonin is among the most popular supplements for treating insomnia, jet lag and other sleep disorders. Melatonin is a natural hormone that's released by the pineal gland at night and readily enters the brain. Unlike many sleep aids, it doesn't render you unconscious or put you to sleep—it causes subtle brain changes that make you "ready" for sleep.

Studies have shown that people who take melatonin in the late afternoon or early evening tend to fall asleep more quickly when they go to bed. The amount of melatonin used in scientific studies ranges from 0.1 mg to 0.5 mg. However, the products in health-food stores typically contain much higher doses—usually 1 mg to 5 mg. Supplemental melatonin also may become less effective over time, which encourages people to increase the doses even more.

Effects on the brain: In people with depression, melatonin may improve sleep, but it may worsen their depression symptoms, according to the National Institutes of Health.

What to do: Melatonin can help when used short term for such problems as jet lag. It is not particularly effective as a long-term solution for other causes of insomnia.

ST. JOHN'S WORT

St. John's wort is probably the most studied herb for treating depression. Researchers who analyzed data from 29 international studies recently concluded that St. John's wort was as effective as prescription antidepressants for treating minor to moderate depression.

St. John's wort appears to be safe, particularly when it's used under the supervision of a physician. However, it can cause unwanted mental changes.

Effects on the brain: St. John's wort may increase brain levels of "feel good" neurotransmitters, including serotonin and dopamine. But unwanted mental changes that may occur in anyone taking St. John's wort include anxiety, irritability and vivid dreams. It may also lead to mania (a condition characterized by periods of overactivity, excessive excitement and lack of inhibitions)—especially in individuals who are also using antipsychotic drugs.

Caution: This supplement should never be combined with a prescription *selective serotonin reuptake inhibitor* (SSRI) antidepressant, such as *sertraline* (Zoloft) or *paroxetine* (Paxil). Taking St. John's wort with an SSRI can cause serotonin syndrome, excessive brain levels of serotonin that can increase body temperature, heart rate and blood pressure—conditions that are all potentially fatal. It also can interact with certain drugs such as oral contraceptives and immunosuppressant medications.

What to do: If you have depression, do not self-medicate with St. John's wort. Always talk to your doctor first if you are interested in trying this supplement.

TESTOSTERONE

Older men whose testosterone levels are declining (as is normal with aging) are often tempted to get a prescription for supplemental "T," which is advertised (but not proven) to improve their ability to get erections. Some women also use testosterone patches or gels (in much lower doses than men) to increase sexual desire and arousal.

Effects on the brain: If your testosterone is low, taking supplemental doses may cause a pleasant—but slight—increase in energy. However, with very high doses, such as those taken by bodybuilders, side effects may include aggression and mood swings. Men and women may experience withdrawal symptoms—such as depression and loss of appetite—when they stop taking it.

Testosterone replacement for men is FDA approved only for those with a clinical deficiency—defined as blood levels under 300 nanograms per deciliter (ng/dL).

What to do: Testosterone has been shown to increase sexual desire in women—it is not FDA approved for women but may be prescribed "off-label." The evidence supporting testosterone's ability to improve sexual function and well-being in normally aging men is weaker—unless they have been proven on more than one occasion to have low testosterone and related symptoms. Both men and women should take testosterone only under the supervision of a doctor.

WEIGHT-LOSS SUPPLEMENTS

Two ingredients that are commonly used in weight-loss supplements, beta-phenylethylamine (PEA) and P-synephrine, are said to increase energy and metabolism and burn extra calories.

Think and Move

Physical-mental exercise slows cognitive decline, we hear from Lawla Law, PhD.

Recent study: Among adults over age 60 with mild cognitive impairment, those who spent a half-hour doing stimulating tasks that worked the body and the mind three times a week (examples include mowing the lawn in a specific pattern or finding items in an unfamiliar supermarket) showed greater improvement in memory and problem-solving skills than those who did only mental exercise.

Explanation: This kind of exercise may stimulate the growth and functioning of new brain cells, slowing cognitive decline.

Lawla Law, PhD, lecturer, University of the Sunshine Coast, Queensland, Australia.

Effects on the brain: Both PEA and P-synephrine (a compound found in supplements made from bitter orange) can make you feel jittery and anxious, particularly when they are combined with stimulants such as caffeine.

Many weight-loss and "energy" products are complicated cocktails of active ingredients that haven't been adequately studied—nor have they been approved by the FDA. They're risky because they've been linked to dangerous increases in blood pressure.

Important: There is little evidence that any of these products is particularly effective as a weight-loss aid.

What to do: Don't rely on weight-loss supplements. To lose weight, you need to decrease your food intake and increase your exercise levels—no supplement can accomplish that!

Necessary Brain Scan

People at high risk for Alzheimer's should have a scan to detect leakage in the barrier between blood vessels and the brain, says Berislav V. Zlokovic, MD, PhD. This barrier can become leaky with age, beginning in the hippocampus—an important learning and memory center. Identifying the leaks before Alzheimer's develops would allow treatment to start earlier and possibly slow development of the disease. Brain scans could be useful for people with symptoms of mild dementia on neuropsychological tests and people with genetic risks for Alzheimer's.

Berislav V. Zlokovic, MD, PhD, professor and chair, department of physiology and biophysics, Keck School of Medicine, University of Southern California, Los Angeles, and leader of a study published in Neuron.

It Might Not Be Alzheimer's

Jacob Teitelbaum, MD, board-certified internist and founder of Practitioners Alliance Network, an organization for health-care providers dedicated to improving communication among all branches of the healing arts. He is the primary investigator on a nationwide study using MIND to treat Alzheimer's and dementia (410-573-5389 for information).

If a doctor says that you or a loved one has Alzheimer's disease, take a deep breath and get a second opinion. Studies have shown that between 30% and 50% of people diagnosed with Alzheimer's turn out not to have it.

Bottom line: The symptoms common to Alzheimer's can be caused by other reversible conditions. Problems with memory and other cognitive functions often are linked to what I call MIND—metabolism, infection or inflammation, nutrition or drug side effects—or a combination of these factors. Addressing these can markedly improve cognitive function. Even people who do have Alzheimer's will see improvements.

METABOLISM

Anyone who is experiencing confusion, memory loss or other cognitive problems should have tests that look at the hormones that affect metabolism. *In particular...*

Thyroid hormone. A low level of thyroid hormone often causes confusion and memory loss. It also increases the risk for Alzheimer's disease. In recent studies, thyroid levels on the low side in the normal range are associated with a 240% higher risk for dementia in women. Borderline low thyroid hormone is associated with as much as an 800% higher risk in men.

My advice: For most people with unexplained chronic confusion and memory loss, I recommend a three-month trial of desiccated thyroid (30 mg to 60 mg) to see if it helps. It is a thyroid extract containing the two key thyroid hormones. (The commonly prescribed medication Synthroid has just one of the two.) If you have risk factors for heart disease—such as high LDL cholesterol and high blood pressure—your doctor should start you with a low dose and increase it gradually.

Testosterone. This hormone normally declines by about 1% a year after the age of 30. But in one study, men who went on to develop Alzheimer's disease had about half as much testosterone in their bloodstreams as men who did not.

Every 50% increase in testosterone is associated with a 26% decrease in the risk for Alzheimer's.

My advice: Men should ask their doctors about using a testosterone cream if their testosterone tests low—or even if it's at the lower quarter of the normal range. Limit the dose to 25 mg to 50 mg/day. More than that has been linked to heart attack and stroke.

INFECTIONS & INFLAMMATION

You naturally will get large amounts of protective anti-inflammatory chemical compounds just by eating a healthy diet and using supplements such as fish oil and curcumin. For extra protection, take aspirin. In addition to reducing inflammation, it's among the best ways to prevent blood clots and vascular dementia, which is as common as Alzheimer's disease. In addition, infections leave us feeling mentally foggy. Have your doctor look for and treat any bladder and sinus infections.

My advice: Talk to your doctor about taking one enteric-coated low-dose (81-mg) aspirin daily to improve circulation and reduce the risk for ministrokes in the brain. Even people with Alzheimer's may have had a series of ministrokes,

---

This Is Your Brain on Sedatives

Sedatives increase the risk for Alzheimer's. Older adults who used benzodiazepine sedatives, such as *lorazepam* (Ativan), *diazepam* (Valium) and *alprazolam* (Xanax), for more than three months within a five-year period had a 51% increased risk for Alzheimer's. These drugs often are prescribed for insomnia or anxiety, but they should not be used long term.

Better approach: The underlying cause of the anxiety or insomnia should be identified and treated without using medicines—for example, with talk therapy.

Malaz Boustani, MD, MPH, chief innovation and implementation officer at Indiana University Health and Richard M. Fairbanks Professor of Aging Research at Indiana University School of Medicine, both in Indianapolis.

---

adding to their cognitive decline. This is especially important when mental worsening occurs in small distinct steps instead of gradually.

NUTRITION

The typical American diet is just as bad for your brain and memory as it is for your heart. Too much fat, sugar and processed food increase cell-damaging inflammation throughout the body, including in the brain.

In one study, Columbia University researchers studied more than 2,100 people over the age of 65 who consumed healthy foods such as nuts, fruits, fish, chicken and leafy, dark green vegetables and who limited their consumption of meat and dairy. They were 48% less likely to be diagnosed with Alzheimer's over a four-year period.

Especially important…

B-12. Millions of older adults don't get or absorb enough vitamin B-12, a nutrient that is critical for memory and other brain functions. You might be deficient even if you eat a healthful diet due to the age-related decline in stomach acid and intrinsic factor, a protein needed for B-12 absorption.

My advice: Take a multivitamin that contains 500 micrograms (mcg) of B-12 and at least 400 mcg of folic acid and 50 mg of the other B vitamins. If you test low-normal for B-12 (less than 400 ng/ml), also ask your doctor about getting a series of 10 B-12 shots.

Helpful: Have one teaspoon of apple cider vinegar with every meal. Use it in salad dressing, or mix it into eight ounces of vegetable juice or water. It will increase B-12 absorption.

Caution: Vinegar is highly caustic if you drink it straight.

Fish oil. The American Heart Association advises everyone to eat fish at least twice a week. That's enough for the heart, but it won't provide all of the omega-3 fatty acids that you need for optimal brain health. Fish-oil supplements can ensure that you get enough.

My advice: I recommend three to four servings a week of fatty fish, such as salmon, tuna, herring or sardines. Or take 1,000 mg of fish oil daily. You will need more if you're already

Caffeine May Improve Memory

Participants given 200 milligrams of caffeine in tablet form—the amount of caffeine contained in a strong cup of coffee—performed better on a memory test than people who were not given caffeine. In the test, participants had to identify pictures that were slightly different from ones they had seen the day before.

Study of 160 people, ages 18 to 30, none of whom consumed caffeine on a regular basis, by researchers at Johns Hopkins University, Baltimore, published in *Nature Neuroscience*.

having memory/cognitive problems. Ask your doctor how much to take.

Curcumin. Alzheimer's is 70% less common in India than in the US, possibly because of the large amounts of turmeric that are used in curries and other Indian dishes.

Curcumin, which gives turmeric its yellow color, reduces inflammation and improves blood flow to the brain. Animal studies show that it dissolves the amyloid plaques that are found in the brains of Alzheimer's patients.

My advice: Unless you live in India, you're not likely to get enough curcumin in your diet to help, because it is poorly absorbed. Use a special highly absorbed form of curcumin (such as BCM-95 found in CuraMed 750 mg), and take one to two capsules twice a day.

Caution: Taking curcumin with blood thinners can increase the risk for bleeding.

TOO MANY DRUGS

Medication side effects are a very common cause of mental decline. This can occur even when you aren't taking drugs with obvious "mind-altering" effects, such as narcotic painkillers. Many drugs—antihistamines, antidepressants, incontinence meds and even simple muscle relaxants—can impair cognitive functions. The risk is higher when you're taking multiple medications and experience drug-drug interactions.

Doctors are far more likely to add medications than to subtract them. Many older adults are taking five or more medications daily.

My advice: Ask your doctor to review all of your medications. Make sure that you're taking only drugs that you absolutely need—not "leftover" medications that might have been prescribed in the past and that you no longer need. Then ask for a three-week trial off each medication that is considered necessary to see if those drugs are contributing to the dementia (substituting other medications or closer monitoring during those three weeks usually can allow this).

Is It a Midlife Crisis... or Frontotemporal Degeneration?

Bradford C. Dickerson, MD, associate professor of neurology, Harvard Medical School, and director of the Frontotemporal Disorders Unit, Massachusetts General Hospital, both in Boston. Dr. Dickerson conducts research on memory disorders, including frontotemporal dementia, and treats patients with the condition.

A loved one turns 50 (or so), impulsively buys a flashy sports car that he can't afford, aggressively propositions women in restaurants, swears at his boss, then lobs insults at you when you suggest that he settle down. You might think that he's having a somewhat tardy midlife crisis…but he's not.

The real problem may be a type of dementia called frontotemporal degeneration (FTD) that leaves memory intact while causing disturbing changes in behavior, personality and/or language. FTD occurs equally in men and women. People with this progressive brain disorder often alienate friends and family, jeopardize their jobs, maybe even get into legal trouble—yet often they're completely unable to recognize that they have a problem. And even if they do see their doctors, they're likely to be misdiagnosed with depression or some other psychiatric problem, at least in the early stages.

That's why they need all of us to be aware of the warning signs…so patients can get the help they need and appropriate plans can be made for their future. *Here's what you should know about FTD…*

RECOGNIZING
AN UNRECOGNIZED DISORDER

One reason why FTD often goes undiagnosed is that it tends to strike earlier than other forms of dementia, typically developing in a person's 50s or 60s—which people may think of as "too young" for dementia. Alzheimer's disease, in comparison, appears 10 to 13 years later, on average. Another source of confusion is the fact that FTD patients usually ace memory tests used to detect Alzheimer's—for instance, they often have no trouble keeping track of day-to-day events and staying oriented to space and time. Also, many people have never heard of FTD (also called frontotemporal dementia or Pick's disease) even though it accounts for up to 20% of all dementia cases.

The term FTD actually encompasses several related disorders, all of which are characterized by progressive damage to the frontal lobe, a brain area associated with decision-making and behavior control...and/or the temporal lobe, which is associated with emotion and language.

Though genetics plays a role in about 15% to 20% of FTD cases, the majority of cases do not appear to be inherited. Doctors aren't sure what triggers FTD, though they do know that in some cases the disorder occurs when a protein called tau degenerates and is no longer able to perform its main function, which is to stabilize the structure of brain cells. Other cases result from changes in other proteins. As a result, neurons die or become shrunken and misshapen...scar tissue forms...and there is an accumulation of abnormal protein within brain cells.

As a consequence of the brain degeneration, patients experience progressive changes in behavior, language and/or motor skills. *Symptoms may include any or all of the following...*

• **Personality changes**—including loss of empathy...heightened aggression...and increasingly inappropriate social behavior (hypersexuality, excessive swearing, laughing at others' misfortunes, etc.).

• **Impulsivity, distractibility, poor judgment and impaired decision-making skills.**

Examples: Impulsive spending or financial risk-taking...inability to plan and prepare a meal...inattention to personal hygiene...driving like a reckless teenager.

• **Compulsive behaviors,** such as repetitive hand clapping, incessant humming or shoplifting...and intense cravings for sweets or other carbohydrates.

• **Apathy, lack of motivation, listlessness, irritability**—symptoms easily mistaken for depression.

• **Increasing problems with language,** such as difficulty naming familiar objects, expressing thoughts and comprehending words. Ultimately, some patients are rendered incapable of speaking...and some lose the ability to comprehend the speech of others.

• **Muscle rigidity, weakness and tremors,** which can lead to trouble balancing and walking. Early on, such symptoms often are misconstrued as signs of Parkinson's disease. Eventually patients become unable to perform daily activities.

Sadly, FTD is ultimately fatal, with the duration of the disease ranging from two years to more than 10 years.

It's tragic to think that, during the early stages, an undiagnosed patient might so alienate his/her family and friends—who are understandably bewildered and upset by the person's disturbing behavior—that he winds up alone during the later stages, with no loved ones to help him. That's one reason why a diagnosis is so crucial.

GETTING HELP

In many people with FTD, the changes in the brain reduce insight and self-awareness to a degree that the patient is not able to recognize his impairments. So if you suspect that a

Alzheimer's–Vitamin Link

Alzheimer's is linked to low vitamin D levels. In a study led by University of Exeter, England, adults over age 65 with very low levels of vitamin D were more than twice as likely to have Alzheimer's as those with normal levels. Boost Vitamin D with supplements, sun exposure and/or dietary changes, such as eating fatty fish and fortified dairy.

Heather M. Snyder, PhD, director of medical and scientific operations at the Alzheimer's Association, Chicago. ALZ.org

loved one has FTD, insist on accompanying him to see his doctor and request a referral to a neurologist with expertise in the disorder. No single diagnostic test exists to confirm or rule out FTD. Diagnosis is based on a detailed cognitive and neurological exam…a neuropsychological exam to assess behavior, language and decision-making functions…and neuroimaging tests such as MRI or PET scans to check for atrophy in various areas of the brain.

There is no known way to cure FTD or stop the progression of the disease, but there are treatments that can help ease some of the symptoms. *For instance…*

•**Antidepressant selective serotonin reuptake inhibitors** may be able to help control aggressive behaviors, impulsivity and carbohydrate cravings.

•**Antipsychotic or mood-stabilizing medications** may be able to help manage irrational or compulsive behaviors and ease agitation. However, these drugs can have serious side effects, including accelerating heart disease, so the benefits need to be carefully weighed against the risks.

•**Speech and language therapy** can help a patient learn alternative ways to communicate (such as with gestures or by pointing to pictures), reducing frustration and improving quality of life.

•**Occupational therapy** makes it easier for a patient to perform basic activities of daily living and to avoid falls.

•**Counseling or psychotherapy rarely helps FTD patients,** but it almost always helps their families.

FTD eventually progresses to the point that patients need 24-hour care. The sooner a patient is properly diagnosed, the sooner plans can be put in place to make his life as secure and comfortable as possible.

info *For additional information:* Visit the website of The Association for Frontotemporal Degeneration (AFTD) at *www.theaftd.org*. This organization can also help you find doctors with expertise in FTD…as well as programs that provide FTD caregivers with invaluable support.

Work Keeps Your Brain Healthy

Analysis of the records of more than 400,000 retired workers in France by researchers at National Institute of Health and Medical Research, Paris, presented at an Alzheimer's Association International Conference.

Delaying retirement may protect your brain. For each additional year that a person worked before retiring, dementia risk dropped by 3%. That means someone who retired at age 60 had a 15% greater chance of developing dementia, on average, than someone who retired at 65.

Theory: The mental stimulation and social connections at work may keep the brain healthy.

Music and Cooking Ease Alzheimer Stress

Pauline Narme, MD, Neuropsychology of Aging, Paris Descartes University, Boulogne-Billancourt, in collaboration with the University of Lille and the University Medical Center of Reims, all in France.

Dealing with a loved one who is agitated and aggressive is never easy—but it's especially tough when that person has Alzheimer's disease and can no longer understand what is "appropriate" behavior and what isn't. Such behavioral issues are very common in Alzheimer's patients…and medication helps little while potentially causing side effects.

So what can be done about these difficult behavioral issues? According to a recent study, activities involving music and cooking can help patients and their caregivers. *Here's why…*

ENGAGING THROUGH SONG AND FOOD

Forty-eight nursing home residents with moderate-to-severe Alzheimer's disease were randomly assigned to one of two group-activity programs—music or cooking. The goal was to see whether either or both programs would help reduce behavioral problems in patients and ease caregiver stress. Though this study

Better Brain Treatment

Tangled blood vessels in the brain, called arteriovenous malformation (AVM), have traditionally been treated because the knotted blood vessels are at risk of bursting and causing a stroke.

Now: A study has found that AVM patients who opted not to remove or block the tangled blood vessels were less likely to suffer a stroke or disability or to die during a 12-year period than those who were treated.

Reason: Treatment itself can cause the tangles to burst and bleed into the brain.

Rustam Al-Shahi Salman, MD, PhD, professor of clinical neurology, The University of Edinburgh, UK.

looked at professional caregivers, it's reasonable to suppose that family caregivers—who typically would have less caregiving training and a deeper emotional attachment—would experience even greater stress when trying to manage a loved one's behavioral problems.

Two one-hour sessions were held each week for four weeks. In the music group, CDs were played featuring classical music and popular songs from the 1950s through 1980s. Participants were encouraged to listen, sing along and/or keep the beat on a small drum. In the cooking group, all participants cooperated in preparing various foods—for instance, by measuring, mixing, etc.—depending on their capabilities. Participants were invited to express their feelings and to recall memories that were evoked by the music or the food preparation.

The results were encouraging. Both programs helped reduce the severity of behavioral disorders and caregiver distress, with the music program being especially effective. *Specifically, in terms of…*

Severity of patients' behavioral problems: In the music group, patients' average score improved by 74% during the program…and four weeks after the program ended, there was still a 37% improvement. In the cooking group, the patients' average behavioral score improved by 57%…and four weeks after the program ended, there was still a 32% improvement.

Caregiver distress levels: Among caregivers of patients in the music group, the average distress score improved by 78% during the program…and four weeks after the program ended, there was still a 44% improvement. In the cooking group, caregivers' average distress score improved by 65% during the program… and four weeks after the program ended, there was still a 34% improvement.

MUSIC TO THEIR EARS

According to the Alzheimer's Foundation of America, music has the power to improve patients' mood and cognitive function and to stimulate positive interaction because the part of the brain that responds to auditory cues requires little cognitive functioning. That's why, even in advanced dementia, the ability to engage in music by singing along may remain intact.

Although this study showed greater benefits from music than from cooking, the benefits from the cooking were significant…and it's possible that a patient who had a lifelong interest in cooking would respond more positively to a cooking activity than to a music activity.

Advice for caregivers: The supervisors who led the programs in this study were not professional music therapists or chefs—and in fact, one of the researchers' goals was to look for nonmedical care strategies that could easily be adapted for use at home by family caregivers. So why not try re-creating the programs' positive effects yourself when you're with the Alzheimer's patient you care for?

For instance, play some CDs when you're together, choosing a style of music that is familiar and soothing, and encouraging your loved one to sing, clap or drum along to the tune. Or spend time together in the kitchen, preparing a simple recipe (such as pancakes) and inviting your loved one to handle safe and easy tasks, such as measuring, mixing and pouring. You might include other family members, too, to more closely duplicate the social aspect of the study's group activities. You may end up doing everyone involved a world of good.

2 New Alzheimer's Drugs Show Promise in Early Studies

Paul Rosenberg, MD, associate professor, psychiatry and behavioral sciences, Johns Hopkins University School of Medicine, and associate director, Memory and Alzheimer's Treatment Center, Baltimore.

Joel Ross, MD, president, Memory Enhancement Centers of America, Eatontown, New Jersey.

Greg Cole, PhD, associate director, UCLA Alzheimer's Center, Los Angeles.

Mark Forman, MD, PhD, senior principal scientist, Merck, North Wales, Pennsylvania.

Alzheimer's Association International Conference, Boston, presentation.

Researchers say two new drugs for Alzheimer's disease have shown promise in early experiments and will likely progress to the next round of clinical trials.

One drug is thought to reduce damaging inflammation. Patients with mild mental impairment who took the drug for over a year saw significant improvements in some measures of memory and thinking.

The second drug, called a BACE inhibitor, has been in development for more than 10 years. In very early tests, it dramatically reduced levels of beta amyloid, a sticky protein that forms plaques in the brains of Alzheimer's patients.

The results of the studies, both sponsored by companies hoping to market the medications, were presented at the recent Alzheimer's Association International Conference in Boston.

STUDY #1

The first study tested a drug called CHF5074 that's made by an Italian company called Chiesi Pharmaceuticals. The drug is believed to turn down inflammation in the brain by modulating microglial cells.

Microglia are the housekeepers of the brain. They keep its connections free of unwanted garbage, but they also produce chemicals that trigger inflammation, which can become toxic over time.

Ninety-six patients took one of three different doses of the drug or a placebo for the first 14 weeks of the study. Then researchers opened the trial, allowing study participants who wanted to continue to keep taking their original drug dosage. Seventy-four people chose to remain on the drug. All the patients had mild cognitive impairment, an early stage of memory loss that sometimes progresses to Alzheimer's disease.

Fourteen patients dropped out of the trial early. Three left because of adverse events. The main side effect reported in the study was diarrhea, which affected 16% of patients on the highest dose of the drug.

After 16 months on the drug, patients who remained on the drug saw significant improvements on some tests of memory and problem solving. The drug appeared to work especially well in patients who carried a gene called APOE4, which confers the highest genetic risk for Alzheimer's. APOE4 carriers saw improvements in test scores that were about one-third to one-fourth higher than before they started the study.

"Our study shows that we may, in some way, help patients with their memory, perhaps because we're keeping the microglia from overactivity," said study leader Joel Ross, MD, president of the Memory Enhancement Centers of America in Eatontown, New Jersey.

Experts who were not involved in the research saw reasons for caution with the results.

"With [74] patients, you can't jump up and down about some symptoms improving in some patients," said Greg Cole, PhD, associate director of the Alzheimer's Center at the University of California, Los Angeles. "It's also not clear what the nature of the microglia modulation is exactly."

Study authors admit they don't know exactly how the drug works, either. But they said they're already planning larger studies to try to confirm their finding.

STUDY #2

Another drug, a BACE inhibitor that's being developed by Merck, has the opposite problem. Researchers know exactly how it does what it does. They don't yet know whether it will help patients.

BACE inhibitors block an enzyme that cleaves a large protein in the brain into smaller pieces of sticky beta amyloid, a substance that forms telltale plaques in the brains of Alzheimer's pa-

An MRI May Show Alzheimer's Risk

By using arterial spin labeling (ASL), which can be done by all modern MRI scanning machines, it may be possible to detect very subtle blood flow changes in parts of the brain linked to memory. Early detection could make it possible to start medicines to slow decline.

Sven Haller, MD, a senior physician in clinical neuroradiology at Geneva University Hospital, Switzerland, and leader of a study published online in *Radiology*.

tients. Blocking the enzyme blocks production of beta amyloid.

In this study, which was mainly designed to check the safety of the drug, researchers assigned 30 patients to take one of three drug dosages or a placebo for seven days. Patients on the highest doses of the drug saw reductions in beta amyloid in their spinal fluid of over 80%. Researchers say they saw no evidence of adverse effects.

"We can reduce amyloid to unprecedented levels," said Mark Forman, MD, a senior principal scientist at Merck, the company that's developing the drug.

The problem, skeptics say, is that medications have been used to reduce beta amyloid before, and those had no clinically meaningful benefits for patients, at least for those already diagnosed with the disease. There have been some signs that lowering beta amyloid may be helpful for people who haven't yet begun to show symptoms of memory loss.

Dr. Forman said he thinks BACE inhibitors have a better chance of working, however.

"BACE inhibitor block the generation of amyloid at the very first step in its production. It's very different from what some of the other studies have done with antibodies that are really promoting the clearance of beta amyloid after it's formed," he said.

Experts agreed that the drug seems to work well to lower beta amyloid.

"It's been an important target. It took the drug companies at least a decade to develop this class of drugs," said Paul Rosenberg, MD, an associate professor of psychiatry and behavioral sciences at Johns Hopkins University School of Medicine, in Baltimore. "It's really compelling that this drug really does what it says it does." Dr. Rosenberg was not involved in the studies

But, "It remains to be seen if it will achieve a useful, clinical benefit," Dr. Cole said. "That's what we don't know and it will be a long time before we can figure that out."

EXPERTS HAVE HEARD THIS SONG BEFORE

Normally, these reports would be cause for optimism in a disease that affects five million people and currently has no effective treatments.

But Alzheimer's experts have heard this song before, and they say they're not holding their breaths that the new drugs will make it to patients.

"It's like that movie *27 Dresses*," said Dr. Rosenberg. "We've been bridesmaids in this field so many times."

So far, the search for a drug that might slow or stop the relentless march of Alzheimer's disease through the brain has proved fruitless.

Closely watched new agents have recently failed in late-stage clinical trials. In May 2013, a Massachusetts pharmaceutical company announced it would close after its experimental Alzheimer's drug ran into unexpected safety problems. In June 2013, Eli Lilly stopped a study of a different BACE inhibitor when patients who were taking the drug showed signs of liver problems.

YEARS OF TRIAL AND FAILURE

Those disappointments come on top of years of trying—and failing—at other promising approaches. The plaques that clog the brains of Alzheimer's patients seem to be accelerated by high cholesterol in the blood. So researchers tried cholesterol-lowering drugs in Alzheimer's patients. That didn't work. Doctors noticed that the brains of people with Alzheimer's are very inflamed, so researchers mounted large trials to test over-the-counter anti-inflammatory medications against memory loss. They were of no help.

Indeed, most drugs in development face long odds of success. Only about 8% of drugs that reach human trials will eventually make it to market, according to the U.S. Food and Drug Administration.

"In the Alzheimer's field, it can be said to be zero, because we haven't had a new drug in over 10 years," said Dr. Rosenberg.

Hard as it is to hold out hope, Dr. Rosenberg continued, "This is way new stuff."

Research presented at medical meetings should be viewed as preliminary until published in a peer-reviewed journal.

info To learn more about medications available to treat Alzheimer's symptoms, visit *http://www.alz.org/alzheimers_disease_standard_prescriptions.asp.*

Anemia Linked to Dementia Risk

Kristine Yaffe, MD, professor of psychiatry, neurology and epidemiology and biostatistics, University of California, San Francisco.

In an 11-year study of more than 2,500 adults, those who had anemia (low levels of healthy red blood cells) were 41% more likely to develop dementia than those who were not anemic.

Theory: Anemia may reduce the amount of oxygen getting to the brain, which over time may adversely affect memory and cognitive skills.

If you have anemia: Be sure to get proper treatment, which may include iron supplementation.

Very Low Blood Pressure Increases Dementia Risk

Majid Fotuhi, MD, PhD, author of *Boost Your Brain* and founder and chief medical officer, NeurExpand Brain Center, Lutherville, Maryland. *NeurExpand.com*

Having high blood pressure (above 140/90 mmHg) throughout midlife is a major risk factor for dementia later in life. But blood pres-

sure that is consistently far below the normal 120/80 in older people can also signal reduced blood flow to the brain, which can also raise risk for cognitive decline and dementia. Older adults' brains are less able to compensate for the reduced blood flow. Similarly, recent research has linked diastolic (bottom number) blood pressure under 70 in adults with cardiovascular disease to increased risk for brain atrophy, which can lead to dementia. Lower pressure in younger adults does not necessarily harm the brain.

Ever Feel "Spaced Out"?

Lara Jehi, MD, a neurologist who specializes in treating epilepsy in adults. She is director of clinical research at the Cleveland Clinic Epilepsy Center and has published more than 60 papers on epilepsy in medical journals, including the *Journal of Neurosurgery.*

The room suddenly looks different...or you "space out" for 30 seconds or longer, staring vacantly into space unaware of your surroundings...or black out and fall to the floor. You may even smell, see or hear something that isn't there.

Do not ignore it. You could be having an epileptic seizure—a hallmark of epilepsy, a widely misunderstood and life-threatening condition that affects one of every 26 people in their lifetimes.

Most people associate epilepsy with lost consciousness, convulsing limbs and twitching—but these generalized tonic-clonic seizures (once known as "grand mal" seizures) are actually less

---

Brain Spice?

Recent discovery: When mice consumed cinnamon, it was converted into sodium benzoate, a compound that may improve motor functions and reverse brain damage caused by Parkinson's disease.

Journal of Neuroimmune Pharmacology

common than more subtle partial seizure episodes, such as those described above.

That's especially true in adults. While epilepsy often starts in childhood, risk progressively increases starting at about age 55.

Why it goes undetected: Because adult-onset seizures are rarely dramatic, most doctors don't think of epilepsy very often—if at all—when evaluating their older patients.

IS IT EPILEPSY?

Many things can cause a seizure—for example, acute infection, fever, low blood sugar, poisoning and medication side effects. What generally makes it epilepsy is repetition—the same experience, reflecting the same abnormal brain activity, unprovoked by outside stimulus, over and over.

Why does it happen? Much of the time, epilepsy in older adults is the result of more generalized brain disease. Stroke is responsible in one-third of the cases with an identifiable cause. When there's an underlying cause, such as stroke, a single seizure can be labeled epilepsy (see next column).

Alzheimer's and Parkinson's disease account for a total of 11% of cases. Head trauma is responsible for 2% of epilepsy in older adults. Tumors—including metastases of cancer originating elsewhere—also may be involved. But often, no underlying cause can be found.

GETTING THE RIGHT DIAGNOSIS

If you think that you may have had a seizure, discuss this with your internist, who may refer you to a neurologist. Diagnosing epilepsy is not always easy. An electroencephalogram (EEG), a test that records electrical activity in the brain, may show abnormal brain activity only when a seizure is occurring, and brain scans, such as an MRI, can look normal.

That's why it takes an expert to identify epilepsy based on the patient's description of the episodes and other aspects of a person's medical history, such as stroke.

Important update: Traditionally, the diagnosis of epilepsy has required at least two seizures. But the International League Against Epilepsy, a prestigious group of researchers and clinicians, recently broadened the definition to include a single seizure when tests and/or history suggest a high risk for recurrence.

Examples: An MRI shows evidence of a prior stroke…or an EEG finds brain wave patterns typical of epilepsy.

Treatment is essential: Epilepsy is a life-threatening condition that requires treatment. With untreated epilepsy, abnormal brain activity can actually stop the heart—a complication that occurs in roughly 1% of epilepsy patients each year.

A diagnosis of epilepsy should prompt further investigation—the seizures may be the first warning of another serious brain condition. For example, a study in *The Lancet* found that the risk for stroke nearly tripled among older adults who had started having seizures without prior strokes, suggesting undetected brain artery disease.

THE BEST MEDICATION

Medication is effective in quelling seizures two-thirds of the time. In older people, epilepsy is more likely to respond to drug treatment, often at a lower dose than a younger person would require. But some side effects of commonly used medications, such as for sedation, bone loss and difficulty concentrating, can be particularly problematic in older adults. Also, most older adults take medication for other chronic medical problems, which can interact with certain antiepileptic drugs.

What often works best: Several of the newer antiseizure medications—*lamotrigine* (Lamictal), *gabapentin* (Neurontin) and *levetiracetam* (Keppra)—appear to be as effective as tried-and-true standbys like *phenytoin* (Dilantin) in older patients, but with fewer side effects and less interaction with other prescriptions. Side effects can include liver problems, thinning hair, dizziness and loss of balance. Medication is usually taken for at least two years.

Note: People with epilepsy can drive as long as they have not experienced seizures within a certain amount of time (which varies by state).

WHEN TO CONSIDER SURGERY

When seizures persist despite medication, surgery should be considered. The most effective procedure, resective surgery, removes the usually tiny segment of the brain where abnormal activity originates.

Cheers to Brain Health!

Light-to-moderate drinking in later life may keep memory strong. Consuming up to one drink a day is associated with better episodic memory—the ability to remember specific events. Episodic memory is the type that usually diminishes in dementia.

Theory: Alcohol may help preserve the hippocampus, a brain area that shrinks in people with dementia.

Faika Zanjani, PhD, associate professor, department of behavioral and community health, University of Maryland School of Public Health, College Park, and leader of a study of 664 people, average age 75 at the end of the study, published in *American Journal of Alzheimer's Disease & Other Dementias*.

A study presented at an annual meeting of the American Epilepsy Society found good results in nine out of 10 patients ages 60 to 74 (one patient died of a brain tumor) who received resective surgery—seven becoming seizure free—with no postoperative complications.

Breakthrough treatment: When the part of the brain responsible for seizures can't be removed—it is too large or too close to critical structures or multiple brain areas are involved—a device can be permanently implanted to modify brain activity electrically. One device, approved by the FDA recently, functions as a kind of pacemaker for the brain. The Neuropace RNS System detects seizure activity as it starts and produces a mild shock to abort the episode.

In a trial of nearly 200 people whose partial seizures couldn't be controlled with medication, the device reduced episode frequency by more than half, after two years of use. There is a small risk for brain bleeding and infection.

Watch Out for Apathy

Lenore Launer, PhD, chief of neuroepidemiology, National Institute on Aging, Bethesda, Maryland.

Apathy may mean your brain is changing. Older adults who show a lack of interest, energy and emotion and drop activities to stay at home have less brain volume than their active peers. That was the finding in a recent study of more than 4,000 healthy adults (average age 76) who underwent MRI brain scans.

The upshot: It's normal to lose some brain volume as you age, but the larger losses found in this study could be a sign of a brain disorder, such as dementia. If you frequently feel apathetic, discuss this with your doctor.

What You Must Know About Unruptured Brain Aneurysm Removal

Seppo Juvela, MD, PhD, neurosurgeon, department of neurosurgery, University of Helsinki, Finland. His study was published in *Stroke*.

What if you had some reason for needing a brain scan? Maybe you got shook up in a car accident or maybe you have ringing and pressure in one of your ears that affects your hearing. *So you get the scan, and the doctor comes back with good and bad news…*

It turns out that you don't have a brain injury or an acoustic neuroma (a tumor in the ear that affects hearing) or whatever you had the brain scan for, but you do have an unruptured intracranial aneurysm (UIA)—a bulging blood vessel smack in the middle of your brain! An estimated six million people in the United States have a UIA, and one of those UIAs bursts every 18 minutes. If you have a UIA and it bursts, causing a hemorrhagic stroke, there's a 40% chance you won't survive more than 30 days. So surgery to remove it before it bursts sounds pretty attractive. Yet, when small UIAs (one-quarter inch or smaller) are found on brain scans, surgeons usually leave them alone, believing that their risk of bursting is small. In fact, the unruptured aneurysm lodged in your brain might not ever burst—but not necessarily because of its size. A Finnish study found that certain telltale characteristics determine whether or not a UIA should be removed. And this is a key point that American doctors have not been in the know about. For them, size is what matters most, even though small aneurysms have been known to burst, too.

TOP REASON TO HAVE THAT UIA REMOVED

So which people with UIAs are really most at risk for a hemorrhagic stroke? Being a cigarette smoker topped the list. Compared with ex-smokers and nonsmokers, smokers had three times the risk. Since most of us don't know if we are walking around with UIAs, the findings of this study make smoking even more of a game of Russian roulette. If warnings about lung cancer, heart disease and premature aging aren't incentive enough to quit, the risk of brain damage or death from hemorrhagic stroke should be.

It also turns out that women, smokers or not, are more vulnerable than men when it comes to a bursting UIA. Age at diagnosis is also a big factor—men and women who were younger than 50 when the UIA was diagnosed were more than three times as likely to suffer a hemorrhagic stroke as people who were older than 50. If nothing else, these findings are clear—if you are a smoker or younger than 50 and told you have a UIA, you ought to have it removed no matter what the size, according to the researchers. If you are a nonsmoker and older than 40, especially if you are a man, you probably can safely take that watch-and-wait approach, they said.

GETTING RID OF UIAS

Microsurgical clipping and endovascular coiling are two common ways that UIA are surgically taken care of. In microsurgical clipping, a hole is drilled through the skull to get to the aneurysm. Then a small metal clip is permanently placed at the base of the aneurysm to stop blood flow into it. Endovascular coiling, on the other hand, doesn't involve open brain surgery. Instead, a microcatheter is snaked through an artery in the groin to the site of the aneurysm in the brain. An x-ray technology called fluoroscopy is used to guide the microcatheter into place and make it release one or more tiny platinum coils attached to it into the aneurysm. The coils cause the blood in the aneurysm to clot, cutting off blood flow into the bulge.

The most serious complication of these procedures is rupture of the aneurysm. Incidence is not that common, occurring 2% to 3% of the time. And, naturally, recovery for microvascular clipping is longer than it is for endovascular coiling because microvascular clipping involves open brain surgery.

After clipping, most patients spend a night in the intensive care unit and then a few days in a private hospital room. Although patients will be able to be up and about after they leave the hospital, they do have to take it easy for the next four to six weeks to fully recover.

After endovascular coiling, patients also spend a night in the intensive care unit but get to go home the next day. Within a few days, they are fully back to all of their normal activities. One drawback to endovascular coiling, though, is that the UIA can come back. So patients having this procedure are required to visit their doctors for imaging tests on occasion to make sure all is well.

In any case, no matter what your health status, sex or age, there's no guarantee that a brain aneurysm won't burst, and it's ultimately up to you to decide whether to have surgery. The Finnish researchers came to their conclusions after they examined 118 people given a diagnosis of UIA before 1979 and followed them until they had hemorrhagic strokes or died of old age or other causes. The Finns were in a unique position to study what happens to people when UIAs, large or small, are just left alone. Up until 1979, instead of removing at least large UIAs, Finnish doctors just left them alone.

Their study found that women, especially women who smoke and have large UIAs (more

---

Harmful Mild Concussions

Even a mild concussion after age 65 can boost risk for dementia. The older brain appears to be particularly vulnerable to traumatic brain injury.

To reduce the risk for dementia once you've recovered from a concussion: Exercise, be mentally active and maintain an active social life.

Raquel Gardner, MD, clinical research fellow, San Francisco Veterans Affairs Medical Center, and leader of a study published in *JAMA Neurology*.

than one-quarter of an inch in size) are most at risk for a hemorrhagic stroke. In fact, the risk of hemorrhagic stroke in women with large UIAs was 73%. If the woman also smoked, her risk increased to 100%. Meanwhile, men who smoked and had an aneurysm of this size had half the risk of their female counterparts...50%. Risk was virtually nil for men who didn't smoke regardless of the size of their aneurysms...and nonsmoking women had a 31% risk.

Importantly for those people who learn that they have a UIA, this information can help them and their doctors make crucial decisions about whether to go through a risky procedure to remove it. If you do not have any of the risky characteristics, your safest option may be to do nothing at all—be sure to have a thorough discussion about this with your doctor.

Unusual Memory Trouble

Louis R. Caplan, MD, professor of neurology, Harvard Medical School, Boston.

If you suddenly cannot remember where you are or how you got there, then your memory came back, what could be happening?

One possibility is that you had a condition called transient global amnesia (TGA). It is a temporary loss of memory that typically lasts for six to 12 hours. People who have TGA can perform physical tasks, such as driving, and can recognize familiar people, but they are unable to remember recent events. They often ask the same questions repeatedly even after those questions have been answered.

Neurologists don't know exactly what triggers TGA, but many believe it to be a type of migraine headache. It usually is a onetime event. Even though TGA is disturbing, it is a fairly benign condition. However, if this happens to you or someone you know, a neurological exam should be administered to rule out anything more serious, such as a stroke.

Handwriting Gives an Early Warning Sign of Parkinson's Disease

Study titled "Handwriting as an objective tool for Parkinson's disease diagnosis," published in *Journal of Neurology*.

Doctors usually diagnose Parkinson's disease after patients complain of the telltale symptoms—tremors, rigidity, slowed movements, impaired balance. These signs typically don't appear until this degenerative neurological disease is at a relatively late stage. In its early stages, however, Parkinson's often goes unnoticed...which is a problem, because early diagnosis maximizes the treatment options.

Breakthrough: There's a simple clue that can help detect Parkinson's in the early stages, long before obvious symptoms appear, a recent study reveals. *All that's required is putting pen to paper...*

SMALL WRITING, BIG CLUES

The study included 20 patients who had been diagnosed with early-stage Parkinson's disease and did not yet have obvious signs of motor impairment...plus 20 healthy people (the control group) who were matched for age, gender, education level and hand dominance. All of the participants were asked to write their names and copy an address. You may think that this is a very simple task, but actually it's quite complex—because it involves manual dexterity as well as cognitive, sensory and perceptual-motor abilities.

For this study, the participants wrote on regular lined paper attached to an electronic tablet that could measure the amount of pressure applied. The writing utensil was a wireless, electronic pen with a pressure-sensitive tip. A computer assessed the pressure applied by the pen, the placement and angle of the pen's tip, and the length of time it took to prepare and place the strokes of the pen. The length, height and width of the letters each person wrote also were measured.

Findings: Compared with the healthy control group, the patients with early-stage Parkinson's…

•**Spent more time with their pens in the air between strokes** (as if strategically planning their next move, the researchers said).

•**Applied less pressure when writing.**

•**Required more time to complete the handwriting task.**

•**Wrote smaller letters.**

Simplest clue revealed: Next, the researchers determined that it was possible to identify, with 97.5% accuracy, which writing samples were produced by people with early-stage Parkinson's based solely on the size of the letters! Researchers who were unaware of which writing samples came from which participant correctly identified 19 out of the 20 Parkinson's patients as having the disease…and correctly identified all 20 of the healthy controls as not having the disease.

People with Parkinson's frequently notice changes in their thinking ability before they notice any loss of motor skills. That's why a handwriting test that also engages cognitive skills—as opposed to one that focuses strictly on motor skills, such as drawing spirals (an assessment test doctors often use)—could well help doctors diagnose the disease in its early stages.

This was a fairly small study, so the results will need to be replicated in larger studies before the handwriting test could become a standard diagnostic tool. But in the meantime, why not test yourself? Write your name and copy several addresses, then compare what you've written to a sample of your handwriting from years ago. If your letters have become noticeably smaller, bring this fact to your doctor's attention, show him/her this article and ask whether you might benefit from being evaluated for Parkinson's.

Stay Away from Chemicals

Erika Sabbath, ScD, assistant professor, Boston College Graduate School of Social Work, Chestnut Hill, Massachusetts.

The brain may never recover from chemical fumes. In a study of more than 2,000 retired industrial workers, those who had high exposure to benzene, petroleum, paint, glue, chlorinated solvents and other chemicals scored worse on tests for cognitive functioning—and impairment was detected in people whose exposure dated back 50 years.

Explanation: Industrial solvents may permanently damage brain cells, so if you're around them, be sure to wear a face mask and keep the area ventilated.

Face Blindness

Galia Avidan, PhD, senior lecturer in psychology, Ben-Gurion University of the Negev, Be'er Sheva, Israel.

Prosopagnosia, also known as face blindness, is a disorder characterized by the brain's inability to perceive and remember faces. Individuals with this condition typically cannot recognize faces, often including familiar ones such as close friends and family members—and in extreme cases one's own face in the mirror.

Face blindness is often an inherited condition but can also result from a stroke or traumatic brain injury. It is not caused by learning disabilities, vision problems or memory loss. Once thought to be rare, face blindness is estimated to occur to some degree in one out of 50 people in the US.

There's currently no cure for the disorder, but people with this condition often learn to compensate by using other cues to recognize people, such as voice, body shape or other characteristics. For an online face blindness self-test, go to the site *FaceBlind.org/facetests*.

Sound Stimulation for Tinnitus

Richard S. Tyler, PhD, professor of otolaryngology at the University of Iowa Carver College of Medicine. He is the founder of the Tinnitus and Hyperacousis Clinic at University of Iowa and director of the Annual Conference on the Management of the Tinnitus Patient.

Are you one of the 12 million Americans who are vexed by a constant, unrelenting and often distracting ringing in the ears? Tinnitus is actually a collection of symptoms, not a "disease" in itself. There is no outright cure... and remedies, such as ginkgo biloba and zinc supplements, and many other treatments advertised on the Internet and elsewhere, have not been shown to be better than placebo. Naturopathic practitioners, however, argue that if the physical source of the tinnitus can be traced to a peripheral neuropathic, circulatory or inflammatory problem, natural treatments can be successful in minimizing or eliminating tinnitus.

The cause of tinnitus is unclear, but it can be related to noise exposure, head injury, aging, general ear problems and problems as unrelated as vascular disease or use of certain medications. This means that the management approach has to be as unique as the person seeking treatment.

IT MIGHT BE IN YOUR HEAD, LITERALLY

Although tinnitus is considered a problem in the ears, the real source of the trouble is probably in the brain. Tinnitus is associated with at least some hearing loss in nearly all (slightly more than 90%) of its sufferers. People with tinnitus lose tiny nerve fibers in the cochlea, the part of the ear that responds to sound vibrations. Recent studies have detected hyperactivity in nerve fibers in the brain that correspond with cochlear nerve fibers in people who constantly hear sound. This hyperactivity may be the brain's way to compensate for the loss of cochlear nerve fibers—the theory being that the brain fills in some of the hearing loss with the sensation of sound—similar to how the brain may create a "phantom limb" when an arm or leg is lost.

OPTIMIZING TINNITUS RELIEF

Although researchers predict that a cure for tinnitus eventually will be found, what should you do about it now? Past advice for people with tinnitus has been to distract themselves from the ringing by listening to pleasant music or to a constant, low-level "ambient" sound—such as recorded sounds of nature (waves lapping, rain falling) or so-called white noise, often generated by tabletop machines or smartphone apps.

But in the past five years or so, new devices—fashioned like in-the-ear hearing aids and promising sound stimulation—have appeared on the market. They can work pretty well—or they can work very well, according to Dr. Tyler, if you know how to optimize their use.

These sound generators work by covering up the tinnitus with a different sound. The so-called "masking" sounds are usually easy to listen to but also easy to ignore. They are ambient noise, whirring or nature-type sounds. These devices break the vicious habit of mentally fighting the tinnitus noise, and it can take several months before a benefit is noticed, so patience is required. Some of the devices combine a hearing aid with sound stimulation technology because studies have shown that addressing any hearing loss associated with tinnitus can help lessen the tinnitus as well.

But these devices can cost anywhere from $600 to several thousand dollars, and they are usually not covered by insurance. If you decide to invest in one, it might be wise not to do it by mail order based on an Internet advertisement. The quality of such devices may be iffy...and even if your device is OK, you might not be able to fit and adjust it for the most benefit. It's well worth paying for the services of a qualified audiologist, who will

Distrust Harms the Brain

People who habitually distrust others, believing that others act mainly in their own self-interest, are three times more likely to develop dementia than those who do not. That was the finding of a recent eight-year study of older adults (average age 71).

Why: Chronic negative emotions can impair cognitive function.

Anna-Maija Tolppanen, PhD, development director of neurology, University of Eastern Finland, Kuopio.

No-Incision Brain Surgery

For the first time, doctors have used focused ultrasound to destroy a brain tumor. The ultrasound beams can destroy cancer cells while patients are awake, without cutting through the skull.

University Children's Hospital, Zurich.

---

help you select a device, fit it and adjust and readjust it, if necessary, until its sound character and level are at their most comfortable and effective for you. You can find an audiologist who specializes in tinnitus through the American Academy of Audiology or the American Tinnitus Association, where you can also find a tinnitus support group in your area.

And if you really want to optimize use of a sound stimulation device and have greater success in tinnitus management, I recommend that you combine use of it with counseling from an audiologist or psychologist who can help you change the way you think about tinnitus to better cope with it.

Sound stimulation devices simply become a part of life for some people—they find that their tinnitus is reduced, but only as long as they wear the devices. Others find that the tinnitus recedes after six months of use and they no longer need the contraption, but, again, results are as individual as each person and his or her tinnitus. So, if you have tinnitus, you don't have to suffer for lack of silence. You can actually learn to live well with it until a surefire cure is found.

Music for the Brain!

Georg Meyer, PhD, professor of psychology, University of Liverpool, UK.

In a recent study of musicians, researchers found that blood flow to the area of the brain responsible for musical skills also improved language skills. Interestingly, brain blood-flow patterns in non-musicians became similar to those of musicians after only 30 minutes of musical training.

Takeaway: Playing a musical instrument or singing also may help keep your verbal skills sharp.

New Treatment for Tinnitus

Jay F. Piccirillo, MD, FACS, professor of otolaryngology—head and neck surgery, Washington University School of Medicine, St. Louis, and leader of a study published in *JAMA Otolaryngology–Head & Neck Surgery*.

In a small pilot study, patients did computer-based exercises focused on improving their processing of sound, speech and memory. Those who also took the drug *d-cycloserine* reported that they were better able to go about their daily lives than those who did only the training. Talk to your doctor about the best treatment for you.

New Treatment Approved for Schizophrenia and Depression

U.S. Food and Drug Administration, news release.

Rexulti (*brexpiprazole*) has been approved by the U.S. Food and Drug Administration to treat schizophrenia, and as an add-on drug for major depressive disorder (MDD) when a first-line drug fails to effectively treat symptoms.

Schizophrenia is a chronic, disabling brain disorder that primary affects people aged 30 and younger. Affecting about 1% of Americans, the disorder is characterized by hearing voices, believing other people are reading your mind, withdrawal and suspicion.

MDD, commonly called clinical depression, is characterized by persistent sadness that interferes with a person's ability to carry out life's daily activities. Other symptoms may include loss of interest in daily life, weight change, insomnia, restlessness, fatigue, feeling guilty or worthless, and inability to concentrate.

Clinical studies evaluating the drug for both disorders involved more than 2,300 people. The most common side effects included weight gain and feeling the need to move.

Rexulti and other drugs approved to treat schizophrenia include a boxed label warning of the increased risk for death if prescribed for the off-label use to treat behavioral problems in older people with dementia-related psychosis.

The boxed warning also expresses caution on the potential for increased suicidal thinking and behavior among children and young adults, a warning common to most antidepressants, the FDA said.

Rexulti is produced by Otsuka Pharmaceutical Co., based in Tokyo.

 The FDA has more about this approval at *www.FDA.gov* (search Rexulti).

Your Thyroid and Your Brain

Kenneth Ain, MD, professor of endocrinology, University of Kentucky College of Medicine, Lexington.

An underactive thyroid can impair driving.
Recent finding: Adults with untreated hypothyroidism took longer to apply the brakes while behind the wheel—a delayed reaction time that was equivalent to that of drivers who were legally drunk.

Why: Thyroid hormone is needed for proper brain function. If you have symptoms of hypothyroidism, such as weakness or cold intolerance, ask your doctor about being tested for the condition, and be sure to take your medication if you have hypothyroidism.

Beware of Internet Tests

Study of 16 online Alzheimer's tests by researchers at British Columbia University, Vancouver, Canada, presented at the Alzheimer's Association International Conference in Boston.

Beware of online tests for Alzheimer's disease.

Recent finding: When 16 online Alzheimer's tests were evaluated by two panels of experts, the tests were found to be misleading and their results invalid…and some of the tests did not disclose that they were associated with companies that market products and services to people who have dementia.

Cancer

Americans Confused About Cancer Risks

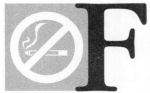

Fewer than half of Americans are aware that some major lifestyle factors can affect their cancer risk, a recent survey suggests.

Instead, many people worry about cancer-causing claims that aren't backed by scientific evidence—such as stress or hormones in foods, according to the survey done by the American Institute for Cancer Research (AICR).

"About half of cancer deaths in the U.S. could be prevented through lifestyle choices—like not smoking, eating a healthy diet, getting regular exercise, and maintaining a healthy weight," said Alice Bender, MS, RD, associate director of nutrition programs for the AICR.

But based on a recent survey, many Americans believe otherwise.

ABOUT THE SURVEY

According to experts, the survey results highlight a troubling lack of public awareness.

Among over 1,100 U.S. adults polled, only a minority were aware of key lifestyle risk factors for cancer—including obesity, physical inactivity and diets high in processed red meat or low in fruits and vegetables.

RISK FACTORS WITHOUT SCIENTIFIC EVIDENCE

More Americans, it seems, are worried about purported risk factors that have little to no scientific evidence to back them up, according to the survey.

Between 54% and 62% of survey respondents believed that psychological stress, hormones in beef, genetically modified foods, and "food additives" raise people's cancer risk.

Alice Bender, MS, RD, associate director, nutrition programs, American Institute for Cancer Research, Washington, DC.

Colleen Doyle, MS, RD, managing director, Healthy Eating, Active Living Environments, American Cancer Society, Atlanta, Georgia.

The AICR 2015 Cancer Risk Awareness Survey Report.

Meanwhile, just over half believed artificial sweeteners cause cancer—which was up by 11 percentage points, versus the same AICR survey done in 2013.

Those beliefs likely reflect popular wisdom, according to Colleen Doyle, MS, RD, managing director of the Healthy Eating, Active Living Environments program for the American Cancer Society.

"There is no good evidence that artificial sweeteners raise cancer risk, but people have heard that they do," Doyle said. "So they'll avoid sweeteners, but not worry about the bacon cheeseburger they're eating—even though there's convincing evidence linking red and processed meats to colon cancer."

So where are Americans getting their information about cancer? This survey did not ask that question, but Bender said that TV and other media are likely sources.

And headlines do get confusing, both she and Doyle said. People may see news stories about individual studies finding a link—or no link—between a lifestyle factor and a given type of cancer.

PROVEN RISK FACTORS

But in science, Doyle noted, no single study is the final word. It's the whole body of evidence that matters. Groups such as the American Cancer Society, the AICR and government health agencies look at the overall evidence and come up with reports and recommendations, Doyle explained.

Bender made the same point. "If you just look at headlines about individual studies, you'll be confused," she said.

Complicating matters, cancer is not one disease—and the risk factors for the various forms differ, Doyle noted. However, lifestyle choices matter in a range of cancers, including colon, breast, lung, kidney and pancreatic cancers.

Some of the survey results were encouraging, according to Bender. Most respondents knew that tobacco and excessive sun exposure can lead to cancer, for example.

On the other hand, about 10% fewer people in 2015 were aware that diets low in fruits and vegetables are linked to elevated risks of certain cancers compared with a 2009 AICR survey.

"That's alarming," Bender said. "Diets with a lot of plant-based foods have many health benefits."

In fact, she noted, all of the measures that can lower cancer risk have wide-ranging benefits.

"They also lower your risks of diseases like type 2 diabetes and heart disease," Bender said. "Plus, they just help you feel better."

Healthy lifestyle choices are no guarantee, Doyle pointed out. "You can do all the 'right' things and, unfortunately, still develop cancer," she said.

"But," she added, "there are very real steps you can take every day to reduce your risk."

Bender agreed. "This is an empowering message," she said. "The risk of developing cancer is not completely out of your control."

 The AICR has advice on reducing cancer risk at *www.aicr.org/reduce-your-cancer-risk*.

4 New (and Delicious) Cancer-Fighting Foods

Alice G. Bender, MS, RDN, associate director for nutrition programs at the American Institute for Cancer Research (AICR), a nonprofit organization that analyzes research and educates the public on the links between diet, physical exercise, weight loss and the prevention of cancer. *AICR.org*

Researchers are continually investigating foods that may help prevent cancer. But which ones have the strongest evidence?

The American Institute for Cancer Research (AICR), a nonprofit group that keeps tabs on cancer and diet research, recently identified the following foods as being among those having the strongest scientific evidence for fighting cancer...*

PUMPKIN

Under the hard rind, orange pumpkin flesh is rich in carotenoids such as beta-carotene, alpha-

*The studies cited in this article are only a small portion of the research supporting these cancer-fighting foods. The AICR and its international panel of experts review a much larger spectrum of research.

carotene, lutein and zeaxanthin. A high intake of foods containing carotenoids has been linked to a lower incidence of many cancers, including those of the esophagus, mouth and larynx. Scientists have recently uncovered another protective compound in pumpkins—*cucurmosin*, a protein that has been shown to slow the growth of pancreatic cancer cells.

Smart idea: Eat pumpkin (plain, canned pumpkin is a convenient option) and the seeds.

What to do: Eat a handful of pumpkin seeds (store-bought are fine) daily as a snack. To prepare your own, rinse fresh seeds in water, air-dry, add a touch of oil and bake at 350° F for 10 to 20 minutes.

GRAPEFRUIT

Grapefruit is a rich source of dietary fiber and vitamin C. The pink and red varieties also contain carotenoids (such as beta-carotene and lycopene) that decrease the DNA damage that can lead to cancer.

Scientific evidence: Strong research shows that foods like grapefruit help reduce risk for colorectal cancer. Other evidence suggests that it reduces risk for such malignancies as those of the esophagus, mouth, lung and stomach.

Helpful: Put red or pink grapefruit slices in a green salad with avocado. The tart grapefruit and creamy avocado are delicious together—and the fat in the avocado boosts the absorption of lycopene.

Caution: Grapefruit contains *furanocoumarins*, compounds that block a liver enzyme that breaks down some medications. (More than 85 medications interact with grapefruit, including cholesterol-lowering statins.) If you're thinking about eating more grapefruit and currently take one or more medications, talk to your doctor first.

APPLES

An apple a day is good for you—but two may be even better!

Scientific evidence: In a study published in the *European Journal of Cancer Prevention*, people who ate an apple a day had a 35% lower risk for colorectal cancer—and those who ate two or more apples had a 50% lower risk.

Apples are protective because they contain several anticancer nutrients (many of them found in the peel), including fiber, vitamin C and flavonoids such as *quercetin* and *kaempferol*—plant compounds that have stopped the growth of cancer in cellular and animal studies. Research does not specify any particular type of apple as being more protective, so enjoy your favorite variety.

A quick and easy apple dessert: Core an apple, stuff it with raisins and cinnamon, top the stuffing with one tablespoon of apple cider or water, cover the apple with waxed paper and microwave for two minutes.

MUSHROOMS
(USED IN A SURPRISING WAY)

When it comes to preventing cancer with diet, it's not only what you eat—it's also what you don't eat.

Scientific evidence: The evidence is convincing that eating too much red meat is linked to colorectal cancer. The AICR recommends eating no more than 18 ounces a week of cooked red meat (such as beef, pork and lamb).

A cancer-fighting meal extender: An easy, delicious way to lower your intake of red meat is to replace some of it in recipes with mushrooms. They're a perfect meat extender, with a savory, meaty taste and texture.

What to do: In a recipe that uses ground meat, replace one-third to one-half of the meat with chopped or diced mushrooms.

In a recent study, people who substituted one cup of white button mushrooms a day for one cup of lean ground beef consumed 123

Less Colonoscopies

Colonoscopy patients with only one polyp removed may need less frequent follow-up. A recent Norwegian study suggested that a follow-up colonoscopy at 10 years may be enough in some cases when a polyp is small and low risk. When more or higher-risk polyps are removed, the follow-up should be in three to five years.

Randall W. Burt, MD, a gastroenterologist at Huntsman Cancer Institute, Salt Lake City.

fewer daily calories and lost an average of seven pounds after one year.

If you're heavier than you should be, losing weight means decreasing cancer risk—the AICR estimates that 122,000 yearly cases of cancer could be prevented if Americans weren't overweight or obese.

A No-Prep Way to Prevent Colon Cancer

Thomas F. Imperiale, MD, professor of medicine, Indiana University School of Medicine and research scientist, Indiana University Medical Center–Regenstrief Institute, both in Indianapolis. His study was published in *The New England Journal of Medicine*.

Have you been screened for colon cancer yet? If you're at least 50 years old, you should be saying, "yes." Then again, only 65% of adults who should be screened are up-to-date about it, and 28% of adults who should be screened never have been.

The good news is that a noninvasive test that screens for colon cancer is now available. It's not the first noninvasive test for colon cancer... it's not entirely pretty...and it does not provide a complete guarantee that you can sidestep a colonoscopy—but it can be a good option for people who want to be assured about colon health but also want to avoid a colonoscopy if at all possible. *See if it's right for you...*

THE OLDER COLON TESTS

A good old-fashioned colonoscopy is still the most thorough and proactive screening for colon cancer, since doctors can not only see what's "up there" in real time but can also snip out any suspicious polyps in the process. But, of course, colonoscopy is expensive and time-consuming, the prep (as we all know!) is fairly horrendous, and the procedure itself is not without risk. The colonoscope can pierce the colon and, although rare, cardiopulmonary problems can result from the anesthesia.

Two other colon-screening options you might have already heard about include sigmoidoscopy and fecal occult blood testing.

Lower Colorectal Cancer Risk

People who regularly use fiber-based laxatives have a 56% lower colorectal cancer risk than people who don't use laxatives. But regular users of nonfiber laxatives have a 49% higher risk. Fiber-based laxatives, which boost the water content and bulk of stool, include Citrucel, Fiberall and Fibercon. Nonfiber or stimulant laxatives, which force the colon to contract, include Correctol, Ex-lax and Dulcolax.

Jessica S. Citronberg, MPH, a predoctoral fellow at Fred Hutchinson Cancer Research Center, Seattle, and leader of a study published in *The American Journal of Gastroenterology*.

Sigmoidoscopy uses a scope that is shorter than the one used for colonoscopy and examines only the lower part of the colon. A fecal occult blood test, also called a fecal immunochemical test, looks for blood in a very small stool sample that the patient collects at home and then mails to a lab in a special envelope. If an abnormality is found with either of these screening tests, a colonoscopy is then done to confirm the diagnosis and continue with next steps, such as removal and biopsy of polyps.

A NEW OPTION

The newest test, called Cologuard, is similar to but more thorough than fecal occult blood testing. It detects colon cancer by examining a stool sample for the presence of blood and also abnormal DNA. To find out whether Cologuard was as good as or better than fecal occult blood testing, its manufacturer sponsored a research study that was conducted at the Indiana University School of Medicine in Indianapolis.

The study included 9,989 men and women from around the United States and Canada. All of them were given a colonoscopy, a fecal occult blood test and a Cologuard test, and the results were compared.

The results: Cologuard was a cut above fecal occult blood testing. Cologuard correctly identified 60 of the 65 cancers detected by colonoscopy and 321 of the 757 advanced polyps detected by colonoscopy. (Advanced polyps are those that are either one centimeter or larger and/or have abnormal cellular DNA.) In comparison, only 48 cancers and 180 advanced polyps were detected by fecal occult blood testing.

On the downside, the Cologuard test was associated with nearly three times more false-positives than fecal occult blood testing. This means that some people who opt for Cologuard because they want to avoid a colonoscopy may end up having to get one anyway to confirm that they do not have colon cancer or precancerous polyps. The false-positives were much more commonly seen in older adults and may have to do with age-related DNA changes or with Cologuard's ability to detect minor polyps, which are very common with increasing age, according to the study's lead scientist, Thomas Imperiale, MD.

IS IT RIGHT FOR YOU?

Dr. Imperiale said that the Cologuard test is for people who do not have risk factors or signs of colon disease but who want to be screened to make sure that all is well and remains so. Folks who have lower gastrointestinal pain or bloody stools, a personal or family history of polyps or colon cancer or who have inflammatory bowel disease (Crohn's disease and ulcerative colitis) aren't eligible and would have to bite the bullet and go for colonoscopy instead.

What's involved in a Cologuard test? You receive a test kit by mail. The kit contains everything you need to collect and package two stool samples, including a special receptacle that fits over the toilet bowl and a liquid preservative. Then you send the samples to the lab in a box that comes with prepaid postage. No special dietary restrictions, preparation or time off from work is required.

If the lab detects blood or abnormal cells in the stool samples, you're told to get a colonoscopy. If all is well, no worries. You repeat the test in another three years instead of annually, which is the frequency required for fecal occult blood testing.

The cost of the Cologuard test is $599, and it is covered by Medicare Part B for people who are 50 to 85 years old. Private insurance companies generally, but not always, cover what Medicare deems is coverable, so if you have private insurance, check in with your provider to find out whether it currently covers or intends to cover Cologuard if you are interested in this colon cancer screening option.

Cologuard seems to be a step up from fecal occult blood testing in its ability to detect nearly as many colon cancers as colonoscopy. It also provides a bit more information than fecal occult blood testing about where a person stands in terms of colon cancer risk—but the fact remains that it can't match the thoroughness of colonoscopy. If you, for whatever reason, simply refuse to have screening colonoscopies, then Cologuard could literally save your life, so be sure to ask your doctor about it. If you are willing to have screening colonoscopies but are considered at low risk for colon cancer, it might also be an option for you—again, discuss it with your doctor.

Danger After a Colonoscopy

Karen Larson, editor of *Bottom Line/Personal*, 281 Tresser Blvd., Stamford, Connecticut 06901. *BottomLinePersonal.com*

What's the best part of a colonoscopy? When it's over, of course. But for one of my colleagues, the end of a colonoscopy was just the start of a medical misadventure—she fainted two days after the procedure and wound up in the emergency room due to dehydration.

That's not uncommon, says Leo Galland, MD, founder and director of the Foundation for Integrated Medicine in New York City. The incident points to a troubling gap in colonoscopy communication—patients are told how to prepare for this procedure but often not what they should do afterward. *Dr. Galland's advice…*

•**Drink eight to 16 ounces of fruit juice right after the procedure.** Ask if the health facility will have juice. If not, bring your own. Any beverage will help with dehydration, but fruit juice also wards off hypoglycemia—low blood sugar. Drink another 48 ounces of fluid during the day and 64 ounces the day after.

•**Eat a light snack as soon as you feel able.** Bring a sandwich or an energy bar with you to the health facility, too. Avoid foods with high fat content—fats are difficult to digest.

•**Take a probiotic supplement.** Take one just before your first meal following the procedure and twice a day for the next 10 days at the start of a meal. Consuming probiotics can reduce bowel irritation and promote good overall digestive health. Try a few different ones well before your colonoscopy to find one that seems to aid your digestion.

New Colon Polyp Removal Method Easier on Patients

Jonathan Buscaglia, MD, director, advanced endoscopy, Stony Brook University School of Medicine, Stony Brook, New York.

Gregory Haber, MD, FRCP, chief, division of gastroenterology, Lenox Hill Hospital, New York City.

Fadi Braiteh, MD, oncologist, Comprehensive Cancer Centers of Nevada, US Oncology Network affiliate, Las Vegas.

Presentation, Digestive Disease Week meeting, Chicago.

A team-based procedure for removing difficult or large precancerous colon polyps is effective and eliminates the need to take out part of a person's colon to reduce their cancer risk, a small clinical trial shows.

In the procedure, a surgeon manipulates the colon from outside the organ so that a second doctor can get to the hard-to-reach polyp and remove it from inside the colon via colonoscopy.

This team procedure, called "laparoscopic-assisted colonoscopy with polypectomy," eliminates the need for a surgeon to remove the entire section of the colon that contains the polyp, a procedure called "laparoscopic hemicolectomy."

A clinical trial comparing the new and old procedures found that laparoscopic-assisted colonoscopy is as safe and effective as surgery to remove part of the colon, but results in shorter hospital stays and less harm done to patients, said lead researcher Jonathan Buscaglia, MD.

"The advantage is that the polyp is removed while sparing that section of colon, which is

A Pill to Detect Cancer?

Researchers at Google are working to create a pill containing magnetic nanoparticles that would travel through the bloodstream searching for cancerous cells. Findings would be sent to a wearable sensor. The cancer-detecting pill is at least a decade away.

Andrew Conrad, head of the Life Sciences team at Google's X lab, Mountain View, California.

important to patients," said Dr. Buscaglia, director of advanced endoscopy at Stony Brook University College of Medicine, in New York. "Patients often can suffer from diarrhea or abnormal bowel movements when they have part of their colon removed."

Dr. Buscaglia presented his team's findings at a recent Digestive Disease Week meeting, held in Chicago.

Colon cancer has decreased about 30% in recent years, mainly because doctors are eliminating the risk by finding and removing precancerous polyps during routine colonoscopies, Dr. Buscaglia said.

In a colonoscopy, a doctor scans the inside of a person's colon using a thin, flexible tube inserted through the anus. A small video camera transmits images of the colon, and if a polyp is found then surgical tools can be sent through the tube so doctors can remove the growth on the spot.

But sometimes these polyps are either very large or located in a fold or bend of the colon, making it tough for doctors to remove them during a colonoscopy, Dr. Buscaglia explained.

In those cases, the alternative has been to remove the section of the colon that contains the polyp, and then sew the colon back together.

TEST DETAILS

Dr. Buscaglia and his colleagues decided to test what they felt would be a better and less invasive way to get at these polyps.

In their team procedure, a surgeon makes a tiny incision in the abdomen and uses a thin, illuminated tube called a laparoscope to move the colon around from the outside of the organ.

By manipulating the organ from the outside, they can move the polyp into a better position for removal from within by a second doctor who is performing a simultaneous colonoscopy.

The recent clinical trial involving 28 patients found that those who underwent the team procedure had an average hospital stay of 2.5 days, while those who had a section of colon removed spent four days in recovery.

Patients treated with the team procedure also lost less blood and required less IV fluid in the operating room. The procedure itself also took much less time, 95 minutes on average compared with 179 minutes for removing part of the colon.

After surgery, team-treated patients were able to resume eating solid foods in less than two days, while the surgical patients had to wait almost four days.

This new procedure could prove very cost-effective, even though it requires two doctors instead of just one, Dr. Buscaglia said.

"Cost, when it comes to operations, is less related to what you're doing in the operating room than how much operating time you're utilizing," he said. "It's also not so much the operation itself, but it's the length of the hospital stay. All of those things go into a heavy cost for someone who has a three-hour surgery and then stays in the hospital for three to five days following surgery."

Dr. Buscaglia and his team plan to conduct a larger, multi-center investigation to confirm these findings.

EXPERT COMMENT

Fadi Braiteh, MD, a Las Vegas oncologist not involved with the study, said such follow-up trials are needed before doctors can begin using this team approach with confidence.

"The use of laparoscopy to assist the operator during colonoscopy for successful resection of the polyp could be a safer and less aggressive measure," said Dr. Braiteh, with Comprehensive Cancer Centers of Nevada, a US Oncology Network affiliate. "These are interesting results, but a larger multi-institutional study is warranted to validate and precisely measure these findings."

Another expert said this new approach appears to have some merit.

"I think it's a very good approach. It's reduced the amount of hospital stay, and it's easier on the patient," said Gregory Haber, MD, chief of gastroenterology at Lenox Hill Hospital, in New York City.

But before calling in a surgeon to collaborate, a doctor ought to consider sending the patient to a physician who is expert at removing tough polyps through colonoscopy, he added.

"If you are not used to doing difficult polyps, rather than thinking about doing a surgery, you should consider sending it to an expert in that area," Dr. Haber said. "This is not necessarily what you have to do when you have a polyp that you have problems with, because you also have the option of going to an expert in polyp removal."

Because this study was presented at a medical meeting, the data and conclusions should be viewed as preliminary until published in a peer-reviewed journal.

 The American Cancer Society has more about colonoscopy at *www.cancer.org*.

This Vitamin Can Prevent Skin Cancer Recurrence

Diona Damian, MBBS, PhD, is professor of dermatology at University of Sydney, Australia, and senior author of a study of 386 skin-cancer patients, presented at a recent meeting of the American Society of Clinical Oncology.

People with a history of multiple skin cancers are less likely to develop new skin cancers if they take a form of vitamin B-3, reports Diona Damian, MBBS, PhD.

Recent finding: 500 mg of nicotinamide (vitamin B-3) taken twice daily cut the risk for nonmelanoma skin cancers (basal and squamous cell carcinoma) by 23%. Other studies have shown nicotinamide may be of benefit to individuals with inflammatory skin conditions. Take only under a doctor's supervision.

Double Trouble

People who use alcohol and tobacco together have nearly twice the risk for esophageal cancer as those who only smoke or only drink. Esophageal squamous cell carcinoma (ESCC) begins in the cells lining the esophagus. Alcohol and tobacco are known ESCC risk factors. A recent study found that using both significantly increases their potency as carcinogens.

Anoop Prabhu, MD, Advanced Endoscopy Fellow, Icahn School of Medicine at Mount Sinai, New York City, and leader of a study published in The American Journal of Gastroenterology.

Alcohol: The Drink That's Linked to Deadly Melanoma Skin Cancer

Study titled "Alcohol drinking and cutaneous melanoma risk—A systematic review and dose-risk meta-analysis," to be published in *British Journal of Dermatology*.

You know that cavorting in the sun without adequate protection from clothing and sunscreen is a big mistake when it comes to preventing melanoma…and you know that this kind of skin cancer can kill. But did you know that what you drink affects your melanoma risk, too? When it comes to alcohol, it's true—in fact, your skin cancer risk rises with as little as one serving of alcohol a day, according to recent research. *Here's the startling connection…*

IMBIBERS BEWARE

It's well-established that the leading cause of melanoma is intermittent, intense, sunburn-causing exposure to the sun's ultraviolet rays. Even sunburns from childhood can come back to haunt you decades later, increasing your skin cancer risk. But other factors (a fair complexion, the presence of moles, advancing age, etc.) enter into the risk equation, too…and researchers decided to see whether alcohol also played a role. To that end, they conducted a meta-analysis, pulling together 16 previous studies that investigated a possible relationship between alcohol consumption and melanoma. The data they examined represented a total of 6,251 cases of this type of skin cancer.

Because the various studies used different measures to describe levels of alcohol consumption, the researchers looked at the grams of ethanol consumed each day, designating one drink as 12.5 grams of ethanol. (For comparison's sake, in the US, one drink is generally defined as 14 grams of ethanol—the equivalent of a 12-ounce beer, a five-ounce glass of wine or a 1.5-ounce shot of 80-proof liquor.) For the recent study, light drinking was defined as no more than 12.5 grams of ethanol per day…moderate-to-heavy consumption was defined as anything in excess of 12.5 grams per day. Although there was limited data on heavy drinking, this level of consumption was defined as more than 50 grams of ethanol (four drinks) per day.

What the researchers discovered: Compared with people who never or seldom drank, people who did drink were 20% more likely to get melanoma. As alcohol intake went up, so did the danger—light drinking was associated with a 10% increase in melanoma risk…moderate-to-heavy drinking was associated with an 18% increase in risk…and heavy drinking was associated with a 55% increase in risk.

What explains the link? You may assume that people who are imbibing at the beach, barbecue or ballgame don't want to interrupt their fun, so they don't bother to refresh their sunscreen…or else they're so buzzed that they're oblivious to how sunburned they're getting. And no doubt that plays a part—in fact, other research suggests that nearly one-fifth of sunburns in American adults are attributable to alcohol consumption.

But drunk-induced sunburns don't tell the whole story, the recent study's authors suggested.

Their theory: Alcohol intake may reduce the strength of the immune system, allowing the sun's UV rays to do greater harm to cells. That's because soon after ethanol is consumed, it's converted to a substance that makes skin even more sun-sensitive and vulnerable to oxidative stress, which in turn damages DNA and increases cancer risk.

Self-defense for your skin: If you plan to drink alcohol when you're outdoors, you'd be wise to slather on the sunscreen beforehand and wear plenty of protective clothing…set a timer on your watch or phone to remind you to refresh your sunscreen every few hours…and limit alcohol consumption to no more than one drink per day. Need even more motivation? Remember that alcohol is linked to numerous other malignancies, including cancers of the mouth, esophagus, stomach, colon, liver, breast and prostate—so in that regard, what's good for your skin is good for the rest of your body, too.

New Drug for Melanoma Beats Out Chemo

Georgina Long, MD, PhD, associate professor of melanoma biology and translational research at Melanoma Institute Australia at University of Sydney. She is coauthor of a study published in *The New England Journal of Medicine.*

A new immunotherapy for advanced melanoma is now available.

Recent finding: Patients who took Opdivo (nivolumab) were 58% less likely to die within one year than patients who used a standard chemotherapy drug. Opdivo, which uses the body's immune system to fight cancer, also has fewer side effects. The U.S. Food and Drug Administration granted accelerated approval to Opidivo for advanced melanoma in December of 2014.

Hyperthermia Therapy Makes Cancer Treatments Work Better

Jennifer Yu, MD, PhD, radiation oncologist and cancer researcher in stem cell biology and regenerative medicine, Cleveland Clinic, Cleveland. She also is the director of the Cleveland Clinic Center for Hyperthermia.

A treatment for cancer used in ancient Egypt is proving to be effective in 21st-century America. The first known mention of therapeutic hyperthermia, which involves using hot water to heat a tumor and the surrounding area, appeared in a 5,000-year-old papyrus! Today, doctors at some cancer centers are using noninvasive mild-heat hyperthermia to boost the effectiveness of other cancer therapies, especially radiation, without increasing the dosage and subsequent risk for unwanted side effects.

How it works: Mild-heat hyperthermia combats cancer several ways. *For instance, it…*

•**Disables certain enzymes,** impairing the cancer cells' ability to repair the DNA damage caused by radiation.

•**Improves blood flow to the area where the tumor is,** bringing more oxygen to the tissues, which in turn increases the effectiveness of radiation.

•**Damages proteins and structures within cancer cells,** causing tumors to shrink—while doing minimal damage to normal tissues.

•**Kills cancer stem cells that often are resistant to radiation.**

•**May enhance the effects of certain anticancer drugs.**

•**Supports the immune system,** increasing the body's ability to fight off the cancer.

What happens during treatment: Hyperthermia is added to a course of radiation. For instance, suppose a patient is scheduled to undergo five radiation sessions per week for four weeks. If he/she is receiving hyperthermia, he also would get two sessions of the mild-temperature hyperthermia therapy, administered immediately before the radiation (the other three days per week, radiation would be administered alone).

Typically hyperthermia is applied with hot-water bags that are carefully positioned and precisely heated with an external microwave unit and temperature monitors. Temperatures are maintained at slightly above "fever range," or around 110° F. The patient lies in a darkened room for an hour during the hyperthermia treatment. It feels like a heating pad. Many patients take a nap during the treatment. Once the hyperthermia session is over, the patient immediately moves on to the radiation.

Risks and side effects are minor. In about 10% of cases, small blisters develop.

Types of cancer treated: Mild-heat hyperthermia is most often used to treat cancers that occur near the surface of the body, such as breast cancer, melanoma, and head and neck cancers. It also is increasingly being used for other types of cancer as well, including cancers of the cervix, prostate, rectum, pancreas, brain, bladder and liver.

Though hyperthermia can help patients who are facing their first bouts with cancer, research suggests that it is especially beneficial for people with recurring cancer where radiation didn't help as much as doctors had hoped initially. For instance, according to one study from Duke University Medical Center that looked at patients with recurrent breast cancer, hyperthermia combined with radiation successfully eradicated tumors in 65% of cases, versus just 42% for radiation alone. For patients whose cancer has metastasized, whole-body hyperthermia may be done using warm-water immersion.

Where to get treatment: Most insurance companies cover hyperthermia therapy. Unfortunately, this safe and effective treatment isn't widely available. Many places do not have the personnel or infrastructure to run these types of facilities, and few young physicians are trained in how to deliver hyperthermia. If you are interested in having a consultation with a doctor who provides this treatment, enlist your oncologist's aid in finding a practitioner.

5 Sunburns = More Risk

Abrar Qureshi, MD, MPH, professor of dermatology, Warren Alpert Medical School, Brown University, Providence.

If you had five or more blistering sunburns before age 20, watch out. This increases lifetime risk for melanoma by 80%, according to a recent study of nearly 109,000 Caucasian women.

Why: Sudden, massive amounts of sun exposure may damage pigment cells in the skin.

If you had many bad sunburns in your youth: Be particularly vigilant about further sun exposure and annual skin exams, which should be performed by a board-certified dermatologist.

Skin Cancer Symptom

Gil Yosipovitch, MD, chair of dermatology at Temple University School of Medicine and director of Temple Itch Center, both in Philadelphia, and leader of a study published in *JAMA Dermatology*.

Pain or itching can be signs of skin cancer, warns Gil Yosipovitch, MD. People often are told to be on the lookout for visual changes to their skin, but it is important not to overlook changes in how skin feels.

Recent findings: More than one-third of skin cancer lesions itch—these can be a sign of basal cell carcinoma. About 30% are painful, and these can indicate squamous cell carcinoma.

Bacteria May Help Battle Cancer, Study Suggests

Symposium on Clinical Interventional Oncology, news release.

Bacteria may offer a new way to treat cancer, a small, preliminary study suggests. Researchers injected a weakened strain of *Clostridium novyi-NT* bacteria spores into tumors in six patients. The bacteria grew in the tumors and killed cancer cells, the investigators reported.

C. novyi-NT, which lives in soil, is a close relative of the bacteria that causes botulism. Before injecting C. novyi-NT into the patients, the researchers weakened it by removing its dangerous toxin.

Five of the six patients are still alive, while one died from unrelated causes several months after receiving the bacteria injection, according to the study that was presented at the annual Symposium on Clinical Interventional Oncology in Hollywood, Florida.

Research presented at medical meetings should be viewed as preliminary until published in a peer-reviewed journal.

"When tumors reach a certain size, parts of them do not receive oxygen, which makes them resistant to conventional therapies such as radiation and chemotherapy," study author Ravi Murthy, MD, a professor of interventional radiology at MD Anderson Cancer Center in Houston, said in a symposium news release.

"C. novyi-NT thrives under these conditions, hones in on the low-oxygen areas and destroys tumors from the inside while sparing normal tissue," Dr. Murthy explained.

C. novyi-NT also triggers an immune response to cancer.

"Essentially, C. novyi-NT causes a potent cancer-killing infection in the tumor," study principal investigator Filip Janku, MD, an associate professor in the department of investigation therapeutics at MD Anderson Cancer Center, said in the news release.

The recent findings are very preliminary. Additional research into the potential therapy is needed, according to study authors.

info The U.S. National Cancer Institute has more about cancer treatments at *http://www.cancer.gov/publications/fact-sheets#therapy.*

The "20-Mole Test"

Giuseppe Argenziano, MD, associate professor of dermatology, Second University of Naples, Caserta, Italy.

If you have a total of 20 or more moles on both your arms, your risk for melanoma is more than six times higher than the risk for people with fewer moles, according to a recent study of more than 2,000 dermatology patients.

Why: Having a lot of arm moles indicates that you may have many on your entire body, raising the risk for DNA changes that can lead to the deadly skin cancer. Only moles were counted—not freckles or age spots.

Singing Bowls: Ancient Vibrational Healing Therapy for Cancer

Diane Mandle, certified in Tibetan Bowl Sound Healing through the state of California and Sacred Sound Workshops, and author of the e-books *How to Clear Space with Sound Using Tibetan Bowls & Tingshas* and *Ancient Sounds for a New Age: Introduction to Sacred Sound Instruments.*

While we Westerners have gotten quite comfortable with the idea of incorporating ancient Eastern healing practices such as yoga and tai chi into our lives, there are other Asian techniques that many find outside their comfort zones.

Case in point: Tibetan singing bowl therapy. The name has a nice, well, ring to it, but are we really to believe that banging on a bowl will help our health, maybe even alter our breath and heart rates to allow speedier healing?

WHY SINGING BOWLS?

When played by a trained practitioner, a singing bowl emits a powerful sound and "tonal" vibration that is felt in the part of the body near where the bowls are placed. This helps to restore normal, healthy "vibratory frequencies" to diseased or out-of-balance points in the body. Each bowl emits a full range of harmonics (a series of overtones produced in addition to the dominant tone). Some we can hear, some we can't. Listening to this tonal vibration also produces the deep, calming brain waves of alpha and theta, as proven by biofeedback equipment. People go into a highly meditative state very quickly. Used this way, the bowls are remarkably helpful for any complaint that relates to stress and pain, including the emotional and physical stress of chemotherapy, fibromyalgia, depression and chronic fatigue.

A SINGING BOWL SESSION

It is not uncommon for the first session to discharge blocked stress, energy and toxins and, as a result, clients are sometimes a little headachy or nauseated afterward. Then again, some go home and sleep incredibly well or may have a surge of new energy. In subsequent sessions, bowls are sounded to produce alignment in clients' areas of need and to reconnect clients to their memories of well-being. Eventually an "anchoring" process ensues where just the memory of the sound experience triggers them into a more peaceful state.

Typically, after four to six weeks of regular sessions, I send my clients off on their own. Some who are undergoing treatment for life-threatening illnesses such as cancer continue to come weekly. It is not uncommon to get follow-up e-mails from happy customers. By then, they have shifted so much that they don't need me any more except for an occasional tune-up. My job is to empower each person to become his/her own healer.

Homework: I give my clients CDs of singing bowl performances that can be used at home.

DO-IT-YOURSELF SINGING BOWL PRACTICE

Using a singing bowl is something anyone can learn to do for themselves. To start you off in singing bowl therapy…

Bowl shopping. You will need a high-quality, authentic bowl, for which you can expect to pay $120 (for a small one) or more. Don't shop for a "bargain." At lower prices, you'd be getting a commercial knockoff made with an alloy that doesn't have quality sound. The ancient bowls were crafted in monasteries by monks who really cared about how they sounded. You can learn more about the different types of bowls and how to ensure that you are buying an authentic one on my website (*SoundEnergyHealing.com*).

Thyroid Cancer: Epidemic or Overdiagnosis?

Juan Pablo Brito, MBBS, assistant professor and healthcare delivery scholar in the division of endocrinology, diabetes, metabolism and nutrition at the Mayo Clinic, Rochester, Minnesota, where he also is coinvestigator of the Knowledge and Evaluation Research Unit.

Any increase in cancer is worrisome, but the dramatic rise in thyroid cancer is particularly troubling. In just 30 years, the

Symptoms of Thyroid Cancer

Thyroid cancer typically doesn't cause any signs or symptoms early in the disease. *As thyroid cancer grows, it may cause…*

- **A lump that can be felt through the skin on your neck**
- **Changes to your voice, including increasing hoarseness**
- **Difficulty swallowing**
- **Pain in your neck and throat**
- **Swollen lymph nodes in your neck**

incidence in the US has more than tripled, from 3.6 cases per 100,000 people in 1973 to 11.6 per 100,000 in 2009.

It is among the fastest-growing diagnoses in the US. This is an alarming trend—but not for the reason you might think.

Experts have concluded that the vast majority of thyroid cancers were there all along. Better imaging tests such as ultrasound and magnetic resonance imaging (MRI) now make it possible to detect minuscule cancers that would have been missed before. What looks like an increase in disease actually is an increase in diagnosis.

Isn't it good to detect cancers when they're still small? Not in this case. The most common type of thyroid cancer grows slowly—if it grows at all. Most patients would never have symptoms or need treatment. But once you know you have cancer, you want that thing out of there. Unfortunately, the treatments often cause more problems than they solve.

MORE SCREENING, MORE CANCER

There's a saying in medicine, "When you have a new hammer, everything looks like a nail."

In the 1980s, ultrasound was the new hammer. Endocrinologists used it routinely during office visits. Even if you came in with vague symptoms that could be caused by just about anything, such as fatigue from insomnia, you would likely be given a neck ultrasound and possibly an MRI or a computerized tomography (CT) scan. These tests can detect nodules as small as 2 millimeters (mm) in diameter.

In many cases, tests that were ordered for other conditions happened to detect a growth in the thyroid. More cases of thyroid cancer are diagnosed incidentally than when doctors actually are looking for them. Doctors call these unexpected findings "incidentalomas."

Does finding small cancers save lives? Despite the tremendous increase in diagnosed thyroid cancers, the death rate has scarcely budged—it was 0.5 per 100,000 people a generation ago, and it is virtually the same today. All that has changed is the ability to detect them.

THE RISK OF KNOWING

About 90% of diagnosed thyroid cancers are small papillary cancers. They usually are indolent—cancers that are unlikely to grow or cause problems. Two Japanese studies and one American study have tracked nearly 1,500 patients who did not receive active treatment for papillary cancers less than one centimeter. After an average of five years, none of these patients has died.

Yet most people who are diagnosed with papillary thyroid cancers opt for treatment—usually a complete thyroidectomy, the removal of the thyroid gland. Once the gland is removed, patients require lifelong treatment with thyroid-replacement medications. Some suffer nerve damage that causes permanent voice changes. When surgery is followed by radioactive iodine therapy, patients face additional risks.

Better Skin Lesion Treatment

Precancerous skin lesions are better treated with photodynamic therapy (PDT) than with cryotherapy, reports Daniel Eisen, MD. In cryotherapy, lesions are frozen with liquid nitrogen. With PDT, the entire treatment area is "painted" with medication and then a special light is directed on it to activate the drug that kills the precancerous cells. Patients may require up to three sessions. Studies show that PDT is 14% more likely to completely clear the area in three months.

Daniel Eisen, MD, clinical professor of dermatology at University of California Davis Health System, Sacramento.

MORE DANGEROUS THYROID CANCERS

There are other types of thyroid cancer—follicular, medullary and anaplastic—that are more serious. These typically require surgery, usually the total removal of the thyroid gland and sometimes the removal of lymph nodes in the neck. Patients with these cancers typically are given postsurgical radioactive iodine to destroy remaining parts of the gland and any cancer cells that were left behind during surgery.

WHAT TO DO

Experts don't recommend widespread screening for thyroid cancer. A neck ultrasound is recommended only for specific patients—people who have a family history of thyroid cancer...had previous exposure to head/neck radiation...or a nodule that can be felt during an exam. If a test reveals a nodule that is one centimeter or more in diameter, a biopsy often is performed to determine the seriousness of the growth.

Also important...

•**Question the ultrasound.** If your doctor recommends neck ultrasonography during a routine checkup or because you're experiencing somewhat vague symptoms (such as fatigue), ask if you really need it and what the benefits and risks are if you do the test or don't do the test. You should clearly understand the goal of doing the test and how you will benefit.

•**Consider a second opinion before agreeing to surgery.** According to data from the US National Cancer Institute, death rates in patients who didn't have immediate surgery for papillary cancers were virtually the same as for those who did have surgery. Watchful waiting—forgoing treatment but getting checkups every six months at the beginning and then every year after that to see if a tumor has grown—usually is the best approach for these cancers.

•**Get the treatment that fits you.** If you have a papillary cancer that does need treatment, ask your doctor if you can have a partial rather than a total thyroidectomy. The partial procedure is safer and, for most papillary cancers, just as effective.

•**Don't agree to postsurgical treatment with radioactive iodine unless your doctor insists that you need it.** It usually is not recommended for low-risk thyroid cancers because it can cause serious side effects, including an altered sense of taste and inflamed salivary glands. The treatment also has been linked to a 5.7-fold increase in the risk for leukemia.

Do Statins Help or Harm Thyroid Cancer Risk?

Study titled "Statin Use and Thyroid Cancer: a Population-based Case-control Study" from the department of otolaryngology, Taipei Medical University, Taiwan, published in *Clinical Endocrinology*.

D o statin drugs lower your risk for certain kinds of cancer? Some doctors think they do. But when a group of Taiwanese researchers recently looked at statin use and a particular kind of common cancer—something never examined before—their findings were especially alarming for women.

THE THYROID CANCER CONNECTION

Researchers from Taipei Medical University reviewed Taiwan's health insurance database to find 500 people in whom thyroid cancer had been diagnosed between 2008 and 2011. They compared each person with five people of the same age and gender who didn't have thyroid cancer. Then, the researchers looked through the medical insurance records of all of these people to see who was ever given a prescription for a statin and how often they took it. They also examined whether high cholesterol itself might be associated with development of thyroid cancer.

The results: The odds of getting thyroid cancer were 40% higher in women who were "regular" statin users—defined as people who were on statins for at least 60 days within six months of getting the cancer diagnosis. Men who regularly used statins and people who used them less often than regularly had no increased risk of thyroid cancer. The researchers could not explain why women were affected and men not.

CAUSE FOR CONCERN?

The role of statins in the development of colorectal, breast and prostate cancers and leukemia has already been studied, with some studies showing that statins decrease the risk of certain cancers and others suggesting that statins have no effect on cancer risk. Although more studies need to be done to better clarify whether statin use puts a person at higher risk for thyroid cancer, the recent study's findings are yet another reason to consider alternatives when a doctor suggests you take a statin—especially if you are a woman.

More Help from Statins...

Statins may reduce risk for Barrett's esophagus, a precursor to esophageal cancer. Barrett's esophagus is mainly caused by long-term gastroesophageal reflux disease (GERD), obesity and/or a family history of GERD.

Recent finding: In older men, the use of statins—mainly *simvastatin*—was associated with a 43% lower risk for Barrett's esophagus. But first-line prevention involves controlling GERD, maintaining a normal weight and eating a balanced diet.

Hashem B. El-Serag, MD, a professor of medicine at Baylor College of Medicine, Houston, and leader of a study of 1,212 men, published in *Gastroenterology*.

High Levels of Cancer-Linked Chemical in E-Cigarette Vapor

James Pankow, PhD, professor, chemistry and civil and environmental engineering, Portland State University, Portland, Oregon.
Gregory Conley, JD, MBA, president, American Vaping Association.
Eric Jacobs, PhD, strategic director of pharmacoepidemiology, American Cancer Society.
New England Journal of Medicine

E -cigarette vapor can contain cancer-causing formaldehyde at levels up to 15 times higher than regular cigarettes, a recent study finds.

Researchers found that e-cigarettes operated at high voltages produce vapor with large amounts of formaldehyde-containing chemical compounds.

This could pose a risk to users who increase the voltage on their e-cigarette to increase the delivery of vaporized nicotine, said study coauthor James Pankow, PhD, a professor of chemistry and civil and environmental engineering at Portland State University in Oregon.

"We've found there is a hidden form of formaldehyde in e-cigarette vapor that has not typically been measured. It's a chemical that contains formaldehyde in it, and that formaldehyde can be released after inhalation," Dr. Pankow said. "People shouldn't assume these e-cigarettes are completely safe."

The findings appear in a letter published in the *New England Journal of Medicine*.

Formaldehyde is a known human carcinogen, according to the U.S. National Cancer Institute. It is a colorless, strong-smelling gas, commonly used in glues for products such as particle board, and in mortuaries as an embalming fluid.

Health experts have long known that formaldehyde and other toxic chemicals are present in cigarette smoke. Initially, e-cigarettes were hoped to be without such dangers because they lack fire to cause combustion and release toxic chemicals, a Portland State University news release said.

But newer versions of e-cigarettes can operate at very high temperatures, and that heat dramatically amps up the creation of formaldehyde-containing compounds, the study found.

"The new adjustable 'tank system' e-cigarettes allow users to really turn up the heat and deliver high amounts of vapor, or e-cigarette smoke," lead researcher David Peyton, PhD, a Portland State chemistry professor, said in the news release. Users open up the devices, put their own fluid in and adjust the operating temperature as they like, allowing them to greatly alter the vapor generated by the e-cigarette.

When used at low voltage, e-cigarettes did not create any formaldehyde-releasing agents, the researchers found.

However, high-voltage use released enough formaldehyde-containing compounds to increase a person's lifetime risk of cancer five to 15 times higher than the risk caused by long-term smoking, the study said.

INDUSTRY RESPONSE

The American Vaping Association, an industry group advocating for e-cigarette makers, argued that the recent study was flawed because e-cigarette users wouldn't operate their devices at such high voltage.

"When the vapor device was used at the realistic setting of 3.7 volts, levels of formaldehyde were similar to the trace levels that are released from an FDA-approved [smoking-cessation] inhaler," association President Gregory Conley said. "However, when the researchers increased the voltage to 5 volts and continued to have their machine take three- to four-second puffs, this caused extreme overheating and the production of formaldehyde."

This is known "in vapor product science as the 'dry puff phenomenon,'" Conley said. "Contrary to the authors' mistaken belief, these are not settings that real-life vapers actually use, as dry puffs are harsh and unpleasant. In the real world, vapers avoid dry puffs by lowering the length of their puff as they increase voltage."

CANCER GROUP REQUESTS OVERSIGHT

Noting that e-cigarettes remain unregulated, a representative with the American Cancer Society said these findings highlight the need for the U.S. Food and Drug Administration oversight.

"This study shows how little we know about toxic exposures that can result from using any one of the many different available types of e-cigarettes at different heating levels," said Eric Jacobs, PhD, the cancer society's strategic director of pharmacoepidemiology.

In April 2014, the FDA proposed federal restrictions that would bring e-cigarettes under the same regulation as tobacco. The proposed federal restrictions are still under review and no schedule has been set for adoption.

"Until these things are monitored and regulated, there's a real potential risk for unexpected exposure to toxic chemicals," Dr. Jacobs said. "We really don't know what kind of exposure the users might get when using any particular product at any particular heating level."

info For more on formaldehyde's cancer risks, visit the U.S. National Cancer Institute at *www.cancer.gov* (search "formaldehyde").

Better Blood Cancer Treatment

A. Keith Stewart, MB, ChB, dean for research, Mayo Clinic, Scottsdale, Arizona.

In a recent study of nearly 800 patients with recurrent multiple myeloma, adding *carfilzomib* to the standard two-drug regimen of *lenalidomide* and *dexamethasone* produced significantly better results. Combined, the three drugs increased the time patients were in remission by almost 50% (26.3 months versus 17.6 months) without additional side effects. More patients responded (87.4% versus 66.9%), and more had no detectable disease after the three-drug treatment (31.8% versus 9.3%).

Theory: Carfilzomib targets proteins that fuel tumor growth.

Mouthwash and Dentures Linked to Oral Cancer

Study titled, "Oral health, dental care and mouthwash associated with upper aerodigestive tract cancer risk in Europe: The ARCAGE study," published in *Oral Oncology*.

You wouldn't dream of leaving the house in the morning or going to bed at night without brushing your teeth. And ideally, you give your pearly whites a good daily flossing, too. But if you're also accustomed to swishing some mouthwash—to sweeten your breath, whiten your teeth, fight infection or make your mouth "feel really clean"—it's important for you to take two specific precautions.

Another alert: If you're a denture wearer, you also need to be on guard. *Here's why...*

RESEARCHERS SINK THEIR TEETH INTO THE DATA

For a recent study, researchers from nine European countries interviewed nearly 2,000 men and women who had been recently diagnosed with oral cancer—malignancies of the mouth, larynx (voice box), pharynx (throat) or esophagus. For comparison's sake, they also interviewed a similar number of age-matched but cancer-free people who served as controls.

All of the participants were asked about various lifestyle and dietary habits...their oral hygiene habits...and their medical and dental history. When the researchers analyzed this data (and adjusted for smoking and alcohol consumption, two known risk factors for oral cancers), they came to some predictable conclusions—for instance, that failing to brush teeth twice daily or to visit the dentist at least annually was associated with significantly increased risk for oral cancer. *But they also found two surprising risk factors...*

•**Wearing dentures.** Even partial dentures were associated with increased risk. And people who wore complete upper and lower dentures had nearly double the risk of people who did not wear dentures. Oral cancer risk was especially high among those who started wearing dentures before they were 55 years old.

•**Frequent use of mouthwash.** Compared with people who did not use mouthwash, those who rinsed their mouths with mouthwash three or more times each day had about triple the risk for oral cancer. However, there was no increased

Dormant Lung Cancer

Lung cancer can lie dormant for more than 20 years and then become aggressive. In a small study of smokers, former smokers and people who never smoked, researchers found that the initial genetic errors that cause cancer can go undetected for many years, and the cancer can become active when triggered by new mutations.

Study by researchers at Cancer Research UK, published in *Science*.

risk found among people who used mouthwash less frequently than three times a day.

Noteworthy: Unfortunately, this study did not distinguish between mouthwash that contained alcohol and mouthwash without alcohol. Some previous, smaller studies suggested that both alcohol-containing and alcohol-free mouthwash may increase oral cancer risk, but other studies found increased risk only with mouthwashes that contain alcohol…and alcohol is a known carcinogen.

Double jeopardy: For people who both wore dentures and used mouthwash three or more times daily, the risk for oral cancer was multiplied more than seven times!

For optimal oral health…

• **Clean your teeth well every day.**

• **Visit your dentist two or more times each year.**

• **If you are a fan of mouthwash,** there's probably no need to stop using it altogether—but it may be wise to stick with brands that are alcohol-free and limit your swishing to no more than once or twice a day.

• **What if you have dentures?** You can't change that—but you can be extra vigilant about watching for possible signs of oral cancer, such as a slightly raised white or red patch in the mouth…an unexplained lump in the neck…discomfort on one side of the throat…subtle changes in voice…unexplained and persistent ear pain…or difficulty or mild pain with swallowing. Remember, as with many diseases, the earlier oral cancer is caught and treated, the better the outcome generally is.

Got Cancer? Here's Help

Mitch Golant, PhD, senior consultant for strategic initiatives at the Cancer Support Community and a clinical psychologist in Los Angeles and coauthor of *The Total Cancer Wellness Guide: Reclaiming Your Life After Diagnosis.*

"You have cancer" are three of the most frightening words a person can hear.

A hidden challenge: While cancer patients are still reeling from the emotions of a potentially life-threatening diagnosis, they are asked to make some of the most important decisions of their lives. Even with the support of loved ones, all the treatment decisions that must be made can feel overwhelming.

Good news: There's now a unique approach that can help cancer patients feel less alone.

WHERE TO START

Most cancer-treatment decisions are made within a few weeks of the initial diagnosis. Patients who aren't thinking clearly are expected to understand what's happening and make difficult decisions.

A resource worth trying: A free, evidence-based counseling program, called Open to Options, is available nationwide. Developed by the Cancer Support Community (CSC), a nonprofit group based in Washington, DC, the program matches cancer patients with paid professional counselors (psychologists, social workers and marriage and family therapists) throughout the country. They are specially trained to help patients better communicate with their doctors by formulating questions about their treatment options during that difficult period between diagnosis and treatment.

What research shows: Studies of nearly 200 patients have found that those who worked with Open to Options counselors were more informed during meetings with their doctors and were less likely to have second thoughts after treatment decisions were made.

HOW IT WORKS

To find professional counselors in their areas, newly diagnosed cancer patients can use the CSC website, *CancerSupportCommunity.org*, or call the Cancer Support Helpline at 888-793-9355. They can meet with counselors face-to-face or communicate by phone or e-mail.

Counselors in this program do not answer medical questions or give medical advice. Rather, the counselors are trained to help patients decide what issues are most important to them and should be discussed with their doctors.

After the counselor and patient meet, the counselor creates a one-page summary agenda that the patient will share with his/her doctor. (The agenda can be faxed or e-mailed to the doctor before the patient's appointment.)

WHAT THE PROGRAM COVERS

When working with a counselor, a patient creates a list of all his questions: "Will I suffer from the mental fog ('chemo brain') that sometimes goes along with chemotherapy?" "How long will I be treated?" "How can I minimize side effects?" "When can I return to work?" "Will my concentration or ability to travel be affected?"

When a patient speaks with a counselor, he'll be guided through a series of steps to answer questions such as…

What's your situation? You already know you have cancer, and your doctor probably has a good sense of how he will recommend treating it. But your personal situation and values will also influence your decisions.

Example 1: Your doctor might be inclined to treat your cancer with a particular form of chemotherapy, one that sometimes causes hand neuropathy as a side effect. If you mention that you're an artist and can't make a living without the use of your hands, he might choose another treatment instead.

Example 2: Your doctor tells you about a new effective oral chemotherapy that costs $20,000 a month. Your insurance covers only 80%. What are the possibilities for payment, financial assistance and therapy?

What are your options? These will depend on your health history and the type of cancer. The counselor will help you formulate some of the most important questions.

Example: You may want to continue working for the next several years. Will you do better with surgery, chemotherapy or radiation? Are the survival rates similar with each treatment? How long will it take to recover from each? What will the side effects be?

Important: Don't forget to ask the doctor whether a clinical trial (a study of a new treatment) is appropriate. Many people avoid clinical trials because they assume that they might be assigned to a "control" group that receives no treatment. However, in a typical clinical trial, participants are assigned to different groups—one is given the current standard care, and the other is given the new treatment being studied. Placebos are never given in place of treatment.

What are your goals? This goes beyond "surviving" or "being healthy." Other factors are equally important—or even more important for some people.

Example: You might want to treat your cancer aggressively but not before you've attended your daughter's wedding. Your objective might be simply to wait a bit before starting treatment. You'll ask your doctor what the ramifications might be.

Who is in your support network? Think about everyone who might be involved in your care—health professionals, your spouse, friends, helpful neighbors, etc.

Will you have someone to help you on the days of your scheduled treatments? Maybe your spouse is available only on certain afternoons. Let your doctor know this—most cancer centers or hospitals have social-work departments that can help you solve logistical problems.

What comes next? You'll probably have many questions as your treatment progresses. Write them down as you go. If you're not sure how to formulate your questions—or you're not even sure what you should know—ask your counselor for help. Even though most patients use the Open to Options program immediately following their diagnoses, they can rely on it anytime a treatment decision must be made. If they like, patients can also work with a specific counselor each time they ask for help.

Important: Even though you may feel inclined to act immediately if you've just gotten a cancer diagnosis, research shows that patients have better treatment outcomes and less anxiety when they are well-informed and partner with their doctors in determining the best treatments for them. This may take a bit longer, but the benefits far outweigh the risks.

Therapy Dogs Help Cancer Patients Cope with Tough Treatments

Stewart Fleishman, MD, retired, founding director, cancer supportive services, Mount Sinai Beth Israel, New York City.

Rachel McPherson, executive director, Good Dog Foundation, New York City.

Journal of Community and Supportive Oncology

People undergoing chemotherapy and radiation for cancer may get an emotional lift from man's best friend, a recent study suggests.

The study of patients with head and neck cancers is among the first to scientifically test the effects of therapy dogs—trained and certified pooches brought in to ease human anxiety, whether it's from trauma, injury or illness.

To dog lovers, it may be a no-brainer that canine companions bring comfort. And therapy dogs are already a fixture in some U.S. hospitals, as well as nursing homes, social service agencies, and other settings where people are in need.

STUDY DETAILS

"We can take for granted that supportive care for cancer patients, like a healthy diet, has benefits," said Stewart Fleishman, MD, the lead researcher on the recent study. "We wanted to really test animal-assisted therapy and quantify the effects."

Dr. Fleishman, now retired, was founding director of cancer supportive services at Beth Israel Medical Center in New York City—now called Mount Sinai Beth Israel.

For the recent study, his team followed 42 patients at the hospital who were undergoing six weeks of chemotherapy and radiation for head and neck cancers, mostly affecting the mouth and throat.

All of the patients agreed to have visits with a therapy dog right before each of their treatment sessions. The dogs, trained by the Good Dog Foundation, were brought in to the waiting room, or hospital room, so patients could spend about 15 minutes with them.

The chemo/radiation regimen in this study was "intense," Dr. Fleishman said.

"These patients get very sick," he noted. "They can't eat well, they have trouble speaking. The treatment becomes more of a burden than the cancer."

But overall, the dogs seemed to make the burden a little easier. Using standard questionnaires, Dr. Fleishman's team found that—as expected—patients' physical well-being deteriorated over the course of their treatment.

Yet their emotional and "social" well-being—which includes feeling supported—actually increased.

"One patient said, 'I would've stopped the treatment, but I wanted to come see the dog,'" Dr. Fleishman said.

The findings, published in the *Journal of Community and Supportive Oncology*, might encourage more hospitals to consider a therapy dog program, Dr. Fleishman said.

POSSIBLE EXPLANATION

Dogs offer something that even the best-intentioned human caregiver can't quite match, said Rachel McPherson, executive director of the New York City-based Good Dog Foundation.

"They give unconditional love," said McPherson, whose organization trains and certifies therapy dogs for more than 350 facilities in New York, New Jersey, Connecticut and Massachusetts.

"Dogs don't judge you, or try to give you advice, or tell you their stories," she pointed out.

Instead, McPherson said, therapy dogs offer simple comfort to people facing scary circumstances, such as cancer treatment. But while that sounds good, doctors and hospitals prefer scientific evidence.

ABOUT THERAPY DOGS

The Good Dog Foundation has been around for 16 years, and McPherson said she's witnessed plenty of evidence that the dogs help a wide range of people—including patients recovering from stroke, nursing home residents, children with autism, and disaster victims.

Still, McPherson said scientific evidence is vital, which is why her foundation partly funded the current study, and plans to be involved in more research.

The foundation finds their good dogs when interested owners volunteer. The dogs go through a screening process; no particular breed is better than others, McPherson said, but the dog does need the "right temperament."

From there, training includes simulations of the settings where they'll work. If the animals are going to visit hospitals, they have to get used to wheelchairs and IV poles, for instance, McPherson noted. They also have to master basic commands and get clearance from a vet.

"We have a strict protocol," McPherson said.

IMPLICATIONS

"It takes time, effort and money for animal-assisted therapy to happen," Dr. Fleishman said. And this study, he added, offers evidence that it's all worth it.

When it comes to cancer treatment, the findings show that the rigors can be lessened, Dr. Fleishman said. "I think patients can take heart," he said. "There are interventions that can make the quality of that time better."

info For more information about animal-assisted therapy, visit the website of The Good Dog Foundation, *http://thegooddogfoun dation.org.*

Consumer Health Alerts

House Calls—They're Back! How to Find a Doctor Who Does In-Home Visits

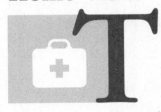

The image of a doctor visiting sick patients at home, black bag in hand, is no longer a part of our past.

What's new: Advances in portable medical equipment, a rapidly aging population and increased payments from Medicare for in-home doctor visits mean that house calls are back. In fact, the number of house calls made to Medicare patients more than doubled in recent years, and private insurers are beginning to cover them as well.

WHY THE COMEBACK?

Until recently, most major tests, like X-rays and ultrasounds, required a visit to a hospital or other medical facility. Now, technology makes possible diagnostic and therapeutic equipment that's portable and accurate. Even a chest X-ray can be done in the comfort of the home. And house-call physicians currently have an arsenal of tools that they can use on the road—such as an ultrasound machine that fits in a pocket…a smartphone case that turns into an EKG machine…and an app for checking drug interactions.

Another driving factor: Most older adults would prefer to remain in their homes as they age and avoid expensive nursing homes. For many, this would not be possible without house calls.

What's more: Studies have shown that doctors visiting patients in the home reduce hospital admission rates, readmission rates and overall costs. In fact, a recent study of Medicare patients found that those cared for at home had 17% lower health-care costs.

Thomas Cornwell, MD, president of the American Academy of Home Care Medicine based in Edgewood, Maryland. Dr. Cornwell has made 31,000 house calls during his 20 years in practice. Based in Wheaton, Illinois, he specializes in family medicine and geriatrics. *AAHCM.org*

The types of doctors most likely to make house calls include family physicians, internists, geriatricians and palliative-care doctors.

THE MANY BENEFITS

Some patients are too sick to come into the doctor's office but don't need to go to an emergency room. Or they simply refuse to go to the doctor's office…or don't have anyone to take them.

Additionally, house calls are typically much longer than the usual office doctor visit. By going into the home, the doctor can assess much more than the current health issue affecting a patient. If the patient is frail, the need for in-home medical equipment, such as grab bars in a shower or bath, can be identified. Plus, safety risks like electrical cords or rugs can be pointed out to help prevent falls.

Patients are encouraged to bring all of their medicines to a doctor appointment, but this is not always done, and often a drug or supplement is forgotten. A home visit is more likely to uncover all the prescriptions and supplements that are being taken. And by investigating other factors like diet and living conditions, a physician can better treat chronic conditions, such as diabetes or heart disease, or determine if the patient should be getting additional at-home assistance.

Finally, by remaining in their homes for medical care, patients are not exposed to the viruses and bacteria common in doctors' offices. This is particularly helpful for those who have weakened immunity.

WHO SHOULD CONSIDER HOUSE CALLS

•**Frail older patients.** For older patients who have difficulty getting out of the house, a home visit can be a literal lifesaver. Home-based primary care for frail older patients can help delay institutionalization or admission to the hospital and allow physicians to assess the quality of help caregivers are able to provide. For patients who are terminally ill, home visits provide palliative care and reduce the chances of dying in a hospital.

•**Patients who have certain disorders/ diseases.** Among patients of all ages, house calls are extremely helpful for those who suffer from neuromuscular diseases like muscular dystrophy, Lou Gehrig's disease or paralysis. With these conditions, getting to an appointment can be an arduous task, and home visits keep the doctor up-to-date on the patient's needs.

OTHER HOUSE-CALL OPTIONS

Some doctors' offices now offer medical concierge services (the patient pays an annual fee or retainer to a primary care doctor). These services may include house calls. Costs range from less than one hundred to several thousand dollars a year. Some employers also offer home visits as part of their employee insurance.

HOW TO ARRANGE A HOUSE CALL

For Medicare recipients and many with private insurance, there needs to be a medically necessary reason for the house call. The patient must also find it physically difficult to leave his/her home in order for Medicare or private insurance to cover some portion of the visit. Medical concierge services may not have this requirement.

To find a doctor who makes house calls: First, check with your primary care doctor to see if he can provide this service or give you a referral. You can also go to the website of the American Academy of Home Care Medicine, *AAHCM.org*, and click on "Locate a Provider."

GETTING THE MOST OUT OF YOUR HOUSE CALL

The length of a house call depends on the patient's specific needs and whether it's a first-time visit or a follow-up. *How to prepare…*

•**As with any doctor appointment,** write down all your questions and concerns beforehand.

•**Before the doctor arrives,** arrange all of your prescription medications, over-the-counter medications and supplements in one place so that they can be reviewed by the doctor.

•**Make sure any family members who help out with your care** are present so the doctor can get an accurate picture of the home environment.

Also: Don't be afraid to reach out to your doctor between visits. Doing so, even if the problem seems minor, such as a lingering cough, may prevent an unnecessary ER visit or hospitalization down the road.

4 Secrets to Avoiding a Misdiagnosis

Trisha Torrey, a Baldwinsville, New York–based patient advocacy consultant, also known as "Every Patient's Advocate," *EveryPatientsAdvocate.com*, and author of *You Bet Your Life! Ten Mistakes That Every Patient Makes*. She is also the founder and director of the Alliance of Professional Health Advocates.

Ten years ago, I noticed a golf ball–sized lump on my torso. My family doctor sent me to a surgeon, who removed the lump and sent it to a lab for testing.

A few weeks later, I got the news from my doctor: "You have a very rare type of lymphoma." I froze with fear. The second blow came when an oncologist told me that if I didn't start chemotherapy right away, I'd be dead within months.

But I didn't feel sick, and my intuition told me that something was off with the diagnosis. So I sought a second opinion from another oncologist, who reviewed my case and had the biopsy analyzed again. As it turned out, I didn't have cancer. The lump was simply an inflamed bundle of fat cells. I didn't need chemo, and 10 years later I'm fine.

So how do you make sure that you or a loved one never experiences a misdiagnosis nightmare? It happens a lot. Twelve million Americans are misdiagnosed each year.

For the past decade, I have dedicated my life to helping people become smarter patients and, in the process, avoid misdiagnoses. Some of what I've learned may sound a little unconventional, but I know from my experience and that of other patients that the steps below work. *How to avoid a misdiagnosis…*

SECRET #1: Track your symptoms. You probably know to write down your questions before seeing a doctor, but I suggest that you first spend at least a little time tracking your symptoms. Medical symptoms can be vague, inconsistent and wax and wane unexpectedly, so patients often don't give their doctors enough facts to ensure a correct diagnosis. Without such details, it's easy for physicians to jump on the most obvious—though sometimes incorrect—diagnosis.

What to do: If you're not dealing with an emergency, keep a diary of your symptoms before you see your doctor. Include a clear description of all your symptoms and when they started. Also, be sure to include any triggers—anything that makes the symptoms worse…or better.

Of course, don't let your symptom tracking become an excuse to delay going to the doctor. Even if your appointment is the next day or so, you can use that time to organize your notes on what you've observed so far. And once you've tracked your symptoms, you'll be better prepared to write down your questions for the doctor.

SECRET #2: Make a list of possible diagnoses. If you've got an unexplained symptom, most doctors tell you to avoid the Internet. You will just confuse yourself, they reason. I disagree. If you've got a weird symptom, you want to know what may be causing it so you can ask the doctor intelligent questions.

When doing research online, just make sure you don't jump to conclusions. And skip websites that are sponsored by pharmaceutical companies or businesses trying to sell you something. Also, disregard comments and forums populated by non–health professionals. Up-to-date and reliable health information is available at such sites as *MedlinePlus.gov…HealthFinder.gov…*and *UptoDate.com* (it's used by many doctors around the world—click on "Patients and Caregivers").

In my own situation, using the Internet helped me to realize that cancer wasn't the only possible diagnosis, and it compelled me to ask many more questions.

Important: Don't try to diagnose yourself… and don't talk yourself out of going to the doctor.

SECRET #3: Ask this crucial question. Your doctor has just given you a diagnosis. Now what? Rather than launching into a discussion about the best treatments for the diagnosis you've just received—as most often occurs—I suggest that you stop and ask the doctor, "What else could it be?"

Specifically, ask the doctor for the "differential diagnosis"—that is, the conditions he/she ruled out. Then ask how he ruled them out. Listen carefully—if there are any gaps in the case he makes for your diagnosis, they are likely to come up at this time. After this explanation, ask about anything you don't understand. Be concise and stay focused. If you start to ramble, your doctor won't stay engaged.

SECRET #4: Don't be afraid of your doctor. There are ways to get what you need and ask your questions without offending anyone.

What you need to know: A good, ethical doctor won't be upset by your desire for additional medical opinions. Getting more than one opinion is crucial, especially if your doctor has recommended any invasive type of treatment such as chemotherapy, surgery or a long-term drug prescription.

Ask for your own medical records and take them to additional opinion appointments. Your goal is to find at least two doctors who give you the same diagnosis, maximizing your odds of getting a correct one. Let new doctors draw their own conclusions about your diagnosis rather than sharing previous opinions they can simply agree with.

If your online research doesn't jibe with what your doctor has told you, don't be confrontational. Instead, ask questions like, "I recently read about this (diagnosis or treatment). Can you tell me why you ruled that out?" This acknowledges your doctor's extensive education and experience but puts him on notice that you've done your homework and need to know more.

Medical Tests That Can Cause More Harm Than Good

Reid B. Blackwelder, MD, FAAFP, president of the American Academy of Family Physicians. He is also a practicing family physician in Johnson City, Tennessee, and professor of family medicine at Quillen College of Medicine at East Tennessee State University, also in Johnson City.

Are you getting cookie-cutter medical care? Too many people are—and one glaring example of this is the number of tests and procedures that are being prescribed regardless of the individual's specific health situation.

In fact, there's more and more evidence that many of the tests that are given so routinely are causing more harm than good.

Here are some popular tests that are often not necessary...*

CT SCANS FOR LOW-BACK PAIN

If your low back is giving you fits, your doctor may order an X-ray or even a more detailed test such as a CT scan to see what's going on.

Problem: Americans are receiving doses of radiation from X-rays and CT scans (not to mention spending enormous amounts of money) to diagnose a problem that will likely go away on its own in a few weeks. In some cases, an incidental finding that's not even related to the pain leads to unnecessary back surgery.

New thinking: Unless you are experiencing worsening nerve damage (such as loss of bladder or bowel control or loss of sensation or muscle power in your legs) or have cancer (which could possibly spread to the back), you probably don't need an imaging test within the first six weeks of your back pain.

Also: There is no medical or legal reason to get X-rays as a "baseline" for work-related back injuries.

BONE-DENSITY TESTS

For years, physicians have been routinely recommending bone-density tests using dual-energy X-ray absorptiometry (DXA). The test estimates the amount of bone in the hip and spine, which is a marker for osteoporosis. Until recently, women have often been advised to have a "baseline" DXA screening at menopause...then periodically after that.

Problem: Being labeled with "preosteoporosis" (commonly known as osteopenia) can start you on a medical journey of repeated DXA testing and use of medications that may be harmful. For example, osteoporosis drugs known as *bisphosphonates—risedronate* (Actonel), *ibandronate* (Boniva) and *alendronate* (Fosamax)—have been shown, in rare cases, to cause an unusual

---

*The tests in this article are evaluated at *ChoosingWisely.org*, a Web site that advises patients and doctors on a wide range of tests and procedures. Developed by more than 50 medical specialty societies, such as the American Academy of Family Physicians and the American College of Surgeons, the information is based on the most current scientific evidence. Remember to check with your doctor for advice that's tailored to your specific needs.

fracture of the thigh bone when one of these medications is taken for longer than five years.

And evidence shows that this test is not always a reliable predictor of fractures even in high-risk patients who are already receiving drug therapy for osteoporosis.

New thinking...

•**Unless you are a woman age 65 or older or a man age 70 or older**—or you have a special risk factor for osteoporosis, such as family history, smoking or alcohol abuse or use of corticosteroid drugs—you probably don't need DXA screening.

•**If your DXA test results show that you have normal bone mass,** you don't need to be tested again for up to 10 years, provided you don't break a bone or show other signs of osteoporosis, such as losing more than an inch in height.

CAROTID ARTERY IMAGING

Your carotid arteries carry blood from your heart through the neck to your brain. If those arteries become narrowed from a buildup of plaque (a condition known as carotid artery stenosis, or CAS), your blood flow is slowed and your risk for stroke increases. Doctors can use ultrasound, magnetic resonance angiography (MRA) or computed tomography angiography (CTA) scans to check for plaque in these arteries.

Problem: If testing does show a blockage, you may be advised to take medication that won't necessarily improve your life expectancy. You may even be urged to undergo surgery (endarterectomy) to clear the artery. However, this is a difficult and complex operation that in rare cases leads to stroke, heart attack or even death.

New thinking: Unless you are experiencing symptoms, such as stroke, transient ischemic attack (a so-called "mini-stroke") or unexplained dizziness, you probably do not need to be screened for CAS. Evidence shows that the harms of screening (and subsequent treatment) in people without symptoms usually outweigh the benefits.

If you do undergo screening for CAS, surgery is generally not recommended unless you have more than 70% blockage in one or both of your carotid arteries and you have had a stroke or ministroke in the previous six months.

EKG AND STRESS TEST

During your routine physical, your doctor may have ordered an electrocardiogram (EKG or ECG) to measure your heart's electrical activity and/or a cardiac stress test to check the same functions but under conditions where you are "stressed" via exercise or medication.

Problem: Unnecessary stress testing can lead to false-positive tests—indicating that something is wrong when you are actually healthy. This can mean more follow-up tests, including CT scans or coronary angiography, both of which expose you to radiation. And in rare cases, an angiography actually leads to a heart attack in people who have the test. Sometimes, after a "bad" EKG or stress test, a doctor may also prescribe unnecessary heart medication.

New thinking...

•**If you don't have any heart-related symptoms (such as chest pain or shortness of breath),** the evidence shows that an annual EKG or other cardiac screening is unlikely to prevent a heart attack, catch a hidden heart problem or otherwise make you any healthier than you already are.

•**If you are getting noncardiac thoracic surgery** (for example, on the lungs, esophagus or other organs in the chest), you do not need to have stress testing before the operation unless you have a history of heart problems. In healthy patients, testing rarely changes how they are treated, so it's generally not necessary.

Are You Taking the Wrong Drug?

Dietrich Stephan, PhD, chairman of the department of human genetics at the University of Pittsburgh Graduate School of Public Health. He leads research in public health genetics at the Institute for Personalized Medicine at the University of Pittsburgh and the University of Pittsburgh Medical Center.

When your doctor writes you a prescription, you may assume that it's just a matter of matching the medication to the condition that's being treated. Not so.

In reality, doctors are trained to narrow down the medication options—sometimes several of them—by taking into account such factors as your age, sex and weight. Until recently, that's all doctors have had to go on.

Now: The medication-choosing process has become far more sophisticated. With pharmacogeno-mics, also known as drug-gene testing, your doctor can use your genetic profile (genotype) to determine in advance if a drug is likely to be effective...the best dose...and how likely you are to have side effects. This breakthrough is now available for many commonly used medications, including heartburn drugs, painkillers, antidepressants, statins and certain cancer drugs.

Here's how to put drug-gene testing to work for you—or a loved one...

PERSONALIZED PRESCRIPTIONS

The genes that you inherited from your parents largely determined what you look like—and even, to an extent, how you act and feel. Are you tall or short? What's your blood type? Are your eyes blue or brown?

Genes, the chemical sets of instructions that the body uses to build proteins, play an important role in making you you—and that includes how you respond to medications. In the future, it's likely that every drug—including over-the-counter standbys such as aspirin—will take genetics into account.

LESS GUESSWORK

Suppose that you have colon cancer and will need chemotherapy. Your oncologist will pick the drugs with the best record of success. For example, two of the most effective drugs for this cancer are *cetuximab* (Erbitux) and *panitumumab* (Vectibix). Yet research has shown that they're not the best choice for about 40% of patients with a particular genetic profile.

Another example: Patients with cardiovascular disease are often given *warfarin* (Coumadin), a blood thinner. It's very effective at preventing clots, but it has a high risk for side effects, such as excessive bleeding—particularly when the dose isn't exactly right. For those with a particular genetic profile, the drug is up to three times more potent than in those with different genes. These patients should be given a much lower dose.

WHAT TO EXPECT

For now, genetic tests are available for more than 150 FDA-approved drugs. (For a complete list of FDA-approved drugs with pharmacogenomic information on the label, go to the FDA website at *snip.ly/P4XQ.*)

If your doctor plans to start you on one of these medications, ask him/her about going to a laboratory to give a blood/saliva sample. This can be used to create your unique genetic profile.

Important: A single test can't predict how you'll respond to all medications. You might need additional tests if you're taking more than one drug—although some test "panels" will include information on multiple medications.

The cost of a drug-gene test can be as little as about $100. More specialized tests—for the drugs used to treat some cancers, for example—can be as high as $7,000. Check with your health insurer to make sure the cost of the test is covered.

CAN YOU BENEFIT?

Genetic variations could account for anywhere from 20% to 95% of the difference in individual responses to various medications, according to a recent review of studies that appeared in *The New England Journal of Medicine.*

Because there's such a high probability that drug-gene testing may yield helpful information, it's wise to discuss with your doctor whether genetic testing is available for any medication he may prescribe for you. *Examples...*

•**Statins.** Depending on the drug, this class of medications can lower LDL "bad" cholesterol by up to 55%—in some people. In others, the results can be quite different. For example, one large study found that more than 13% of participants who took the statin *pravastatin* (Pravachol) failed to lower their LDL by even 10%.

Reason: Some genetic variations make people "poor responders" to statins. They might require a higher-than-normal dose...or a different drug altogether, such as a fibrate like *gemfibrozil* (Lopid). Other genetic variations cause people to metabolize statins too quickly, which increases the risk for muscle pain or other side effects.

•**Proton pump inhibitors (PPIs).** Drugs in this class, such as *omeprazole* (Prilosec) and *lansoprazole* (Prevacid), inhibit the production of stomach acid and are widely used to treat heartburn and stomach and duodenal ulcers. Researchers have identified a number of genetic variations that affect how well these medications work.

Patients who are "extensive metabolizers," for example, will require a higher dose than those who have genetic factors that cause them to metabolize the drugs more slowly.

•**Selective serotonin reuptake inhibitor (SSRI) antidepressants.** SSRIs require a lot of trial and error. About half of patients with depression don't improve on their first drug. Their success on second and third drugs is even lower.

With genetic tests, psychiatrists can make more than an educated guess about which drug and doses to try. An analysis of studies presented at a meeting of the International College of Neuropsychopharmacology found that genetics-based prescribing for SSRIs doubled response rates as well as the rate of remission.

•**Painkillers.** Codeine is among the most effective (and least expensive) analgesics, but some individuals have a genetic variation that inhibits their ability to convert it into morphine (the mechanism that provides its pain-relieving effect). They usually require a higher dose—or sometimes a different medication, such as fentanyl or hydromorphone.

Another genetic variation causes codeine to be metabolized much more rapidly than normal. These patients are more likely to suffer serious side effects, including impaired breathing, when they're given a standard dose.

How to Find a (Good) Doctor Online

Charles B. Inlander, a consumer advocate and healthcare consultant based in Fogelsville, Pennsylvania. He was founding president of the nonprofit People's Medical Society, a consumer advocacy organization credited with key improvements in the quality of US health care, and is author or coauthor of more than 20 consumer-health books.

Y ou can pretty much shop for anything online. But a doctor? Yes, you can even find a good doctor online—if you know what information is trustworthy (and what might not be). The appeal of sites such as *HealthGrades.com*, *RateMDs.com* and *Vitals.com* is that they offer the kind of firsthand feedback that we used to get only from family and friends. How's a doctor's bedside manner? Is it tough to get an appointment? Even though these sites provide good information, they do have their limits. *Here are the advantages and disadvantages of using such websites…*

PRO: **The basics are all in one place.** Most doctor-rating sites give helpful biographical information, such as the doctor's age…where he/she went to school…if he is board-certified in a particular specialty…and how long he's been in practice. Some sites also list the hospitals where the doctor has admitting privileges or is employed.

Excellent feature: Most doctor-rating sites let you search doctors by specialty anywhere in the US. This is a great service if you're looking for a doctor for a family member in another locale.

CON: **High ratings don't always mean good medical care.** While the actual reviews provided by patients give some telling details about a doctor's willingness to answer questions and other aspects of his patient care, remember these are only opinions. A patient may write a negative review simply because a doctor wouldn't prescribe an antibiotic for a cold or held off on ordering an MRI in favor of another test. Meanwhile, a good review might have been submitted by a practitioner's relative or friend (even though some sites have systems to screen phony reviews). That's why I advise trying to find multiple reviews of a doctor (which may mean checking more than one site) in case the feedback is skewed for one of these reasons. But you must realize that these sites don't review a doctor's medical competence. In fact, studies show that patients tend to give higher ratings to doctors who prescribe more drugs and tests and run up more costs.

To find out about a physician's skill level: You need to consult resources beyond doctor-rating websites. If you are looking for a skilled orthopedic surgeon, for example, go to *US News & World Report's* well-respected hospital ratings (*USNews.com/best-hospitals*) to find the best hospital in your region that is known for its orthopedic department. Check that hospital's website to review its roster of doctors. You can even check the rosters of nationally ranked hospitals outside your region and call one of the top doctors there. It's been my experience that those doctors often can refer patients to highly skilled doctors in other locales. In addition, many states, such as California, Massachusetts, New York, Pennsylvania and Texas, have their own physician outcome data for certain procedures and make it available to the public. Contact your state's Health Department for information. Medicare also has information on physician outcomes on its website. Go to *Medicare.gov/physiciancompare*.

Is Your Doctor Scamming You with "Self-Referrals"?

Jean Mitchell, PhD, economist and professor of public policy, McCourt School of Public Policy, Georgetown University, Washington DC.

I *magine:* Your knee hurts. Your orthopedist says that he needs to do an MRI…and for your convenience, he has an MRI machine just down the hall. After checking your scan, the orthopedist recommends surgery, which can be done at an adjoining outpatient surgery center…after which you'll attend physical therapy, again conveniently located in the doctor's office complex.

Hassle-free, one-stop medical care for the patient? Or a money-making racket for the doctor?

Consider: If your doctor owns or leases the MRI machine used to examine your knee or if he owns part of the surgery center and/or physical therapy center, he is making money on every phase of your examination and treatment. He not only collects his professional fees for your office visit, but he also shares in any profits generated by the scan, the surgery or the physical therapy.

Those are huge monetary incentives.

Of course, it's quite possible that you really need the MRI, the operation and the physical therapy. But the doctor's financial involvement in so many of your health-care services creates a serious conflict of interest that makes it hard to know whether he is protecting your well-being or his own bottom line.

A TOOTHLESS LAW

The process described above is called self-referral, and in many circumstances, it's illegal. The federal government prohibits doctors from referring patients to facilities in which they have a financial interest. This regulation, known as the Ethics in Patient Referrals Act or the Stark Law (after the congressman who sponsored the bill), applies only to Medicare and Medicaid patients, but about half of the states have similar laws that apply to privately insured patients.

The loophole problem: The law is simply not enforced…and there are loopholes so big you can fit an MRI machine through them. The biggest loophole is the in-office ancillary services exception, which allows doctors to self-refer if the service is provided by them or by members of their practice in their office—which pretty much takes the teeth right out of the law.

Doctors have figured out other ways to circumvent the law, too. For example, a medical practice can enter into a contract with an independent imaging facility and agree to pay the facility a reduced, set fee for each service performed (a practice called payment per click). The referring doctor then bills the insurance company for the full-price service—and pockets the difference between what he collects from the insurance company and what he pays the imaging facility.

OVER-EVERYTHING

The biggest problems with self-referral involve three types of overutilization of health care…

Overtesting: Self-referral can lead to a lot of unwarranted tests, many of which carry risks. For instance, CT scans and X-rays involve radiation…the contrast materials used in some CT and MRI scans can cause kidney problems or allergic reactions…biopsies can be painful and can leave scars…and testing is highly stressful, particularly as anxious patients await the results.

Does ownership really affect doctors' decisions about the amount of testing to do? You bet it does. *Consider this evidence from recent studies…*

Self-Defense Against Self-Referral

As patients, we don't have the clinical expertise to know whether we truly need a particular procedure, so we rely on our physicians to act as our agents. Until the Stark Law is fixed and enforced, what can you do to protect your own health and wallet rather than the doctors' financial interests?

• **Ask your doctor directly whether he/she is self-referring.** When your doctor recommends a test or treatment, you can say point-blank, "Doctor, do you have any financial interest in this test or treatment?" If the answer is yes, inquire whether the results of the test will affect the treatment decision (if it won't, there's no reason to get the test)…and whether a particular treatment is the gold standard for your condition (if it isn't, the doctor should have a darn good explanation for why he's recommending it). You can keep your eyes open for subtler clues, too. If the service you're being sent for, such as physical therapy or imaging, is offered right in the doctor's office, it's quite likely that your doctor is self-referring. Or you can look at the doctor's website to see if it advertises the doctor's own imaging, surgery or radiation center.

• **Get a second opinion.** Consulting a second physician, especially before having an operation or starting a treatment program, is always a good idea. Just be sure that second doctor is not in the same practice as the first doctor—and again, ask this second doctor whether he's self-referring.

• **Feel free to go elsewhere for services.** Consider seeing a doctor who's on staff at a hospital associated with a university—these practitioners may be more likely to follow established guidelines on testing and treatment. Doctors on hospital staffs are frequently on salary, so although they may feel some indirect pressure from their institutions, they are less likely to be motivated by direct financial incentives.

Bottom line: If you have explored your options and decided that the convenience of a self-referral outweighs the downside, that's your right. Just don't let yourself be unwittingly herded into tests or treatments that do little more than create revenue for your doctor.

• **Doctors who owned imaging centers** or leased imaging equipment referred their patients for imaging tests more than twice as often, on average, as doctors in the same specialties but without this financial interest.

• **Patients of doctors who owned or leased MRI machines** were 33% more likely to have normal MRIs than patients of doctors who didn't have MRI machines—because owner-doctors were less selective in determining which patients really needed the test.

• **Male patients who had prostate biopsies** performed by doctors with an ownership interest in the pathology lab had 72% more specimens examined than patients of doctors without a financial interest—yet the patients of the lab-owning doctors were less likely to actually have cancer.

Overtreating: As if unwarranted tests weren't bad enough, self-referring doctors on average provide more unneeded treatments, too. *Examples from recent studies…*

• **Surgeons who were partial or full owners of surgery centers** performed at least twice as many of five studied procedures (such as knee arthroscopy and carpal tunnel surgery) as non-owner surgeons in the same specialties.

• **Prostate cancer patients being treated by urologists** who owned the equipment needed to perform intensity-modulated radiation therapy (IMRT) were nearly three times more likely to undergo this expensive treatment than men treated by urologists who did not own IMRT equipment.

• **Doctors who purchased IMRT equipment** more than quadrupled their use of this treatment after acquiring the equipment, on average—even though studies show that for low-risk disease (which accounts for the vast majority of prostate cancers), IMRT is no better than other treatments that cost about half as much. However, before these urologists purchased their IMRT equipment, they were no more likely than non-owner urologists to refer patients for IMRT.

Overcharging: Even when a test or procedure is necessary, the "convenience" of self-referral comes at a price. For instance, a recent study showed that for imaging tests, with the exception of X-rays, fees are higher, on average, when doctors self-refer patients rather than sending patients elsewhere for services. Even if you don't pay directly for those medical expenses, the excess costs still affect you—and everyone else—in the form of increased insurance premiums and copays.

How can consumers protect themselves in this era of self-referral?

Is the Blood Supply Safe?

Richard Benjamin, MD, PhD, chief medical officer, American Red Cross, Washington, DC.

Blood transfusion is safer than it has ever been but should be used only when absolutely necessary. Blood donors must be healthy and are screened by a detailed questionnaire, an interview and a brief physical exam. Prescription medications are not in themselves a reason for deferral from donation unless they indicate an underlying medical condition that is of concern. Donors are required to list all medications and are asked about specific drugs that may harm the recipient, such as *finasteride* (Proscar), often used for enlarged prostate. This drug (and some others) would result in a donation deferral. Other drugs are likely to be present in such small amounts that the risk to the person getting the blood is insignificant. If you are still worried, talk to your doctor about storing some of your own blood prior to the surgery.

Don't Let What Happened to Joan Rivers Happen to You

David Sherer, MD, an anesthesiologist and former physician-director of risk management for a major HMO in the metropolitan Washington, DC, area. He is author, with Maryann Karinch, of *Dr. David Sherer's Hospital Survival Guide.* DrDavidSherer.com

Ever since Joan Rivers died after a routine surgical procedure at an outpatient center in Manhattan, people have been wondering if they're better off having surgery in a hospital.

The reality is that the vast majority of outpatient procedures go off without a hitch. But you can reduce your risk by getting involved before the procedure. *Important steps...*

CHECK YOUR PHYSICAL STATUS

Ask your doctor about your "physical status classification." The American Society of Anesthesiologists uses a numerical scale to assess a patient's surgical risks. Patients with higher physical status (PS) scores (four or five) because of health problems should have procedures done in hospitals because their risk for complications is higher.

Example: A patient who needs a knee replacement also might have poorly controlled diabetes, kidney insufficiency and nerve damage. His/her PS might be rated as four—too high to safely have a major procedure at an outpatient center.

In general, patients with PS scores of one through three—with one being generally healthy and three indicating that they have serious diseases that aren't life-threatening—are good candidates for outpatient procedures.

PICK YOUR SURGEON CAREFULLY

Don't assume that every surgeon in an outpatient center has the same experience—or the same credentials.

Suppose that you're planning to get Botox or Restylane injections. These are not as simple as most people think. For the best results—and the lowest risk for complications—you should have the procedure done by a physician who is board-certified in plastic and reconstructive surgery.

Caution: In many states, many procedures can be done by any physician who has undergone minimal training in these procedures, such as a weekend course or three-day seminar. These doctors might be board-certified in something but not necessarily in the field that concerns you.

Also important: The amount of experience. Studies have clearly shown that doctors who do a lot of procedures have better results, with fewer complications, than those who do them less often.

Example: If I were planning to have LASIK eye surgery, I wouldn't feel comfortable seeing a surgeon who had done the procedure 50 times. I would want someone whose total cases numbered in the hundreds or even thousands.

INSIST ON PAIN CONTROL

Most people assume that their surgeons will do everything possible to minimize postoperative pain. Not true. Some doctors are reluctant to order strong painkillers on an ongoing basis because they worry that the patient will become addicted. Or they mainly use narcotics (opioids, such as codeine and morphine) that dull pain but can cause unpleasant and sometimes dangerous side effects, including impaired breathing, constipation, itching, nausea and vomiting.

Poorly controlled pain is among the most serious postoperative complications. It impairs immunity and increases the risk for infection… slows healing times…and can increase the risk for blood clots when patients hurt too much to move normally.

My advice: Tell your surgeon that you're terrified of pain. Ask what he/she plans to use to relieve your pain—and emphasize that you would like to avoid narcotics if at all possible.

Also, ask about *bupivacaine* (Exparel), a nonnarcotic anesthetic that was recently approved by the FDA. The active ingredient is encapsulated in liposomal (fat-based) particles and slowly released over 72 hours. When injected into the surgical area, it relieves pain as effectively as narcotics with fewer side effects.

BEWARE OF SUPPLEMENTS

Tell your doctor about everything that you're taking. Surgeons and anesthesiologists routinely ask patients about medications that they're using. They don't always think to ask about supplements.

This is a dangerous oversight because many supplements—along with garden-variety over-the-counter medications such as aspirin—can interact with the drugs that are used during and after surgery.

Examples: Garlic supplements increase the risk for excessive bleeding, particularly when they're combined with aspirin. The herbs ephedra and kava can interfere with anesthetics.

Patients who are taking natural remedies—including vitamin E, echinacea, ginseng, valerian and St. John's wort—should ask their doctors if they need to quit taking them. You may need to stop two weeks or more before the procedure. Aspirin should be discontinued two to three days before.

PLAN FOR THE WORST

Even routine procedures sometimes go south. Most outpatient surgical centers are equipped with crash carts (used for cardiac emergencies) and other equipment and drugs for handling serious complications—but some don't have these on hand.

Ask the surgeon if a crash cart will be available. *Also ask…*

•**Is there *dantrolene* (Dantrium)?** It can reverse a rare but deadly complication from anesthesia known as malignant hyperthermia. The drug is always stocked in hospitals, but an outpatient center might not have it.

•**Is there succinylcholine (Anectine, Quelicin)?** It's a fast-acting paralytic agent that assists doctors in quickly intubating patients who can't breathe—one of the most dangerous complications of anesthesia. It has been reported that Joan Rivers might have lived if this drug had been available.

DON'T PUT UP WITH NAUSEA

It is estimated that 30% of all postsurgical patients will experience nausea, retching or vomiting. These are among the most common surgical complications.

My advice: Tell your anesthesiologist/surgeon if you've suffered from surgery-related nausea in the past. He/she can administer *granisetron* (Kytril) or *ondansetron* (Zofran), which helps prevent nausea in most patients.

GET MOVING

Try to get moving as soon as you can. Surgeons used to recommend lengthy bed rest for postsurgical patients. They now know that it's better to move around as soon as possible to prevent constipation, urinary retention and muscle weakness, among other common complications.

As soon as you're able, get up and walk (with your doctor's permission, of course). If you can't stand right away, at least move in bed. Stretch your legs. Move your arms. Roll over, sit up, etc. Any kind of physical movement increases blood flow and improves recovery times. It also improves the movement of your lungs, which can help prevent postsurgical pneumonia.

Doctors and Hospitals Are Adding Sneaky Fees

Charles Inlander, consumer advocate and health-care consultant based in Fogelsville, Pennsylvania. He is co-author of more than 20 consumer-health books.

Many doctors and hospitals are adding on sneaky fees for services that used to be included with routine visits and treatments. And the fees typically are not covered by insurance.

EXAMPLE #1: A patient who went to see a mental health therapist was billed an additional $100 "facility" fee for the room in which the visit took place.

EXAMPLE #2: A woman who walked into an emergency room after a bicycle accident was charged a "trauma activation" fee of $2,457 for the hospital to alert trauma personnel, including a surgeon, none of whose services were ever used.

If you are covered by Medicare, the medical provider is required by law to clearly inform you in advance about any service that may not be covered and to estimate what the cost to you will be. However, private insurers are under no such obligation if patients don't ask for this information.

Self-defense...

Speak to your doctor and the person in charge of billing before you are treated.

Ask: "Is everything you are going to do for me covered by my insurance? If not, you need to tell me in advance." If they disclose an unexpected fee, check ahead of time whether your insurer will agree to cover it as part of the general treatment. If not, tell your doctor, "I'm not able to afford to pay anything beyond my co-pay and

Eye Contact with Your Cereal

Cereal-box characters are designed to make eye contact to build brand loyalty. Characters on cereals intended for adults, which usually are placed on upper store shelves, generally look straight ahead or slightly up to make eye contact with adults. Characters on child-oriented cereals look slightly downward to make eye contact with kids.

Study by researchers at Cornell Food and Brand Lab, Ithaca, New York, published in *Environment and Behavior.*

deductibles," and ask to have the fee removed or reduced. Many doctors will comply.

Refuse to pay a bill if there's a fee that was not disclosed even though you asked. File a report with the state insurance department requesting that it launch a fraud investigation. Many providers would rather dismiss a miscellaneous charge than endure an investigation.

Kidney-Donation Caution

Dorry Segev, MD, PhD, associate professor of surgery, The Johns Hopkins University School of Medicine, Baltimore.

A recent study of more than 1,000 kidney donors found that 7% had difficulties obtaining health insurance, and 25% reported problems getting life insurance. New guidelines under the Affordable Care Act should make getting health insurance easier for organ donors, since insurers are not supposed to deny coverage or charge higher rates, but unfortunately it still seems to be happening in some cases.

Insurance companies could be rejecting claims because of misinterpreted blood work in medical records—for example, serum creatinine (a measure of kidney function). Organ donors should call insurance companies and clarify that they donated a kidney after passing a detailed health screening and that the creatinine level in a record is only a reflection of the fact that they have one kidney, not that they have kidney disease. If the insurer still refuses to cover or tries to charge a higher premium, ask the transplant center to call on the donor's behalf.

Is the Cheaper Store-Brand Supplement Really as Good?

Edgar Dworsky, creator of the consumer advocate websites *ConsumerWorld.org* and *MousePrint.org*. Formerly, he served as consumer education consultant for the Federal Trade Commission and was a Massachusetts assistant attorney general.

S tore-brand vitamins and supplements can save you money, but they may not be as perfect a match to national brands as you often are led to believe.

Examples…

•**Walgreens One Daily Women's 50+ Multivitamin** (about $13) may seem like a good substitute for Centrum Silver Women 50+ Multivitamin/Multimineral Supplement (about $16). But the Walgreens supplement contains only 23 specific vitamins, minerals and nutrients, while Centrum has 31, including boron and potassium, which are not in the Walgreens version, and higher daily doses of vitamins A, C and E. Which is better? That may depend on an individual shopper's nutritional needs. But what's clear is that the Walgreens version isn't an exact substitute for the national brand.

•**CVS Advanced Eye Health softgel tablets** (about $17) say on the label that they're "comparable" to the AREDS 2 study formula softgels popularized by Bausch & Lomb PreserVision (about $35). The Bausch & Lomb product contains all six ingredients that were used in that study by the National Institutes of Health, which resulted in slower progression of age-related macular degeneration, a very serious eye condition that could lead to partial blindness. The CVS product contains only two of the six ingredients—lutein and zeaxanthin—while leaving out all of the study's proven vitamins and minerals (vitamin C, vitamin E, copper and zinc).

Bottom line: Compare ingredients carefully.

Are Your Herbal Supplements Contaminated or Fake?

Stefan Gafner, PhD, chief scientific officer, American Botanical Council, Austin, Texas. He has served as a peer reviewer for many scientific journals including *Journal of Agricultural and Food Chemistry* and *Journal of Natural Products*.

Steven Newmaster, PhD, professor, botanical director, Biodiversity Institute of Ontario and Centre for Biodiversity Genomics, University of Guelph, Guelph, Ontario, Canada. His research on DNA barcoding of herbal supplements was published in *BMC Medicine*.

A ccording to a recent Canadian study, more than half of herbal products tested (44 products from 12 companies) were contaminated with ingredients other than what was on the labels…and about one-third contained absolutely none of the material that was on the labels.

If valid, these findings are outrageous! But what if the researchers are wrong…?

The study has attracted a lot of attention from supplement naysayers, who point to it as evidence that dietary supplements are worthless… and from supplement-industry supporters, who say that the study had serious flaws.

Among the critics of this study is Stefan Gafner, PhD, chief scientific officer of the American Botanical Council (ABC), a trade group that promotes the use of herbal supplements. Dr. Gafner does not deny that adulteration in supplements is a problem. In fact, he is a member of a consortium focused on identifying and eliminating intentional and accidental adulteration of plant-based health products. However, he contends that this study has too many flaws to be credible.

Dr. Gafner contested the idea that the supplement industry is clueless about what's in its products, saying that several reputable organizations have published research on various microscopic, macroscopic and chemical methods for authenticating botanical raw materials. And he added that all supplement manufacturers and importers in the US are required to comply with the rules of the current "good manufacturing practices" in the federal Dietary Supplement Health and Education Act of 1994, which includes use of adequate testing. Still, he conceded that currently there is no single uniform method for authenticating herbal products.

Part of the problem is that although the Food and Drug Administration (FDA) is responsible for oversight of the supplement industry, it does not routinely test supplement ingredients nor frequently inspect manufacturing facilities. This means that supplement manufacturers are largely left to operate on the honor system.

TELL US THE BRANDS!

Of the 12 companies with products that were tested, only two provided authentic products with no fillers or substitutions—and the names of those two companies were not revealed by the researchers. In fact, the researchers did not provide the brand names of any of the products they tested…which is a big criticism of the Canadian study. Supplement consumers want to know which brands passed muster and which did not! So why was this information omitted from the study?

Steven Newmaster, PhD, professor and botanical director at the Biodiversity Institute of Ontario and Centre for Biodiversity Genomics at the University of Guelph, is the lead author of the study.

Here's his response: "We provide an unbiased 'watchdog' service. The herbal industry has been alerted to a problem, and now it has the ability to take action."

Without access to the desired information on specific brands, consumers are left to wonder how to buy supplements without worrying that we're getting a bottle full of useless rice—or worse—instead of the health aid we wanted. It may be just a matter of time before the technique used in this study (DNA barcoding) is used routinely on all products made from living materials, including herbal supplements, helping to make products safer and of higher quality. *Until then, here are some tips for consumers…*

•**Do your research,** suggested Dr. Gafner—but don't rely on Google or other basic search engines, or you might be misled by the thousands of hits that aren't associated with clinical trials.

Better: Search PubMed, which is a search engine for medical literature…or Google Scholar, which provides a search of scholarly literature across many disciplines and sources. In the search bar, type in the brand and product name

of any product you are considering using to help you find out whether a particular manufacturer has invested in clinical research.

•**If an herbal product you currently are using is working for you,** stick with it, suggested Dr. Newmaster. Otherwise, try a different brand. If a product makes you feel at all unwell, stop using it immediately!

•**Order your supplements through a licensed naturopathic doctor rather than buying them over the counter.** These physicians have access to professional-grade supplements that are likely to have undergone quality-assurance testing and/or that have been shown to be effective for the doctors' other patients…so you can feel more confident that what you're swallowing actually is what it claims to be. Or try the professional-grade brands that naturopathic physicians prescribe—Douglas Laboratories, Eclectic Institute, Priority One, Pure Encapsulations, Thorne Research and Wise Woman Herbals.

Is That Newfangled Coffeemaker Safe?

Patricia Hunt, PhD, researcher, School of Molecular Biosciences, Washington State University, Pullman.

The individual packages (called K-Cup and Vue packs) used to brew beverages in Keurig coffee machines do not contain bisphenol A (BPA), according to the manufacturer. BPA, a chemical used in many plastic containers and metal cans, is believed to disrupt the endocrine system and has been linked to reproductive disorders, heart disease, diabetes and some forms of cancer.

However, researchers continue to study other chemicals in plastics to see if they might possibly leach into food and water and create health problems. Until more is known, old-fashioned stainless steel percolators and ceramic pour-over models may be the safest coffeemakers, since they contain no plastic.

Surgery Danger for People With Anemia

Anemic patients had a 42% greater risk of dying within 30 days of noncardiac surgery than patients with normal levels of healthy red blood cells.

Self-defense: If surgery can be delayed, talk to your doctor about iron replacement and the use of erythropoietin to boost preoperative hemoglobin levels.

Faek R. Jamali, MD, FACS, program director, general surgery residency at American University at Beirut Medical Center, Lebanon. He led a study of 69,229 people with preoperative anemia, published online in *The Lancet*.

The Dark Side of Superfoods

Jamison Starbuck, ND, naturopathic physician in family practice and a guest lecturer at the University of Montana, both in Missoula. She is past president of the American Association of Naturopathic Physicians and a contributing editor to *The Alternative Advisor: The Complete Guide to Natural Therapies and Alternative Treatments*.

Most of us who watch what we eat know that whole, nutritious food functions as medicine. But advertisers have now gotten in on the act by co-opting the term "superfood" for one-sided campaigns to sell grocery items—and not in a way that's always healthful! While there's certainly plenty of truth to the health benefits conferred by superfoods, it's only fair that any downsides of these highly touted foods get equal airtime. *Some not-so-super facts about four enormously popular superfoods…*

•**Kale.** This slightly bitter, leafy green is rich in vitamin K, folic acid and calcium. It also contains indole-3-carbinol, a compound thought to lower cancer risk. All that sounds great. But there can be some problems if certain people consume too much kale. If you take a blood thinner, such as *warfarin* (Coumadin), all that vitamin K will interact with the drug. Kale also contains oxalates that may contribute to kidney stones, and raw kale can act as a goitrogen,

meaning it reduces thyroid function. Additionally, when eaten raw, kale can cause intestinal gas and bloating in some people.

Bottom line on kale: If you are on a blood thinner or have had oxalate-type kidney stones, avoid kale. If you have hypothyroidism (low thyroid function), don't consume concentrated, juiced kale. Cooking kale deactivates some of its goitrogenic properties, so it's OK to enjoy a couple of servings per week. For everyone else, it's safe and healthy to eat kale once a day.

•**Goji berry.** Goji is believed to improve physical stamina, promote sleep and help confer a longer life. The downside? Well, goji isn't all that unique from a nutritional standpoint—in fact, it's similar to many red-colored fruits and berries. Goji is rich in vitamins, particularly beta-carotene and vitamin C, and it's a good source of calcium. However, there have recently been reports of pesticide-laden goji being imported from Asia. That's why you must read labels and inquire about sources when you purchase goji. To play it safe, avoid goji from Asia—it may contain pesticides. Buy organic goji from the US or grow it yourself. Enjoy goji as you would raspberries or blackberries.

•**Chia seeds.** Rich in fiber, antioxidants and calcium, chia seeds (like flaxseeds) have a mild, nutty flavor. They are a good plant source of omega-3s and make a nice addition to oatmeal, baked goods and protein-rich snack bars. The problem with chia seeds? Some promoters sell chia seeds as a weight-loss aid, but this has not been proved.

•**Quinoa.** Gluten-free and high in protein, quinoa is often called the superfood of grains. However, quinoa contains saponins, foamy, bitter chemical compounds that can create indigestion in some people. Food manufacturers know this and often prewash quinoa before processing it to be sold to consumers. Even so, some saponins slip through. So if you like quinoa but it gives you indigestion, be sure to rinse it thoroughly before cooking.

6 Surprising Places Where Mold Lurks

Jeffrey C. May, a certified indoor air-quality professional (CIAQP) and founder and principal scientist of May Indoor Air Investigations, LLC, an air-quality-assessment company located in Tyngsborough, Massachusetts. He is also author of several books, including *The Mold Survival Guide. MayIndoorAir.com*

We all know that mold thrives in obvious places such as damp basements, steamy bathrooms and storage areas with piles of old books and/or clothing. But there are plenty of other spots you'd never suspect that also can harbor these nasty fungal spores.

For the 10% to 15% of Americans who are allergic to mold, inhaling (or ingesting) the spores can trigger symptoms such as sneezing, runny nose, swollen eyelids, an itchy throat and wheezing.

Six surprising mold hot spots...

HOT SPOT #1: Your coffeemaker. In one study, mold was found in the water reservoirs of about half of the tested drip-type coffeemakers.

What to do: Once a month, fill your coffeemaker's reservoir with a 50/50 mixture of water and white vinegar. Turn the coffeemaker on, just as you would if you were brewing a pot of coffee. When the reservoir is half emptied, turn off the coffeemaker. Wait 30 minutes and then finish the brewing cycle. Rinse the machine by running plain, cool water through the cycle twice (or check manufacturer's instructions). When you finish your coffee each day, allow the reservoir to dry completely by leaving the lid open.

HOT SPOT #2: Your washing machine. Mold has no problem growing inside the rubber gaskets on the doors of front-loading machines. Those gaskets prevent water from pouring through the door, but water is often trapped inside the rubber folds. In all kinds of machines, detergent trays can stay damp between cycles, and the agitators of top-loading machines can be an area for mold growth, too.

What to do: Keep the door and detergent tray open when you're not using the washing machine. For front-loaders, wipe the inside of the gasket bottom with a rag or paper towel to dry it if no more loads will be done that day.

If you think you have mold, run an empty cycle with the machine on its hottest setting, using a mixture of one cup of baking soda, one cup of bleach and one-half cup of powdered dishwasher detergent. Some front-loading washers have a separate cycle for washing the inside of the machine. If a top-loading washer smells musty, the agitator may have to be removed and the shaft and agitator cleaned.

HOT SPOT #3: Under your refrigerator. Keep an eye on frost-free refrigerators and freezers.

Here's why: Your freezer section isn't actually frost-free. Frost is automatically melted during a heating cycle, and then the water accumulates in a pan at the bottom. The heat released from the condenser coils is supposed to speed up this evaporation, but often there is standing water in the pan. This water allows bacteria, yeast and mold to grow in the dust in the pan, and air movement can disperse these organisms into your kitchen.

What to do: Keep the condenser coils on your refrigerator clean by removing the grille at the bottom or back of the appliance and vacuuming the dust from the coils. A 36-inch Flexible Crevice Tool is available at *Amazon.com* for

The Truth About Salt Lamps

Himalayan salt lamps carved from large salt crystal rocks are touted as natural generators that emit healthy negatively charged oxygen ions. Negative ions attract mold, dust, pollen and other irritants and have been shown to improve mood. The lamps are beautiful, but there is no evidence that they provide any health benefits. The fresh air you feel after a storm or at the beach is due to a high concentration of ionized oxygen that has been created in the atmosphere. Salt lamps are supposed to replicate that same kind of clean air, but it has not been shown that salt lamps actually ionize oxygen.

Michael Terman, PhD, president, Center for Environmental Therapeutics, New York City.

$12.99. Cleaning the coils once a year improves the efficiency of the refrigerator and can eliminate dust-containing pollen, mold spores and pet dander.

Cleaning the drip pan might not be as easy—with some refrigerator models, the pan is accessible only from the back of the fridge and/or may be attached to the condenser. Check the refrigerator manufacturer's instructions for proper cleaning of the condenser coils and drip pan.

HOT SPOT #4: The underside of the toilet tank. You probably don't look, but moisture often lingers here—and so does mold.

What to do: If it's easy enough, get on the floor (otherwise, use a mirror and flashlight) and take a look at the underside of each toilet tank in your home. If there's mold, mix one cup of bleach with one gallon of water, open a window or door for ventilation and scrub the moldy areas with gloved hands. Clean these areas with a nonabrasive bathroom cleanser once a month during times of high outdoor humidity.

HOT SPOT #5: Your Waterpik and toothbrush. The water reservoir of your Waterpik or other water-jet appliance may not dry out between uses, and mold may grow on rubber gaskets and/or the water reservoir. Toothbrushes generally dry too fast for mold to grow, but it can grow inside the hollow heads of electric toothbrushes.

What to do: After each use of your Waterpik, remove the water reservoir, invert it and let it dry. To drain the pump, lower the sprayer in the sink so that it is below the level of the pump. Gravity will allow the water to drain. To clean electric toothbrush heads, soak in diluted bleach, 3% hydrogen peroxide or vinegar for a few minutes once a month.

HOT SPOT #6: Your dehumidifier. Dehumidifiers are designed to remove moisture and help prevent mold. But condensed water accumulates on cooling coils and can lead to mold growth in any dust trapped on the cooling-coil fins.

What to do: Empty the water basin at least weekly. During hot, humid weather, empty it daily. A few times a year, wash the plastic filter in a sink, scrub the inside of the bucket with nonabrasive cleanser (use diluted bleach if it is moldy) and spray any dust off the fins with water. Before storing the dehumidifier when it's not in use, wash and dry all of the parts carefully. Follow the manufacturer's instructions for cleaning the machine.

No Need to Overpay for Good-Looking Glasses

ConsumerReports.org.

With name-brand eyeglasses, you are paying for the name, but the glasses usually are made by the same firms that make less expensive ones.

Example: Luxottica makes Chanel, Prada and Versace glasses, which can cost $350 or more—and also ones for LensCrafters, Pearle Vision, Sears Optical and Target Optical, which can be less than $100. Instead of buying from an eye doctor or optometrist, shop discount stores. Costco gets especially high satisfaction ratings. Also look online at sites such as *SimplyEyeglasses.com* and *LensesRx.com*. Stores and websites sometimes have coupons and half-price deals that can cut costs. You may have to buy two pairs, which can be a good idea in case one pair gets lost or broken.

Hazardous Hair Dyes

Exposure to *toluidines* and other potential carcinogens in dye and perm products could explain the higher risk for bladder cancer in hairdressers. Always wear gloves when using these products.

British Medical Journal

Do Fitness Trackers Really Work?

Jung-Min Lee, PhD, assistant professor, Physical Activity and Health Promotion Laboratory, University of Nebraska, Omaha. His study was published in *Medicine and Science in Sports and Exercise.*

Fitness trackers are relatively inexpensive devices that promise to tell you how much exercise you're getting and how fit you are. The idea is that you wear one of these lightweight, computerized sensors (also called activity trackers) on your body or clothing, and it records when you're moving and how you're moving, so that you can learn whether you're getting enough exercise and burning enough calories…or if you should raise the bar on your activity level.

But do they really work?

Not precisely, according to several different studies that evaluated different models. But that doesn't mean they're useless. Researchers from the University of Nebraska conducted a study that evaluated eight different fitness trackers that claim to use a technology called indirect calorimetry, a measurement of energy—or calorie—expenditure that uses oxygen consumption as a gauge. The eight trackers included BodyMedia FIT, which is a band worn on the upper arm, DirectLife, which can be worn around the neck (or carried in a pocket or attached to a belt), the Fitbit One, Fitbit Zip and ActiGraph, which are all belt clips, and the Nike+Fuel Band, Jawbone UP and Basis B1 Band, which are wristbands.

These eight commercially manufactured trackers were compared with a professional indirect calorimetry device (a unit used in university, government and commercial research) in 60 healthy men and women who wore all of the trackers and the indirect calorimetry device simultaneously. The study participants, decked out in their array of trackers, performed a series of activities that lasted for a total of 69 minutes. They walked on a treadmill at different speeds, reclined, used a computer, ran at different speeds, went up and down stairs, played basketball and rode a stationary bike. All this time, each device was (supposedly) measuring how many calories the participants burned.

The results: According to the professional-grade indirect calorimetry device, the average energy expenditure was 356.9 calories, but the average of readouts from the various consumer fitness trackers ranged from 271.1 calories for the Basis B1 Band to 370.1 calories for the Fitbit Zip. Although no consumer tracker hit the nail on the head, all except the Basis B1 Band came within a relatively acceptable margin, with error ratings ranging from 9% to 13%. The BodyMedia Fit, Nike+Fuel Band and Fitbit Zip were closest in accuracy to the indirect calorimetry device.

LESS ABOUT PRECISION, MORE ABOUT MOTIVATION

Although the above study proved that these consumer-grade fitness trackers are only "OK" when it comes to accurately counting calories burned, they can be worth the money, but with certain caveats.

Reason: Trackers are great motivational tools. Almost all trackers have goal-setting features that allow you to program your desired activity level into them. The tracker will then give you feedback, via communication with your smartphone or whatever other electronic device you've synced it with, to keep you motivated. For example, if you've set a goal to walk 6,000 steps in a day but the monitor determines that you're sitting down, you might get a gentle reminder via e-mail or smartphone to get moving.

Even if your tracker is off by 5% or 10% or so on your calories burned, it's OK because you are also going to use your eyes and your common sense when it comes to assessing your fitness. If your tracker tells you that you are burning the same number of calories that you believe you are eating, but you are still gaining weight, you know. You need to eat less and/or exercise more.

There's also a style factor. Most wristbands look more like high-tech watches or jewelry than fitness gadgets. And some trackers, such as Misfit, are waterproof so that they can literally be worn all the time.

Recommendations for anyone who wants to use a fitness tracker: Get as much information as possible about different models. Carefully peruse online reviews of actual users to get the pros and cons, and comparison shop at sites such as TopTenReviews.com, which list and rate features, side by side, of the most popular models. Then go to a store that carries several brands to try them on and see how they feel.

Fluoride in Drinking Water Tied to Higher Rates of Underactive Thyroid

Edmond Hewlett, DDS, American Dental Association spokesman and professor and associate dean for outreach and diversity, University of California, Los Angeles School of Dentistry.

Terry Davies, MD, Florence and Theodore Baumritter Professor of Medicine, Icahn School of Medicine, Mount Sinai, and endocrinologist, The Mount Sinai Hospital, New York City.

Spyros Mezitis, MD, endocrinologist, Lenox Hill Hospital, New York City.

Journal of Epidemiology & Community Health.

A British study finds a correlation between the amount of fluoride in public drinking water and a rise in incidence of underactive thyroid.

According to the U.S. National Institutes of Health, the thyroid is a butterfly-shaped gland near the base of the neck that produces hormones. Thyroid hormones control the rate of many body activities, including how fast calories are burned and how fast the heart beats. If the thyroid gland isn't active enough, it does not make enough thyroid hormone to meet the body's needs.

STUDY DETAILS

Led by Stephen Peckham of the University of Kent in Canterbury, England, researchers compared national data (from 2012) on levels of fluoride in drinking water to trends for hypothyroidism (underactive thyroid) as diagnosed by family physicians across England during the year span 2012-13.

They found that in locales where tap water fluoride levels exceeded 0.3 milligrams per liter, the risk for having an underactive thyroid rose by 30%.

Peckham's team also found that hypothyroidism rates were nearly double in urbanized regions that had fluoridated tap water, compared with regions that did not.

"Consideration needs to be given to reducing fluoride exposure," the researchers wrote. They believe that public efforts to strengthen dental health should move away from fluoridated water and instead "switch to topical fluoride-based and non-fluoride-based interventions."

EXPERT COMMENT

While the study is only able to establish an association, not cause-and-effect, experts say the link deserves serious investigation.

"Clinicians in the United States should emphasize to patients this association and should test patients for underactive thyroid," said Spyros Mezitis, MD, an endocrinologist at Lenox Hill Hospital in New York City.

"Patients should probably be advised to drink less fluoridated water and consume less fluoridated products, including [fluoridated] toothpaste," added Dr. Mezitis, who was not involved in the study.

Dr. Mezitis also noted that, while "fluoridation of the water supply is important for dental health, studies have also shown that iodine deficiency that may be caused by extra ingestion of fluoride is related to hypothyroidism."

He added that "drinking water is fluoridated in the United States, where hypothyroidism is a highly prevalent disorder—affecting over 15 million individuals mainly female and greater than 40 years old."

Another thyroid expert agreed that attention should be directed at fluoride in the drinking supply.

"This dramatic increase in thyroid dysfunction associated with fluoridation of the water supply adds to previous studies indicating that fluoride has an inhibitory effect on the thyroid gland," said Terry Davies, MD, a professor of medicine at the Icahn School of Medicine at Mount Sinai, in New York City.

The study "supports the argument that our water supply should be pure water and nothing else," said Dr. Davies, who is also an endocrinologist at The Mount Sinai Hospital.

RESPONSE FROM DENTAL INDUSTRY

But a representative of the American Dental Association took issue with the British report.

"Public health policy is built on a strong base of scientific evidence, not a single study," said Edmond Hewlett, DDS, ADA spokesman and a professor at the UCLA School of Dentistry. "Currently, the best available scientific evidence indicates that optimally fluoridated water does not have an adverse effect on the thyroid gland or its function.

"A far more rigorous systematic evaluation of human studies conducted by the Scientific Committee on Health and Environmental Risks at the request of the European Commission does not suggest a potential thyroid effect at realistic exposures to fluoride," he said. "Additionally, the 2006 Report by the U.S. National Research Council found no adverse effects on the thyroid even at levels more than four times greater than that used in fluoridation."

And fluoride in the water supply protects dental health, Dr. Hewlett added. "Even with the widespread availability of fluoride toothpaste, studies show that community water fluoridation prevents at least 25% of tooth decay in children and adults throughout the lifespan," he said.

The findings are published online in the *Journal of Epidemiology & Community Health*.

info For more on water fluoridation, visit the U.S. National Institute for Dental and Craniofacial Research at *http://www.nidcr.nih.gov*.

You're Cooking Chicken Wrong!

Christine Bruhn, PhD, director, Center for Consumer Research, University of California at Davis.

Forty percent of people undercook chicken.

Best: Always use a meat thermometer—slicing through the meat is not a good guide to whether chicken is properly cooked to 165°F.

Better Nose Jobs

Due to its strength, a patient's own rib cartilage is the preferred material to build up the bridge of the nose in rhinoplasty, but its use has been criticized because of side effects, such as a collapsed lung.

Recent finding: An analysis of 10 studies found that long-term complication rates of using rib cartilage were actually very low—including a less than 1% risk for infection or a collapsed lung. Synthetic materials, such as silicone, which are used in place of rib cartilage, have a higher risk for side effects, including infection.

Hong-Ryul Jin, MD, professor of otorhinolaryngology, Seoul National University College of Medicine, South Korea.

Also: Do not wash chicken before cooking it—washing uncooked chicken can spread bacteria around the kitchen.

And: Wash your hands for at least 20 seconds before handling anything else after you touch raw chicken. Use a separate cutting board exclusively for chicken, and clean that board in the dishwasher.

Toss Those Products with Dyes

Jamison Starbuck, ND, naturopathic physician in family practice and a guest lecturer at the University of Montana, both in Missoula. She is past president of the American Association of Naturopathic Physicians and a contributing editor to *The Alternative Advisor: The Complete Guide to Natural Therapies and Alternative Treatments*.

Peek inside the typical American's medicine cabinet, and you're likely to see a virtual rainbow of brightly colored products that contain potentially harmful dyes. Among the most popular are intensely colored cold and flu formulas and cough syrups.

Scientists have long suspected that dyes can be dangerous for human consumption. In the early 20th century, metals used for coloring, such as arsenic, lead and mercury, were banned from use in foods and medicines. Coal-tar derivatives then became the new dye source—bright, almost fluorescent colors with numbers for names—Blue 1 and 2...Yellow 5 and 6...Red 3 and 40. Over the years, some coal-tar dyes (but not all) have been banned due to health concerns. Now, scientists have become increasingly concerned about research linking food dyes to allergies and attention deficit hyperactivity disorder. In animal studies, dyes have been linked to tumors. Some manufacturers now produce dye-free products. Interestingly, however, the European Union requires warning labels on products that contain many dyes that the US Food and Drug Administration (FDA) still allows. Armed with the right information, you can be smarter than the FDA by stocking your home medicine chest with dye-free natural remedies for the following conditions...*

•**Cold and flu.** *What to skip:* Theraflu, which contains such dyes as Blue 1 and Red 40.

Better choices: Botanical antivirals (in tincture or capsule form), such as echinacea, Oregon graperoot, osha and elderberry.

•**Cough.** *What to skip:* Delsym, which contains Yellow 6 or other dyes.

Better choices: Effective herbs for cough include ivy leaf, wild cherry bark, olive leaf and

*Check with your doctor before trying these remedies—especially if you take any medication or have a chronic medical condition.

elecampane—all of which are available in syrups made with honey or stevia.

•**Gas and indigestion.** *What to skip:* Pepto Bismol, which contains Red 22 and Red 28.

Better choice: Gas, bloating and acute diarrhea respond well to activated charcoal, which binds toxins from the gastrointestinal tract. It's inert and will pass through the gastrointestinal tract without being absorbed into the blood. Activated charcoal can be found in drugstores. Follow label instructions.

•**Sleep.** *What to skip:* NyQuil PM, which contains Green 3, Blue 1 and other dyes.

Better choices: For occasional insomnia, take 50 mg of 5-HTP, an amino acid that plays a role in the production of sleep-promoting serotonin, at bedtime. (Do not try this remedy if you take an antidepressant.) When you use 5-HTP, it also helps to take Rescue Remedy, a Bach flower remedy that relaxes the nervous system.

What to do: Add two drops of Rescue Remedy to the water you use to take the supplement, and keep some of this water next to your bed to sip on if you awaken during the night.

Caution: To make their products appear more visually appealing, some manufacturers have begun adding dyes to herbal medicines. If a packaged natural product is overly bright—beware! Check labels on all medicines, and avoid dyes whenever you can.

Diabetes

The Secret Invasion That Causes Diabetes

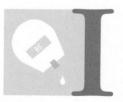

I t's easy to get the impression that diabetes is all about blood sugar. Most people with diabetes check their glucose levels at least once a day. Even people without diabetes are advised to have glucose tests every few years—just to make sure that the disease isn't creeping up on them.

But glucose is only part of the picture. Scientists now know that chronic inflammation increases the risk that you'll develop diabetes. If you already have insulin resistance (a precursor to diabetes) or full-blown diabetes, inflammation will make your glucose levels harder to manage.

A common mistake: Unfortunately, many doctors still don't test for inflammation even though it accompanies all of the main diabetes risk factors, including smoking, obesity and high-fat/sugar diets. *What you need to know about this important aspect of diabetes care…*

SILENT DAMAGE

You hear a lot about inflammation, but what exactly is it—and when is it a problem? Normal inflammation is protective. It comes on suddenly and lasts for just a few days or weeks—usually in response to an injury or infection. Inflammation kills or encapsulates microbes…assists in the formation of protective scar tissue…and helps regenerate damaged tissues.

But chronic inflammation—caused, for example, by infection or injuries that lead to continuously elevated levels of toxins—does not turn itself off. It persists for years or even decades, particularly in those who are obese, eat poor diets, don't get enough sleep or have chronic diseases, including seemingly minor conditions such as gum disease.

The diabetes link: Persistently high levels of inflammatory molecules interfere with the ability of insulin to regulate glucose—one cause of

George L. King, MD, research director and chief scientific officer of Harvard's Joslin Diabetes Center and coauthor, with Royce Flippin, of *The Diabetes Reset: Avoid It, Control It, Even Reverse It—A Doctor's Scientific Program.*

high blood sugar. Inflammation also appears to damage beta cells, the insulin-producing cells in the pancreas.

Studies have shown that when inflammation is aggressively lowered—with *salsalate* (an anti-inflammatory drug), for example—glucose levels can drop significantly. Inflammation is typically identified with a blood test that measures a marker known as CRP, or C-reactive protein.

HOW TO FIGHT INFLAMMATION

Even though salsalate reduces inflammation, when taken in high doses, it causes too many side effects, such as stomach bleeding and ringing in the ears, to be used long term. *Safer ways to reduce inflammation and keep it down…*

•**Breathe clean air.** Smoke and smog threaten more than just your lungs. Recent research has shown that areas with the highest levels of airborne particulates that are small enough to penetrate deeply into the lungs have more than 20% higher rates of type 2 diabetes than areas with the lowest levels of these particulates.

Air pollution (including cigarette smoke) increases inflammation in fatty tissues and in the vascular system. In animal studies, exposure to air pollution increases both insulin resistance and the risk for full-fledged diabetes.

My advice: Most people—and especially those who live in polluted areas—could benefit from using an indoor HEPA filter or an electrostatic air filter.

Products such as the Honeywell Long-Life Pure HEPA QuietCare Air Purifier (available at Amazon.com) will trap nearly 100% of harmful airborne particulates from indoor air.

If you live in a large metropolitan area, avoid outdoor exercise during high-traffic times of day.

•**Take care of your gums.** Even people who take good care of their teeth often neglect their gums. It's estimated that almost half of American adults have some degree of periodontal (gum) disease.

Why it matters: The immune system can't always eliminate infections that occur in gum pockets, the areas between the teeth and gums. A persistent gum infection causes equally persistent inflammation that contributes to other illnesses. For example, research shows that people with gum disease were twice as likely to develop diabetes as those without it.

My advice: After every meal (or at least twice a day), floss and brush, in that order. And clean your gums—gently use a soft brush.

It's particularly important to follow these steps before you go to bed to remove bacteria that otherwise will remain undisturbed until morning.

•**Get more exercise.** It's among the best ways to control chronic inflammation because it burns fat. When you have less fat, you'll also produce fewer inflammation-promoting cytokines.

Data from the Nurses' Health Study and the Health Professionals Follow-Up Study found that walking briskly for a half hour daily reduced the risk of developing diabetes by nearly one-third.

My advice: Take 10,000 steps per day. To do this, walk whenever possible for daily activities, such as shopping, and even walk inside your home if you don't want to go out. Wear a pedometer to make sure you reach your daily goal.

•**Enjoy cocoa.** Cocoa contains a type of antioxidant known as flavanols, which have anti-inflammatory properties. Known primarily for their cardiovascular benefits, flavanols are now being found to help regulate insulin levels.

My advice: For inflammation-fighting effects, have one square of dark chocolate (with at least 70% cocoa) daily.

•**Try rose hip tea.** Rose hips are among the richest sources of vitamin C, with five times as much per cup than what is found in one orange. A type of rose hip known as *rosa canina* is particularly potent because it may contain an additional anti-inflammatory compound known as *glycoside of mono* and *diglycerol* (GOPO). It inhibits the production of a number of inflammatory molecules, including chemokines and interleukins.

My advice: Drink several cups of tangy rose hip tea a day. It's available both in bags and as a loose-leaf tea. If you're not a tea drinker, you can take rose hip supplements. Follow the directions on the label.

•**Season with turmeric.** This spice contains curcumin, one of the most potent anti-inflammatory agents. It inhibits the action of eicosanoids, "signaling molecules" that are involved in the inflammatory response.

My advice: Eat more turmeric—it's a standard spice in curries and yellow (not Dijon) mustard. You will want something more potent if you already have diabetes and/or elevated CRP. I often recommend Curamin, a potent form of curcumin that's combined with boswellia, another anti-inflammatory herb.

Important: Be sure to talk to your doctor before trying rose hip or turmeric supplements if you take medication or have a chronic health condition.

CHECK YOUR CRP LEVEL

An inexpensive and accurate blood test that is often used to estimate heart attack risk is also recommended for people who have diabetes or are at increased risk for it. The blood test measures C-reactive protein (CRP), a marker for inflammation, which can lead to heart disease and impair the body's ability to regulate glucose.

Doctors may recommend the test for patients beginning in their 30s. It's wise to get it earlier if you have diabetes risk factors, such as obesity or a family history.

A high-sensitivity CRP (hsCRP) test typically costs about $20 and is usually covered by insurance. A reading of less than 1 mg/L is ideal. Levels above 3 mg/L indicate a high risk for insulin resistance and diabetes as well as for heart attack.

If the first test shows that your CRP level is elevated, you'll want to do everything you can to lower it—for example, through exercise, a healthful diet and weight loss. Repeat the test every four to six months to see how well your lifestyle improvements are working.

Prediabetes Link with Cancer

Prediabetes is linked to 15% higher risk for cancer overall. Prediabetes, which is increasingly common, is indicated by a blood sugar level between 100 mg/dL and 125 mg/dL. Prediabetes is associated with a 100% higher risk for liver cancer...60% for endometrial cancer...55%, stomach/colorectal cancer...19%, pancreatic cancer...and 19%, breast cancer. It does not increase risk for bladder, kidney, lung, ovarian or prostate cancer.

Self-defense: Cut blood sugar levels with diet and exercise.

Joel Zonszein, MD, professor of clinical medicine at Albert Einstein College of Medicine and director of the Clinical Diabetes Center at Montifiore Medical Center, the Bronx, New York.

Low Levels of Vitamin D Linked to Type 2 Diabetes Risk

The Endocrine Society, news release.

People with low levels of vitamin D appear to have an increased risk for type 2 diabetes, even if they aren't overweight or obese, a recent study suggests.

Exposure to sunlight triggers the body to produce vitamin D, which is also found in certain foods. The researchers say more than one billion people worldwide have low vitamin D levels due to limited exposure to sunlight.

The study included a small group of participants (about 150) in Spain. Their vitamin D levels were checked, as was their body mass index (BMI—an estimate of body fat based on height and weight). They also had tests for diabetes, prediabetes or other blood sugar (glucose) metabolism disorders.

Obese people who didn't have diabetes or related disorders had higher vitamin D levels than those with diabetes. Lean people with diabetes or related disorders were more likely to have low vitamin D levels than those without such disorders.

The results show that vitamin D levels were more closely linked to blood sugar levels than BMI, according to the study.

What the study wasn't able to tease out, however, was whether or not vitamin D played a role in causing diabetes or other disorders that affect the metabolism of glucose. The study was only designed to find an association between these factors.

The findings were published recently in the *Endocrine Society's Journal of Clinical Endocrinology & Metabolism*.

"Our findings indicate that vitamin D is associated more closely with glucose metabolism than obesity," study author Manuel Macias-Gonzalez, PhD, of the University of Malaga in Spain, said in a society news release.

The study suggests that vitamin D deficiency and obesity may work together to heighten the risk of diabetes. "The average person may be able to reduce their risk by maintaining a healthy diet and getting enough outdoor activity," he said.

Previous research has found that people with low vitamin D levels are more likely to be obese and to have diabetes, prediabetes and related disorders, according to the society.

info The U.S. National Library of Medicine has more about vitamin D at *http://www.nlm.nih.gov/medlineplus/vitamind.html*.

Thin People Get Diabetes, Too

Mercedes Carnethon, PhD, associate professor of preventive medicine and epidemiology at Northwestern University Feinberg School of Medicine in Chicago, where she specializes in population studies of diabetes, obesity, cardiovascular disease and fitness.

It's widely known that type 2 diabetes tends to strike people who are overweight. In fact, about 85% of people with diabetes are carrying extra pounds. But what about those who aren't overweight?

A popular misconception: It's commonly believed—even by many doctors—that lean and normal-weight people don't have to worry

New Insulin Gets FDA Nod

The new diabetes drug Afrezza is a fast-acting inhalable insulin that comes in a small inhaler that looks like a whistle. No needles are required.

How it works: At the beginning of each meal, the user inhales powder from the device. People with chronic obstructive pulmonary disease (COPD) or other lung conditions should not use Afrezza.

Osama Hamdy, MD, PhD, medical director, Obesity Clinical Program, Joslin Diabetes Center, Boston.

about diabetes. The truth is, you can develop diabetes regardless of your weight.

An unexpected risk: For those who have this "hidden" form of diabetes, recent research is now showing that they are at even greater risk of dying than those who are overweight and have the disease.

What you need to know about diabetes—no matter what you weigh…

THE EXTRA DANGER NO ONE EXPECTED

No one knows exactly why some people who are not overweight develop diabetes. There's some speculation that certain people are genetically primed for their insulin to not function properly, leading to diabetes despite their weight.

Still, because diabetes is so closely linked to being overweight, even researchers were surprised by the results of a recent analysis of 2,600 people with type 2 diabetes who were tracked for up to 15 years.

Startling finding: Among these people with diabetes, those who were of normal weight at the time of diagnosis were twice as likely to die of non–heart-related causes, primarily cancer, during the study period as those who were overweight or obese.* The normal-weight people were also more likely to die of cardiovascular disease, but there weren't enough heart-related events to make that finding statistically significant.

*Normal weight is defined as a body mass index (BMI) of 18.5 to 24.9…overweight is 25 to 29.9…and obese, 30 or above. To calculate your BMI, go to *NHLBI.NIH.gov* and search for "BMI Calculator."

Possible reasons for the higher death rates among normal-weight people with diabetes...

•**The so-called obesity paradox.** Even though overweight and obese people have a higher risk of developing diabetes, kidney disease and heart disease, they tend to weather these illnesses somewhat better, for unknown reasons, than lean or normal-weight people.

•**Visceral fat, a type of fat that accumulates around the internal organs, isn't always apparent.** Unlike the fat you can grab, which is largely inert, visceral fat causes metabolic disturbances that increase the risk for diabetes, heart disease and other conditions. You can have high levels of visceral fat even if you're otherwise lean. Visceral fat can truly be measured only by imaging techniques such as a CT scan (but the test is not commonly done for this reason). However, a simple waist measurement can help indicate whether you have visceral fat (see below).

•**Lack of good medical advice.** In normal-weight people who are screened and diagnosed with diabetes, their doctors might be less aggressive about pursuing treatments or giving lifestyle advice than they would be if treating someone who is visibly overweight.

HOW TO PROTECT YOURSELF

It's estimated that about 25% of the roughly 29 million Americans with diabetes haven't been diagnosed. *Whether you're heavy or lean...*

Treatment for Diabetic Retinopathy

The first treatment for diabetic retinopathy has been approved. The FDA recently approved injections of the drug Lucentis—also used to treat macular degeneration in older adults—for diabetic retinopathy in patients with macular edema (swelling that occurs when fluid builds up in the eye). Diabetic retinopathy, which causes bleeding and/or abnormal blood-vessel growth in the retina, is the leading cause of blindness in Americans with diabetes.

Deeba Husain, MD, a retina specialist and associate professor of ophthalmology at Harvard Medical School, Boston.

•**Get tested at least once every three years starting at age 45**—regardless of your weight. That's the advice of the American Diabetes Association (ADA). You may need even earlier testing and/or more frequent tests if you have risk factors, such as a family history of diabetes and/or a sedentary lifestyle. Talk to your doctor.

Remember: If your weight is normal, your doctor may have a lower clinical suspicion of diabetes—a fancy way of saying he/she wouldn't even wonder if you have the condition. As a result, the doctor might think it's OK to skip the test or simply forget to recommend it. Ask for diabetes testing—even if your doctor doesn't mention it.

A fasting glucose test, which measures blood sugar after you have gone without food for at least eight hours, is typically offered.

Alternative: The HbA1c blood test. It's recommended by the ADA because it shows your average blood glucose levels over the previous two to three months. Many people prefer the A1c test because it doesn't require fasting. Both types of tests are usually covered by insurance.

•**Pull out the tape measure.** Even if you aren't particularly heavy, a large waist circumference could indicate high levels of visceral fat. "Abdominal obesity" is defined as a waist circumference of more than 35 inches in women and more than 40 inches in men. Even if you are under these limits, any increase in your waist size could be a warning sign. Take steps such as diet and exercise to keep it from increasing.

To get an accurate measurement: Wrap a tape measure around your waist at the level of your navel. Make sure that the tape is straight and you're not pulling it too tight. And don't hold in your stomach!

•**Watch the sugar and calories.** The Harvard Nurses' Health Study found that women who drank just one daily soft drink (or fruit punch) had more than an 80% increased risk of developing diabetes.

Research has consistently linked sweetened beverages with diabetes. But it's not clear whether the culprits are the sweeteners (such as high-fructose corn syrup) or just the extra calories, which lead to weight gain. Either way, it's smart no matter what you weigh to eliminate soda and other supersweet beverages from your diet—or if you don't want to give them up, have no more than one soft drink a week, the amount that wasn't associated with weight gain in the study.

Remember: A single soft drink often contains hundreds of calories.

•**Get the right type of exercise.** People who want to lose weight often take up aerobic workouts, such as swimming or biking, which burn a lot of calories. But if you don't need to lose weight, strength training might be a better choice. When you add muscle, you significantly improve insulin sensitivity and enhance the body's ability to remove glucose from the blood.

Walking may not sound very sexy, but it's one of the best exercises going because it has both aerobic and muscle-building effects. In fact, walking briskly (at a pace that causes sweating and mild shortness of breath) for half an hour daily reduces the risk for diabetes by nearly one-third. That's pretty impressive!

Shocking Diabetes Trigger

Hyla Cass, MD, a board-certified psychiatrist and nationally recognized expert on integrative medicine based in Los Angeles. She is author of 10 books, including *8 Weeks to Vibrant Health* and *The Addicted Brain and How to Break Free. CassMD.com*

Everyone knows about high blood sugar and the devastating effects it can have on one's health and longevity. But low blood sugar (hypoglycemia) can be just as dangerous—and it does not get nearly the attention that it should.

Simply put, hypoglycemia occurs when the body does not have enough glucose to use as fuel. It most commonly affects people with type 2 diabetes who take medication that sometimes works too well, resulting in low blood sugar.

Who gets overlooked: In other people, hypoglycemia can be a precursor to diabetes that is often downplayed by doctors and/or missed by tests. Having low blood sugar might even make you think that you are far from having diabetes...when, in fact, the opposite is true.

Hypoglycemia can also be an underlying cause of anxiety that gets mistakenly treated with psychiatric drugs rather than the simple steps (see below) that can stabilize blood sugar levels. That's why anyone who seems to be suffering from an anxiety disorder needs to be seen by a doctor who takes a complete medical history and orders blood tests. When a patient comes to me complaining of anxiety, hypoglycemia is one of the first things I test for.

What's the link between hypoglycemia and anxiety? A sudden drop in blood sugar deprives the brain of oxygen. This, in turn, causes the adrenal glands to release adrenaline, the "emergency" hormone, which may lead to agitation, or anxiety, as the body's fight-or-flight mechanism kicks in.

THE DANGERS OF HYPOGLYCEMIA

Hypoglycemia has sometimes been called carbohydrate intolerance, because the body's insulin-releasing mechanism is impaired in a manner similar to what occurs in diabetics. In people without diabetes, hypoglycemia is usually the result of eating too many simple carbohydrates (such as sugar and white flour). The pancreas then overreacts and releases too much insulin, thereby excessively lowering blood sugar.

The good news is that hypoglycemia—if it's identified—is not that difficult to control through diet and the use of specific supplements. Hypoglycemia should be considered a warning sign

Fake Sugar Warning

Artificial sweeteners may increase diabetes risk in some people.

Recent finding: Studies in mice and people show that some users of artificial sweeteners have different gut bacteria from those of non-users—and have higher glucose intolerance, which puts them at increased risk for diabetes.

Eran Segal, PhD, is a professor in the department of computer science and applied mathematics, Weizmann Institute of Science, Rehovot, Israel. He is coauthor of a study published in *Nature*.

Fruits That Fight Diabetes

Reduce risk for type 2 diabetes with blueberries, grapes and apples.

Recent finding: People who ate at least three servings of these fruits per week were up to 26% less likely to develop type 2 diabetes than people who ate less of these fruits. Eat the whole fruit, not just the juice. Fruit juice increases risk for diabetes.

Study of 187,382 health professionals by researchers from the US, UK and Singapore, published in *BMJ*.

that you must adjust your carbohydrate intake or risk developing type 2 diabetes.

Caution: An episode of hypoglycemia in a person who already has diabetes can be life-threatening and requires prompt care, including the immediate intake of sugar—a glass of orange juice or even a sugar cube can be used.

Common symptoms of hypoglycemia include: Fatigue, dizziness, shakiness and faintness…irritability and depression…weakness or cramps in the feet and legs…numbness or tingling in the hands, feet or face…ringing in the ears…swollen feet or legs…tightness in the chest…heart palpitations…nightmares and panic attacks…"drenching" night sweats (not menopausal or perimenopausal hot flashes)…constant hunger…headaches and migraines…impaired memory and concentration…blurred vision…nasal congestion…abdominal cramps, loose stools and diarrhea.

A TRICKY DIAGNOSIS

Under-the-radar hypoglycemia (known as "subclinical hypoglycemia") is difficult to diagnose because symptoms may be subtle and irregular, and test results can be within normal ranges. Technically, if your blood sugar drops below 70 mg/dL, you are considered hypoglycemic. But people without diabetes do not check their blood sugar levels on their own, so it is important to be aware of hypoglycemia symptoms.

If you suspect that you may have hypoglycemia, talk to your physician. Ideally, you should arrange to have your blood glucose levels tested when you are experiencing symptoms. You will then be asked to eat food so that your blood

glucose can be tested again. If this approach is impractical for you, however, talk to your doctor about other testing methods.

THE RIGHT TREATMENT

If you have been diagnosed with diabetes, hypoglycemia may indicate that your diabetes medication dose needs to be adjusted. The sugar treatment described earlier can work in an emergency but is not recommended as a long-term treatment for hypoglycemia. Left untreated, hypoglycemia in a person with diabetes can lead to loss of consciousness and even death.

In addition to getting their medication adjusted, people with diabetes—and those who are at risk for it due to hypoglycemia—can benefit from the following…

•**A high-protein diet and healthful fats.** To keep your blood sugar levels stabilized, consume slowly absorbed, unrefined carbohydrates, such as brown rice, quinoa, oatmeal and sweet potatoes. Also, get moderate amounts of healthful fats, such as those found in avocado, olive oil and fatty fish, including salmon…and protein, such as fish, meat, chicken, soy and eggs.

Recommended protein intake: 10% to 35% of daily calories. If you have kidney disease, get your doctor's advice on protein intake.

•**Eat several small meals daily.** Start with breakfast to give your body fuel for the day (if you don't, stored blood sugar will be released into your bloodstream) and then have a small "meal" every three to four waking hours.

•**Avoid tobacco and limit your use of alcohol and caffeine.** They cause an excessive release of neurotransmitters that, in turn, trigger the pancreas to deliver insulin inappropriately.

The supplements below also help stabilize blood sugar levels (and can be used in addition to a daily multivitamin)…*

•**Chromium and vitamin B-6.** Chromium helps release accumulated sugars in the liver, which can lead to a dangerous condition called fatty liver. Vitamin B-6 supports chromium's function and helps stabilize glucose levels.

*Consult your doctor before trying any supplements, especially if you take prescription medicine and, or have a chronic condition, including diabetes.

Typical daily dose: 200 micrograms (mcg) of chromium with 100 mg of vitamin B-6.

•**Glutamine.** As the most common amino acid found in muscle tissue, glutamine plays a vital role in controlling blood sugar. Glutamine is easily converted to glucose when blood sugar is low.

Typical daily dose: Up to four 500-mg capsules daily...or add glutamine powder to a protein drink or a smoothie that does not contain added sugar—these drinks are good options for your morning routine. Glutamine is best taken 30 minutes before a meal to cut your appetite by balancing your blood sugar.

If You Have Diabetes... How to Fast Safely for a Medical Test

Paula Vetter, RN, MSN, a diabetes educator, holistic family nurse practitioner, personal wellness coach and former critical care nursing instructor at the Cleveland Clinic. *CrazyDiabetesMyths.com*

Recently, an employee at *Bottom Line Health* was scheduled for a colonoscopy, the screening test for colon cancer. The medical test turned into medical mayhem.

The day before the test, the woman followed her doctor's orders to start ingesting a "clear liquid" diet, which includes soft drinks, Jell-O and other clear beverages and foods. But when she drank the "prep"—the bowel-cleaning solution that is consumed the evening before a colonoscopy (and sometimes also the morning of)—she vomited. Over and over. As a result, her colon wasn't sufficiently emptied to conduct the test, which had to be postponed.

WHAT WENT WRONG?

The woman has diabetes—and her glucose (blood sugar) levels had become unstable, triggering nausea and vomiting. Yet not one medical professional—not a doctor, not a nurse, not a medical technician—had warned her that people with diabetes need to take special precautions with food and diabetes medicine whenever they have any medical test that involves an extended period of little or no eating. Unfortunately, this lack of diabetes-customized instruction about medical tests is very common. *What you need to know...*

DO IT EARLY

If you're undergoing a test that requires only overnight fasting, which includes many types of CT scans, MRIs and X-rays, make sure that the test is scheduled for early in the morning—no later than 9 am. That way, you will be able to eat after the test by 10 am or 11 am, which will help to stabilize your blood sugar as much as possible

Don't expect your blood sugar levels to be perfect after the test. The important thing is to keep them from getting too high or too low.

THE RIGHT CLEAR LIQUIDS

Conventional dietitians and doctors specify clear liquids and foods that reflect the conventional American diet, such as regular soda, sports drinks, Popsicles, Kool-Aid and Jell-O (no red or purple). But the pH of these products is highly acidic. And that could contribute to diabetic ketoacidosis, a potentially life-threatening condition where the body burns fat instead of glucose for fuel, producing ketones, substances toxic to the liver and brain.

When my clients with diabetes are on a clear-liquid diet before a test, I recommend that they consume liquids with essential nutrients and a more balanced pH, such as apple juice, white grape juice and clear, fat-free broth (vegetable, chicken or beef). A typical "dinner" could include

---

Yogurt May Protect Against Diabetes

People who ate at least four-and-a-half servings of low-fat yogurt weekly—one serving equals 4.4 ounces—had 28% lower risk for diabetes than people who did not eat yogurt. The calcium, magnesium and vitamin D in fortified, fermented dairy products such as yogurt may have a protective effect.

Nita Forouhi, PhD, group leader, nutritional epidemiology program, University of Cambridge, UK, and leader of a study of 4,255 people, published in Diabetologia.

up to three-quarters cup of juice (to limit sugar) and any amount of broth. A bedtime "snack" could include one-half cup of juice and any amount of broth. Plenty of good pure water between "meals" also is important to stay well-hydrated.

CHECK BLOOD SUGAR OFTEN

Many people with diabetes check their blood sugar a few times a day—typically right before a meal and again one to two hours afterward. But if you're on a clear-liquid diet or fasting before a medical test, you should check your glucose level every two to three hours. If it's too low, correct it with a fast-acting carbohydrate, such as four ounces of 100% fruit juice or a glucose gel (a squeezable, over-the-counter product).

Important: Take fruit juice or a glucose gel with you to the test—if the test is delayed for any reason, you can ingest the carb and keep your blood sugar on track.

STOP TAKING METFORMIN

Your doctor likely will recommend that you stop taking the diabetes medication *metformin* 24 hours before the test. Metformin (Glucophage) also can contribute to acidosis and typically is stopped 24 hours before and up to 72 hours after any test that requires a contrast agent (an injected dye often used in an X-ray, CT scan or MRI that helps create the image). Talk to your doctor about when to stop taking your medication and when to resume or about the possible need for an alternative diabetes drug during this period.

An unexpected threat: Metformin is a component of many multi-ingredient diabetes drugs—so you may not realize you're taking it and therefore may need to discontinue it. Drugs that include metformin are Actoplus Met and Actoplus Met XR…Avandamet…Glucovance…Janumet and Janumet XR…Jentadueto…Kazano…Kombiglyze XR…Metaglip…and PrandiMet. New drugs are being developed constantly, so check with your pharmacist to see if yours contains metformin.

Also important: Many X-rays, CT scans and MRIs utilize an injected dye or a contrast agent that can damage the kidneys in people with diabetes (contrast-induced nephropathy). Before restarting metformin, have a kidney function test (such as BUN, which requires a blood sample, and creati-

nine clearance, which requires a urine sample and a blood sample) that confirms that your kidneys are working normally. These tests are recommended 24 to 48 hours after your procedure is completed and usually are covered by insurance.

DECREASE INSULIN

Insulin is the hormone used by the body to regulate blood sugar—and many people with advanced diabetes give themselves shots of short- and/or long-acting insulin to keep glucose levels steady. But if you're consuming only clear liquids or fasting before a medical test, you likely will need to take less insulin.

Excellent guidelines for insulin use before a medical procedure have been created by the University of Michigan Comprehensive Diabetes Center. *In general, it recommends…*

•**Take one-half of your usual dose of long-acting insulin the evening before the procedure.**

•**Take one-half of your usual dose of long-acting insulin the morning of the test and no short-acting insulin the morning of the test.**

You can find the complete guidelines in downloadable PDF form at *Med.UMich.edu/1libr/MEND/Diabetes-OutpatientProcedure.pdf.* Print them out, and discuss them with your doctor.

REDUCE ANXIETY

Anxiety triggers the release of the stress hormone cortisol, which in turn sparks the production of glucose. *To keep blood sugar balanced before a test, use these two methods to keep anxiety in check…*

•**Get all your questions answered.** Fear of the unknown is the greatest stress. Before your procedure, create a list of questions to ask your doctor or nurse practitioner.

Examples: What is going to happen during the procedure? What is it going to feel like? What are the potential side effects from the test, and how can I best avoid them? When will I be informed of the test results? How will the test results affect future decision-making about my health?

•**Breathe deeply.** Deep breathing is the easiest and simplest way to reduce anxiety. My recommendation, based on the approach of Andrew Weil, MD…

Repeat this breathing exercise three times, and do it three times a day every day: Inhale for a count of four…hold for a count of seven…exhale for a count of eight. (Don't worry if you can't do the entire count—shorter counts also work.) Do this exercise when you get up in the morning, at midday and at bedtime. You can do it more often, but most people find three times simple and easy to integrate into their routines.

Also, you can use this breathing technique in any situation that you find anxiety-producing, such as before and during the test itself. Breathe deeply three times every 10 or 15 minutes, and be sure to keep the 4:7:8 ratio—inhale for four, hold for seven, exhale for eight.

Diabetes Drug Affects Thyroid

Laurent Azoulay, PhD, assistant professor of cancer epidemiology, McGill University, Montreal, Quebec, Canada.

Diabetes drug may affect thyroid levels, we hear from Laurent Azoulay, PhD.

Recent large study: People taking *metformin* for type 2 diabetes while being treated for hypothyroidism (underactive thyroid) were 55% more likely to have low thyroid-stimulating hormone (TSH) levels than those taking sulfonylurea diabetes drugs. Low TSH is associated with hyperthyroidism (overactive thyroid).

Implication: Hypothyroidism patients on metformin may need to have their TSH levels monitored and thyroid medication adapted.

Ease Diabetic Nerve Pain

Anne Bunner, PhD, associate director of clinical research, Physicians Committee for Responsible Medicine, Washington, DC.

A plant-based diet eases diabetic nerve pain. In a 20-week study of people with diabetic neuropathy (which often leads to pain and numbness in the legs and feet), half ate a low-fat vegan diet and took a vitamin B-12 supplement (diabetes patients are often deficient in B-12), and the other half took only the supplement.

Result: The group eating the plant-based diet had significantly greater pain relief and lost more weight than the other group.

How to Beat the 3 Big Mistakes That Worsen Diabetes

Osama Hamdy, MD, PhD, medical director of the Joslin Diabetes Center's Obesity Clinical Program and an assistant professor of medicine at Harvard Medical School, both in Boston. He also is coauthor of *The Diabetes Breakthrough*.

Despite what you may have heard, type 2 diabetes doesn't have to be a lifelong condition. It can be controlled and even reversed in the early stages or stopped from progressing in the later stages—with none of the dire consequences of out-of-control blood sugar.

Sounds great, right? What person with diabetes wouldn't want to do everything possible to help prevent serious complications such as coronary heart disease, kidney disease, blindness or even amputation?

The problem is, even people who are following all the doctor's orders may still be sabotaging their efforts with seemingly minor missteps that can have big consequences. Among the most common mistakes that harm people with diabetes are oversights in the way they eat and exercise. *For example…*

MISTAKE #1: Skimping on protein. The majority of people with type 2 diabetes are overweight or obese. These individuals know that they need to lose weight but sometimes fail despite their best efforts.

Here's what often happens: We have had it drummed into our heads that the best way to lose weight is to go on a low-fat diet. However, these diets tend to be low in protein—and you need more protein, not less, if you have type 2 diabetes and are cutting calories to lose weight.

105

What's so special about protein? You need protein to maintain muscle mass. The average adult starts losing lean muscle mass every year after about age 40. If you have diabetes, you'll probably lose more muscle mass than someone without it. And the loss will be even greater if your diabetes is not well controlled.

Muscle is important because it burns more calories than other tissues in your body. Also, people with a higher and more active muscle mass find it easier to maintain healthy blood-glucose levels, since active muscle doesn't require insulin to clear high glucose from the blood.

My advice: Protein should provide 20% to 30% of total daily calories. If you're on an 1,800-calorie diet (a reasonable amount for an average man who wants to lose weight), that's about 90 g to 135 g of protein a day. If you're on a 1,200- to 1,500-calorie diet (a sensible amount for an average woman who is dieting), that's about 60 g to 113 g of protein a day.

Examples: Good protein sources include fish, skinless poultry, nonfat or low-fat dairy, legumes and nuts and seeds. A three-ounce chicken breast has about 30 g of protein...a three-ounce piece of haddock, 17 g...one-half cup of low-fat cottage cheese, 14 g...and one-quarter cup of whole almonds, 7 g of protein.

Note: If you have kidney problems, you may need to limit your protein intake. Check with your doctor.

MISTAKE #2: Not doing resistance training. It's widely known that aerobic exercise is good for weight loss and blood sugar control. What usually gets short shrift is resistance training, such as lifting weights and using stretch bands.

When you build muscle, you use more glucose, which helps reduce glucose levels in the blood. If you take insulin for your diabetes, toned muscles will also make your body more sensitive to it.

An added benefit: People who do resistance training can often reduce their doses of insulin or other medications within a few months.

My advice: Do a combination of resistance, aerobic and flexibility exercises. Start with 20 minutes total, four days a week—splitting the time equally among the three types of exercise. Try to work up to 60 minutes total, six days

a week. An exercise physiologist or personal trainer certified in resistance training can help choose the best workout for you.

MISTAKE #3: Ignoring hunger cues. Many individuals are so conditioned to eat at certain times that they virtually ignore their body's hunger signals. Learning how to read these cues can be one of the best ways to achieve (and maintain) a healthy body weight.

The key is to recognize that there are different levels of hunger. It's easy to overeat when you do not acknowledge the difference between feeling satisfied and stuffing yourself.

My advice: Imagine a five-point hunger scale—1 means you're feeling starved...2 is hungry...3 is comfortable...4 is full...and 5 is stuffed. Before you start eating, rate your hunger between 1 and 5. Halfway through the meal, rate it again.

Here's the secret: Stop eating when you rate your hunger somewhere between "comfortable" and "full." If you give your hunger a ranking of 4 and you still want to eat, get away from the table and do something else!

Note: It can take up to 20 minutes for the "satiety signal" to kick in, so eat slowly. If you eat too quickly, you may miss the signal and overeat.

After just a few weeks of eating this way, it usually becomes second nature.

Statins Help with Diabetes

According to recent research, in addition to lowering risk for heart attack and stroke, statins lowered risk for diabetes complications. People with diabetes taking statins were 34% less likely to be diagnosed with diabetes-related nerve damage (neuropathy)...40% less likely to develop diabetes-related damage to the retina...and 12% less likely to develop gangrene than diabetics not taking statins.

Børge G. Nordestgaard, MD, DMSc, is chief physician at Copenhagen University Hospital, Herlev, Denmark, and leader of a study of 60,000 people, published in *The Lancet Diabetes Endocrinology*.

IF YOU TAKE DIABETES MEDS

Sometimes, diet and exercise aren't enough to tame out-of-control blood sugar. *Traps to avoid...*

•**Drug-induced weight gain.** Ironically, the drugs that are used to treat diabetes also can cause weight gain as a side effect. If you start taking insulin, you can expect to gain about 10 pounds within six months—with oral drugs, such as *glipizide* (Glucotrol), you'll probably gain from four to seven pounds.

My advice: Ask your doctor if you can switch to one of the newer, "weight-friendly" medications.

Examples: A form of insulin called Levemir causes less weight gain than Lantus, Humulin N or Novolin N. Newer oral drugs called DPP-4 inhibitors, such as Januvia, Onglyza and Nesina, don't have weight gain as a side effect.

Important: The newer drugs are more expensive and may not be covered by insurance. But if they don't cause you to gain weight, you might get by with a lower dose—and reduced cost.

•**Erratic testing.** You should test your blood sugar levels at least four to six times a day, particularly when you're making lifestyle changes that could affect the frequency and doses of medication. Your doctor has probably advised you to test before and after exercise—and before meals.

My advice: Be sure to also test after meals. This will help determine the effects of different types and amounts of foods.

Better Glucose Meter Accuracy

Katherine O'Neal, PharmD, assistant professor, The University of Oklahoma College of Pharmacy, Tulsa.

Glucose meters that check blood sugar should be tested for accuracy every time users open a new pack of test strips, get a new meter or suspect a malfunction. A recent survey found that only 23% of patients with diabetes who use glucose meters said they followed these manufacturer recommendations.

Here's how to test a glucose meter: Use one drop of the control-solution liquid on the test strip (just like you would check your own blood sugar) to test the accuracy of both the meter and packages of test strips.

Insulin Not Always the Answer

Sandeep Vijan, MD, professor of internal medicine, University of Michigan Medical School, Ann Arbor.

Some diabetics may be better off not starting insulin. For adults over age 50 who have type 2 diabetes but a low risk for complications because their glucose levels are under control (A1C level of 8% to 8.5%), the side effects of taking a daily insulin shot or other diabetes medications may do more harm than good, a recent study reports. Common side effects such as low blood sugar may be worse than the small benefit of the medication. Diet and exercise may be better for these patients.

Caution: Do not stop taking insulin or other diabetes drugs without first consulting your doctor.

Diabetes Overtreatment Scandal

Kasia Joanna Lipska, MD, MHS, assistant professor of medicine (endocrinology), department of internal medicine, Yale School of Medicine, New Haven, Connecticut. Her study was published in *JAMA Internal Medicine*.

Bringing blood sugar down with diabetes drugs might be too simple an approach and, worse, ineffective and even harmful for some of us, especially those of us who are 65 or older. What's more, the reason why so many Americans have diabetes might not be because their blood sugar levels are dangerously high but because the system that defines what constitutes diabetes is rigged. And even doctors might not realize it!

Here's how to really protect your health and protect yourself from overtreatment when a doctor tells you that your blood sugar is high…

FOLLOW THE MONEY

Diabetes management has become big business, amassing billions of dollars in annual sales. In 2014, sales of diabetes drugs alone reached $23 billion. For this we can thank, in part, the changing definition of what exactly diabetes is. Since 1997, the American Diabetes Association and other professional endocrinology groups have twice lowered blood sugar thresholds for type 2 diabetes and prediabetes. Each time they did this, millions more Americans were suddenly considered, by definition, diabetic or prediabetic.

But the doctors making these blood sugar threshold changes have strong incentives to do so that have nothing to do with your well-being, according to a recent exposé published by the medical news outlet MedPage Today and the *Milwaukee Journal Sentinel*. Many of these doctors receive speaking and consulting fees from diabetes-drug manufacturers. In one analysis, the authors of the exposé found that 13 of 19 members of a committee responsible for diabetes guidelines accumulated a combined sum of more than $2 million in speaking and consulting fees from companies that make diabetes drugs. Whether doctors responsible for diabetes guidelines are intentionally and systematically basing their decisions on their bank account balances isn't known, but the findings do reveal an obvious and material conflict of interest.

EFFECTIVENESS OF THERAPIES QUESTIONED

The authors of the exposé also pointed out that although they reduce blood sugar, none of the 30 diabetes drugs approved since 2004 has been definitively proven to reduce the risk of heart attack and stroke, blindness or any other diabetes-related complication. "In order to approve a new diabetes drug, the FDA requires evidence that the drug effectively reduces hemoglobin A1C levels—a measure of blood glucose—and that it doesn't result in an unacceptable increase in heart disease risk. The evidence that the drug reduces the risk of complications of diabetes,

such as heart attacks and stroke, is not required," explained endocrinologist Kasia Lipska, MD, assistant professor of medicine at Yale School of Medicine. She is the leader of a recent, related study that showed that mature adults are being treated too aggressively for diabetes, sometimes with dangerous consequences. The study population of nearly 1,300 adults, selected from the National Health and Nutrition Examination Survey database, represents a cross section of senior Americans with diabetes.

Similar to a recent study showing that tight blood pressure control may not be beneficial in older adults, prior studies suggest that tight blood sugar control in people 65 and older who have serious health problems actually may do more harm than good. Tight blood sugar control is defined by the American Diabetes Association as a hemoglobin A1C level of less than 7%.

DANGEROUS SIDE EFFECTS

Insulin and sulfonylurea drugs such as *glipizide* (Glucotrol), *glyburide* (Micronase) and *glimepiride* (Amaryl) have been associated with dangerously low blood sugar (hypoglycemia), and other drugs, such as *pioglitazone* (Actos), with risk of fluid retention and fractures. Some drugs, such as *saxagliptin* (Onglyza), may be associated with heart failure, while, for very new drugs, such as *canagliflozin* (Invokana), the risks are not yet known.

Although the American Diabetes Association and other professional groups have been lowering the threshold for what constitutes "diabetes"

Drug for Diabetes and Kidney Disease

For diabetes patients with kidney disease, the benefits of *metformin* may outweigh the risks. The drug metformin is very effective for type 2 diabetes, but an FDA label dating to 1994 restricts its use in patients with kidney problems. Evidence now shows that metformin is safe for patients with mild-to-moderate kidney disease.

James H. Flory, MD, MSCE, a fellow in endocrinology at Weill Cornell Medical College, New York City.

(and, thereby, driving the market for diabetes drugs, at least according to the Medpage exposé), the American Diabetes Association and the American Geriatrics Society discourage tight blood sugar control in older adults. They acknowledge that older adults whose blood sugar is too aggressively controlled are more vulnerable to the dangerous side effects mentioned above. One treatment standard does not fit all in older adults, because their health and treatment preferences vary greatly. Tight control may be safe and appropriate for one person and not another.

AVOID OVERTREATMENT

To avoid overtreatment for diabetes, you should make the necessary lifestyle changes and work together with doctors and other healthcare providers on a personalized approach to your specific health needs and safety. You need to be engaged and part of the plan. The plan should involve much more than simply prescribing a diabetes drug if your blood sugar is above the recommended threshold.

Injectable Diabetes Drug Available

Ralph A. DeFronzo, MD, deputy director, Texas Diabetes Institute, San Antonio.

A new weekly diabetes drug is available. Recently approved by the FDA, *dulaglutide* (Trulicity) is a once-a-week injectable, single-dose pen that has been shown to safely improve blood sugar levels in six separate trials of more than 3,300 people with type 2 diabetes. The medication, which requires no mixing (as do competing drugs), can be used alone or in combination with other diabetes medication, including *metformin* and mealtime insulin. Potential side effects include nausea, diarrhea and abdominal pain. People at risk for thyroid or endocrine gland tumors should not take dulaglutide.

New Eye Implant

Joel Zonszein, MD, professor of clinical medicine at Albert Einstein College of Medicine and director of the Clinical Diabetes Center at Montefiore Medical Center, the Bronx, New York.

A nyone with type 1 or type 2 diabetes is at risk for vision loss caused by diabetic macular edema (DME), which affects up to 28% of diabetics. Once the Iluvien implant is in place, it slowly delivers a submicrogram dose of the corticosteroid *fluocinolone acetonide* for 36 months—which helps to control inflammation in the eye. Possible side effects include cataracts and increased intraocular pressure.

Diabetes-Related Foot Condition Often Missed

American College of Foot and Ankle Surgeons, news release

A debilitating condition called Charcot foot is often missed among the nearly 30 million Americans with diabetes, doctors say.

The condition is highly treatable, but if left alone it can lead to permanent deformity, disability, surgery and even amputation, according to the American College of Foot and Ankle Surgeons (ACFAS).

Charcot foot can occur in the one-third of diabetes patients who lose feeling in their feet and other lower extremities, a condition called peripheral neuropathy.

In the early stages of Charcot foot, bones in the foot may weaken and break. Casts can help the bones heal and special orthopedic footwear can protect the feet once the bones have healed, doctors say.

But if the condition isn't diagnosed early, the foot continues to be damaged and can become abnormal in shape. Many patients don't know they have Charcot foot until it's in this late stage.

"People think they don't have a problem because they feel no pain, but that isn't the case,"

Valerie Schade, MD, a foot and ankle surgeon in Tacoma, Washington, said in an ACFAS news release.

"Anyone at risk for neuropathy, including diabetics, alcoholics and some chemotherapy patients, should see a foot and ankle surgeon early and at least once every year, even if they are considered low-risk," she added.

Monitoring for changes in the feet is the single most important way to prevent Charcot foot.

"Anyone who notices a difference—discomfort, unexplained swelling or redness, or changes to the shape of the foot—should seek care right away," Dr. Schade said.

info The U.S. National Institute of Diabetes and Digestive and Kidney Diseases has more about diabetes and the feet at *http://diab etes.niddk.nih.gov/*.

A Great "Whey" to Control Blood Sugar

Study titled "Incretin, insulinotropic and glucose-lowering effects of whey protein pre-load in type 2 diabetics: a randomized clinical trial," published in *Diabetologia*.

For people with type 2 diabetes, eating isn't the problem…it's what happens after eating that can be dangerous. Glucose accumulates in the bloodstream, where levels go way up after a meal. This phenomenon, called "spiking," irritates blood vessels and throws your metabolism out of whack, increasing risk for cardiovascular disease, eye and kidney damage, and possibly Alzheimer's disease and cancer, too.

A short, brisk exercise session before meals helps prevent post-meal blood glucose spiking. Here's another, even easier (and surprising) trick for keeping your blood sugar where it should be—it involves using whey…

WHEY TO GO!

It turns out that whey protein—yes, that stuff you see sold in giant tubs in the bodybuilder and sports section of health-food stores—is a great pre-meal tonic for glucose control. Whey protein products are powdered, concentrated milk protein—made from the watery stuff that accumulates and rises to the surface of containers of cottage cheese and yogurt that you probably drain off. Studies have shown that beginning a meal with a whey protein drink helps get post-meal insulin secretion into action, which, in turn, helps reduce glucose spiking.

This effect was recently confirmed in a small international study that also pinpointed how whey protein does its magic. The study took 15 people with type 2 diabetes, divided them into two groups, and fed them a sugary breakfast—with the difference being, one group drank 50 grams (about three-and-a-half tablespoons) of whey protein dissolved in water before eating breakfast…and the other group drank just plain water. Each group took a turn at drinking the whey protein on different days so that the effect could be gauged on every participant.

Results: When participants drank whey protein before breakfast, they accumulated an average 28% less blood glucose after the meal. And the whey had a strong and protective impact—insulin levels nearly doubled in whey drinkers within the first half-hour after eating and remained high. This happened because, in the whey drinkers, an insulin-stimulating hormone, called *glucagon-like peptide-1* (GLP-1), didn't degrade as quickly as it normally would. The presence of additional GLP-1 gave insulin a better chance of doing its job.

Here's the kicker: The researchers pointed out that the effect of whey on glucose control and insulin secretion was better than what would be expected from using diabetes drugs such as *glipizide* (Glucotrol), *glyburide* (Glynase) and *nateglinide* (Starlix).

Whereas the side effects of diabetes drugs can include headaches, joint aches, nasal congestion, back pain and flu-like symptoms, whey protein is well-tolerated in doses of up to 50 grams per day.

WHEY FOR YOU

Although 50 grams per day taken before breakfast was looked at in the research study, how much daily whey protein do you need in an ordinary life setting to control blood sugar spiking? *Daily Health News* medical advisor Andrew L. Rubman, ND, founder and director of the Southbury Clinic for Traditional Medicines in Southbury, Connecticut, recommends using up to 800 milligrams per kilogram of body weight. That's a daily dosage of about 44 grams for a 120-pound person…54 grams for a 150-pound person…and 91 grams for a 250-pound person. These dosages refer to products that are whey isolate, not whey concentrate. Whey isolate provides more protein and significantly less lactose than whey concentrate, said Dr. Rubman.

The daily dosage should be adjusted so that you are taking the least amount you need to best control symptoms associated with blood sugar spiking—and this will differ from one person to another, said Dr. Rubman. People who have chronic kidney problems should seek medical supervision before supplementing their diets with any dose of whey protein.

Side effects of whey were not reported in the study, but high doses of more than 50 grams per day, particularly of whey concentrate, can cause digestive troubles such as increased bowel movements, nausea, thirst, bloating, cramps and lack of appetite, said Dr. Rubman. These effects are mostly caused by the lactose in whey products. Other possible side effects include tiredness and headache, low blood pressure and low blood sugar. So, everything in moderation if you decide to include a whey protein supplement in your diet.

Also, people with allergies to milk should avoid whey (it is milk protein, after all). It can also interfere with certain drugs, such as *levodopa* for Parkinson's disease, *alendronate* (Fosa-max) for osteoporosis, and quinolone antibiotics (such as Cipro) and tetracycline antibiotics such as *doxycycline*—so if you take any such drug, speak with your doctor or pharmacist for guidance on whether (and when) you can safely take whey protein and at what dosage.

A brand of whey isolate that Dr. Rubman recommends is NOW Foods Whey Protein Isolate.

Control Blood Sugar and Keep Fit with Prebiotic Sunchokes

Tamara Duker Freuman, RD, CDN, registered dietitian in private practice and a clinical preceptor for the Dietetic Internship Program at Columbia University's Teacher's College, both in New York City. *TamaraDuker.com*

Although nutritionists know that the sunchoke—a root vegetable that looks like a cross between a knob of ginger and a potato, also known as the Jerusalem artichoke—is great for glucose control, scientific studies to back up this idea have been few and far between. Now, a team of researchers from Japan has demonstrated that sunchokes may help prevent type 2 diabetes and fatty liver disease (a condition that often goes with diabetes and that can lead to life-threatening liver cirrhosis and hepatitis). But even if the researchers' claim is too ambitious, there are plenty of reasons to get familiar with sunchokes, their many health benefits and delicious recipes.

LESSONS FROM FAT RATS

The Japanese researchers fed rats a diet that was either 60% fructose (fruit sugar) or 60% fructose and 10% sunchoke powder to see whether sunchokes could prevent diabetes in the rodents. That is, they regularly fed the rats lots of sugar to get their blood sugar levels to spike (hyperglycemia) and their innate blood sugar controller—their insulin-producing pancreas—to malfunction. After four weeks of these diets, the blood and livers of the rats showed that, although signs of diabetes and fatty livers developed in all of them from all that fructose, the effects were milder in the rats that were

Diabetes and Heart Attack Risk

Low blood sugar levels overnight may trigger prolonged slow heart rates during sleep in people with diabetes. This could lead to abnormal heart rhythms, which increase risk for heart attack.

If you have diabetes (especially if you also have cardiovascular disease): Talk to your doctor about ways to stabilize your blood sugar overnight, such as adjusting the timing, dose and/or type of medication you take.

Simon Heller, MD, professor of clinical diabetes, The University of Sheffield, UK.

This Nut Helps Diabetes

Walnuts seem to dramatically cut risk for diabetes.

Recent finding: Women who eat at least eight ounces of walnuts a month are 24% less likely to develop type 2 diabetes than women who eat none.

Possible reason: Walnuts are especially rich in polyunsaturated fats, which may help prevent diabetes. They also have high amounts of dietary fiber, antioxidants and other beneficial substances.

The results most likely apply to men, too.

Frank Hu, MD, PhD, professor of nutrition and epidemiology, Harvard School of Public Health, Boston, and senior author of a study published in *Journal of Nutrition*.

---

also eating sunchokes. The sunchoke eaters did so much better, in fact, that the researchers suggested that at least 10% of the daily diet of people at risk for diabetes and fatty liver disease should consist of sunchokes.

Similar tests would need to be performed in humans to really know whether eating sunchokes could similarly lessen risk of diabetes in people, and if so, how much would be needed to cut diabetes off at the pass. Besides, rather than overloading your diet with sunchokes in quest of glucose control, it would be more reasonable to simply add them, in moderation, to the list of healthful nondrug food and remedies that you already know help prevent diabetes.

Until human studies can confirm the findings of these Japanese researchers, here are more health-boosting reasons to enjoy the little tubers.

A PREBIOTIC POWER FOOD

Sunchokes are the tuberous root of a type of sunflower that's native to North America. They provide generous amounts of iron and potassium and help the body absorb certain minerals, such as calcium…and they are rich in fiber, which helps prevent certain types of cancer, such as colon cancer.

In fact, sunchokes are packed with an important type of fiber called inulin, which is a prebiotic. Inulin is a carbohydrate, but because your body can't digest it, it doesn't affect your blood sugar. This characteristic gives the sunchoke its low glycemic effect. But even though you can't digest inulin, the healthful probiotic bacteria in your gut feast on it and, in fact, need it to provide their health benefits to you, explained Tamara Duker Freuman, RD, CDN.

But inulin does have one unfortunate downside—which also puts a crimp in the advice of the Japanese researchers to load your daily diet with sunchokes. Eating too much inulin—more than 10 grams a day—can make you gassy. Since one-half cup of sunchokes has 18 grams of inulin in it, Freuman suggests eating no more than one-quarter cup at a time if you are new to this root vegetable but want to add it to your diet. Within six to eight hours—the amount of time it takes for the sunchokes to travel from your mouth to your colon—you'll know whether your body tolerates the inulin well or not. As your body gets used to this new food, you may be able to increase how much you eat without the gassy side effect.

DELICIOUS WAYS TO EAT SUNCHOKES

Cooking sunchokes, rather than eating them raw, lessens the inulin's gassy effect. So instead of chomping on your first chokes raw, try some of these ways to prepare them (no need to peel the sunchokes—just scrub them well)…

• **Roasted sunchokes.** Roughly cut sunchokes into one-inch chunks, and toss them in olive oil and salt. Roast at 400°F for about 40 minutes until they are tender and golden brown.

• **Sunchoke chips.** Slice the chokes thinly using a mandoline or sharp knife. Toss the slices in oil, salt, pepper and any of your favorite spices (such as garlic powder or thyme) and spread them in a single layer on a baking sheet. Bake at 400°F for 15 minutes, flip them over and bake for another 10 to 15 minutes or until crisp. Freuman warns that these chips are addictive, so don't dive into a giant batch until you've made friends with inulin!

• **Sunchoke mash.** Steam or boil sunchokes as you would potatoes, and season them with butter, salt and pepper. Or boil and mash them with potatoes to add a new taste sensation to an old standard.

• **Sunchoke soup.** After roasting sunchokes, simmer them in a saucepan with onions and garlic sautéed in olive oil along with broth or water.

Season with thyme or rosemary. Stir in one-quarter cup of milk, cream or yogurt. Then purée.

•**Sunchoke salads and snacks.** Slice or shave raw sunchokes, and add to salads (toss them in lemon juice or vinegar first, since the cut sides will discolor) or just eat out of hand.

So, certainly, if you are looking for new healthy foods to keep your blood sugar on an even keel as well as optimize the health of your friendly gut bacteria, look for sunchokes at farmers' markets and your grocery (they are in season from late fall to early spring).

Diabetic? Stop Blood Sugar from Spiking with Red Ginseng

Andrew L. Rubman, ND, founder and medical director, Southbury Clinic for Traditional Medicines, Southbury, Connecticut. *SouthburyClinic.com*

Adult-onset (type 2) diabetes is so common that it ultimately impacts a whopping one in four people age 65 and older. In this type of diabetes, blood sugar can go way up—or "spike"—after a meal. You'll know your blood sugar is spiking because instead of feeling energized and fit after nourishing yourself, you'll just crash. More than just wanting to take a nap—you won't be able to do anything but. That's right. You'll have to take a rest after eating a meal because you will feel sleepy…exhausted. Your eyes may even blur. If this happens often enough, hardening of the arteries can occur, which, as you know, can lead to a heart attack. But you can prevent this from happening naturally. Red ginseng extract may be just the thing to keep blood sugar on an even keel.

Why is it called "red" ginseng? Tonics, extracts and teas of Asian white ginseng (also called Chinese or Korean white panax ginseng) are natural powerhouses of health and vitality made from the raw dried root of the plant. They increase energy and stamina, reduce cholesterol and blood pressure and fight cancer and aging. But steaming the root before drying it starts a fermentation process that supports well-

ness even more. Once fermented, the ginseng is called red ginseng, and this is the kind that is especially good for people with diabetes and others who have problems with glucose control. Korean researchers have recently confirmed that red ginseng significantly reduces blood glucose levels and increases insulin levels after meals. That makes it especially helpful in preventing dangerous spikes in blood sugar that can happen after diabetics or borderline diabetics have a meal.

The researchers recruited 42 healthy men and women between the ages of 20 and 75 for their study. Nineteen of these participants had type 2 diabetes and the remaining 23 had prediabetes. Half of the group received capsules of fermented red ginseng extract, and half received capsules of a placebo. They were instructed to take one capsule three times a day for four weeks. The total daily dose of red ginseng for the treatment group was 2.7 grams (0.1 ounces).

The researchers found that red ginseng was able to regulate glucose and insulin after meals, thus preventing blood sugar spikes. Compared with the placebo group, insulin increased and glucose decreased after meals. And no serious side effects were reported in the Korean study, although one person in the treatment group had to drop out because hypoglycemia (low blood sugar) developed.

This Spice Stops Diabetes

There is a common spice that can stop diabetes from developing.

A study showed that when given a curcumin extract (1.5 grams daily) for nine months, participants at risk for diabetes did not develop the disease. Among a similar group given a placebo, 16.4% developed the disease.

Curcumin is the main compound in turmeric, a spice used in curry powders and mustards.

Study by researchers at Srinakharinwirot University, Bangkok, Thailand, published in *Tufts University Health & Nutrition Letter*.

NATURAL BUT POTENT DIABETES CARE

"Red ginseng extract may be a good addition to a natural, broader approach to controlling, limiting or getting rid of type 2 diabetes," said Andrew Rubman, ND, a naturopathic physician and founder of the Southbury Clinic for Traditional Medicine in Southbury, Connecticut. In his opinion, however, alpha-lipoic acid, a powerful antioxidant that helps the body use glucose more efficiently, may be a better choice. Plus, it relieves pain, inflammation, burning, tingling and numbness in people who have peripheral neuropathy (nerve damage) caused by diabetes. But because it can reduce blood glucose levels (leading to hypoglycemia), it should not be used without the supervision of a health-care professional who can monitor your blood sugar levels.

Another readily available herbal supplement recommended by Dr. Rubman for type 2 diabetes is Gymnema extract, used in Ayurvedic medicine for centuries.

As for red ginseng, most people can use it daily with no side effects, according to Dr. Rubman. He cautioned that people who are taking several medications, especially antacids or statins, or who have liver or gastrointestinal diseases should hold off on taking ginseng extracts, since they can put an added burden on the liver. He also said that anyone who wants to try red ginseng for diabetes should do so under the supervision of a naturopathic doctor or clinically trained nutritionist—or at least let your doctor know that you are taking the extract so that he or she can monitor and interpret your physical exams and blood tests. Minor side effects include decreased energy, irregularity and/or intestinal gas.

Red ginseng is widely available online, in Asian-food stores and at large health-food and nutrition shops.

Diet, Nutrition and Fitness

The Eat-What-You-Want Diet

S ome people fast to "rest" the digestive tract, while others do so as part of religious tradition. The last time you fasted may have been before a medical test, such as a colonoscopy.

But as a weight-loss technique, fasting has always been controversial. Its detractors claim that it shifts the body into a starvation mode that makes unwanted pounds even harder to drop.

What's gaining favor: More and more scientists are now studying fasting as a method for losing extra pounds and fighting disease. But does it work?

As one of the few scientists worldwide who has studied fasting in humans, I consider it to be the most effective—and healthful—method for most people to lose weight.* *How it works...*

*Check with your doctor before trying this diet—especially if you have diabetes. Fasting is not recommended for pregnant women.

THE SIMPLE FORMULA

With intermittent fasting, you eat a reduced number of calories every other day. Scientifically, this is called alternate-day modified fasting.

The principle is simple: Most people find it easier to stay on a diet in which they can eat whatever they want half of the time. In the eight clinical studies I have conducted involving about 600 people (including an ongoing three-year study funded by the National Institutes of Health), intermittent fasters typically have lost 1.5 to 3 pounds per week, depending on how much weight they had to lose.

People lose weight by eating just 500 calories one day ("fast day") and all they want and anything they want the next day ("feast day")—alternating fast days with feast days until their weight-loss goal is reached. Goal weight is maintained by increasing calories on fast days to 1,000 three days a week and enjoying feast days the rest of the time.

Krista Varady, PhD, associate professor of kinesiology and nutrition at the University of Illinois at Chicago. She is also coauthor of *The Every-Other-Day Diet.*

WHY IT WORKS

Key points about using this method to lose weight...

•**Why 500 calories?** Animal studies showed that consuming 25% of the normal calorie intake on fast days produced the best results in preventing and reversing disease.

Translating this finding to people, I calculated 25% of daily recommended calories, which resulted in a general recommendation of 500 calories on fast day using foods with optimal nutrients.

Those 500 calories are consumed with one 400-calorie meal and a 100-calorie snack, since people tend to overeat if calories are broken up throughout the day. Lunch or dinner works best for the meal—if you eat your 400-calorie meal for breakfast, you'll be too hungry later in the day.

Example of a lunchtime meal: A turkey and avocado sandwich (two slices of turkey, one slice of Swiss cheese and one-quarter of an avocado on one slice of multigrain bread) and fruit (such as one-half cup of strawberries) for dessert.

Before or after your meal, you can have a snack such as a smoothie.

Tasty option: In a blender, mix one cup of unsweetened chocolate almond milk with one-half cup of unsweetened frozen cherries and one cup of ice.

•**Hunger disappears.** After two weeks of alternate-day modified fasting, hunger on fast day disappears for most people. During those

As a Disease-Fighter

People who have followed alternate-day modified fasting not only lose weight but also improve their overall health. In weight-loss studies of 600 people that lasted up to one year, average reductions in risk occurred for...

•**Heart disease.** Total cholesterol dropped 21%...and LDL "bad" cholesterol dropped 20 points. Triglycerides fell from 125 mg/dL (considered "normal") to 88 mg/dL (defined as "optimal").

•**Type 2 diabetes.** Glucose (blood sugar) levels dropped by up to 10% after eight weeks on the diet.

Animal studies have shown that intermittent fasting may help prevent...

•**Cancer.** The diet may also slow the growth of existing malignancies.

•**Cognitive decline.** Intermittent fasting helped protect the brains of mice genetically programmed to develop Alzheimer's... stopped the early development of nervous system problems in mice programmed to develop Parkinson's...and helped animals recover from stroke.

two weeks, ease your fast-day hunger by drinking eight to 10 eight-ounce glasses of water and other no-cal beverages such as coffee and tea and chewing sugar-free gum. Some people reported mild constipation, weakness and irritability, which subsided after two weeks.

•**You won't overeat on feast day.** My studies show that people almost never overeat on feast day—on average, they consume 110% of their normal caloric intake. Over the two-day fast/feast cycle, that's an average of 67.5% of normal caloric intake—a perfect formula for safe, steady weight loss but without the nonstop deprivation of everyday dieting.

•**Add exercise—and lose twice as much weight.** Every-other-day fasters can exercise on fast day without feeling weak or light-headed. Exercising before the fast-day meal is best because you'll feel hungry afterward—and can eat.

Good news: People who go on an intermittent fast and exercise (45 minutes of brisk aerobic exercise, three times a week) lose twice as much weight, on average, as people who only fast. You can exercise on both fast and feast days.

•**You won't lose muscle.** Five out of six conventional dieters who lose weight gain it all back. That's probably because the typical dieter loses 75% fat and 25% muscle—and never regains that calorie-burning muscle mass after the diet is over.

But people who lose weight using alternate-day modified fasting lose only about 1% muscle—a unique and remarkable result. And my one-year maintenance studies show that these alternate-day fasters maintain their weight. Longer-term studies are also needed.

Why You Need the Type of Fat That Babies Have

George King, MD, professor of medicine at Harvard Medical School, Boston, where he heads the Vascular Cell Biology research section. He also is research director and chief scientific officer of Harvard's Joslin Diabetes Center, Boston, and author of *The Diabetes Reset: The Revolutionary Plan to Reverse, Control, and Avoid Type 2 Diabetes.*

Fight fat at all costs! For decades, this has been the prevailing message from medical experts. But cutting-edge research suggests that you actually can benefit from having more fat—as long as it's the right kind of fat.

What's new: Scientists have discovered that many adults have small amounts of brown fat. Brown fat is more active than any other tissue in the body. In fact, when fully activated, brown fat generates 300 times more heat than any other tissue in the body.

A few ounces of this high-octane fat can burn as much as 200 to 300 calories a day, the equivalent of 30 minutes of brisk walking.

PURE ENERGY

Most of us think of "fat" as the white stuff that stores calories and tends to accumulate, pound after unwelcome pound, on the belly, thighs and hips. White fat has caused the nation's obesity epidemic along with the attendant risks, including higher rates of medical problems such as heart disease, diabetes and cancer.

Brown fat does the opposite. It doesn't store calories—it burns them at a very rapid rate, thus boosting weight loss. It also improves insulin sensitivity and prevents excess glucose (blood sugar) accumulation in the blood.

A NEW DISCOVERY

Until recently, brown fat was thought to exist only in newborns and babies. They have small amounts of brown fat between their shoulder blades—this fat generates heat and protects them from cold.

MRIs and other imaging tests now have revealed that some people retain brown fat—along with an "intermediary" form known as beige fat—throughout their lives. In adults, it's located around the neck, in between the collarbone and shoulder, and in parts of the spine.

People with generous amounts of brown fat tend to be leaner than those without it.

It's clear that brown fat is beneficial. The million-dollar question is whether it can be manipulated—either by increasing the amount in one's body or making it more metabolically active—to prevent diabetes, improve glucose control and help with weight loss.

The preliminary answer seems to be yes. Research has shown that it may be possible to transform white fat into the beneficial brown and beige forms and to make them burn even more calories and regulate blood sugar more efficiently.

COLD IS THE KEY

Since brown fat is meant to keep infants warm, it makes sense that it would be more active at cold temperatures.

Recent study: For four months, researchers exposed men to different temperatures—one temperature for an entire month. Participants went about their normal lives during the day but slept in temperature-controlled rooms at night. After one month of sleeping in 66°F temperatures, the men's stores of brown fat almost doubled. They burned more calories and had improvements in insulin sensitivity. When the heat was turned up (to 81°F), their brown fat diminished.

In another study, researchers found that sitting in a 59°F room for two hours wearing summer clothing stimulated brown fat to burn an extra 100 to 250 calories, depending on the individual.

LIGHT THE FIRE

Here's what you can do to increase and activate brown fat…

•**Keep it cold.** Lowering the thermostat of your home to the mid-60s or below may be enough to stimulate at least some brown-fat activity. That's chillier than the temperature at which most people keep their homes, but it's easy to get used to.

Bonus: Cool temperatures also may overcome the set-point phenomenon, the discouraging tendency of the body to slow down and burn fewer calories when you're dieting.

•**Dress lightly.** During the cold months, go outside a few times a day while wearing only the basics—a sweater, a light jacket or even just a T-shirt. Any exposure to cold will help you burn more calories. A study in northern Finland found that people who worked outdoors had more brown fat than those who worked inside.

Alternative: Cooling vests, which use cold water or refrigeration to lower body temperature, are available online. Exposing even small parts of the body to cold—with a cooling band wrapped around an arm or a leg, for example—activates brown fat.

•**Regular workouts.** In addition to the obvious benefits—better cardiovascular health, improved blood sugar, weight loss, etc.—exercise causes an increase in irisin, a hormone that appears to convert white fat into the beige form. Beige fat isn't quite as active as brown fat, but it still has a high metabolic rate.

I advise patients to get a mix of aerobic and strength-training workouts, preferably for 30 to 45 minutes, most days of the week.

•**Forget hot yoga.** It makes no sense to exercise in a hot room. People think that the extra perspiration is a sign of weight loss. It's not—and a hot environment inhibits brown-fat activity.

More helpful: Exercise in relatively cool temperatures—62°F to 64°F or lower. And exercise with your skin exposed by wearing a T-shirt and shorts, for example. The evaporation of sweat during workouts has a cooling effect.

•**Less fat, more carbohydrates.** Preliminary evidence suggests that people who cut back on dietary saturated fat and eat healthful carbohydrates, such as leafy greens, cruciferous vegetables and whole grains—not processed carbohydrates such as sugar and bread—may have an increase in brown-fat activity. I recommend a traditional Asian diet, which is about 15% fat and 65% to 70% healthful carbohydrates, with the rest from protein with an emphasis on nuts, seeds and soy.

Special Spinach Extract Puts an End to Mindless Eating

Study titled "Body weight loss, reduced urge for palatable food and increased release of GLP-1 through daily supplementation with green-plant membranes for three months in overweight women," published in *Appetite*.

Some people just can't stop eating and eating no matter what—and it's not because they're hungry. They simply like to eat. If you thought a visit to a psychiatrist or gastric-banding surgeon were the only ways to fix that, hold on. A dietary supplement made from a certain leafy green vegetable may be the answer to curing even the most voracious appetite naturally. But there's a catch. Not any old green-food supplement will do—and, beware, some green-food supplements are already riding on the coattails of the new product although they may not deliver the promised effect. Here's the information.

IT'S NOT EXACTLY THE LEAVES

Before we talk about the new diet supplement, it will help to think about what really makes people overweight. Portion control is often at the top of the list when we talk about weight management, and, sure, we also struggle with food cravings and ways to beat them. But the biggest problem when it comes to keeping a healthy weight is something called hedonic eating. That's not the same as actually craving a food. It's "mindless eating," and it's often done out of stress or boredom…tends to bring very little pleasure (especially in relation to the calories)…and becomes true gluttony when overdone.

It's appetite, not hunger.

It turns out that spinach and similar leafy green vegetables, such as kale and collards, can significantly control appetite and, specifically, keep you from reaching for the box of cookies, chips, chocolate covered pretzels or whatever your between-meal edible is. The magic ingredients in spinach and some other greens are thylakoids, which make up the plants' cell membranes. Rich in vitamins A, E and K and antioxidants, thylakoids include compounds that slow down the digestion of fat…and they impact hormones that affect how the pancreas and intestines trigger appetite, especially hormones that tickle our yens for sweet and fatty foods.

But you would have to eat a pound of spinach (and/or other greens) a day to get its appetite-suppressing effects. Commercially available spinach extracts, which generally are powdered concentrates of spinach leaves, do contain thylakoids and other nutrients, but the new formulation that's creating the Internet stir about spinach extracts is a powder specifically made from the cell membranes of baby spinach leaves—not the whole leaf…just the part that contains the thylakoids. Called Appethyl, it is standardized to contain specific proportions of the naturally occurring vitamins and other compounds in thylakoids that affect how the pancreas processes fat and affects appetite.

The most recent study included 38 volunteers—all overweight women between the ages of 40 and 65—who took part in a three-month experiment. Each volunteer was supplied with a small, two-ounce blueberry smoothie to drink every morning before breakfast. For half of the women, chosen randomly, the smoothies included a teaspoon of the thylakoid extract.

The results: Cravings, particularly for sweets, were significantly reduced among those who got the extract. Also, weight loss was 43% greater in the women receiving the thylakoid extract than in women whose smoothies did not contain the extract (the placebo group). Also, the body's hormone that suppresses appetite, GP-1, was higher after meals in women receiving the thylakoid extract. No side effects were reported.

All in all, this study is extremely promising for those who want to lose weight or who seem to have to work hard to maintain their weight. You can purchase Appethyl online at *appethyl sale.com* (844-748-2669). It is also available as one of many ingredients in an appetite suppressant called Hydroxycut Appetite Control Plus Appethyl. The manufacturer doesn't say how much Appethyl is in each serving, however.

Surprising Restaurant Tricks That Keep You Slim

Brian Wansink, PhD, John Dyson Professor of Marketing, director, Cornell Food and Brand Lab, Dyson School of Applied Economics and Management, Cornell University, Ithaca, New York. He is author of *Slim by Design: Mindless Eating Solutions for Everyday Life*.

Nobody goes to a restaurant to stress over every bite. We go to have fun. But a recently published study found that fun translates into significantly more calories, saturated fat, sugar and sodium, whether you're grabbing a burger or dining at a four-star establishment.

Using info from the National Health and Nutrition Examination Survey—a huge, long-term government project that collects and interprets data on health and nutrition—two days' worth of eating habits of more than 12,000 people were analyzed. It found that if you only eat one fast-food and one restaurant meal each week, the calories alone add up to an extra six pounds a year—year after year. So much for winning the battle of the bulge!

But you can dine out without sabotaging your health or denying yourself pleasure. The trick is to tilt the dining-out experience in your favor. A few small tweaks will help you eat less when dining out without even knowing it.

•**Seat yourself.** Believe it or not, where you sit in a restaurant affects how much you eat. People seated at tables near a window or in a well-lit section of the high-end restaurant order lighter items than folks who sit in dark corners. People seated on stools at high-top tables order more salads and fewer desserts. Select seating that jibes with the dietary behaviors you want to have rather than the behaviors you unconsciously give in to.

People sitting in loud, brightly lit areas of fast-food restaurants tend to eat more quickly. Also, unlike the scenario that plays out in fancy restaurants, fast-food patrons who sit in dimmer, mellower areas of the restaurant eat 18% less than other patrons.

•**Plan ahead with a "doggie bag."** In one experiment, people who considered getting a doggie bag before ordering were 40% more likely to take food home than those who considered it after being served the food. As you walk into the restaurant, say to yourself, *Portions are huge here. I could get two meals out of this. What a bargain.* If your hotel room has a refrigerator (and many even have microwaves), commit to yourself to take at least some portion of your meal back with you. Otherwise, do not feel compelled to clean your plate.

•**Read the fine print.** Menu design secretly and sneakily influences what we order—it's a science unto itself. Designers know that when we read menus, our eyes automatically scan from the top left to the top right, zoom straight past the middle to the bottom left, then across to the bottom right. As a result, the top and bottom corners of the menu are where designers place the crowd-pleasers or the items that make the most money for the restaurant. Items that are bolded, boxed or in a different color also attract our attention. Usually they're not the healthy choices.

Make it a point to read all the items in between the top and bottom of the menu. Take notice of items that are in plain print instead of the ones in bold, bright and fancy type. The ordinary listing is where the healthier menu options hide.

•**Smart tie-breaking trick.** When you can't decide between two items, ask yourself, "What would Batman eat?" No kidding. This tip comes from an experiment that I did with kids to see whether they would choose a healthier option without an adult suggesting it. After considering what Batman might want, the majority of children in these studies opted for apple slices instead of French fries.

This trick works for grown-ups, too—just substitute the name of someone you admire or want to impress. Stopping to think about what somebody else wants is a great way to break yourself out of the moment. That pause might be all you need to choose the better option.

Free Weight-Loss Counseling

Medicare offers free weight-loss counseling, but fewer than 1% of Medicare's 50 million beneficiaries use it—even though 30% of seniors are obese and eligible for counseling.

Problem: Many of the most knowledgeable providers, such as weight-loss specialists, are not allowed to participate, because Medicare reimburses only primary-care providers, nurse practitioners and physician assistants working in doctors' offices.

Also: Medicare requires that counseling be given during a separate appointment, not when patients come in for other services. For information, go to *Medicare.gov*.

Roundup of experts on senior obesity and Medicare requirements, reported at *MedPageToday.com*.

The Truth About Soy: Healthy or Dangerous?

Donald R. Yance, CN, clinical master herbalist and medical director at the Mederi Centre for Natural Healing in Ashland, Oregon. He is author of *Adaptogens in Medical Herbalism* and *Herbal Medicine, Healing & Cancer. DonnieYance.com*

O ver the past few years, soy seems to have gone from one of the healthiest foods to one of the least healthy, with some health professionals accusing the bean of causing a wide range of problems, from thyroid damage to pancreatic cancer. Are they right? Should you avoid soy?

My viewpoint: Eating traditional soy foods such as miso, tofu and others in amounts eaten by Asian peoples for thousands of years not only poses no threat to health…but (according to thousands of scientific studies) may help protect you from many chronic diseases, including heart disease, cancer, osteoporosis and kidney disease.

On the other hand, eating some of the recently invented foods that are made from soy— and there are thousands of these—is a different story altogether.

What you need to know…

HOW MUCH TO EAT

I recommend eating (or drinking) three-to-four weekly servings of traditional "good" soy foods (see below). That amount delivers the daily amount of isoflavones eaten in traditional Eastern cultures and the amount that matches the level in studies that show benefits from soy intake.

However, certain soy foods are bad for you. Here, the worst and the best…

BAD SOY

The worst soy products are margarines and shortenings made from partially hydrogenated soybean oil. These contain trans fat, which hardens and clogs arteries, increasing the risk for heart attack and stroke. And many packaged foods—crackers, cookies, canned food, frozen entrées—contain partially hydrogenated soybean oil. Minimize or eliminate them all from your diet.

Another bad-for-you type of soy is processed soy protein, such as soy protein isolate, soy protein concentrate, texturized vegetable protein and hydrolyzed vegetable protein—ingredients that you will find in many processed foods ranging from nutritional powders to energy bars to veggie burgers.

GOOD SOY

Traditional soy foods are good choices. When possible, look for foods that are organic and do not contain genetically modified organisms (GMOs). No one really knows what effects GMO foods might have on our health, and animal studies link them to infertility, immune problems, digestive disorders and other issues. Human studies show that they may increase the incidence of food allergies. *Traditional soy foods include…*

•**Miso (fermented soybean paste).** Soybeans contain "antinutrients" such as enzyme inhibitors that can interfere with digestion. But Asian cultures discovered thousands of years ago that soaking, sprouting or fermenting soybeans neutralizes the antinutrients. Miso—fermented soybean paste—is such a food. And miso soup—a nourishing broth of fermented soybean paste and seaweed, often with vegeta-

Allergic to Soy?

Symptoms develop within minutes to hours after eating soy and include mouth tingling, hives or itching, swelling of the tongue, lips or vocal cords, trouble breathing, diarrhea, nausea or vomiting. A severe reaction to soy (anaphylaxis) is rare—symptoms include constriction of airways, rapid pulse and dizziness—and warrants emergency treatment.

You might not be allergic to soy, but you might be sensitive to it. The symptoms of food sensitivity such as nausea, vomiting and diarrhea appear gradually—even days after ingestion—and usually happen when you eat too much or too often. If you have a soy sensitivity, determine the amount you can eat without symptoms (see also page 123).

bles and tofu—is a dietary mainstay for many Japanese people.

Important scientific evidence: Research from Japan's National Cancer Center showed that women who ate three or more bowls of miso soup daily had a 54% lower risk for breast cancer than women who ate one bowl.

•**Tempeh** (fermented soybeans formed into a burgerlike patty). This soy food is a rich source of protein.

Recent research: In an animal study, rats were protected from drug-induced neurological damage and memory loss when they ate tempeh.

•**Natto** (boiled soybeans fermented with the bacterium *Bacillus subtilis*). This soy food is rich in vitamin K-2, a must for healthy bones. It's also loaded with nattokinase, an enzyme that thins the blood and may help protect against heart attack and stroke.

•**Tofu** (soybean curd). Tofu is coagulated soy milk pressed into soft white blocks. My favorite way to eat it is to marinate it and make a wrap sandwich with some veggies and plum sauce.

Important scientific research: In one study of more than 1,500 women, published in *Cancer Epidemiology, Biomarkers & Prevention*, every additional weekly serving of tofu lowered the risk for breast cancer by 15%.

●**Soy milk.** Look for an organic, non-GMO brand, such as Pacific.

●**Tamari.** Tamari is made from fermented soybeans and is similar to soy sauce but has more soy and less wheat and is thicker and less salty.

●**Edamame** (green, immature soybeans, generally steamed and eaten out of the pod). Edamame contains fewer toxins than mature beans.

If You Can't Eat Fish, Nuts, Soy or Dairy or Gluten...

David Grotto, MS, RDN, founder and president of Nutrition Housecall, LLC, a Chicago-based nutrition consulting firm. He is author of *The Best Things You Can Eat*. *DavidGrotto.com*

You may know about all the health benefits of fish, nuts, soy, dairy and whole wheat. But what if you're allergic to those foods or for various other reasons cannot eat them? How can you get the same nutritional benefits?

Here, common food sensitivities—and the best substitutes...

FISH

Fish is among the healthiest foods you can eat. It is high in protein and healthful fats and rich in vitamin D, selenium and zinc.

It is the healthful fats—long-chain omega-3 fatty acids—that fish is best known for. People who eat as little as three to six ounces of fish a week can reduce their risk of dying from heart disease by more than one-third.

The problem: Many people are allergic to fish.

What to eat instead: There are plenty of choices if you can't eat fish. The alpha-linolenic acid (ALA) in plant foods is converted to healthful omega-3s in the body.

Examples: Walnuts, flaxseeds, pumpkin seeds and canola oil contain ALA. The catch is that ALA isn't efficiently converted to long-chain omega-3s. When you eat ALA-rich plant foods, you get only about 10% to 25% of the beneficial fats that you would get from fish.

My advice: Get these fats from as many different sources as you can. Snack on nuts during the day. Cook tofu in canola oil or soybean oil. Add some ground flaxseed to your morning cereal.

NUTS

A recent study found that people who ate nuts seven or more times a week were 20% less likely to die from any cause during the study period than those who didn't eat nuts. Nuts are high in zinc as well as phytosterols, compounds that reduce cholesterol and may protect against cancer. Recent research suggests that they also help relieve symptoms in men with enlarged prostate glands.

The problem: You potentially can be allergic to any one type of nut or to all of them. And peanuts—which technically are a legume, not a nut—are a serious (in some cases, life-threatening) allergen for some people.

What to eat instead: Pumpkin or sunflower seeds. You can eat them raw, roasted or salted. These seeds are just as healthful as nuts, and they have the crunch, rich flavor and grab-and-go convenience of nuts. *In my house, we enjoy this recipe for roasted pumpkin seeds...*

Take one cup of seeds, rinse them off and pat dry. Melt one tablespoon of butter (or no-trans-fat margarine spread) in a saucepan. Add one tablespoon of Worcestershire sauce. Toss the seeds and the butter sauce in a bowl. Spray a cookie sheet with nonstick cooking spray. Spread the seed mixture on the cookie sheet, and bake at

---

You Can Leave the Water Bottle Behind

Drinking water before meals does not help you eat less. The body has different satiety points for food and water, and one doesn't translate to the other.

Also: You don't need to drink eight glasses of water a day...and being thirsty does not mean that you are dehydrated.

Psychology Today. PsychologyToday.com

Trick to Lose Weight

To lose weight, get into daylight before noon.

Recent finding: People who spent 20 minutes outdoors in bright light in the morning had a lower body mass index (BMI) than people who got most of their light exposure later in the day.

Study of 54 people by researchers at Northwestern University Feinberg School of Medicine, Chicago, published in *PLOS ONE*. The influence of light on body weight was independent of physical activity level, caloric intake, sleep timing and age.

350°F for about 30 minutes, turning the seeds occasionally so that they brown on both sides.

DAIRY

There are plenty of reasons to enjoy milk, cheese and other dairy foods. The calcium is good for your bones. Dairy is high in protein. Even the fats seem to be beneficial. Studies have shown that people who eat dairy tend to lose more weight than people on low-dairy diets even when they get the same number of calories.

The problem: Millions of Americans don't produce enough lactase (an enzyme) to completely digest dairy. Others have a true allergy—they get symptoms such as a rash or hives when they consume one or more dairy proteins.

What to eat instead: You can buy milk and cheeses that are spiked with extra lactase. Also, research has shown that you can increase your natural supply of lactase. People who give up dairy for a few weeks and then slowly reintroduce it—say, by consuming an ounce a day for a week, then slowly adding to that amount over time—can boost their production of lactase.

It's tougher if you are allergic.

My advice: Give up cow's milk, and switch to soy milk or almond milk. These have many of the same nutrients that are found in cow's milk, and most people like the taste. Goat's milk is another possibility. People who are allergic to cow's milk usually can drink goat's milk without discomfort—but the musky taste isn't for everyone.

SOY

Tofu and other soy foods have long been the go-to protein source for people who don't eat meat. Soy also is rich in isoflavones, antioxidants that help balance hormones, increase bone strength and reduce the risk for some cancers.

The problem: Soy allergies are common, and they aren't limited to tofu. If you are allergic, you have to avoid a lot of different foods, including soy sauce, miso, soy milk, tamari, edamame, etc.

What to eat instead: Other beans, such as lentils, pinto beans, kidney beans and chickpeas. All of these legumes have healthful amounts of protein, fiber and antioxidants. If you're not sensitive to gluten, try seitan. It's a form of wheat gluten that's popular in Asia (and in some Asian restaurants) that mimics the texture—and the protein content—of meat. Just make sure that your seitan dish isn't made with soy sauce!

IF YOU CAN'T EAT GLUTEN...

Whole grains are high in fiber, B vitamins, vitamin E and other antioxidants. A diet that includes whole wheat and other whole grains can significantly reduce your risk for diabetes, cancer, heart disease and digestive problems.

The problem: About 5% to 6% of Americans are sensitive to gluten, a protein in wheat, barley and rye. A smaller percentage suffers from celiac disease, a serious autoimmune disease triggered by gluten.

What to eat instead: Gluten-free grains, such as rice, quinoa and amaranth, have similar nutritional benefits. I recommend teff, an African grain that has a mildly nutty flavor and about the same amount of fiber that you would get from wheat.

Unfortunately, gluten-free breads often are dry and crumbly—they lack the chewiness and mouth feel that comes from gluten. But manufacturers of gluten-free breads are getting better.

Example: The Udi's brand makes gluten-free bread that tastes (and feels) almost like traditional bread.

Caution: Oats don't contain gluten, but products such as oatmeal often are tainted when they are processed with the same machinery that is used for other grains or when oat crops are grown too close to wheat fields. Look for oats that are guaranteed to be gluten-free. It will be noted on the label.

Is Sprouted Garlic Still Edible?

John La Puma, MD, ChefMD, a professionally trained chef with a private nutritional medical practice in Santa Barbara, California. *DrJohnLaPuma.com*

Yes! A garlic sprout is a new seedling and will eventually develop into a whole garlic plant. It has greater flavor and pungency than the clove itself. Garlic that has been sprouted for five days has twice as many antioxidants as unsprouted garlic and knocks back free radicals better, too, probably because the seedling is creating natural defenses designed to protect the up-and-coming plant. So enjoy the garlic clove and the sprout.

Got This? Don't Eat That

Michael T. Murray, ND, a naturopathic physician and leading authority on natural medicine. Dr. Murray serves on the Board of Regents of Bastyr University in Kenmore, Washington, and has written more than 30 books, including *The Encyclopedia of Natural Medicine* with coauthor Joseph Pizzorno, ND. *DoctorMurray.com*

Let's say you've got arthritis…heartburn… heart disease…or some other common health problem.

You follow all your doctor's suggestions, but you still don't feel better. It could be that you're not getting the right medication or other treatment, but there's an even stronger possibility.

What often gets overlooked: Your diet. Far too many people sabotage their treatment—and actually make their health problems worse—by eating the wrong foods. Meanwhile, you could be helping yourself by eating certain foods that ease whatever is ailing you.

Common health problems that foods can worsen—or help…

ARTHRITIS

Both osteoarthritis and rheumatoid arthritis involve inflammation that causes joint pain and/or swelling.

What hurts: Refined carbohydrates (sugar, white bread, white rice and most pasta). They cause a spike in glucose (blood sugar) that leads to inflammation.

What helps: Raw, fresh ginger. It's a potent inhibitor of prostaglandin and thromboxanes, inflammatory compounds involved in arthritis. And unlike anti-inflammatory medications, ginger doesn't cause an upset stomach. Be sure to use fresh ginger—it's better than powdered because it contains higher levels of active ingredients. For pain relief, you need to eat only about 10 g (about a quarter-inch slice) of raw, fresh ginger a day.

Smart idea: You can add raw ginger to any fresh fruit or vegetable juice with the help of a juice extractor. Ginger mixes well with carrot, apple, pear or pineapple juice. You also can grate fresh ginger and add it to any hot tea.

CARDIAC ARRHYTHMIAS

Everyone notices occasional changes in the way the heart beats at certain times—during exercise, for example. But persistent irregularities could be a sign of arrhythmias, potentially dangerous problems with the heart's electrical system. The heart can skip beats or beat too slowly or too quickly—all of which can signal heart disease.

What hurts: Too much caffeine. Whether it's in coffee, tea or chocolate, caffeine stimulates the heart to beat more quickly, which triggers arrhythmias in some people.

What helps: Berries. All types of berries, including cherries, blackberries, raspberries and blueberries, are rich in procyanidins, plant pigments that reduce arrhythmias and improve blood flow through the coronary arteries. Aim for one cup of fresh berries daily (frozen are fine, too).

Also helpful: Concentrated extracts made from hawthorn. This herb contains the same heart-healthy compounds as berries. In Germany, it is commonly used to treat arrhythmias and congestive heart failure. If you have heart problems, a hawthorn extract containing 10% procyanidins (100 mg to 200 mg three times daily) is often recommended. Hawthorn can interact with heart medications and other drugs, so check with your doctor before trying it.

HEARTBURN

Also known as gastroesophageal reflux disease (GERD), heartburn is usually caused by the upward surge of digestive juices from the stomach into the esophagus. People who suffer from frequent heartburn can get some relief with lifestyle changes, such as not overeating and staying upright for a few hours after eating. But most people with heartburn don't pay enough attention to their diets.

What hurts: Alcohol and coffee are widely known to trigger heartburn. Many people, however, don't consider the effects of chocolate, fried foods and carbonated drinks, which also may weaken the esophageal sphincter (the muscle that prevents acids from entering the esophagus) or increase the intra-abdominal pressure that pushes acids upward.

What helps: Fresh (not bottled) lemon juice—two to four ounces daily in water, tea or apple or carrot juices. Lemon contains D-limonene, an oil-based compound that helps prevent heartburn. Also, use the peel if you can. It's an especially good source of D-limonene.

EYE DISEASE

Age-related macular degeneration (AMD) is a leading cause of vision loss, but it (as well as cataracts) can often be prevented—or the effects minimized—by eating carefully.

What hurts: Animal fat and processed foods. A study of 261 adults with AMD found that people who ate a lot of these foods were twice as likely to have a worsening of their eye disease compared with those who ate less of the foods. Animal fat also increases risk for high cholesterol, which has been linked to increased risk for cataracts.

What helps: Cold-water fish. The omega-3 fatty acids in fish can help prevent AMD and cataracts—or, if you already have one of these conditions, help prevent it from getting worse. Try to eat three to four weekly servings of cold-water fish, such as salmon or sardines.

Also helpful: Tomatoes, watermelon and other red fruits and vegetables (such as red peppers) that are high in lycopene. Green vegetables are also protective. Foods such as spinach and kale are high in lutein and other plant pigments that concentrate in the retina to help prevent eye disease.

ROSACEA

Some 16 million Americans have rosacea, a chronic skin condition that causes bright-red facial flushing for at least 10 minutes per episode, along with bumps and pustules.

What hurts: Hot foods. "Hot" can mean temperature (a hot bowl of soup or a steaming cup of coffee or tea) or spicy (such as chili powder, cayenne or curry). Alcohol also tends to increase flushes.

What helps: If you have rosacea, ask your doctor to test you for H. pylori, the bacterium that causes most stomach ulcers and has been linked to rosacea. If you test positive, drink cabbage juice (eight to 12 ounces daily). It's not the tastiest juice, but it inhibits the growth of H. pylori. Make your own cabbage juice in a juicer (add some apples and/or carrots to improve the taste). If you have thyroid problems, check with your doctor—fresh cabbage may interfere with thyroid function.

Better Lunch Choices

Rhonda Sebastian, MA, nutritionist, Beltsville Human Nutrition Research Center, Maryland.

In a survey of nearly 6,000 adults, those who ate at least one sandwich daily got considerably more calories and sodium than those who didn't eat sandwiches.

Why: Typical sandwich ingredients, such as bread, cheese and processed meat, tend to be high in calories and sodium. For adults over age 50, one sandwich had about half of the daily recommended dietary allowance of sodium.

Better options: Sandwiches made with healthier ingredients, such as fresh meat and vegetables, or salad...fruit...or low-sodium tuna.

Are Your Grandmother's Prunes the New Superfood?

Maria Stacewicz-Sapuntzakis, PhD, professor emerita, department of kinesiology and nutrition, University of Illinois at Chicago.

What comes to mind when you hear the word "prunes"? You probably think of one of two things—laxatives or senior citizens. That's why the prune industry is trying to change the name to "dried plums."

Prunes are actually very good for everyone. They are nutrient-rich…inexpensive…they can satisfy a sweet tooth without the horrid effects of processed sugar…they can even help you get going with a healthy slimming diet. But there's a lot more to this simple, inexpensive superfood—yes, superfood—that could make you healthier and get you thinking about prunes in a whole new way…

A MAGIC INGREDIENT

Prunes have a unique combination of nutrients that aren't found in other foods, not even other dried fruits. They're very high in a sugar alcohol called sorbitol, which is the key magic ingredient to the prune's health benefits.

On its own, too much dietary sorbitol can cause gas and unwanted laxative effects, and 50 grams or more a day is considered excessive. In fact, the FDA makes companies add warning labels about the laxative effect of sorbitol to food products that contain it. But you'd have to eat more than a half a pound of prunes in one sitting to total 50 grams—and if you do try that at home, you sure will be "sitting." Five prunes contain a modest 7 grams of sorbitol, which combines with other nutrients in the fruit to pump up its nutritional and health-enhancing powers.

Two daily servings of prunes (that's 10 to 12) can help your body…

•**Lose weight.** Research recently reported at the European Congress on Obesity found that dieters who ate prunes lost more pounds and more inches and felt fuller longer than dieters who didn't eat them.

•**Regulate blood sugar.** Although prunes are sweet, they rate relatively low on the Glycemic Index scale, which measures how fast and how much a certain food raises blood sugar levels. This makes prunes a good food choice for folks with hyperglycemia or diabetes. Sorbitol itself has a low glycemic value, which may explain why something that tastes so much like candy keeps blood sugar levels on an even keel instead of making them spike.

•**Strengthen bones.** Prunes contain several nutrients, including boron, copper, vitamin K and, as mentioned, potassium that help prevent bone loss. Plus, sorbitol—that secret ingredient—increases absorption of calcium from prunes and other foods.

•**Prevent or slow arteriosclerosis.** Studies in animals and humans suggest that compounds in prunes can lower blood levels of cholesterol and, thereby, prevent or slow the progression of arteriosclerosis—or hardening of the arteries—caused by buildup of cholesterol and other debris on artery walls.

•**Prevent colon cancer.** The fiber, phenolic compounds (which are antioxidant substances found in fruits) and sorbitol help prunes move waste through the colon quickly enough to keep bile acid by-products from injuring the lining of the colon, which can be cancer-causing.

THE BEST WAYS TO EAT PRUNES

If you eat the whole fruit, you get the benefits of all the great nutritional compounds in prunes. Some of these compounds become lost in prune juice. But if you have never eaten prunes and now have an interest in adding them to your diet, start slow with four or five a day. Once you're sure that your body can tolerate them without an unwanted laxative effect, work up to 10 to 12 each day. That racks up 240 calories, but you'll feel full longer than if you ate the same amount of calories in the form of, say, bread and cheese.

And prunes can be a lot more than wrinkled things you pluck from a box. *Consider these tasty ways to enjoy them…*

•**Homemade no-bake energy bars**—Place a handful of prunes in a food processor along with any combination of your favorite nuts and seeds, such as almonds, walnuts, and sesame, sunflower or pumpkin seeds. You can add some shredded coconut, too…maybe even sprinkle in some unsweetened cacao to sate a chocolate craving. Process the ingredients into a paste, and then press the mixture into a baking dish. Chill until firm and cut into squares for a perfect on-the-go energy boost and healthy sweet-tooth satisfier.

•**Prunes in a blanket**—Wrap individual prunes in paper-thin slices of prosciutto—or do the same using turkey bacon if you prefer—then roast at 400°F until crisp on the outside, sweet and gooey inside. I dare you to eat just one!

•**Spicy moroccan-style stew**—Simmer prunes with lamb, beef or chicken and aromatic Moroccan spices, such as ginger, saffron, cinnamon and pepper, to serve up a traditional Moroccan stew called tagine.

Bon appétit and healthy eating with prunes!

The Three Supplements Everyone Should Take

Alan R. Gaby, MD, contributing medical editor for *Townsend Letter*, contributing editor for *Alternative Medicine Review*, and chief science editor for *Aisle 7*. His most recent book is the comprehensive textbook *Nutritional Medicine*, widely used by natural practitioners as a reference manual. *DoctorGaby.com*

Vitamin supplements have taken a beating lately. And plenty of people who use them to help ensure their good health are now left wondering whether these pills should be dumped in the trash.

But before you do that, there's another side to the vitamin question that you should know—most of the negative findings are misreported and/or the studies are flawed. After decades of research (backed by more than 26,000 medical journal articles and 19 years of clinical practice treating thousands of patients), I am confident that supplements can and often do work. The question is, which supplements?

WHAT EVERYONE NEEDS

In an ideal world, we'd get all our nutrients from foods—there's a powerful synergistic effect when vitamins and minerals are found in foods. But the reality is, most people don't get enough of these crucial nutrients. That's why certain individual supplements can help.

Even if you take a standard, over-the-counter multivitamin, such as Centrum or One A Day, you may benefit from the following supplements because most multis don't contain enough of these nutrients.

Exception: If you use a high-potency multivitamin (it has megadoses of nutrients and is usually labeled "high potency"), you're most likely getting enough of the necessary nutrients and probably don't need to add the supplements below. But you may still need these additional supplements if you have any of the health conditions described in this article.

THREE KEY SUPPLEMENTS

Supplements everyone should consider taking…*

•**B-complex.** The B vitamins—thiamine, riboflavin, niacin and several others—are a must for the body's production of energy. They also play a key role in the health of the brain and nervous system.

But when foods are refined—for example, when kernels of whole wheat are stripped of their outer covering of fibrous bran and inner core of wheat germ and turned into white flour, as commonly occurs in American manufacturing practices—B vitamins are lost.

New scientific evidence: A study of 104 middle-aged and older adults, published this summer, showed that taking three B vitamins (folic acid, B-6 and B-12) lowered levels of the amino acid homocysteine in people with very high levels (such elevations are linked to heart disease) and improved several measurements of mental functioning, such as memory.

Typical dose of B vitamins: Look for a B-complex supplement that contains at least 20

---

*Be sure to check with a nutrition-savvy health practitioner before taking any supplements. To find one near you, consult the American Holistic Medical Association, *HolisticMedicine.org,* or the American Association of Naturopathic Physicians, *Naturopathic.org.*

Add-On Supplements You May Need...

Certain people may need additional supplements to protect or improve their health. *Two key "add-on" supplements...*

• **Fish oil.** A large body of scientific research shows that fish oil can help prevent and treat heart disease.

Typical dose: About 1 g daily for people who want to reduce heart disease risk...and 2 g to 6 g daily for people diagnosed with the condition. People with coronary heart disease need 360 mg to 1,080 mg daily of eicosapentaenoic acid (EPA) and 240 mg to 720 mg of docosahexaenoic acid (DHA). Talk to a health practitioner before taking fish oil—it may increase bleeding risk.

• **Vitamin D.** Vitamin D deficiency is common, and it can increase risk for bone loss (osteoporosis), falls in older people (frailty), the flu, autoimmune diseases (such as rheumatoid arthritis, lupus and multiple sclerosis) and even cancer.

New thinking: 400 international units (IU) daily was once thought to preserve bone and prevent falls, but studies now show that 800 IU daily is preferable. An even higher dose (up to 1,200 IU daily) may be needed, depending on age (older people may need more)...weight (the obese are at greater risk for deficiency)... and skin color (people with dark skin produce less vitamin D when exposed to the sun). Ask your doctor for advice on the best dose for you, and use vitamin D-3 (the type derived from sunlight and animal sources).

mg of most of the B vitamins, including B-6, thiamine and niacin...and at least 50 micrograms (mcg) each of B-12 and biotin.

• **Magnesium.** Without this mineral, your body couldn't produce energy, build bones, regulate blood sugar or even move a muscle. But most Americans don't get enough of this mineral in their diets.

Magnesium is used by nutritionally oriented clinicians to treat many health problems, including insomnia, chronic muscle pain, headache, heart disease, diabetes, osteoporosis and hearing loss. Overall, magnesium is the most beneficial supplement I have seen in my patients.

Typical dose of magnesium: 200 mg, twice a day. A capsule or a chewable or liquid form is preferable to a tablet, because it is more easily absorbed. But all types of magnesium—including magnesium oxide, magnesium citrate and magnesium aspartate—are equally effective for most conditions. If you develop diarrhea, reduce the dose until diarrhea eases.

• **Vitamin C.** This vitamin is an antioxidant—a nutrient that protects you from oxidation, a kind of inner rust that destroys cells. A low level of oxidation is normal, but it's increased by many factors—such as stress and chronic disease.

Recent finding: A review of 13 studies involving nearly 4,000 people with colorectal adenoma (a benign tumor that can turn into colon cancer) found that people with the highest levels of vitamin C were 22% less likely to develop colon cancer.

Typical dose of vitamin C: 100 mg to 500 mg daily, for general nutritional support. If you have a family history of colon cancer (for example, in a first-degree relative, such as a parent or sibling), consider taking 1,000 mg, three times daily.

How to Choose the Perfect Omega-3 Supplement

C. Leigh Broadhurst, PhD, a physical chemist with a major government agricultural research laboratory in Beltsville, Maryland. Dr. Broadhurst has conducted peer-reviewed research on omega-3 fatty acids for nearly 20 years.

Millions of Americans now pop omega-3 supplements as routinely as they shower and brush their teeth. And with good reason. Omega-3s help fight everything from arthritis and depression to macular degeneration and high triglycerides.

But with so many of these supplements on the market, how do you know which is best for you? *C. Leigh Broadhurst, PhD, a chemist* *and leading expert on omega-3 supplements, provides some answers...**

DO YOU NEED MORE?

Omega-3s are essential fatty acids. As such, these nutrients cannot be manufactured by the body, so they need to be obtained from foods or supplements.

As with most nutrients, it's preferable to get your omega-3s from food, which also provides a slew of beneficial vitamins and minerals. For example, the richest omega-3 food sources, including oily fish such as salmon, sardines and trout, are also high in immune-supporting vitamin D and selenium.

What you may not know: Getting enough omega-3s from one's diet is tough. In fact, the US Dietary Guidelines Advisory Committee has estimated that about 70% of Americans are deficient in this crucial nutrient.

Unless your daily diet includes marine sources of omega-3s, you should consider taking omega-3 supplements. Walnuts, flaxseed and other plant sources have the omega-3 alpha-linolenic acid, which the body does not convert very efficiently to *eicosapentaenoic acid* (EPA) and *docosahexaenoic acid* (DHA)—the two main types of omega-3s. Therefore, plant foods don't provide nearly as much of these crucial omega-3s as do the fish listed earlier.

WHICH IS RIGHT FOR YOU?

Several omega-3 sources are available in supplement form, including fish oil, krill oil and algae (see descriptions of each below). To ensure that you're getting an adequate dose of EPA and DHA, look for an omega-3 supplement that is labeled "concentrated."

My advice: Take two 1,000-mg capsules of fish oil daily (at least 400 mg of EPA...and 200 mg of DHA in each capsule).**

Good product for general health: Jarrow Formulas' EPA-DHA Balance, *Amazon.com.* This is a highly concentrated, purified fish oil (made with anchovies and sardines), produced by a reputable manufacturer.

*Dr. Broadhurst has been a consultant in the natural products industry but has no financial interest in any of the products mentioned in this article.

**Consult your doctor before starting an omega-3 regimen.

When larger doses of omega-3s may be needed: Individuals who suffer from severe rheumatoid arthritis or who have heart disease should eat seafood at least twice a week. In addition, the National Institutes of Health recommends that rheumatoid arthritis sufferers get 3.8 g of EPA and 2 g of DHA daily via supplements...those with heart disease should get up to 6 g of EPA and up to 3.7 g of DHA daily.

Caution: Taking 3 g or more daily of omega-3s may cause excessive bleeding in some people, so this much fish oil should be taken only when recommended by a physician for a specific purpose.

To avoid taking multiple capsules, consider trying a pourable variety of omega-3s—a single teaspoon contains about 2 g of omega-3s, which is the equivalent of two 1,000-mg capsules. Liquids are generally more cost-effective, too.

If you're worried about the taste of an omega-3 liquid: Try a flavored fish oil (such as lemon, orange or mint) or mix your omega-3 dose in orange juice or pineapple juice. Good liquid omega-3 products are available from Twinlab and Nordic Naturals.

If you're allergic to fish or you are a vegetarian: Many algae-based omega-3 products are available. DSM Nutritional Products makes life'sDHA, which is a highly purified and concentrated source of DHA (available at *lifesDHA.com*).

What about krill oil? This omega-3 product is derived from krill—tiny, shrimplike crustaceans that are normally eaten by whales, penguins and seals. Some people find that krill oil helps relieve joint pain faster than fish oil does.

Good krill oil supplements are available from Twinlab, Jarrow, Nature's Way and Natrol.

MAKE SURE IT'S PURE

A final point to consider in choosing an omega-3 supplement is the quality of the manufacturing process. To ensure that the company is complying with high manufacturing standards, choose omega-3 products that are labeled with the Good Manufacturing Practices (GMP) certification. This certification, granted by the Natural Products Association, shows that the company's manufacturing facility has been inspected every

Fatty Acid Face-Off: EPA vs. DHA

There are two main types of omega-3 fatty acids—eicosapentaenoic acid (EPA) and docosahexaenoic acid (DHA). Each of these fatty acids plays a different role in keeping our bodies healthy.

EPA inhibits a key enzyme that fuels the production of inflammatory hormones. As a result, it is slightly more effective than DHA against certain types of inflammatory conditions, such as arthritis and joint and tendon problems. DHA, on the other hand, will boost the health of your brain's neurotransmitters.

For the greatest benefit: It's wise to choose an omega-3 supplement that contains both EPA and DHA. Just as calcium and vitamin D work synergistically, so do EPA and DHA.

two years by an independent third-party auditor who checks production processes and that the product meets specifications in such areas as purity and strength. For a list of GMP-certified companies, go to the Web site of the Natural Products Association, *NPAinfo.org.*

An alternative to look for: Certification from NSF International, an independent testing organization, *NSF.org*, indicates that an independent accredited lab has confirmed that the product contains what is on the label and on-site inspections have been made at the manufacturing facility.

Secret Weight-Loss Weapon

Cyril Kendall, PhD, nutrition researcher, University of Toronto, Canada.

What if there were a food that had an incredible power to help you lose weight or avoid gaining weight? You'd try it, right? Well, a recent study shows exactly what that food is. It's beans and other legumes! To see what new benefits these nutrient-packed foods might have, researchers tracked adults who ate a daily

serving (three-quarters cup) of beans, lentils, peas or chickpeas.

Result: They felt 31% fuller after meals than those who didn't eat legumes.

If you're trying to lose weight: Add legumes to your daily diet.

Juice for Healing Power

Michael T. Murray, ND, a naturopathic physician who has written more than 30 books, including the *The Complete Book of Juicing: Your Delicious Guide to Youthful Vitality. DoctorMurray.*com

Juice has gotten a bad rap. We're often advised to eat whole fruits and vegetables—for the fiber and because they are lower in calories than an "equal" amount of juice. But for the many Americans who don't eat the recommended three to five servings of vegetables and two to three servings of fruit daily, juice can be a lifesaver—literally. Juice is loaded with nutrients that protect against heart disease, cancer, diabetes, arthritis, Alzheimer's and other chronic conditions.

We can pack in a day's worth of fruits and vegetables in just 12 to 16 ounces of juice. *How to do it right…*

•**Opt for fresh juice, not packaged.** Packaged juices, whether in a can, bottle, carton or frozen, are lower in nutrients. And packaged juices have been pasteurized, which destroys health-giving compounds.

Example: Fresh apple juice contains ellagic acid, an anticancer nutrient that shields chromosomes from damage and blocks the tumor-causing action of many pollutants. In contrast, commercial apple juice contains almost no ellagic acid.

•**Use a quality juicer.** If you juice once or twice a week, try a high-speed centrifugal juicer. They're relatively inexpensive, ranging from $100 to $400. (*Examples:* Juice Fountain Duo or Juice Fountain Elite, both from Breville.)

If you juice more frequently, consider investing in a "slow juicer" ($300 and up) that typically operates at 80 revolutions per minute (RPM), compared with the 1,000 to 24,000 RPM of a centrifugal model. (I use The Hurom Juicer.) A slow juicer expels significantly more juice and better preserves delicate nutrients. And because the damaged compounds produced by a centrifugal juicer taste a little bitter, a slow juicer provides better-tasting juice.

Follow this basic juice recipe: Use four unpeeled carrots and two unpeeled, cored apples cut into wedges as a base for creating other juice blends by adding such things as a handful of kale, spinach, radishes and/or beets. Ideally, use organic fruits and vegetables. If not, be sure to wash them thoroughly.

•**Keep blood sugar balanced.** Fruit and vegetable juices can deliver too much natural sugar, spiking blood sugar levels, a risk factor for heart disease, diabetes and other chronic conditions.

What you need to know: The metabolic impact of the sugar in a particular food can be measured using the glycemic index (GI)—how quickly a carbohydrate turns into glucose (blood sugar). But a more accurate way to measure this impact is with the glycemic load (GL)—a relatively new calculation that uses the GI but also takes into account the amount of carbohydrate in a specific food. Beets, for example, have a high GI but a low GL—their carbohydrate is digested quickly, but there's not a lot of it. Charts providing the GI and the GL are available on the Internet. I like those at *Mendosa.com*.

Bottom line: Limit the intake of higher-GL juices such as orange, cherry, pineapple and mango. You can use them to add flavor to lower-GL choices such as kale, spinach, celery and beets.

Healthier Frozen Yogurt

Franci Cohen, MS, CDN, nutritionist and fitness specialist in Brooklyn, New York. *FranciCohen.com*

Frozen yogurt generally has some healthful probiotics, such as acidophilus, but not as much as regular yogurt. However, not all frozen yogurt is created equally. For example, some brands are made with heat-treated yogurt,

which kills active cultures, and some freezing processes destroy healthful bacteria.

To find a frozen yogurt that contains probiotics, look for the "Live & Active Cultures" seal on the label (or ask the clerk at a frozen-yogurt shop). This seal, established by the National Yogurt Association, ensures that frozen yogurt contains at least 10 million live and active cultures per gram (100 million for regular yogurt) at the time it is manufactured.

Correct Way to Take Calcium

Dennis Goodman, MD, board-certified cardiologist and director of integrative medicine, New York University School of Medicine, New York City. He is author of *Magnificent Magnesium: Your Essential Key to a Healthy Heart & More.*

Do calcium supplements cause heart failure?

Calcium supplements can be dangerous if not taken with magnesium. On its own, calcium causes contraction of heart cells—one study found that it doubles heart attack risk. Magnesium counters calcium's contracting effect and also stops calcium from forming plaque and causing atherosclerosis (hardening of the arteries). The ratio of calcium to magnesium should be 2:1 or lower—that is, 1,000 mg of calcium to 500 mg or more of magnesium. Use magnesium dimalate so that the supplement does not cause diarrhea. Jigsaw is a good slow-release formula available through *Amazon.com*.

5 Weird Fruits with Amazing Health Benefits

Chris Kilham, an instructor of ethnobotany at University of Massachusetts, Amherst. He is author of *Kava: Medicine Hunting in Paradise. MedicineHunter.com*

If you crave something new and want to get the most nutritional bang for your buck, try these "weird" fruits. They often are available at natural-foods markets such as Whole

Foods—and even at some "regular" supermarkets. These fruits may look a little strange—and the flavors definitely will be unfamiliar. But they have some remarkable health benefits—and you will discover some fascinating flavors that you never knew existed.

ARONIA

Even though it is native to the US, most people have never heard of aronia. Its nickname, chokeberry, suggests why it's more obscure than other berries. It's tart!

Don't let a little mouth-pucker put you off. The chokeberry has more antioxidant activity than any of the regular "superberries," including cranberries (see box), blueberries and strawberries. Research suggests that chokeberries may lower blood sugar and increase the body's production of insulin—helpful even for people who don't have diabetes because stabilizing blood sugar reduces the tendency for weight gain. Compounds in the berries have been linked to tumor inhibition, including tumors of the breast, colon and skin.

Chokeberries also are high in *catechins*, one of the high-powered substances in green tea. Catechins and related compounds have been shown to be very good for cardiovascular health, in part because they reduce arterial inflammation and the risk for clots.

The berries sometimes are available fresh but most often are frozen. Add them to yogurt or smoothies. If you wish, you can sweeten them with a touch of sugar, honey or agave nectar. The sugar offsets the tartness—it "opens up" the flavor and makes it more satisfying.

BURITI

This fruit is harvested from Amazonian palm trees that can tower more than 100 feet. Buriti can be peeled and eaten raw, although the firm flesh is somewhat similar to a sweet potato. It is tastier and softer when soaked in water and then put in a food processor or blender with a little water and sugar to make a creamy drink.

Buriti provides high levels of carotenoids that transform to vitamin A in the body, along with tocopherols, forms of vitamin E. Research has shown that people who get plenty of vitamin E from foods (not from supplements) tend to have lower rates of heart disease and some cancers.

Not So Weird But Super-Good for You: Cranberries

Cranberries contain *proanthocyanidins* (PACs), compounds that help prevent infection-causing bacteria from adhering to tissues in the urinary tract, thus helping to prevent urinary-tract infections.

Men, take note: Cranberries can make life a little easier if you have benign prostatic hyperplasia, enlargement of the prostate gland that can make urination difficult—and way too frequent.

A study of men in their 60s found that those who were given a cranberry extract had improved urinary symptoms, including improvements in their flow rate. The men also had lower levels of prostate-specific antigen (PSA), an enzyme associated with prostate cancer.

Regarding drinking cranberry juice, I feel that there is not enough good data to support that the juice works for urinary tract problems or for prostate disorders. It's better to eat whole cranberries. Simmer the cranberries in a little water…add a little sugar to subdue the tartness…and continue cooking until the berries burst.

—Chris Kilham

DRAGON FRUIT

You might recoil the first time you see this exotic-looking fruit. It looks like a cross between a pomegranate and an iguana. Once you slice through the fleshy protrusions on the skin, you will see that the ugliness is on the surface. The flesh inside might be white, yellow or blue, freckled with generous amounts of what appear to be poppy seeds. It has a delicate taste that some compare to kiwifruit or some melons and can be eaten raw. Dragon fruit is a rich source of antioxidants, including catechins and lycopene. Lycopene is especially important for men because it reduces risk for prostate cancer.

GAC

Gac, which is native to Vietnam, is a mango-size fruit with deep reddish-orange flesh. The color indicates very high levels of beta-carotene, the same potent antioxidant that you get from carrots—except that gac has about 10 times more. The zeaxanthin (another antioxidant) in gac has been linked to a reduced risk for macular degeneration, a serious eye disease. The fruit is loaded with lycopene, with about 70 times more than that in a tomato.

The flavor of the raw fruit has been compared to that of a slightly sweet cucumber. In Vietnam and other Asian countries, the pulp and seeds usually are cooked with a gelatinous form of rice and served during special events.

You can make the same dish with glutinous rice (available in Asian markets), gac fruit, coconut milk, sugar and a dash of red wine. For a recipe, search for "xoi gac" at *TheRavenous Couple.com*.

AÇAÍ BERRY

You may have heard of this one, but it is so good for you that it bears repeating. The most common form of açaí is the juice. But in Brazil, its home country, açaí (ah-sa-yee) is eaten fresh. The fruits are mashed to separate the seeds from the flesh. The mashed fruit is mixed with the Brazilian equivalent of granola, sweetened with a little sugar and served with banana slices.

Açaí is rich in anthocyanins, antioxidants that help reduce premature cell aging and may reduce the intestinal inflammation that accompanies inflammatory bowel disease. Anthocyanins are common in fruits with red and purple colors such as grapes and berries, but açaí has far more than any other food.

You might find fresh or frozen açaí berries in specialty stores, but if all you can find is the juice, look for one where açaí is the first ingredient on the label.

The Quick, Powerful Workout You're Probably Not Getting

Wayne L. Westcott, PhD, a professor of exercise science at Quincy College in Quincy, Massachusetts, and a strength-training consultant for the American Council on Exercise and the American Senior Fitness Association. He is also coauthor of several books, including *Strength Training Past 50*.

Until recently, fitness gurus have advised people to "take the stairs" mainly as a substitute for do-nothing elevator rides.

Now: Stair-climbing is becoming increasingly popular as a workout that's readily accessible (stairs are everywhere)…often climate-controlled (indoor stairs)…and free.

It burns more calories than walking…strengthens every muscle in the legs…and is good for your bones as well as your cardiovascular system. It may even extend your life span.

Compelling research: A study found that participants who averaged eight flights of stairs a day had a death rate over a 16-year period that was about one-third lower than those who didn't exercise—and more than 20% lower than that of people who merely walked.

A CONCENTRATED CLIMB

Walking is mainly a horizontal movement, with an assist from forward momentum. Stair-climbing is a vertical exercise. Your body weight is lifted straight up, against gravity. Climbing stairs also involves more muscles—in the calves, buttocks and the fronts and backs of the thighs—than walking. Even the arms get a workout. Canadian researchers found that it required double the exertion of walking on level ground—and 50% more than walking up an incline.

As a weight-loss tool, stair-climbing is hard to beat. An hour of climbing (for a 160-pound person) will burn about 650 calories. That compares with 400 calories an hour for a 15-minute-mile "power walk"…and 204 calories for a leisurely stroll.

Eating a Big Breakfast Spurs Weight Loss

Over a 12-week period, obese women who consumed most of their 1,400 allotted daily calories during breakfast lost an average of 17.8 pounds and three inches from their waists. Women who consumed most of their calories during dinner lost an average of 7.3 pounds and 1.4 inches from their waists. Breakfast eaters also showed better glucose control and decreased triglyceride levels.

Study of 93 obese women by researchers at Tel Aviv University, Wolfson Medical Center, Holong, Israel, and Hebrew University of Jerusalem, published in Obesity.

IT'S EASY TO START

Inconvenience is one of the biggest barriers to exercise. It sometimes feels like a hassle to change into workout clothes and drive to a health club...or even exercise at home. But you can always find a set of stairs—in your neighborhood, at work, at the mall or at home.

You don't need fancy workout gear to climb stairs (uncarpeted stairs are preferred). Because it doesn't involve side-to-side movements, you don't necessarily need to invest in specialized shoes. You can do it in any pair of athletic shoes or even work shoes, as long as they don't have high heels.

HOW TO CLIMB

When getting started, begin with a single flight of stairs. When that feels easy, take additional flights or increase the intensity by going a little faster. Work up to five minutes, then slowly increase that to 10, 15 and 20 minutes, if possible, three times a week. *Other tips...*

•**Keep your upper body straight.** There's a natural tendency to lean forward when you climb stairs, particularly because a forward-leaning position feels easier. Remind yourself to stand straight when you're climbing and descending. It will give your legs a better workout...strengthen your abdominal and other core muscles...and help improve your balance.

Stair-Stepping Without a Staircase

If you want to climb stairs without using a staircase, consider buying a commercial "stepper," such as those from StairMaster. Some have components that work the arms as well as the legs. Stair-steppers, however, don't provide the benefit of actual stair-climbing, which uses more muscles because of the descents. These machines can be costly (at least $2,500 for a new one but much less for a used one on Craigslist or eBay). They typically hold up for years of hard use.

Caution: I avoid "mini-steppers" that sell for as little as $60. They have hydraulics, bands or other systems that cause the steps to go up and down, but the equipment usually breaks quickly.

Better Way to Get Protein

Healthy adults whose protein intake was spread evenly throughout the day had 25% higher levels of muscle growth and repair than those who ate most of their daily protein with dinner—a typical eating pattern. The recommended dietary allowance (RDA) for protein is at least 46 g daily for women and 56 g for men. (If you have kidney disease, ask your doctor for advice on protein intake.)

Douglas Paddon-Jones, PhD, professor of nutrition, The University of Texas Medical Branch at Galveston.

•**Swing your arms.** You don't need an exaggerated swing, but keep your arms moving—it helps with balance and provides exercise for your arms and shoulders. You'll often see stair-climbers with their hands or arms on the rails. It's OK to use the rails if you need the support, but it reduces the intensity of the exercise. It also causes the stooped posture that you want to avoid.

•**One step at a time.** Unless you're a competitive stair-climber, you'll probably do best by taking just one step at a time. Ascending stairs is a concentric exercise that increases muscle power...it's also the part of the workout that gives most of the cardiovascular benefit.

Coming down the stairs is an eccentric (also called "negative") movement that puts more stress on the muscles and increases strength.

Important: Descend the stairs slowly, and keep "jolts" to a minimum. It sounds counterintuitive, but the descents cause more muscle soreness than the climbs.

You can take two steps at a time on the ascent—if your balance is good and you're bored with single-step plodding. The faster pace will increase the intensity of your workout, particularly when you give your arms a more exaggerated swing. To minimize jolts and maximize safety, however, stick to single steps on the descent.

TO END YOUR WORKOUT

The "Figure 4" stretch is a great way to conclude a stair-climbing workout. It stretches the calves, hamstrings, gluteals, low back and upper back.

What to do: While sitting on the floor with your right leg straight, bend your left leg so that your left foot touches your right thigh. Slowly reach your right hand toward your right foot. Then grasp your foot, ankle or lower leg, and hold for 20 seconds. Repeat on the other side.

Caution: Stair-climbing should be avoided if you have serious arthritis or other joint problems. It's less jarring than jogging, but it's still a weight-bearing exercise that can stress the joints. People with joint issues might do better with supported exercises, such as cycling, rowing or swimming.

Before taking up stair-climbing as a form of exercise, check with your doctor if you're middle-aged or older, have arthritis, a history of heart or lung disease or if you've been mainly sedentary and aren't confident of your muscle strength—or your sense of balance.

You Can Exercise Less and Be Just as Healthy

Barry A. Franklin, PhD, director of Preventive Cardiology and Cardiac Rehabilitation at William Beaumont Hospital in Royal Oak, Michigan. He is coauthor, with Joseph C. Piscatella, of *109 Things You Can Do to Prevent, Halt & Reverse Heart Disease.*

Do you struggle to fit the recommended amount of exercise into your busy schedule?

Well, what if we told you that the amount of exercise needed to reap health benefits might be less than you think? Maybe you could free up some of your workout time for other activities that are important to you and beneficial to your health—like playing with your kids or grandkids, volunteering for a favorite charity or cooking healthful meals.

THE LATEST IN EXERCISE RESEARCH

A recent study published in the *Journal of the American College of Cardiology* found that people lived longest when they ran, on average, for 30 minutes or more, five days a week. Surprisingly, that research also showed that people who jogged at an easy pace for as little as five to 10 minutes a day had virtually the same survival benefits as those who pushed themselves harder or longer.

Also surprising: A study recently done at Oregon State University found that one- and two-minute bouts of activity that add up to 30 minutes or more per day, such as pacing while talking on the telephone, doing housework or doing sit-ups during TV commercials, may reduce blood pressure and cholesterol and improve health as effectively as a structured exercise program.

HOW TO EXERCISE SMARTER, NOT HARDER

Here are four strategies to help you exercise more efficiently...

• **Recognize that some exercise is always better than none.** Even though exercise guidelines from the Centers for Disease Control and Prevention (CDC) call for at least 150 minutes of moderate exercise each week, you'll do well even at lower levels.

A *Lancet* study found that people who walked for just 15 minutes a day had a 14% reduction in death over an average of eight years. Good daily exercises include not only walking but working in the yard, swimming, riding a bike, etc.

If you're among the multitudes of Americans who have been sedentary in recent years, you'll actually gain the most. Simply making the transition from horrible fitness to below average can reduce your overall risk for premature death by 20% to 40%.

Breakfast Before a Workout

While vigorous exercise after a full meal might cause you to feel nauseated or bloated, you can certainly grab a banana, a handful of trail mix or a granola bar to eat before a morning workout. Or you can eat part of your breakfast before you exercise and enjoy the rest afterward.

Some people think they'll burn more body fat if they avoid eating before working out, but that's not true. You will lose body fat if you use more calories than you consume by the end of the day.

Nancy Clark, RD, sports nutritionist in private practice in Boston, and author of Nancy Clark's Sports Nutrition Guidebook. NancyClarkRD.com

•**Go for a run instead of a walk.** The intensity, or associated energy cost, of running is greater than walking. Therefore, running (or walking up a grade or incline) is better for the heart than walking—and it's easier to work into a busy day because you can get equal benefits in less time.

For cardiovascular health, a five-minute run (5.5 mph to 8 mph) is equal to a 15-minute walk (2 mph to 3.5 mph)…and a 25-minute run equals a 105-minute walk.

A 2014 study of runners found that their risk of dying from heart disease was 45% lower than nonrunners over a 15-year follow-up. In fact, running can add, on average, three extra years to your life.

Caution: If you take running seriously, you still should limit your daily workouts to 60 minutes or less, no more than five days a week. (See below for the dangers of overdoing it.) People with heart symptoms or severely compromised heart function should avoid running. If you have joint problems, check with your doctor.

•**Ease into running.** Don't launch into a running program until you're used to exercise. Make it progressive. Start by walking slowly—say, at about 2 mph. Gradually increase it to 3 mph…then to 3.5 mph, etc. After two or three months, if you are symptom-free during fast walking, you can start to run (slowly at first).

•**Aim for the "upper-middle."** I do not recommend high-intensity workouts for most adults. Strive to exercise at a level you would rate between "fairly light" and "somewhat hard."

How to tell: Check your breathing. It will be slightly labored when you're at a good level of exertion. Nevertheless, you should still be able to carry on a conversation.

Important: Get your doctor's OK before starting vigorous exercise—and don't ignore potential warning symptoms. It's normal to be somewhat winded or to have a little leg discomfort. However, you should never feel dizzy, experience chest pain or have extreme shortness of breath. If you have any of these symptoms, stop exercise immediately, and see your doctor before resuming activity.

TOO MUCH OF A GOOD THING?

Most people who run for more than an hour a day, five days a week, are in very good shape. Would they be healthier if they doubled the distance—or pushed themselves even harder? Not necessarily. *Risks linked to distance running include…*

•**Acute right-heart overload.** Researchers at William Beaumont Hospital who looked at distance runners before and immediately after marathon running found that they often had transient decreases in the pumping ability of the right ventricle and elevations of the same enzymes (such as troponin) that increase during a heart attack.

•**Atrial fibrillation.** People who exercise intensely for more than five hours a week may be more likely to develop atrial fibrillation, a heart-rhythm disturbance that can trigger a stroke.

•**Coronary plaque.** Despite their favorable coronary risk factor profiles, distance runners can have increased amounts of coronary artery calcium and plaque as compared with their less active counterparts.

Watch out: Many hard-core runners love marathons, triathlons and other competitive events. Be careful. The emotional rush from competition increases levels of epinephrine and other "stress" hormones. These hormones, combined with hard exertion, can transiently increase heart risks.

Of course, all this doesn't mean that you shouldn't enjoy a daily run…or a few long ones—just don't overdo it!

When to Lift Weights

Don't lift weights before cardio exercise. People who did upper-body exercises before cycling had a 35% decline in endurance.

Possible reason: Working the shoulders, arms, chest and back may also tire the legs as lactate and other fatigue-related substances move through the bloodstream.

Study by researchers at Nottingham Trent University, Nottingham, England, published in *Medicine & Science in Sports & Exercise.*

Emotional Well-Being

Are You "Almost Depressed"?

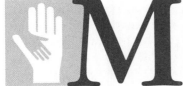

Most people know if they're suffering from deep depression. But what's that vaguely uncomfortable, empty feeling you may have had lately? You're not miserable, but it's as if the vitality has been sucked out of your life.

Though it often goes undiagnosed, so-called "almost depression" may have snuck up on you. It can prevent you from enjoying your leisure activities and leave you feeling unsatisfied with your family life, friendships and work.

Don't pooh-pooh it: You may be tempted to ignore these often subtle, though persistent, feelings of discontent. But don't. Almost depression can throw you into a downward spiral that deepens into serious depression—a condition that may increase your risk for chronic physical ailments such as heart disease and dementia.

The good news is that almost depression responds well to some surprising, life-affirming strategies that don't necessarily involve the conventional treatments (such as medication and/or therapy) that are usually prescribed for depression.

What you need to know about almost depression…

LOOKING FOR CLUES

If you have almost depression, life may generally seem bland and gray. You haven't stopped eating, but nothing tastes very good. You still laugh at jokes…but just to be polite. These are red flags that the brain circuits responsible for processing your feelings of pleasure (the brain's "reward system") may have shifted into low gear—this is widely considered to be an underlying cause of almost depression.

Often, close friends and family members can see changes first. If you think you may be

Jefferson Prince, MD, an instructor in psychiatry at Harvard Medical School, Boston, and director of child psychiatry at MassGeneral Hospital for Children in Salem, Massachusetts. He is coauthor of *Almost Depressed: Is My (or My Loved One's) Unhappiness a Problem?*

almost depressed, ask someone you trust for his/her candid opinion. For more signs of almost depression, see the self-test box.

GETTING BACK ON TRACK

If you're like most people, you can pull yourself out of almost depression—the trick is to take steps to rev up your brain's sluggish reward system. *The best ways to do that...**

• **Get up and at 'em.** Idleness due to illness or an emotional setback is a common trigger of almost depression. Fortunately, scientists are now finding more and more evidence that exercise improves mood, possibly by altering brain chemistry. In several studies, regular workouts were as effective as antidepressants. But of course, the longer you are inactive, the harder it is to get going—and a trip to the gym may sound impossible.

Best approach: Start by adding just a bit more activity to your day...the 10-minute walk you take is far better than the strenuous workout you avoid. Tomorrow, you may want to take a longer walk or do some gardening. Put yourself in motion...add a bit more activity week by week...and see what happens. It will be good!

• **Put more meaning in your life.** Do you often wonder, "What's all this for?" Almost depression can be a sign that you lack a sense of purpose for your life. Take a good look at

---

Almost Depressed? Take the Self-Test

Do any of the following statements apply to you?

- **I get more frustrated than usual over little things.**
- **Instead of having fun with friends, I avoid them.**
- **I haven't been sleeping well lately.**
- **Nothing tastes very good.**
- **I would like to "stop the world" and take a break from everything.**
- **Nothing seems very funny (or interesting or exciting) these days.**
- **I get irritated more easily than I used to.**
- **I'm less interested in sex.**
- **I just want to be left alone.**
- **I have trouble concentrating on books or TV.**
- **I feel tired for no reason.**

If two or more of these statements apply to you, you're likely almost depressed.

---

your values. For some people, family comes first, and for others, it's career, spiritual growth or health. The key is, any of these can give you a sense of purpose.

Best approach: Identify your two or three top values. And be honest with yourself. You may think "helping others" should be your ultimate concern, but if, say, financial security actually takes priority, there's nothing wrong with making that your goal.

Then start including activities to promote these two or three values every day. Also look for small actions that promote your values. To "improve the lives of others," you don't have to volunteer at a soup kitchen—a smile or doing a favor for a stranger counts, too. Give yourself credit for these moments.

• **Let your creativity run wild.** When you scratch beneath the surface, most people with almost depression have bottled-up emotions. Expressing these dark feelings through a creative outlet is liberating—and healing.

Don't worry about being talented...just allow yourself to tap into your creative side.

To express yourself: Set aside 20 minutes to write on a computer or by hand about something that's bothering you. Don't edit your feelings—no one will see this but you. In fact, you don't ever need to look at your writing again... the benefit is in the process, not the product.

The next day, write down a story about your life. It's human nature to see life as a narrative with heroes, villains and victims. Being almost depressed puts you in a story that isn't going so well. So go ahead and rewrite your personal narrative. Create a story where the main character has problems like yours but works things out—perhaps through personal change

---

*If you suspect that you're almost depressed, and there's no improvement after trying the strategies in this article, see your doctor for advice. Many physical conditions (such as diabetes, lung disease and cancer) can cause depressive symptoms, as can some blood pressure and cholesterol drugs, antibiotics and other medications. If none of these apply to your situation, your doctor may refer you to a mental-health professional, such as a psychiatrist or psychologist.

or new insights. The character you invent may teach you some useful strategies—and you will emerge happier.

If you're more of a visual person, you can draw or paint images that will help unleash trapped emotions. Whatever approach you choose, allow your creativity to flourish.

Loneliness Harms Your Health

Gregory T. Eells, PhD, associate director of Gannett Health Services and director of Counseling and Psychological Services at Cornell University in Ithaca, New York.

O h, those long, lonesome days…and nights! Most of us occasionally feel that way. But what if you are lonely more often than not? Plenty of people are.

Why loneliness deserves our attention: While loneliness has long been known to exact a psychological toll, studies are increasingly showing that persistent loneliness also has a profound effect on one's physical health.

Important recent finding: Persistent loneliness is being linked to a growing list of health problems, including insomnia, cardiovascular disease and Alzheimer's disease. Even more startling is the fact that loneliness raises the risk for premature death among adults age 50 and older by 14%.

So for the sake of your health—and happiness—here's what you need to know about loneliness…

ARE YOU LONELY?

While it's easy to assume that anyone who is struggling with loneliness would know that he/she is lonely, that's often not the case. For many people, that extreme sense of social disconnection—the feeling that no one really knows you and what your life is like—is so familiar and constant that they don't even realize that they're lonely. And friends and family might not necessarily recognize that a friend or loved one is lonely.

Of course, most of us do need some time by ourselves, and solitude—the opportunity to think and feel quietly without the distraction and demands of other people—is rightly valued. But loneliness is very different.

Here are some red flags that you may be lonely: You spend hours of alone time on the computer (perhaps surfing the Internet or following the activities of "friends" on social media sites)…you have pangs of anger or envy when others around you are happy…and/or you feel a vague sense of dissatisfaction even when you are spending time with other people.

But just as you can be alone without being lonely, you can be lonely without being alone. Someone who looks happy and well connected from the outside—the person who invites 20 of his/her closest friends to a party—may still feel empty and isolated inside. Nor are romantic relationships or marriage a surefire defense against loneliness. Feeling uncomfortably alone and alienated is a frequent complaint of troubled couples.

WHY IT'S BAD FOR YOU

The connection between loneliness and depression has been established for quite some time. But only recently have researchers discovered that loneliness itself is linked to elevated blood pressure, increased stress hormones and impaired immune function.

Loneliness also exacts a huge toll when people turn to unhealthy behaviors to avoid the pain it brings—if we don't try to drink it away, for example, then we might spend far too many hours at work to busy ourselves rather than face painful time alone.

HOW TO OVERCOME LONELINESS

Alleviating loneliness is like falling asleep or growing a garden—you can't force it to happen, but you can create conditions that encourage it to unfold. *Here's how…*

SECRET #1: Share more about yourself. Sharing the details of your life with others and showing vulnerability will foster deep connections and minimize loneliness. This may feel risky. After all, you might run up against rejection or disapproval, but such fears are usually groundless. Nothing ventured, nothing gained!

Example: You might ask a friend to have coffee and share with him/her discipline problems you are having with your teenage daughter.

SECRET #2: Make room for "small" connections. While quantity doesn't replace quality in relationships, momentary contacts do add to your sense of being part of the social world around you.

Exchange a few extra words with the clerk at your local convenience store, and smile at those you pass on the street. These pleasant interactions will prime you for deeper, more meaningful ones with close friends and family.

SECRET #3: Be part of something big. Meaningful activity will bring you in contact with like-minded others. OK, so maybe volunteering in a hospital or soup kitchen isn't your thing. Perhaps you would rather get involved with your local political party…tutor a child who is struggling in school…join a gardening club…or get involved at your house of worship.

Your local newspaper and websites such as *Meetup.com* and *Groups.Yahoo.com* are great resources for finding local groups involved in a wide variety of activities that might interest you.

Show up for whatever new activity you choose for several weeks, and if you're not feeling more connected by the end of that time, then look for something else that might be more to your liking.

SECRET #4: Don't hole up by yourself when your life changes. For most people, significant changes such as job loss, the death of a loved one, divorce or retirement provide a good excuse to shut out others—and the perfect setup for loneliness. But don't let the natural tendency to withdraw at such times go on for more than a few months.

Challenge yourself to set up two outings a week with a friend, neighbor or family member to get yourself out of the house.

SECRET #5: Consider getting a pet. Pets are more than mere company…dogs, cats, birds and even guinea pigs are, after all, fellow creatures that have their own feelings and are often responsive to ours. These are real connections, too.

If you don't have the time to care for a pet full time, consider sharing a pet. There are several sites (such as *CityDogShare.org*) that enable you

---

Better Depression Treatment

In a recent finding, among people with both depression and insomnia, 87% of those whose insomnia was successfully treated with cognitive behavioral insomnia therapy also recovered from their depression, whether they were taking an antidepressant or not.

Possible explanation: Regular sleep-wake cycles are necessary to regulate neurotransmitters in the brain and stave off depression.

Colleen E. Carney, PhD, director, Sleep and Depression Laboratory, Ryerson University, Toronto, Ontario, Canada.

---

to meet people near you who are interested in doing this. Or volunteer at your local animal shelter.

Both of these activities are great ways to connect with animals and animal lovers.

Mental Health Care Is Now More Affordable

Money.com

Insurance plans that are bought on state insurance exchanges must include mental health care as one of the 10 mandated benefits under the Affordable Care Act. Large employers' health plans that include mental health coverage must treat it like other medical care in terms of prior authorizations, number of annual visits and other factors. Companies' employee-assistance programs (EAPs) often provide five or six sessions of no-cost counseling—and about three-quarters of companies offer EAPs. But finding a therapist on your own still can be challenging and costly. Because of low reimbursement rates and billing issues, only 55% of psychiatrists accept private insurance, compared with 89% of doctors in all other medical specialties. Coverage under Medicare also has improved. Medicare beneficiaries pay 20% of mental health care costs in 2014, down from 50% in earlier years.

PTSD: A Hidden Danger After a Serious Illness

Robert London, MD, practicing physician/psychiatrist for more than three decades, who is on the professorial staff of NYU School of Medicine in New York City. *Dr RobertLondon.com*

If you've been successfully treated for a serious illness, you're likely to feel so much relief at having dodged a bullet that you may downplay or dismiss the emotional trauma following your medical care.

An overlooked problem: Survivors of a traumatic medical situation—for example, a stay in the intensive care unit (ICU) or treatment for a heart attack or cancer—are at increased risk for post-traumatic stress disorder (PTSD).

Surprising fact: PTSD can strike weeks— or even years—after an illness. Symptoms may include nightmares, flashbacks, irritability and feeling detached (depersonalization) and emotionally numb. Ignoring PTSD after a serious medical situation carries its own risks. Without treatment, symptoms worsen, impacting the sufferer's social, family and work relationships.

HOW TO FIGHT PTSD

Anyone who suffers PTSD after a serious illness—or wants to help prevent it—can benefit from one or more of the following…*

• **Cognitive behavioral therapy** typically involves weekly visits with a therapist for several months during which sufferers learn to reprocess the traumatic events by gaining a new perspective on the past trauma and improving skills to cope with the distressing thoughts that arise from it.

• **Prolonged exposure therapy** involves the patient revisiting the specific trauma in a safe environment through guided imagery until it's no longer distressing.

To find a psychologist or psychiatrist trained in these therapies, consult the Association for Behavioral and Cognitive Therapies, *ABCT.org.*

• **Hypnosis** helps people reprocess traumatic memories first by using relaxation strategies and

*These therapies are generally covered by health insurance. Check with your insurer.

then a series of visual images to slowly reintroduce the trauma. This is usually coupled with pleasant visualizations that reduce the anxiety of the traumatic memory. Patients generally require four to 16 sessions. To find a qualified hypnotherapist near you, consult the American Society of Clinical Hypnosis, *ASCH.net.*

Other therapies to consider…

• **EMDR.** With eye movement desensitization and reprocessing (EMDR), the therapist asks the patient to perform certain eye movements, such as following the therapist's finger from side to side, while the patient talks about the trauma. The exercise is then repeated, this time focusing on positive memories to help the brain reprocess the trauma so that the emotional distress is decreased. EMDR usually requires four to 12 sessions and has been approved as a PTSD treatment by the US Department of Defense. To find an EMDR-trained practitioner, consult the EMDR International Association, *EMDRIA.org.*

• **Medications.** Antidepressants known as selective serotonin reuptake inhibitors (SSRIs), which work by raising the level of the mood-boosting chemical serotonin in the brain, have been shown to help with PTSD, especially if depression is present. *Sertraline* (Zoloft) and *paroxetine* (Paxil) are two SSRIs that have been approved by the FDA specifically for PTSD.

• **Support groups.** Most PTSD sufferers find it helpful to join a support group of other people who have had similar experiences. Family members may also find comfort from support groups aimed at those caring for someone with PTSD. To find a support group near you, check the psychology/psychiatry department at your local hospital.

SPECIFIC STEPS THAT HELP

In addition to the steps above, the following strategies help prevent or treat PTSD in patients after…

• **An ICU stay.** Even though most ICU patients receive lifesaving care, ICUs are high-intensity settings with constant noise and bright lights, which can further traumatize an already vulnerable, perhaps disoriented patient. One-quarter of those admitted to a hospital ICU have symptoms of PTSD after their stays.

To prevent PTSD in ICU patients: Unlike most PTSD survivors, who have flashbacks about actual events, ICU patients often suffer flashbacks about delusions or hallucinations that occurred during their stays—a relatively common problem among these patients.

What helps...

ICU diaries, in which nurses and family members record what's happening daily while the patient is hospitalized, are one way to reduce the risk for PTSD. After discharge, the patients are given the diary to review with a nurse or family member whenever the patient feels anxious. This process helps establish what actually occurred during the patient's stay rather than focusing on the frightening details of their misperceptions.

Music therapy, which relaxes and distracts seriously ill patients during the hospital stay, helps reduce the likelihood of lasting psychological trauma. If permitted, a patient could listen to favorite music through headphones.

•**Heart attack.** Around 12% of heart attack sufferers develop PTSD, and those who do are more likely to experience a second heart attack. Some heart attack survivors may go into a state of anxiety or panic whenever they feel shortness of breath, fearing that another heart attack is on the way. This often creates a vicious circle of symptoms and worry.

To prevent heart-related PTSD: Heart patients should seek counseling to learn calming strategies such as relaxation techniques. Heart patients who have a lot of support from their families and friends—especially so that the patient can ask for help when needed—are also less likely to develop PTSD. Having this type of readily available assistance appears to reduce the feelings of vulnerability and helplessness, which so often occur in heart attack survivors.

•**Cancer.** PTSD can follow treatment for any type of cancer. As with other conditions, the more intense or frightening the situation, the higher the chance for PTSD.

To prevent cancer-related PTSD: For some patients, learning all the specifics of their disease from their doctors can help reduce anxiety, while others prefer to know as little as possible. In either case, talk to your doctor about your risk for recurrence and steps you can take to monitor for any early signs that the cancer may be returning.

As with other serious illnesses, family support is crucial in helping cancer patients readjust psychologically after treatment.

A Surprising Way to Handle Difficult People

Judith Orloff, MD, assistant clinical professor of psychiatry at UCLA. She is author of the national best-seller The Ecstasy of Surrender: 12 Surprising Ways Letting Go Can Empower Your Life *upon which this article is based. DrJudithOrloff.com*

When faced with difficult behavior at work or with family and friends, most people tend to revert to automatic reactions. They cave in...get defensive or aggressive...or dig in their heels and refuse to budge.

None of these reactions produces satisfying results, but they are the only alternatives most of us are aware of.

A more effective way to deal with difficult people is to surrender—to let go of the need to control a situation and let go of the illusion that you can compel someone to change. Surrendering means accepting a person or situation as is. This is very different from caving in, which means giving up your needs simply to make peace without any effort to try to create positive change.

Surrender is an active choice to accept what life brings you, to be flexible rather than rigid and to see past a momentary block to a greater breakthrough beyond. Surrendering allows you to let go of overthinking and second-guessing.

PRACTICING SURRENDER

Surrender often needs to be learned and practiced and is easier to do when you are only mildly stressed. With practice, you can learn to let go even in more challenging encounters. Simple ways to practice...

•**Drink a glass of water or juice—slowly.** Savor the sensation of quenching your thirst.

Enjoy the fact that there is nothing you have to do but sip and be refreshed.

• **Observe water.** Watch the water in a fountain or creek. Notice how water doesn't keep bumping into the same boulder over and over again—it flows around the obstacle. Water can teach you how to flow.

• **Appreciate your body's natural joyful responses.** Let out a hearty laugh. Put on your favorite music, and dance around the living room. Let yourself feel awe at a sunset or laughing child. Don't choke off those urges—enjoy them.

DIFFICULT SITUATIONS

In most cases, difficult people aren't trying to make your life miserable—they are just preoccupied with their own frustrations and needs. *Guidelines for dealing with difficult behavior...*

• **Pause.** If you feel yourself getting angry or tense, don't say anything. Let go of the urge to express your immediate reaction. Instead, take a few slow breaths to calm your stress. Count to 10 or 20 if it helps you postpone action.

• **Listen without interrupting.** Let go of the need to direct the discussion. Hear the other person out.

Exception: If the person is being verbally abusive, cut off the abuse at once. Verbal abuse includes personal attacks that target your worth—such as *You're a terrible mother* or *You can't do anything right*. In cases like these, break in and set boundaries in a calm voice.

PTSD Link to Food Addiction

Post-traumatic stress is linked to food addiction. Women with the largest number of symptoms of post-traumatic stress disorder (PTSD) are almost three times as likely to develop addictions to food as women without the symptoms. PTSD symptoms include flashbacks, nightmares, difficulty relaxing and extreme anxiety. Mental health–care professionals who are aware that PTSD and food addiction may occur together can better tailor treatment to patients.

Study of 49,408 women by researchers at University of Minnesota, Minneapolis, published in JAMA Psychiatry.

Example: "That kind of statement is unacceptable. If you continue like this, I will leave the room."

• **Don't argue.** You may have the strong desire to state all the evidence that shows you are right, but defensiveness in charged situations doesn't change anyone's mind—it just fuels the conflict.

• **Empathize.** Make a genuine effort to see the situation from the other person's point of view. People who behave badly are suffering in some way. This doesn't excuse their behavior, but once you recognize that they are trying to avoid pain or anxiety, letting go becomes easier.

• **Be willing to concede a point.** Even if you agree with only 1% of what the person is saying, acknowledge that point of agreement. You can say, "That's a good point, and I'm going to think about it."

Also be willing to apologize for your own difficult behavior.

Example: "I'm sorry I snapped at you. I didn't act with love." Too many relationships disintegrate because no one will give ground. Let go of the need to protect your turf. Look at the larger picture—which is more important, this battle or the relationship?

• **Use a pleasant, neutral tone.** No matter how carefully you choose your words, they will get you nowhere if your voice has an edge of irritation, condescension or sarcasm. Practice a neutral tone by role-playing with a friend until you are able to keep the edge out of your voice.

THREE DIFFICULT TYPES

Here's how to deal with three common types of difficult people...

• **The Guilt Tripper.** Blamers and martyrs activate your insecurity to get what they want. Their sentences often start with, "If it weren't for you..."or "I'm the only one..." *What to do...*

• Make a matter-of-fact statement. Tell guilt trippers that those comments hurt your feelings and that you would be grateful if they would stop making them. If you don't get emotional, most guilt trippers will lose interest in baiting you.

•**The Control Freak.** Control freaks micromanage, give unsolicited advice, voice strong opinions relentlessly and are rarely satisfied. *What to do…*

•Don't try to control a controller or win over the person to your way of thinking—it's a waste of time. Say, "Thank you for your input. I'll take it into consideration" or "I value your advice, but I want to work through this myself."

Be patient. Control freaks don't give up easily, so repetition is key.

•**The Anger Addict.** Let go of the impulse to cower or to lash out in return. The more impulsively you react to someone else's rage, the more you reinforce the anger addict's aggressive behavior. Even if you are upset, stay as neutral as you can. Get centered before you respond.

If the anger addict is your boss, acknowledge the person's point of view. Say, "I can see why you would feel that way." Then bring the discussion back to a solution focus. Say in a calm tone, "I have a different take that I'd like to share" or "That's fine—tell me what you need, and I'll do it."

Look for another job if you can, because being the recipient of chronic anger takes a physical and mental toll. In the meantime—or if changing jobs is not possible—remind yourself that the rage is about the other person, not you.

If the anger addict is a spouse or family member, set limits. Say, "Your anger is hurting me. We have to find a better way to communicate" or "I care about you, but I shut down when you raise your voice. Let's talk about this when we can hear each other better." Later, when you are both calm, request a small, doable change.

Example of a small, doable change: "When we are in the midst of a disagreement, I propose that we each wait five seconds before saying anything. Would you be willing to try that?"

If the person doesn't try to change, observe how your health is affected. You may need to let go of the relationship to protect your well-being.

How to Break a Bad Habit

Richard O'Connor, PhD, a psychotherapist in private practice in Canaan, Connecticut, and New York City. He is author of *Rewire: Change Your Brain to Break Bad Habits, Overcome Addictions, Conquer Self-Destructive Behavior. UndoingDepression.com*

•**Spend a few days studying a bad habit you want to change.** Take note of the triggers of this habit—time of day, level of hunger, something someone has said, a memory, etc. Ask yourself what you can do about these triggers. Can you avoid some? Prevent some? Knowing your triggers can help you take positive actions (such as starting a new project) rather than negative actions (such as overeating).

•**Practice daily meditation to calm yourself** and help you shut out negative thoughts.

•**Practice willpower.** This is a skill, not a trait. Imagine it as a muscle in your brain that gets strengthened each time you use it.

Banish a Bad Mood—in Just Minutes!

Pierce Howard, PhD, managing director of research and development at the Center for Applied Cognitive Studies in Charlotte, North Carolina, a firm that provides consulting services in leadership. He is author of *The Owner's Manual for the Brain: The Ultimate Guide to Peak Mental Performance at All Ages. CentACS.com*

Depression is serious business and should be treated by a professional. But what if you're not depressed—perhaps just feeling a little blue or in a funk?

With the steps below, most people can escape a bad mood in a matter of minutes instead of toughing it out for hours or even an entire day or more. *To get started…*

CHECK IN WITH YOURSELF

•**How's your physical state?** Are you hungry? Thirsty? Tired? You may not think to ask yourself these questions, but any of these conditions can make you feel out of sorts.

• **Do a gut check.** Once your physical needs are taken care of, take a minute to ask yourself why you might be feeling down. An honest assessment of what's bugging you may reveal a way to actively address the problem.

Even if you identify the cause of your bad mood—maybe you're overworked, for example, or worried about a loved one's health—and can take steps to address the issue, your dark cloud might not lift immediately. *Other steps you can take to boost your mood…*

QUICK FEEL-GOOD TRICKS

• **Turn on some minor-key tunes.** Research shows that people who are bordering on depression tend to feel better after listening to music in a minor key—perhaps because happier, major keys prove too jarring to their emotional state.

Good choices: "Hey Jude" by The Beatles… "Bad Romance" by Lady Gaga…and *Piano Concerto in A Minor* by Edvard Grieg. If you find that this type of music doesn't lift your mood, switch to some up-tempo music such as Aaron Copland…most big-band music…and "Born to Run" by Bruce Springsteen. According to recent research, people are happier in both the short term and long term after listening to up-tempo music.

• **Take a brisk, five-minute walk outdoors.** Brisk walking gets your blood moving, which means more oxygen and energy-boosting glucose are getting to your brain. Five minutes is the minimum time needed, according to research, to produce mood-enhancing changes.

Walking outside helps most. That's because sunlight suppresses the production of the sleep hormone melatonin (making you feel less sluggish and more alert) and gives you a dose of energy-boosting vitamin D. The fresh air also may contain negative ions that attach themselves to particles in the atmosphere and act as air purifiers, allowing you to get more oxygen to your brain with each breath.

• **Eat a hamburger (really!).** "Comfort foods," such as ice cream, chocolate, cheese and pasta, produce a quick mood boost by encouraging the release of the neurotransmitter serotonin. But if you overdo it, you'll end up feeling bloated and tired.

What works better: When you're feeling down, eat some protein or complex carbohydrates. Good protein choices include a hamburger without the bun…nuts…eggs…and beans. Good complete carbohydrates include dark berries…bananas and a salad full of vegetables.

• **Use your words.** Using language triggers the pleasure pathway in the brain, but you don't need to have a gabfest if that's not in your nature. While some people find that having a conversation with a friend elevates their mood, others might prefer writing in a journal or composing a letter. Research has shown that the act of using language is soothing whether you're focusing on whatever is causing your bad mood or something unrelated.

• **Tweak your posture.** If you're slouching in your chair or staring down at the sidewalk while walking, you may be inadvertently prolonging the blues by inhibiting the blood and oxygen circulation in your body.

What to do: Pull your shoulders back and balance your head over your spine. When you are in perfect alignment, your ear, shoulder, hip, knee and ankle should form a vertical line when viewed from the side.

An App for Recovery

New smartphone app helps recovering alcoholics stay sober. Study participants who used the Addiction-Comprehensive Health Enhancement Support System (A-CHESS) were 65% more likely to abstain from alcohol in the year following their release from a treatment facility than people who did not use the app. A-CHESS issues daily support messages and asks questions that help counselors assess the person's sobriety. It also tracks users' locations and issues warnings when users are near familiar bars or liquor stores. Other apps are available, but A-CHESS is the first to undergo a large-scale clinical trial.

Study of about 350 people by researchers at University of Wisconsin, Madison, published in JAMA Psychiatry.

Join the Trees

Living in areas with fewer trees increases risk for depression. People living in areas with less than 10% "tree canopy" were much more likely to feel unhappy and anxious. In fact, poorer people living in greener areas generally were happier than richer people living in areas with few trees.

If you do not live near trees: Bring live plants into your office and home.

Survey of 2,500 people in 229 neighborhoods by researchers at University of Wisconsin School of Medicine and Public Health, Madison, published in *International Journal of Environmental Research and Public Health*.

•**Ditch the alarm clock.** Most people sleep in cycles lasting around 90 minutes, progressing from a light to deep sleep and back again. If you have your alarm set to go off in the later stages of your cycle, chances are you'll awaken in a disoriented, grumpy mood.

What to do: Try experimenting with your bedtime so that you wake naturally without using an alarm. If you go to bed early enough, you'll wake up on your own feeling refreshed after an optimal number of complete sleep cycles.

6 Foods Proven to Make You Happy

Tonia Reinhard, MS, RD, a registered dietitian and professor at Wayne State University in Detroit. She is author of *Superfoods: The Healthiest Foods on the Planet* and *Superjuicing: More Than 100 Nutritious Vegetable and Fruit Recipes*.

You can eat your way to a better mood! Certain foods and beverages have been proven to provide the raw materials that you need to feel sharper, more relaxed and just plain happier. *Best choices…*

HAPPY FOOD #1: CHOCOLATE

Chocolate contains specific chemical compounds known as *polyphenols*, which interact with neurotransmitters in the brain and reduce anxiety. An Australian study found that men and women who consumed the most chocolate polyphenols (in the form of a beverage) felt calmer and more content than those who consumed a placebo drink.

Chocolate also boosts serotonin, the same neurotransmitter affected by antidepressant medications. It triggers the release of dopamine and stimulates the "pleasure" parts of the brain.

Then there's the sensual side of chocolate—the intensity of the flavor and the melting sensation as it dissolves in your mouth. The satisfaction that people get from chocolate could be as helpful for happiness as its chemical composition.

Recommended amount: Aim for one ounce of dark chocolate a day. Most studies used dark chocolate with 70% cacao or more.

HAPPY FOOD #2: FISH

The omega-3s in fish accumulate in the brain and increase "membrane fluidity," the ability of brain-cell membranes to absorb nutrients and transmit chemical signals.

A study in *Archives of General Psychiatry* looked at patients diagnosed with depression who hadn't responded well to antidepressants. Those who were given 1,000 mg of EPA (a type of omega-3 fatty acid) daily for three months had significant improvements, including less anxiety and better sleep.

Recommended amount: Try to have at least two or three fish meals a week. Cold-water fish—such as sardines, mackerel and salmon—have the highest levels of omega-3s. Or choose a supplement with 1,000 mg of EPA and DHA (another omega-3 fatty acid) in total.

HAPPY FOOD #3: DARK GREEN VEGGIES

Dark green vegetables such as spinach, asparagus, broccoli and Brussels sprouts are loaded with folate, a B-complex vitamin that plays a key role in regulating mood. A Harvard study found that up to 38% of adults with depression had low or borderline levels of folate. Boosting the folate levels of depressed patients improved their mood.

Dark green vegetables are particularly good, but all vegetables and fruits boost mood. Researchers asked 281 people to note their moods on different days. On the days when the participants consumed the most vegetables and fruits, they reported feeling happier and more energetic. Folate certainly plays a role, but self-satisfaction may have something to do with it as well. People feel good when they eat right and take care of themselves.

Recommended amount: The minimum you should have is five servings of vegetables and fruits a day.

Bonus: Middle-aged men who had 10 servings a day showed reduced blood pressure.

HAPPY FOOD #4: BEANS (INCLUDING SOYBEANS)

Beans are rich in tryptophan, an essential amino acid that is used by the body to produce serotonin, the neurotransmitter that affects feelings of calmness and relaxation.

Beans also are loaded with folate. Folate, as mentioned in the veggies section, plays a key role in regulating mood.

In addition, beans contain manganese, a trace element that helps prevent mood swings due to low blood sugar.

Recommended amount: For people not used to eating beans, start with one-quarter cup five days a week. Build up to one-half cup daily. This progression will help prevent gastrointestinal symptoms such as flatulence.

HAPPY FOOD #5: NUTS

Nuts are high in magnesium, a trace mineral involved in more than 300 processes in the body. People who don't get enough magnesium feel irritable, fatigued and susceptible to stress.

The elderly are more likely than young adults to be low in magnesium—because they don't eat enough magnesium-rich foods and/or because they tend to excrete more magnesium in their urine.

Also, many health problems can accelerate the depletion of magnesium from the body.

Examples: Gastrointestinal disorders (or bariatric surgery), kidney disease and sometimes diabetes.

Recommended amount: Aim for one ounce of nuts a day. Good choices include almonds, walnuts, cashews, hazelnuts and peanuts (the latter is technically a legume). If you don't like nuts, other high-magnesium foods include spin-

ach, pumpkin seeds, fish, beans, whole grains and dairy.

HAPPY FOOD #6: COFFEE

The caffeine in coffee, tea and other caffeinated beverages is a very beneficial compound. One study found that people with mild cognitive impairment were less likely to develop full-fledged Alzheimer's disease when they had the caffeine equivalent of about three cups of coffee a day.

Caffeine can temporarily improve your memory and performance on tests. It enhances coordination and other parameters of physical performance. When you feel energized, you feel happier. Also, people who feel good from caffeine may be more likely to engage in other happiness-promoting behaviors, such as seeing friends and exercising.

Recommended amount: The challenge is finding the "sweet spot"—just enough caffeine to boost mood but not so much that you get the shakes or start feeling anxious. For those who aren't overly sensitive to caffeine, one to three daily cups of coffee or tea are about right.

5 Toxic Misconceptions About Grief

Alan D. Wolfelt, PhD, CT (certified thanatologist, which indicates an expertise in strategies for coping with death), founder and director of the Center for Loss and Life Transition in Fort Collins, Colorado. Dr. Wolfelt is author of several books, including *Understanding Your Grief* and *Healing a Spouse's Grieving Heart. CenterforLoss.com*

When someone you love dies, it's natural to feel the pain of your loss—and to grieve. But too many people try hard not to feel the pain. While it's understandable to want to avoid pain, it's a mistake to do so. People who appear to be "doing well" with their grief sometimes develop chronic, low-grade depression, anxiety and/or addiction to alcohol or drugs as they self-treat their emotional pain.

Recent developments: An increasing body of research is now also linking this type of unreconciled grief (meaning an inability to move forward in life without the person who died)

Perfectionism Can Kill

Perfectionism is a bigger risk for suicide than previously thought and could require intervention. Perfectionists tend to feel hopeless and hide their pain from others. Researchers note that doctors, attorneys and architects, in particular, are at increased risk for perfectionism-related suicide because their occupations emphasize precision.

Conclusion: If you're troubled by your own perfectionism, consider seeing a therapist.

Gordon Flett, PhD, professor of psychology, York University, Toronto, Ontario, Canada.

to a wide range of physical ailments, including fatigue, headache, high blood pressure and heart disease.

For many people, grief is prolonged and unresolved because there are so many misconceptions surrounding it. *Among the most common—and dangerous—misconceptions about grief...*

MISCONCEPTION #1: Grief and mourning are the same thing. People tend to use the words "grieving" and "mourning" interchangeably, but they have different meanings.

Grief is the constellation of internal thoughts and feelings you have when someone you love dies. Mourning is when you take the grief you have on the inside and express it outside yourself.

Examples of mourning: Talking about the person who died. Crying. Expressing your thoughts and feelings through art or music. Celebrating anniversary dates that held meaning for the person who died.

Many people grieve but don't mourn. When you don't honor a loss by acknowledging it—first to yourself, and then to others—your grief will accumulate. The denied losses then come flowing out in other ways, such as depression and physical problems...all of which compound the pain of your loss.

MISCONCEPTION #2: You should move away from grief, not toward it. Our society does not give people much time to grieve. They're expected to get "back to normal" in short order. People who continue to express grief outwardly are often viewed as weak or

self-pitying. The resulting message is, "Shape up and get on with your life."

This attitude leads many people to either grieve in isolation or attempt to run away from their grief through various means, such as overworking or abusing alcohol or drugs. Masking or moving away from your grief creates anxiety, confusion and depression.

What to do: Continually remind yourself that leaning toward—not away—from the pain will help you heal. To lean toward the pain, when you are feeling bad, stop and allow yourself to feel the emotion by talking to someone or writing about it.

MISCONCEPTION #3: Grief is mainly about the physical loss of the person who died. The death of a loved one creates many secondary losses—such as connections to yourself and the world around you.

Examples: You can lose the self ("I feel like a part of me died")...identity (such as your role as a spouse or child)...security (for example, a widow may not feel as safe in her home)...and meaning (when dreams for the future are shattered).

Important: Understanding the range and depth of your personal losses can help you be more self-compassionate. This involves showing sensitivity toward yourself for what you're going through.

Physical self-compassion can include eating well, exercising regularly and getting enough sleep.

Emotional self-compassion can include claiming your right to feel a multitude of emotions and the right to talk about your grief.

Mental self-compassion can mean asking yourself two questions on a daily basis that will help you survive the difficult months of grieving and learn to love life again...

1) What do I want? (now that the person you love is gone). Ask yourself what's doable and what you'd like to accomplish today.

2) What is wanted of me? (Who depends on you? What skills and experience can you bring to others?)

Social self-compassion can include finding a grief "buddy"—a friend who has also had a loss—and/or joining a grief support group. To find a group near you, check with local hospices and funeral homes.

Grief forces us to consider what life is about and what greater purpose there might be for our lives. Spiritual self-compassion can mean starting each day with a meditation or spending time in nature.

MISCONCEPTION #4: After a loved one dies, the goal should be to "get over" your grief as soon as possible. Grief is not a problem that you can solve or an illness from which you recover. Rather, you become reconciled to your grief—you integrate the new reality of moving forward in life without the person who died. With reconciliation comes a renewed sense of energy and confidence, an ability to fully acknowledge the reality of the death and a capacity to become re-involved in the activities of living.

MISCONCEPTION #5: When grief and mourning are fully reconciled, they never come up again. Grief comes in and out like the tide. Sometimes heightened periods of sadness occur even years after the death.

Example: My dad loved Frank Sinatra's music—and I have bursts of grief almost every time I hear Frank's voice.

You will always, for the rest of your life, feel some grief over a loved one's death. It will no longer dominate your life, but it will always be there, in the background, reminding you of the love you had for the person who died. And you needn't think of that as a bad thing.

info If you follow the advice in this article but are still struggling with grief, consider seeing a compassionate grief counselor. To find one, consult the Association for Death Education and Counseling (*ADEC.org*).

Grieving for a Beloved Pet

Phyllis Kosminsky, PhD, clinical social worker in private practice in Pleasantville, New York, and author of *Getting Back to Life When Grief Won't Heal.*

Pets provide us with unconditional love and companionship, so it's only natural to grieve the loss of this beloved family member. There is no timetable for the grieving process, so be patient with yourself during the time it takes to heal.

Computer Time Beats the Blues

The Internet prevents depression in older people. After controlling for various factors, researchers found that people over age 50 who used the Internet were one-third less likely to be depressed than nonusers. The reduced rate of depression was greatest among those who lived alone, leading researchers to believe that Internet use counters feelings of loneliness and isolation.

University of California, Berkeley Wellness Letter. BerkeleyWellness.com

Sometimes when we experience a loss, it can bring up feelings about other losses, such as the death of a parent, sibling or friend. If you think that old grief might be adding to what you're feeling about losing your dog, you might want to work with a grief therapist. To find one, go to *GoodTherapy.org*.

What It Means If You Talk to Yourself...

Linda Sapadin, PhD, a psychologist in private practice in Valley Stream, New York, and author of *How to Beat Procrastination in the Digital Age. PsychWisdom.com*

For the overwhelming majority of people, there is nothing wrong with talking to yourself. It not only may relieve loneliness, it also may help you clarify your thoughts and firm up your decisions.

There's only one proviso: You must speak respectfully to yourself. Cut out any negative self-talk, such as "You idiot! You should have known better...done it this way...or thought of it sooner."

For productive self-dialogue: Give yourself compliments ("I'm so proud of you!") when you accomplish even a small thing like turning down a rich dessert. Motivate yourself in a kind way with language like, "Hey, guy, you've got time to organize your desk. How about it?"

For enhanced decision-making: Running through the pros and cons of a big decision

Let the Computer Help You Quit

Puzzles, games and hobbies with your partner can lower nicotine cravings and make it easier to quit smoking. Smokers who engaged in new "self-expanding" activities with their partners had significantly greater activation of a reward center in their brains than smokers who did not take part in such activities. Such activities appear to activate the reward center associated with addictive behaviors and replace the craving for nicotine.

Arthur Aron, PhD, research professor, department of psychology, Stony Brook University, Stony Brook, New York, and leader of a study of 20 couples who engaged in two-player cooperative games with their relationship partners, published in PLOS ONE.

out loud can help you clarify your choices and figure out what decision is best.

For goal-setting: Articulating your goal by saying it out loud focuses your attention, reinforces the message, controls any runaway emotions and screens out distractions.

Whether you're living alone or with others, you're always living with yourself. So converse, chatter and communicate respectfully with yourself. It can be a sign of good health!

In only rare cases, when you're unaware of what you're doing or talking incoherently, is talking to yourself an indication of a mental disorder.

New Treatment for Bipolar Depression

Robert Rowney, DO, is a psychiatrist in the department of psychology and psychiatry at the Cleveland Clinic.

Bipolar depression is difficult to treat, so a new treatment—the antipsychotic drug Latuda (*lurasidone*)—offers another valuable option. Latuda can be used on its own for patients who respond well to it. Other patients may have only a partial response, in which case Latuda can be combined with medications such as *lithium* or *valproate*. Latuda is well-tolerated by most peo-

ple who take it. However, some patients develop side effects such as restlessness, nausea, drowsiness, muscle twitching and slowed movements.

Bad News for Healthy Eaters

Thomas M. Dunn, PhD, an associate professor in the department of psychology at University of Northern Colorado in Greeley.

Sometimes it seems as if everyone is on a special diet—gluten-free…dairy-free…sugar-free…vegetarian…vegan.

That's not surprising. There are numerous health benefits to eating right. But mental-health experts have noticed a disturbing trend—people are becoming obsessed with the perfect diet. There's even a name for the condition—orthorexia nervosa, which, roughly translated, means "correct eating," explains Thomas M. Dunn, PhD, an associate professor in the department of psychology at University of Northern Colorado in Greeley.

At what point does the desire to eat healthier start to become an unhealthy obsession? *Dr. Dunn offers these warning signs…*

•**You're often or always anxious about what you eat.** You feel shame when you don't live up to the ideal—after munching a single chip, for example.

•**Your list of "no" foods and ingredients keeps getting longer.**

•**Your social life suffers.** You think twice about going out with friends. You avoid events involving food or you bring your own.

If you think that you have orthorexia…

•**Understand that eating a "no" food now and then is OK.** Balance is what matters.

•**If you're at a restaurant or party where you think there's nothing to eat,** remind yourself that there's always a fallback position. Choose foods that you think are reasonably healthy even if they're not on your "A" list.

•**See a therapist who specializes in eating disorders.** To find a referral or support group, go to *NationalEatingDisorders.org.*

Binge-Watching TV May Be Sign of Depression, Loneliness

International Communication Association, news release.

Binge-watching television is linked with feeling lonely and depressed, a recent study suggests.

"Even though some people argue that binge-watching is a harmless addiction, findings from our study suggest that binge-watching should no longer be viewed this way," study author Yoon Hi Sung said in a news release from the International Communication Association.

The study included more than 300 people. They were between the ages of 18 and 29. The researchers asked about their TV viewing habits and their moods.

The more lonely and depressed people were, the more likely they were to binge-watch TV. And people binge-watched in an attempt to distract themselves from their negative feelings, according to the University of Texas at Austin researchers.

The researchers also found that people who lacked self-control were more likely to binge-watch TV. They were unable to stop even when they knew they had other tasks to complete.

"Physical fatigue and problems such as obesity and other health problems are related to binge-watching and they are a cause for concern. When binge-watching becomes rampant, viewers may start to neglect their work and their relationships with others. Even though people know they should not, they have difficulty resisting the desire to watch episodes continuously," Sung said.

"Our research is a step toward exploring binge-watching as an important media and social phenomenon," Sung concluded.

The study was presented at the International Communication Association's annual meeting in 2014. Findings from meetings are generally considered preliminary until they've been published in a peer-reviewed journal.

info Mental Health America outlines how to live your life well at *http://www.mentalhealthamerica.net/live-your-life-well*.

Cheap Natural Compound May Help Smokers Quit

Natalie Walker, PhD, associate director, Center for Addiction Research, University of Auckland, New Zealand.
Nancy Rigotti, MD, professor, medicine, Harvard Medical School, Boston.
New England Journal of Medicine

The naturally occurring plant compound cytisine may be more effective than nicotine replacement therapy in helping smokers quit, a recent study suggests.

Cytisine, an acid-like chemical found in the seeds of the golden rain tree, has been used in Eastern Europe for decades to help smokers quit, researchers say. But it's not widely available.

"Cytisine is one of the most affordable smoking cessation medicines available," said lead researcher Natalie Walker, PhD, an associate director of the Center for Addiction Research at the University of Auckland in New Zealand.

"It is much cheaper than nicotine patches, gum and/or lozenges and other smoking cessation medicines," she said. "However, currently cytisine is only sold in a number of countries in Eastern and Central Europe. It is important that cytisine become more widely accessible and available."

STUDY DETAILS

For the study, Dr. Walker and her colleagues randomly assigned more than 1,300 men and women who called a national smoking quit line in New Zealand to 25 days of treatment with cytisine or eight weeks of nicotine replacement therapy with patches, gum and/or lozenges. All participants also received telephone support.

After a month, 40% of those taking cytisine pills said they hadn't smoked, compared with 31% of those who used nicotine replacement therapy, the researchers found.

The findings were published in the *New England Journal of Medicine*.

HOW CYTISINE WORKS

Cytisine mimics nicotine so smokers get the same satisfaction as if they smoked, the experts said.

"To the brain, cytisine looks a little like nicotine, and so it works to alleviate any urges to smoke and reduces the severity of nicotine withdrawal symptoms," Dr. Walker explained.

"Plus, if you do smoke while using cytisine, it will be less satisfying—making quitting easier," she said.

Cytisine was more effective than nicotine replacement therapy in helping smokers stay off cigarettes in the first week, and after two and six months, the researchers found.

However, cytisine can cause side effects, Dr. Walker said. "Three out of every 10 people who used cytisine had a side effect, compared with two out of every 10 that used nicotine patches, gum and/or lozenges," she said. The side effects didn't last long and weren't serious. "Some people felt nauseous or sick and some had sleep disturbances, such as bad dreams," Dr. Walker said.

EXPERT COMMENT

Nancy Rigotti, MD, a professor of medicine at Harvard Medical School and author of an accompanying journal editorial, said she supports cytisine's use as a smoking cessation tool.

"Cytisine is an old medication, and studies like this one have shown that it is effective," she said. "We need to find a way to make treatment of tobacco use accessible and affordable to all of the world's smokers."

The challenge, Dr. Rigotti said, is to figure out how to get cytisine licensed as a tobacco treatment in all countries, including the United States, while still keeping it affordable.

Tobacco use is the leading preventable cause of death worldwide, she noted.

"A majority of smokers now live in low- and middle-income countries," she added. "We have effective treatments to help smokers, but they are generally too expensive for smokers in low- and middle-income countries to afford."

info For more about quitting smoking, visit the American Cancer Society at *http://www.cancer.org/healthy/stayawayfromtobacco/guidetoquittingsmoking/index.*

Medication for Recovery

Fewer than 9% of alcoholics get medication that could help them stop drinking. In a recent 12-week study, alcohol-dependent patients taking the anticonvulsant drug *gabapentin* were four times more likely to stop drinking altogether than those taking a placebo. The medication helps people to better cope with alcoholic cravings by improving sleep and mood.

Barbara J. Mason, PhD, is codirector of Pearson Center for Alcoholism and Addiction Research, Scripps Research Institute, La Jolla, California. She led a clinical trial of gabapentin, published in *JAMA Internal Medicine.*

The Difference Between Excessive Drinking and Alcoholism

Not everyone who drinks heavily is an alcoholic. Many people who drink too much at one time or over the course of a week are considered to be "excessive drinkers" but are not physically or mentally addicted to alcohol, which defines "alcoholism."

Twenty-nine percent of the US population meets the definition for excessive drinking—five or more drinks in one sitting or 15 or more during a week for men...four or more drinks at one time or eight or more during a week for women. But 90% of them are not addicted to alcohol.

Excessive drinking is responsible for 88,000 deaths each year. About 3,700 alcohol-dependent people die each year, according to the U.S. Centers for Disease Control and Prevention.

Survey of 138,100 adults by researchers at the Centers for Disease Control and Prevention, Atlanta, reported in *The New York Times.*

Walk This Way to Get Happy

Hirofumi Tanaka, PhD, professor and director, Cardiovascular Aging Research Laboratory, University of Texas at Austin. His study was published in *The Journal of Alternative and Complementary Medicine*.

When you are feeling blue, do you ever take a stroll to walk it off? If you do, you may be just a few proverbial steps away from practicing something called walking meditation. Not only does this walking technique have the power to beat depression that is deep enough to send you to a psychiatrist, it is actually more heart-healthy, more stress-busting and a lot less strenuous than traditional aerobic fitness walking. No special equipment or exercise clothing is required either. *Just put on a pair of comfortable shoes and go...*

BETTER THAN POWER WALKING

Here's how the participants in a recent study practiced walking meditation...

•**Stand tall with your arms at your sides.**

•**Let your gaze be softly directed at the ground six feet in front of you, and begin to walk.** Walk slowly...as if you're stopping to smell the roses. And really let yourself do that. Forget about the cares of the day. In fact, focus instead on the sole of each foot as it makes contact with the ground.

•**While you slowly walk,** let your arms gently swing in unison forward and back—yes, that means both arms forward at the same time and both arms back at the same time, which is different from the way we normally walk but not difficult to do...and as you walk this way, repeatedly say or think, in rhythm with your movements, a word or short phrase that is personal and inspiring to you.

In the Thai study, participants repeated a term that, as Thais, was meaningful to them—"Budd" with each upward swing of the arms and "Dha" (Buddha) with each downward swing. For you, if you happen to be a spiritual type, you might want to choose a word or term from your own tradition. If not, choose any word or phrase that is uplifting for you, such as "Peace and serenity," "Easy breezy," "It's all good," "Sunshine and rainbows"—even the name of a pet or someone dear who gives you joy.

•**If your mind wanders to worries and concerns, that's OK.** Catch yourself at it...take a relaxing breath...and return to focusing on your walk and your inspiring phrase.

•**Walk this way for 20 minutes at a time when you first begin,** and aim to lengthen the time up to a maximum of an hour.

The study recruited 45 women between the ages of 60 and 90 who all received full physical examinations and then were divided into three groups. One group received no supervised walking activity. Another group learned and practiced traditional aerobic fitness walking, which involved brisk walking and arm swinging that was intensified as the study progressed. (That's the sort of energetic, chin-up, no-guts-no-glory exercise walking that many of us do in America.) The third group learned and practiced the walking meditation described above, and this was intensified as the study progressed not by having participants quicken their pace, but by having them hold weights in the form of filled water bottles.

Both walking groups practiced their walking regimens three times a week for 12 weeks. Participants in both of the walking groups also did the same warm-up and cool-down stretching exercises before and after each walking session. Walks were 20 minutes long for the first six weeks and increased to 30 minutes for the last six weeks.

At the end of the program, there were some really fantastic benefits seen in the walking meditation group...

•**Weight loss.** While both groups lost about 3% of body mass, members of the walking

Nasal Spray Relieves Depression

A 50-milligram dose of the intranasal spray *ketamine*, an FDA-approved anesthetic, was found to alleviate depressive symptoms within hours with few side effects in people with treatment-resistant major depressive disorder.

Study by researchers at Icahn School of Medicine at Mount Sinai, New York City, published in *Biological Psychiatry* meditation group had a 5% decrease in body fat, while the fitness walkers did not lose any.

•**Blood and cardiovascular health.** The degree of ease of blood flow improved by 72% in the fitness walking group—that's very good—and by 88% in the walking meditation group—that's great.

•**Fitness.** Compared with prestudy timed walking scores, the fitness walking group improved by 29%…while the walking meditation group improved by 84%. Amazing!

•**Happiness.** A significant drop in depression scores, based on psychological testing, was seen only in the meditation walking group, with the average score dropping below that signifying a depression diagnosis. In comparison, the participants in the fitness walking group had very mild reductions in depression test scores and those not doing any walking exercise at all had a slight increase in their depression scores.

The findings from this study were similar to those reported in other studies of mind-body exercise regimens, such as tai chi and yoga.

So, if you need to lighten and brighten your day and want to stay fit without breaking a sweat, here's a kind of light and relaxing walk you can take with a happy song in your heart.

A Conversation Boost

Study of 253 people, ages 18 to 45, by researchers at University of Connecticut, Storrs, published in *Communication Monographs*.

Orgasms improve communication. After orgasm, people are more likely to share important information with their partners.

Possible reason: Orgasm increases the body's production of the hormone oxytocin, which is linked to social bonding and increased trust. This may make people feel safe about disclosing information.

But: Alcohol, which is widely thought to cause people to tell more of their secrets, does the opposite—immediately after sex, people who have been drinking may say things they had not planned to disclose, but what they reveal is less important and less positive. Alcohol, combined with failing to have an orgasm, produces even more negativity.

To Stop Worrying…

Psychology Today

Tone down extremes by writing your worries down and rewording them—instead of "Nobody likes me," you might write, "My boss does not like my report." Think of worries as trains posted on the departure board at a station—they all are there, but you need not board any of them, and as they depart, you can let them go. Set aside 20 "worry minutes" a day, and refuse to think about troubling matters at any other time—when your thoughts do drift toward something that causes anxiety, write the concern down and come back to it at the scheduled time. Make monotony your friend by slowly repeating worrying notions to yourself—expressing a negative to yourself over and over should soon make your mind wander to more enjoyable thoughts.

Family Matters

How to Truly Help Someone Who Is Depressed

Robin Williams's recent suicide has started a national conversation about depression. And now, many people are still left wondering—What would I do if a loved one were seriously depressed?

We'll never know whether more could have been done to save Williams. But it is important for everyone to realize that there are practical and effective ways to help a loved one who is depressed—whether or not he/she is suicidal.

UNDERSTANDING DEPRESSION

Depression causes many well-known symptoms, such as lethargy, insomnia, loss of interest in work and hobbies, hopelessness and despair. But perhaps the most difficult behavior to cope with in a loved one who is depressed is the person's tendency to withdraw. Your loved one's depression is likely to leave him feeling deeply alone and misunderstood.

That's why it's crucial that you respond appropriately when your loved one shares any of his feelings—even if they sound angry, illogical or accusatory.

FINDING THE RIGHT WORDS

Here are the approaches that will allow you to help a loved one with depression…

•**Use the "observer's mind."** With this approach, you detach yourself from the situation so that you respond to the feelings behind your loved one's words rather than their literal content. Pay close attention to the person's facial expressions, hand gestures, body language and tone of voice rather than focusing so much on what the person is saying. You might think to yourself, *It looks like my husband is angry*…or *My wife seems lost and confused.*

Mitch Golant, PhD, a psychologist in private practice in Los Angeles and coauthor of seven books, including *What to Do When Someone You Love Is Depressed.*

This way, you don't take your loved one's comments personally—and you avoid being drawn into an argument neither of you wants. Instead, you simply look and listen without responding immediately to what the person with depression is saying—you are silently calm, receptive and empathetic—and then you respond with support and help, using the next step…

•**Validate your loved one's feelings.** Try a technique known as "mirroring." With this approach, you verbally reflect back what your loved one is saying on an emotional level, not necessarily on a content level—this process validates his emotions and helps him feel heard and understood (the experience that a person with depression wants the most). *Two examples…*

Example #1: Your loved one says: "I'm all alone."

Don't say: "No, you're not. I'm sitting here with you right now."

Do say: "I know that you're feeling alone right now. Is there anything I can do to help? Together, we'll get through this lonely feeling."

Example #2: Your loved one says: "Why bother? Life isn't worth living. There's no point in going on."

Don't say: "How can you think that? You have two beautiful children and a great job. I love you. You have everything to live for."

Do say: "I know it feels that way to you right now, but I want you to know that you matter to me and to the children. We'll get through this hopeless feeling together."

Very important: Notice that these "do say" examples all include statements that validate your loved one's feelings and a second state-

If Your Loved One Is Suicidal...

If a loved one makes statements that suggest he/she may be thinking about suicide (for example, "You'd be better off without me"…or "I just want to check out"), this is an emergency. It's a myth that people who talk about suicide don't actually follow through. What you say and do in these situations can be vital to your loved one's survival.

What to say: "I know things look hopeless right now, and I'm taking this very seriously. We need to get help"…or "I'm here with you, and I'm not going to leave. You're not alone. We're going to the hospital right away." *For advice on assessing the problem…*

•**Call your local suicide-prevention center.** Or call the National Suicide Prevention Lifeline at 800-273-8255.

If the situation is dire…

•**Call 911 or the police.** Emergency workers and police are trained to deal with mental health emergencies. They will come and determine if your loved one should be hospitalized. The key is whether he is a danger to himself or others.

ment that reminds him of your dependability—and of hope for the future.

GETTING HELP FOR YOUR LOVED ONE

Research shows that 80% of people with depression can be helped with psychotherapy with or without medication. Even though depression can make it difficult for the sufferer to motivate himself to reach out for help, you can play an active role in encouraging your loved one to get the care he needs. *What to do…*

•**Take charge.** Assisting your loved one in getting professional help is crucial—even if he protests.

•**Enlist support.** Call your family doctor, clergyman, therapist or another health-care professional, and ask for advice in creating a realistic plan of action to help the person with depression.

•**Schedule an appointment for your loved one to see his doctor,** who may refer him to a psychiatrist or psychologist. (If you think your loved one would prefer scheduling this appointment himself, consider allowing him to do so.)

•**Call a meeting.** Include the person with depression and any other friends or family members whose support you can count on.

Tell your loved one: "Honey, we're all here because we're worried about you and don't want you to suffer. We've scheduled an appointment with the doctor. You and I can go together and figure this out." (As an alternative, you can simply give your loved one the doctor's phone number and offer to go with him to the appointment.) Most people who are suffering with depression are grateful that they are no longer emotionally invisible. When all of these elements are in place—especially your emotional resolve—there's a good chance your loved one will respond appropriately.

How to Convince a Loved One to Get a Hearing Aid

Richard E. Carmen, AuD, an audiologist and editor, co-author or author of several books, including editor of *The Consumer Handbook on Hearing Loss & Hearing Aids*, and author of *How Hearing Loss Impacts Relationships: Motivating Your Loved One.*

About 36 million Americans suffer from hearing loss—but only one in five people who would benefit from a hearing aid actually wears one.

How does untreated hearing loss affect the sufferer's loved ones? Over time, it can seriously strain—even destroy—a marriage or parent-child relationship due, for example, to misunderstandings and frayed nerves in the person who must constantly repeat himself/herself. Fortunately, you can motivate your loved one to take action...

MORE THAN JUST HEARING LOSS

Understanding the full extent to which hearing loss impacts your loved one will strengthen your resolve to motivate him to get treatment. The psychological effects are huge. People with untreated hearing loss tend to become withdrawn and are significantly more prone to depression and anxiety than those with adequate hearing. Anger, confusion, discouragement, loss of self-esteem and shame often occur as well.

Important recent discovery: Researchers at Johns Hopkins University and the National Institute on Aging found that even mild hearing loss was associated with twice the risk for dementia, while people with severe hearing loss were five times more likely to develop the condition—a link that gives sufferers yet another reason to consider getting hearing aids.

BREAKING THROUGH DENIAL

More than two-thirds of people who refuse hearing aids do so because they think "my hearing isn't bad enough," according to research conducted by the National Council on Aging. It is also easy for the person with hearing loss to blame other people ("you're just mumbling").

The most direct way to respond to this situation is to use "tough love." This means that you must stop being your loved one's ears. Take sensible steps to optimize communication—for example, speak clearly and face to face, not from another room. However, do not repeat yourself every time your loved one asks what you said and don't shout yourself hoarse just so he can hear. If you stop filling in the information that your loved one isn't hearing, he will be more likely to get treated.

Helpful: Tell your loved one that you're going to begin this practice out of love and concern and to make both your lives better. It is not a step that you're taking out of anger or vindictiveness.

If it feels too extreme to stop helping your loved one when he doesn't hear something, try this: Keep repeating yourself and/or conveying what others are saying, but preface it each time with the phrase "hearing help." This reminds your loved one of the hearing problem without cutting off communication.

Important: If you can't bear to try one of these approaches with your loved one, take an honest look at your own feelings about the situation. Is it possible that you find some degree of satisfaction in being your spouse's or parent's link to the world and having that person depend on you so much? Wanting to help is a wonderful human trait, but when you need to help your loved one, it locks you both into a pattern of codependence. If you suspect that you're caught in such a cycle, seeing a therapist can help—even in just a session or two.

KNOWLEDGE IS POWER

If your loved one recognizes his hearing problem but still won't get treated, here are some possible reasons why—and how to respond...

Vanity. Research shows that 20% of those who refuse to have their hearing corrected said the following about using a hearing aid: "It makes me feel old"..."I'm too embarrassed to wear one"...or "I don't like what others will think of me."

What to do: Tell your loved one that the inability to hear is far more noticeable than a hearing aid and may well be interpreted as a cognitive problem or other illness. Then ask your loved one if he is familiar with modern hearing devices, which are much smaller and far less intrusive than those used years ago.

Expense. Even many people who can well afford the cost of a hearing aid use price as an excuse to avoid treatment.

What to do: Ask if your loved one knows exactly how much hearing aids cost. Mention that many different devices are available and that costs vary widely.

Then remind your loved one how hearing loss impacts his life, yours and other family members'—and ask, "What's it worth for you to keep these relationships intact?"

Inferior equipment. Many people say, "I've been told that hearing aids don't work so well."

What to do: Ask for the source of your loved one's information to determine how reliable it is. Then ask whether he's willing to take a 30-day trial to test the effectiveness of hearing aids. Most state laws mandate a trial period. Check local laws by contacting your state's Department of Consumer Affairs. If your state does not require a 30-day trial, ask that it be written into any hearing-aid sales agreement—reputable sellers will agree to this.

If a loved one says, "I tried hearing aids and they didn't work," find out when and where the devices were purchased and suggest that he go to another audiologist. To find one near you, check with the American Academy of Audiology, *Audiology.org.*

STRONG MEDICINE

If you try these approaches and your loved one still won't address his hearing loss, even stronger actions may be necessary. Be sure to consider your loved one's personality—can he deal with more direct confrontation, even if done in a gentle, loving way?

If so, you might try…

Videotape. Make a videotape of your loved one in a situation where he struggles to hear, such as a family get-together. Then sit down and view the tape with him privately to prevent embarrassment.

Intervention. Without prior warning to the loved one, family members meet with him for 10 to 15 minutes to talk about how the problem has affected them. The overall message of the meeting should be how much the family members care…and want a higher quality of life for the person with hearing loss (and for themselves).

Four Steps to Improve Life for Dementia Patients and Caregivers

Helen C. Kales, MD, professor of psychiatry, director, section of geriatric psychiatry and Program for Positive Aging, University of Michigan, Ann Arbor. Her study appeared in the *Journal of the American Geriatrics Society.*

Some of you are undoubtedly caring for other adults who are slipping into the abyss of Alzheimer's disease. Although we casually think of Alzheimer's as memory loss, any caregiver will tell you that it's far more than that—depression, anxiety, agitation, delusions, hallucinations and apathy are all symptoms, and they all can take a great toll on the caregiver. How to cope with this often martyring challenge?

A new strategy that goes by the acronym DICE and is forged by a partnership between patient, caregiver and health-care provider is getting a lot of buzz right now in the health-care community. The Centers for Medicare and Medicaid Services are even planning to include DICE in their training and resource modules for health-care providers. But if you are the caregiver of someone with dementia, can DICE really improve life for you and the person you care for?

FOUR STEPS TO WORK IT OUT

DICE is a four-step process in which the patient, caregiver and a health-care provider—it could be a geriatrician, geriatric psychiatrist, nurse practitioner or physician assistant, social worker or similar professional trained in dementia care—work as a team to identify the real causes of a patient's "bad behavior" in any given situation and come up with solutions. The four steps are…

•**D…escribe.** Encouraged by the health-care provider, the caregiver describes a specific event that exemplifies the patient's behavior problems to the health-care provider in a way that gets the caregiver to relive the episode with all its details and feelings. One way of doing this is to describe the event as if it were a movie scene. This conversation may take place in person or over the phone, and the patient may also be present. The caregiver may be encouraged to record episodes of problem behavior in a journal so that one or another episode can be easily remembered and discussed when meeting with the health-care provider. Unless dementia in the person being cared for is so severe that he or she can't communicate anymore, the health-care provider also gets that person's version of the story. The provider then helps the caregiver think about what led up to the event being discussed and its aftermath to get insight about the context and patterns underlying it.

•**I…nvestigate.** The health-care provider then investigates the cause of the problem. Issues to be probed include whether another medical or psychiatric condition is at play, whether the patient's behavior is related to side effects of medications, whether he or she is in pain or not getting enough sleep or is frightened, depressed, bored, etc. or whether the dementia is simply getting worse. Much of this can be learned from a physical and psychiatric exam. Follow-up laboratory work may also help shed light on underlying causes (such as a urinary tract infection). The caregiver's expectations and any social or cultural issues, such as economic status, education level, ethnic traditions and religious beliefs, of the caregiver and patient might also be examined.

•**C…reate.** Together, the caregiver and health-care provider—with participation from the patient, if possible—create a plan for positive change. The plan begins with the health-care provider addressing problems discovered during the investigation. For example, a medication might be discontinued if it is thought to be

---

Signs an Elderly Person Should Give Up Driving

Signs that it is time to discuss an elderly person's driving include scrapes on the person's car, a garage door or a mailbox. If you notice these signs, ride with the driver to evaluate how well he/she drives and whether it is time to give up driving. In 2012 (latest data available), 17% of traffic deaths in the US involved people age 65 and older who made up only 14% of the population, according to the US Department of Transportation.

Survey conducted by Liberty Mutual Insurance of 1,007 adults ages 40 to 65 with at least one parent who drives, reported in *USA Today*.

---

causing a behavioral side effect…pain management might be started if pain is the issue…more intensive psychiatric care might begin and any other newly discovered health need of the patient will be attended to.

The caregiver will be directed toward education resources and support groups, and the caregiver and health-care provider will work together to improve communication with the patient, simplify caregiver tasks, create structured routines and establish meaningful activities for the patient (such as revival of a hobby or participation in an adult day-care program) to help minimize his or her boredom, frustration, fear or other difficult emotions.

•**E…valuate.** The health-care provider then evaluates the plan as time goes by. Is the caregiver using it? Is it working? If so, great! If not, a reassessment takes place to tweak and optimize the plan.

PLAYING WITH THE DICE APPROACH

The DICE approach is just now being rolled out in a formal way, with training for health-care personnel being developed and a clinical trial under way. Its real value and feasibility won't be fully known until its use becomes more widespread and clinical trials are completed to scientifically prove its value, ease of use and cost effectiveness. If you would like to try the DICE approach, start by asking your loved one's health-care providers whether they are famil-

159

iar with it—they may be able to refer you to a specialist or a practice that provides a similar service. You could also contact a geriatric psychiatrist, whose training makes it more likely that he or she will apply an approach similar to DICE when working with dementia patients and their caregivers. You might even find that some or all of this is covered by insurance, depending on your loved one's coverage.

How to Argue with Your Spouse

Laurie Puhn, JD, a couples mediator in private practice in New York City. She is author of Fight Less, Love More: 5-Minute Conversations to Change Your Relationship without Blowing Up or Giving In. *LauriePuhn.com*

You can argue and still have a happy marriage—if your arguments lead to solutions rather than lingering bitterness. *Four ways to encourage this...*

•**Alter argument patterns.** Many couples have fallen into argument patterns that lead to more anger instead of a peaceful resolution. Maybe she criticizes, he gets defensive, she dredges up an old disagreement, he insults her, then she storms off—again and again.

Making even a minor change near the outset of an argument could prevent this pattern from recurring, improving the odds of a positive outcome.

Example: As soon as an argument begins, stop and say, "Let's sit down at the kitchen table and talk this through." Sitting is a particularly useful suggestion because it helps the brain remain calm and rational during arguments rather than shifting into panic-driven fight-or-flight mode.

•**Ask neutral questions when you feel wronged by your spouse.** Married people sometimes see nefarious intent in their spouses' missteps where none truly exists.

When you feel you have been wronged, ask calm, nonaccusatory questions that encourage your spouse to explain his/her actions. Imagine that you're a dispassionate detective trying to get to the bottom of the situation, not the aggrieved party.

•**Stop arguing about pointless stuff.** Don't argue about what your adult children should do or over facts that you easily can check. Alternatively, you could turn the disagreement into a lighthearted low-stakes bet—"I bet you a dollar that I've got this one right!"

•**Team up to find a solution.** People are more likely to live up to the terms of an agreement when they feel that they had a role in crafting it. Thus the best way to prevent a problem from recurring in a marriage isn't thinking up a solution—it's sitting down with your spouse to think up a solution together.

Example: Don't tell your spouse, "Keep a cell-phone charger in your car so you can call the next time you're going to be late." Ask your spouse, "What could be done to avoid this happening again?" If your spouse doesn't think up the car-charger solution, raise it yourself in the form of a question—"How about we keep cell-phone chargers in our cars?"

How to Cope If Your Loved One Is a Narcissist

Wendy T. Behary, LCSW, founder and clinical director of the Cognitive Therapy Center of New Jersey and the New Jersey Institute for Schema Therapy, both in Springfield. She is author of Disarming the Narcissist: Surviving & Thriving with the Self-Absorbed.

He's boastful, arrogant, the center of attention and gets angry when anyone questions his authority. She's outwardly unassuming but equally self-centered and touchy. Both feel entitled to whatever they want. These people have the classic personality traits of a narcissist.

If you have a friend or coworker who is a narcissist, you know how stressful it can be. And living with a narcissist can be hazardous to your mental and emotional health and your overall well-being.

What's new: A growing body of research is uncovering key aspects of the narcissist's personality—and showing how best to cope with such a person.

LIVING WITH A NARCISSIST

Good relationships are based on reciprocity—you listen attentively and empathetically to the other person's joys and sorrows, for example…and he/she listens to yours. With narcissists, it's a one-way street. A steady diet of this can be toxic to your sense of self.

Important recent finding: In a study recently published in *Personality and Individual Differences*, researchers found that narcissism is closely tied to perfectionism, making narcissists extremely demanding and hypercritical of others.

If your partner or spouse is a narcissist, this means you may well be subjected to insults and admonishments for always doing something wrong and never measuring up. Belittling you makes the narcissist feel bigger.

THE NARCISSIST'S STORY

So what's the source of all this self-centeredness? Some people become narcissists because they were spoiled from early on. Taught that they were special and that others exist to serve them, narcissists carry these beliefs into adulthood.

Ironically, though, narcissists usually do not feel good about themselves. Their earliest emotional needs often went unmet. They may have never gotten the love, support and approval that nourishes true self-worth, so they ache deep inside with emptiness. Beneath the boasting and arrogance is likely a very wounded person.

Having insight into the narcissist's suffering soul isn't going to change his behavior—and certainly doesn't excuse it. But this understanding can relieve you of the often painful burden of taking it personally. It's not your fault.

WHAT YOU CAN CHANGE

Because narcissism is deeply rooted in one's personality, it's not something that you alone can change in another person. What you can change is the way that you respond to situations as they arise.

Helpful: With the use of empathic confrontation, you demonstrate that you appreciate how the other person feels while making an

Old School Best for Sex

Traditional gender roles lead to more sex. In marriages where chores were divided based on traditional stereotypes—women did the housework and men handled car care and lawn mowing, for example—couples had sex an average of 4.8 times a month. When both partners helped with everyday chores, the frequency dropped to 3.9 times a month.

Study of data led by researchers at Juan March Institute, Madrid, Spain, and University of Washington, Seattle.

unambiguous statement of how you feel and what you need.

Example one: Your spouse comes home an hour after you were planning on dinner—again—and says, "So I'm late, OK? I'm tired, and I don't want to hear any of your complaints…let's eat."

What not to say: "Don't you dare talk to me that way!"

What to say: "I know that you're the boss at work, but I'm not one of your subordinates…our relationship doesn't work that way. And I know you're exhausted and you've had a tough day, but I'm allowed to be disappointed when you're late. It's been three times this week."

Example two: Your partner talks at length about a series of frustrating encounters with a friend, then starts reading e-mail on her cell phone when you start to describe your day.

What not to say: "I can't believe how selfish you are!"

What to say: "It sounds like you had a lot to deal with today, and I know you like to stay on top of your e-mail. But our relationship is a two-way street. I care about you and would like to feel that you're caring for me, too."

SHOULD YOU STAY OR GO?

Whether this approach can help your relationship evolve so that you feel more empowered ultimately comes down to a question of leverage. Does your partner care enough to change the way he acts? Will your partner respect reasonable limits on selfish, entitled and inconsiderate behavior?

If you're not sure whether your change in behavior is improving your relationship enough to stay in it, consider trying psychotherapy. It can help you clarify your feelings and give you the strength to stay strong in a taxing environment…or make an informed decision to leave the relationship.

With or without professional help, it is crucial to take care of yourself.

What to do: Spend as much time as possible with friends and family who value and care about you. Cultivate healthy distractions such as exercise and reading…and pursue self-soothing pleasures such as music, yoga and meditation.

Also helpful: Journaling. Writing out your feelings of frustration and anger can help keep your appraisals of the situation as objective and accurate as possible.

Warning: Don't be tempted to escape into alcohol, overeating or drugs. This will only fuel the self-blame and insecurity you're likely feeling and exacerbate any depression you may be experiencing.

Are You Your Family's Food Police?

Bonnie Taub-Dix, RDN, CDN, director and owner, BTD Nutrition Consultants New York City and Long Island, New York. She is the author of *Read It Before You Eat It* and a blogger for EverydayHealth.com and the *US News & World Report* "Eat + Run" column. *BetterThanDieting.com*

Remember what the road to hell is paved with? Yep, good intentions. So even though your intentions are good when you "encourage" family members and friends to eat more healthfully, if you overstep and start to seem like the self-appointed Food Police, there could be a very damaging backlash. *For instance…*

• **The people you're trying to help may assert their independence** by obstinately doing the opposite of what you're pushing for.

• **Your criticism may wound a loved one's self-esteem.**

Kids Naturally Hate the Green Stuff

Kids have a natural aversion to vegetables. Most children are wary of plant foods—which stems from our ancestors, who had to be cautious because many plants were poisonous or covered with spines or thorns.

Study of 47 children 18 months old to age eight by researchers at Yale University, New Haven, Connecticut, published in *Cognition*.

• **Relationships can be damaged or destroyed** if other people decide to tune you out or avoid you altogether to escape your proselytizing.

• **Food Police are all too common.** "In my practice, I routinely counsel couples and families in which one person has unwittingly offended another in an effort to help that person eat better," said Bonnie Taub-Dix, RDN, CDN, owner of BTD Nutrition Consultants in New York City and Long Island, New York, and author of *Read It Before You Eat It*.

Here's what to do—and what not to do—to help those you cherish clean up their eating habits…

• **Focus on health, not on weight.** Harping on body size is likely to backfire and even may contribute to eating disorders.

Evidence: In a recent study of almost 1,300 adults, people whose partners strongly pressured them to lose weight during the previous year were much more likely to engage in binge eating, regardless of their weight. Bingeing occurred among 25% of women and 14% of men whose partners pushed them to slim down, versus 14% of women and 4% of men whose partners did not do so.

The problem, Taub-Dix explained, is that by emphasizing weight, you sound judgmental rather than supportive. "Saying something like, 'I thought you were trying to lose weight, so why are you eating that cake?' only makes the other person resentful. She may even think to herself, 'I'll show you—not only am I going to eat cake, I'm going to have two slices!' Or she may start to angrily sneak food when you're not around," Taub-Dix said.

Better strategy: Gently remind your loved one that you care for her and want her to be healthy…so you can enjoy each other's company for many years to come. Expressing concern about another person's health does not carry the same sense of censure as expressing dissatisfaction with her weight. Then share information, such as articles on good nutrition, so that information comes across as objective and helpful rather than judgmental.

•**Pick the right time and place.** It may seem logical to talk about food while you and the other person are actually eating—such as when you see your loved one eating that slice (or two!) of cake mentioned earlier. But in fact, that's the worst time to initiate such a discussion, Taub-Dix said.

Reasons: Once the person has the food on his plate (or at least in his sights), he may already be too emotionally invested in eating it to hear your message…and he may feel defensive and resentful about being "caught in the act." This is especially likely to happen if there are other people at the table, because having additional witnesses will increase his embarrassment.

Instead: Bring up the subject of healthful eating when you're both involved in some pleasant, nonfood-related activity. This way, the conversation is less emotionally charged…and the other person can better absorb your message.

•**Speak about your own struggles with food and how you solve them.** By relating eating issues to yourself rather than to the other person, you avoid the kind of finger-pointing that makes others self-conscious or angry.

For instance: You might say, "This bread on our table isn't good for us, but it's hard for me to resist. Do you mind if we ask the waiter to take it away?"

•**Setting a good example can be very powerful.** Research from the Framingham Heart Study, which followed more than 3,400 people for many years, showed that eating behaviors—good and bad—tend to spread among family members and social networks. So keep your kitchen stocked with nutritious foods, and let your loved ones see how much you enjoy eating healthfully. Do not moan about how much you crave tiramisu as you eat your salad!

Remember, in the end it's not up to you. If your loving encouragement and role modeling don't succeed in changing another person's eating habits, you need to accept that he simply isn't ready to make a change. You cannot do it for him…and if you keep pushing, you may succeed only in pushing him away. Poisoning the relationship won't help him get any healthier—it will only hurt you both. Let it go, at least for now. You can always try again later…and by then, your loved one may be more open to your message.

Dentists' Group Expands Recommended Use of Fluoride for Kids

American Dental Association, news release.

Children should begin using toothpaste with fluoride as soon as they get their first tooth, according to updated American Dental Association (ADA) guidelines.

To help prevent cavities, parents should use a smear (an amount about the size of a grain of rice) of fluoride toothpaste for children younger than three years old and a pea-sized dab for those aged three to six, the association recommends.

Previous guidelines recommended using water to brush the teeth of children younger than age two and brushing the teeth of children aged two to six with a pea-sized amount of fluoride toothpaste.

Divorce Can Be Fattening

Children of divorced parents are 54% more likely to be overweight than those with married parents.

Possible reason: More convenience foods in single-parent households.

Norwegian Child Growth Study.

"For half a century, the ADA has recommended that patients use fluoride toothpaste to prevent cavities, and a review of scientific research shows that this holds true for all ages," said Edmond Truelove, DDS, chairman of the ADA's Council on Scientific Affairs.

"Approximately 25% of children have or had cavities before entering kindergarten, so it's important to provide guidance to caregivers on the appropriate use of fluoride toothpaste to help prevent their children from developing cavities," Dr. Truelove said.

The ADA said the updated guidelines are meant to help prevent cavities in children while limiting their risk of fluorosis, which is a mild discoloration of the teeth.

Tooth decay is the most common chronic childhood disease in the United States, and more than 16 million American children have untreated cavities, according to the U.S. Centers for Disease Control and Prevention.

The recommendations appeared in a February 2014 issue of *The Journal of the American Dental Association*.

info The American Academy of Pediatrics has more about children's oral health at *www.aap.org*.

Prenatal Exposure to Common Chemicals Linked to Lower IQs

Andrew Adesman, MD, chief, developmental and behavioral pediatrics, Cohen Children's Medical Center of New York, New Hyde Park, NY.
Pam Factor-Litvak, PhD, associate professor, epidemiology, Columbia University Medical Center, New York City.
PLOS ONE, online

Children exposed in the womb to higher amounts of two chemicals commonly found in plastics may be at higher risk for lower IQ, a recent study suggests.

The two compounds, *di-n-butyl phthalate* (DnBP) and *di-isobutyl phthalate* (DiBP), are part of a class of chemicals called phthalates and are found in a variety of household goods.

"This study adds to the small but growing body of research linking children's prenatal exposure to phthalates and later development," said Andrew Adesman, MD, chief of developmental and behavioral pediatrics at Cohen Children's Medical Center of New York, who was not involved with the study. "This is the first prospective study to identify an association between prenatal phthalate exposure and IQ in school-age children."

ABOUT PHTHALATES

Phthalates are added to plastics to make them more flexible and harder to break, according to the U.S. Centers for Disease Control and Prevention. But they serve other purposes as well, said study author Pam Factor-Litvak, PhD, an associate professor of epidemiology at the Columbia University Medical Center in New York City.

"Depending on the specific phthalate, they are used to make plastic flexible, as adhesive and as additives to cosmetics, air fresheners and cleaning products, as several 'hold' scents," Dr. Factor-Litvak said.

STUDY DETAILS

Dr. Factor-Litvak and her colleagues gave IQ tests to seven-year-old children of 328 inner-city mothers whose urine had been tested for phthalates exposure during late pregnancy.

The children of women in the highest quarter of exposure to DnBP and DiBP had IQs an average seven points lower than children of mothers in the lowest quarter of exposure, the investigators found.

The children also had poorer processing speed, perceptual reasoning and working memory if they were exposed to higher levels of these two chemicals, the findings showed. Perceptual reasoning refers to a person's ability to visualize and understand non-verbal information. In addition, verbal comprehension was lower among children with the greatest exposure to DiBP.

The researchers had also looked at exposure to three other phthalates—*butylbenzyl phthalate* (BBP), *di-2-ethylhexyl phthalate* (DEHP) and *diethyl phthalate* (DEP)—but did not see any differences among the children, with the exception of lower perceptual reasoning linked to BBP exposure.

The findings were published in the journal *PLOS ONE*.

IMPLICATIONS

"Although we cannot conclusively deduce that phthalates are responsible for the adverse effects on children's development, the growing body of research certainly suggests that phthalates may not be as safe as previously thought and that steps should be taken at a national level to reduce exposure to these chemicals," Dr. Adesman said.

Congress has already banned three phthalate types when they occur in concentrations greater than 0.1% in children's toys and specific child care articles, according to Dr. Factor-Litvak. Those include BBP, DEHP and dibutyl phthalate (which includes DiBP and DnBP), all of which were studied in this paper.

"While these regulatory actions were taken to protect young children, there have been no regulatory actions to protect the developing fetus in utero, which is often the time of greatest susceptibility," Dr. Factor-Litvak noted. "There are some replacement compounds on the market, but to our knowledge, they have not been studied extensively."

Dr. Adesman pointed out that the 2013 CDC fact sheet on phthalates states that human health effects from exposure to low levels of phthalates are unknown.

"Several studies now suggest that there may be adverse effects on children from prenatal phthalate exposure," Dr. Adesman said. "The CDC needs to encourage more research in this area and consider revising these fact sheets to reflect recent research. Likewise, the government should consider mandating changes to product labels to indicate which products have phthalates and/or consider restrictions on which types of products can include phthalates."

HOW TO REDUCE EXPOSURE

Dr. Factor-Litvak said it's difficult for individuals to completely avoid exposure to phthalates since the compounds are so widely used in consumer products, but there are steps people can take to reduce their exposures.

"Avoid microwaving food in plastic and avoid scented products, such as cleaning supplies, air fresheners and personal care products as much as possible," Dr. Factor-Litvak said. "Avoid use of plastics labeled as #3, #6 and #7 as these contain phthalates as well as BPA (bisphenol A), and store food in glass rather than plastic containers as much as possible."

info For more information on phthalates, visit the U.S. Centers for Disease Control and Prevention at *www.cdc.gov* and search "phthalate factsheet."

How Bullying Lasts Beyond School Years

The National Child Development Study, which followed almost 8,000 children born in England, Scotland and Wales, led by researchers at Kings College London, published in *The American Journal of Psychiatry*.

Researchers found that men who were bullied as children made less money and were more likely to be unemployed. Adults who suffered from childhood bullying had greater physical and mental health issues, lower levels of education and more social awkwardness when compared with those who were not bullied.

Best: Keep an open dialogue with your child so that there is a greater chance that he/she will tell you if he is being bullied. Anti-bullying awareness and laws are more common now but can help only if the bullying is reported.

No Link Seen Between Oxytocin-Assisted Labor and ADHD

Mette Juhl, PhD, MPH, midwife and associate professor, Midwifery Department, Metropolitan University College, Copenhagen, Denmark.
Glen Elliott, MD, PhD, chief psychiatrist and medical director, Children's Health Council, Palo Alto, California.
Pediatrics

Mothers who get an extra boost during labor with the medication *oxytocin* don't face a higher risk of having a child with attention-deficit/hyperactivity disorder (ADHD), a recent study says.

If a woman giving birth stops progressing during labor, she might receive oxytocin (brand name Pitocin) as "augmentation." This drug is a synthetic version of the oxytocin hormone involved in birth. It helps push labor along, increasing the likelihood that the cervix will continue dilating. But the hormone may have other effects, too.

"Oxytocin has many functions, including affecting social interactions," said Glen Elliott, MD, PhD, chief psychiatrist and medical director of Children's Health Council in Palo Alto, California. "Earlier studies were divided as to whether use of oxytocin to help labor progress increased the risk of the child later having a diagnosis of ADHD."

Children with ADHD, a brain disorder, tend to be inattentive, impulsive and hyperactive. These symptoms can make it hard to succeed in school and get along with others.

The original concern that ADHD and oxytocin might be linked arose from nonhuman studies, study author Mette Juhl, PhD, explained.

"Animal studies have found that oxytocin is passed on from mother to fetus via the placental barrier, and that the fetal brain has been affected by exposure to oxytocin," said Dr. Juhl, an associate professor of midwifery at Metropolitan University College in Copenhagen, Denmark.

It was possible, she said, that oxytocin might have some direct effect on the brain of the baby being born.

Bad Medicine for Kids

Giving children the wrong medicine and dosage is common. Nearly 700,000 children under age six experienced a medication error between 2002 and 2012. One-fourth of the errors involved children under a year old. Errors led to 25 deaths.

Statistical study by researchers at Center for Injury Research and Policy, Nationwide Children's Hospital, Columbus, Ohio, published in *Pediatrics*.

"According to the U.S. Institute for Safe Medication Practices, oxytocin is a drug that should be used with caution," Dr. Juhl said. "In light of the extensive use of labor augmentation in healthy young women, it is important to find out if augmentation treatment is associated with adverse effects, such as ADHD."

STUDY DETAILS

Dr. Juhl's team looked at children who had received either an ADHD diagnosis or a prescription for an ADHD medication among more than 546,000 Danish mothers.

Then they compared the 26% of children born to mothers who received oxytocin for labor augmentation with the children of mothers who did not.

The results showed that 0.9% of the children exposed to oxytocin had been diagnosed with or treated for ADHD. Overall, however, children exposed to oxytocin were no more likely to have ADHD than those not exposed, the study found.

EXPERT COMMENT

"One of the ongoing concerns physicians and parents alike have is that actions taken early on, especially during pregnancy and delivery, may cause unanticipated problems later on," said Dr. Elliott, who was not involved in the study. "But using a large registry of births, the authors found no evidence to support an increased risk of ADHD when oxytocin was used during labor."

This study's finding that ADHD and oxytocin augmentation are unrelated is important, Dr. Elliott said, because past research has found that complicated deliveries are related to a higher risk of various developmental problems later on.

"This study, hopefully, will reassure the obstetrician and mother-to-be that if oxytocin seems appropriate to ease delivery, it will not lead to markedly higher risk of the child having ADHD later in life," Dr. Elliott said.

The study, published online in *Pediatrics*, was funded by the Tryg Foundation and the Danish Medical Research Council. The authors reported no financial ties related to this research.

info The Nemours Foundations has tips on preparing for childbirth at *www.kids health.org/parent* (search "birthing classes").

States Are Getting Stricter on Child Vaccine Exemptions

Saad Omer, PhD, MPH, associate professor, global health, Rollins School of Public Health, Emory University, Atlanta.
Paul Offit, MD, chief, infectious diseases, and director, Vaccine Education Center, Children's Hospital of Philadelphia.
Journal of the American Medical Association

Legislative skirmishes over childhood vaccines are still happening in many states, but there are signs of a shift in the US toward limiting "personal belief" exemptions, a recent study finds.

All states require children to receive routine vaccines against diseases such as polio, measles, mumps and whooping cough before starting day care or public school. But most states allow parents to forgo vaccines for religious reasons, and 20 states permit "personal belief" exemptions for parents with philosophical objections.

In the recent study, researchers found that although lawmakers in other states have tried to introduce personal belief exemptions in recent years, none has been successful.

On the other hand, three states that allow the exemptions—California, Vermont and Washington—have recently passed laws to curb them. Basically, the states have increased the red tape parents face when applying for an opt-out on philosophical grounds.

"I think the bottom line is that while the advocacy efforts of pro-vaccine stakeholders have been successful in some states, there are still substantial efforts to weaken school immunization mandates," said study author Saad Omer, PhD, MPH. "Therefore, those who believe in the value of vaccines need to continue their advocacy efforts in their respective states."

Dr. Omer, an associate professor of global health at Emory University, in Atlanta, and colleagues reported their findings in a February 2014 issue of the *Journal of the American Medical Association*.

VACCINE FEARS AND EXEMPTIONS

An expert not involved in the study called the results "good news."

"I think what you're seeing now is the pendulum swinging in the other direction," said Paul Offit, MD, chief of infectious diseases at Children's Hospital of Philadelphia.

Dr. Offit said personal belief exemptions got their start in the 1970s and 1980s as a backlash against childhood vaccination mandates.

In recent years, a growing number of parents have been using the exemptions to shun vaccines over safety concerns. In a 2006 study, Dr. Omer's team found that the number of children in states with the opt-out who went unvaccinated for non-medical reasons more than doubled between 1991 and 2004—from about 1% to 2.5%.

Vaccine fears were set off in 1998, when a small study linked the measles-mumps-rubella vaccine to autism. That research was later found

Antibiotics Better for Appendicitis

Antibiotics treat appendicitis better than surgery. A recent study found that the majority of children with uncomplicated acute appendicitis who received antibiotics alone showed improvement within 24 hours, had less pain and missed fewer days of school.

Study by researchers at Nationwide Children's Hospital, Columbus, Ohio, published online in *Journal of the American College of Surgeons*.

to be fraudulent, but some parents' worries over vaccine safety persist.

EXEMPTIONS AND OUTBREAKS

Despite parental fears, lawmakers seem to be trying to rein in personal belief exemptions, Dr. Offit said.

That's at least partly in response to concerns about disease outbreaks. In 2010, for example, California had an outbreak of whooping cough that sickened more than 9,000 people and killed 10 infants—most of whom were too young to be vaccinated.

In a recent study of that outbreak, researchers at Johns Hopkins University found that whooping cough cases tended to concentrate in areas of the state with the highest rates of personal belief exemptions.

For the recent study, Dr. Omer's team looked at a legislative database maintained by the advocacy group Immunization Action Coalition.

The researchers found that between 2009 and 2012, 18 states introduced at least one bill on vaccine exemptions. Most of the bills—31 in all—were aimed at launching or expanding personal belief exemptions. None of them passed.

There were only five bills intended to restrict the exemptions, but three of them were signed into law.

Dr. Omer and his colleagues emphasized that success rate. "All of the legislative efforts to expand exemptions failed," they said. "However, the majority of bills to restrict exemptions passed."

Dr. Offit agreed. "If three out of five passed, that's pretty good," he said.

And although there were many more bills trying to expand personal belief exemptions, Dr. Offit said he saw that as "a last flicker, because they all failed."

"Previous studies have shown that high vaccine refusal rates tend to increase the risk of vaccine-preventable disease in the whole community—including for those who are vaccinated," Dr. Omer said. "So it is in everyone's interest to ensure that their community has high vaccination rates."

info The U.S. Centers for Disease Control and Prevention has more on childhood vaccinations at *http://www.cdc.gov/vaccines*.

School Lunches More Nutritious Than Home-Packed Lunches

Alisha Farris, MS, RD, PhD candidate, Virginia Tech University, Blacksburg.
Connie Diekman, MEd, RD, director of university nutrition, Washington University, St. Louis.
Journal of Nutrition Education and Behavior

Lunches packed at home are generally not as nutritious as school lunches, a recent study shows.

About 50 million children go to elementary and secondary public schools in the United States every day, according to background information in the study. About 60% eat the school lunch; the other 40% bring their lunch.

STUDY FINDINGS

Researchers compared more than 750 school meals with more than 560 packed meals given to pre-K and kindergarten students in three schools, analyzing them for nutritional value over five days.

"We found that packed lunches were of less nutritional quality than school lunches," said lead researcher Alisha Farris, a registered dietitian and a PhD candidate at Virginia Tech University.

The packed lunches had more fat, and included more desserts and sugary drinks than the school lunches did, the researchers found.

As a whole, the packed lunches overall had more calories, fat, saturated fat, sugar, vitamin C and iron than school lunches. In addition, meals brought from home generally had less protein, fiber, vitamin A and calcium than school lunches, according to the study.

"There was a spectrum," Farris said. "There were some really healthy packed lunches. But overall, they were pretty unhealthy."

The study is published in the *Journal of Nutrition Education and Behavior*.

PACKED VERSUS SCHOOL LUNCHES

To analyze the nutritional content of the lunches, the researchers used the National School Lunch Program Standards as a guide.

The school lunches had about 512 calories on average and the packed meals about 608, the researchers found. The protein content of the school meals was about 26 grams, compared with 18 in packed lunches.

The researchers also found that packed lunches were less likely than school lunches to have fruits, vegetables, sugar-free juice and milk.

Packed lunches had more snacks such as chips and crackers, she found.

Farris found that sodium was higher in school lunches than packed, probably due to the entree items found in school lunches. School lunches had about 1,000 milligrams (mg) of sodium; packed lunches about 880 mg.

One limitation in the study, Farris said, is that actual consumption wasn't measured, only observations about the contents of the lunches.

EXPERT REACTION

The findings are no surprise to Connie Diekman, MEd, RD, director of university nutrition at Washington University in St. Louis. "This study provides outcomes that are similar to other studies that show the positive benefits of school lunch," she said.

"While it is surprising to see the higher sodium content in the school lunch, the nutritional pluses of the school lunch—more fiber, vitamin A and less sugar and saturated fat—make the [nutritional] value aspect of school lunch better," Diekman said.

HOW TO PACK A NUTRITIOUS LUNCH

Diekman has served on her school district's wellness committee and has visited schools to observe lunch programs. Involving the kids

in the planning helps improve children's food choices, she said.

For parents who want to pack lunches for their kids, Farris has these tips. "Include a fruit, a vegetable, protein and dairy," she said. "Pack a sandwich. Put in an apple and carrot sticks." For dairy, she said, choose what your child likes, such as yogurt, milk or cheese, and put in a cold pack to keep it chilled.

info For more strategies for packing a healthy lunch, visit the Academy of Nutrition and Dietetics website, *www.eatright.org*, and search "nutritious lunchbox."

Pizza Takes a Slice Out of Kids' Health

Lisa M. Powell, PhD, professor, health policy and administration, and director, Illinois Prevention Research Center, University of Illinois at Chicago School of Public Health.
Yoni Freedhoff, MD, CCFP, assistant professor, family medicine, University of Ottawa, and founder and medical director, Bariatric Medical Institute, Ottawa.
Connie Diekman, MEd, RD, director, university nutrition, Washington University in St. Louis.
Pediatrics

On the days your kids eat pizza, they likely take in more calories, fat and sodium than on other days, a recent study found.

On any given day in the United States in 2009-10, one in five young children and nearly one in four teens ate pizza for a meal or snack, researchers found.

THE STUDY

Study author Lisa M. Powell, MD, a professor of health policy and administration at the University of Illinois at Chicago and her team analyzed data from four U.S. National Health and Nutrition Examination Surveys from 2003 to 2010. Families of nearly 14,000 children and teens, aged two to 19, reported what their kids had eaten in the previous 24 hours.

From the first survey in 2003-2004 to the last survey in 2009-2010, calories consumed from pizza declined by one-quarter overall among children aged two to 11. Daily average calo-

---

Caffeine Can Harm Children

Even low doses of caffeine—the equivalent of what is found in a half can of caffeinated soda or a half cup of coffee—slow children's heart rates and increase their blood pressure. It is not yet known what the long-term effects of repeated exposure to caffeine would be.

Study of 52 children, ages eight and nine...and 49 children, ages 15 to 17, by researchers at University at Buffalo School of Public Health and Health Professions, New York, published in *Pediatrics*.

Soap Packs Look Like Candy

Ten thousand children were poisoned by laundry and dishwasher detergent packs in 2014. Many of the single-dose detergent capsules look like candy. When ingested, they can cause digestive and breathing problems, especially in young children.

The New York Times. www.nytimes.com

ries from pizza also declined among teens, but slightly more teens reported eating pizza.

The proportion of younger kids eating pizza at dinner and from fast food dropped over the period studied. When they did eat it, however, it bumped up their total average calories eaten that day, especially if it was eaten as a snack or from a fast-food restaurant.

On the days children ate pizza, they consumed 84 more calories, 3 grams more saturated fat and 134 milligrams more sodium than average, the investigators found. Teens took in an extra 230 calories, 5 grams saturated fat and 484 mg sodium on pizza days.

"There were no differences in impact on calories and nutrients between whether youths ate pizza from stores or from fast food, suggesting that efforts to improve the nutritional content of pizza should include pizza from all sources," Dr. Powell said.

The only time pizza did not increase kids' daily caloric intake were days they ate it from the school cafeteria. That could mean school pizzas are healthier, or it could mean other school lunches are equally high in calories, Dr. Powell said.

The findings were reported in the journal *Pediatrics*.

IMPLICATIONS

"Given that pizza remains a highly prevalent part of children's diet, we need to make healthy pizza the norm," said Dr. Powell.

"Efforts by food producers and restaurants to improve the nutrient content of pizza, in particular by reducing its saturated fat and sodium [salt] content and increasing its whole-grain con-

tent, could have quite broad reach in terms of improving children's diets," Dr. Powell said.

Pizza's popularity comes largely from being tasty and inexpensive, but it's also because children have so many opportunities to eat it, said Yoni Freedhoff, MD, an assistant professor of family medicine at the University of Ottawa in Canada.

"It's constantly being thrust at them," he said. "From school cafeterias to weekly pizza days in schools without cafeterias to birthday parties to group events to pizza night with the parents to pizza fund-raising—it's difficult to escape," Dr. Freedhoff said.

"But of course, that doesn't make it healthy," he added.

When pizza is consumed, it makes up more than 20% of the daily intake of calories, the study authors said. Poor eating habits—too many calories, too much salt and too much fat—raise children's risks for nutrition-related diseases, including type 2 diabetes, high blood pressure and obesity, the study authors added in background notes with the study.

HOW TO MAKE PIZZA MORE HEALTHFUL

Connie Diekman, MEd, RD, director of university nutrition at Washington University in St. Louis, said "The big take-away is that the overall balance of kids' diets is not as healthful as it needs to be. If kids love pizza, assess how it fits into the whole day so that it doesn't take calories away from other food groups."

She said ways to make pizza healthier can include using whole-wheat or white whole-wheat for the crust, using more fruits and vegetables instead of meat, and using less cheese or stronger-flavored cheeses.

Dr. Freedhoff has his own low-calorie pizza recipe. By skipping the meat and sticking to part skim-milk mozzarella, basil, onion and garlic, a pizza can still total less than 200 calories a slice.

Dr. Freedhoff said store-bought pizza can be enjoyed in moderation. But frequently eating pizza at school may lead children to think of fast-food pizzas as a regular meal rather than a treat, a habit that could carry over into adulthood, he said.

"There's often a world of difference between doing what's right and doing what's easy," he added. "By leaning on pizza because we can, we're normalizing a culture of convenience that isn't in our children's or their health's best interest."

info For guidelines on healthy eating for children, visit the American Heart Association at *www.heart.org* and search "Dietary Recommendations for Healthy Children."

Pediatricians' Group Opposes Legal Marijuana

American Academy of Pediatrics, news release.

Marijuana shouldn't be legalized because of the potential harm it can cause children and teens, the American Academy of Pediatrics says.

However, the group's updated policy statement does support the compassionate use of marijuana for children with debilitating or terminal illnesses.

The academy supports decriminalizing marijuana, which means offenses would result in civil penalties or lesser criminal charges than they currently carry. But, the AAP recommends this be done in conjunction with programs to prevent marijuana use and provide early treatment for teens with marijuana use problems.

The statement also includes steps to protect children in states that have legalized marijuana for recreational or medicinal use.

The AAP policy statement was published online in *Pediatrics*.

"We know marijuana can be very harmful to adolescent health and development," Seth Ammerman, MD, FAAP, a member of the AAP Committee on Substance Abuse and an author of the policy statement, said in an academy news release.

"Making it more available to adults—even if restrictions are in place—will increase the access for teens. Just the campaigns to legalize marijuana can have the effect of persuading adolescents that marijuana is not dangerous, which can have a devastating impact on their lifelong health and development," Dr. Ammerman said.

HOW MARIJUANA IS DANGEROUS

In teens, marijuana can cause memory and concentration problems that may lead to difficulties in school. Also, the drug can impair motor control, coordination and judgment, leading to an increased risk of accidental injury and death, according to the AAP.

What's more, the AAP pointed out that regular use of marijuana can lead to poorer lung health, psychological problems and a greater chance of drug dependence in adulthood.

"It is true we do not yet have data documenting changes to child health in response to the legalization of marijuana in Washington and Colorado, though there have been reports of child ingestion and injuries," said Sharon Levy, MD, FAAP, chair of the AAP Committee on Substance Abuse.

"It took several generations, millions of lives and billions of dollars to establish the harms of tobacco use on health, even though these harms are overwhelming. We should not consider marijuana 'innocent until proven guilty,' given what we already know about the harms to adolescents," Dr. Levy said.

info The U.S. National Institute on Drug Abuse has more about marijuana at *http://www.drugabuse.gov/publications/drug facts/marijuana*.

Important Parent-Teen Talk

Teens whose parents told them they were against underage drinking are more than 80% less likely to drink than teens whose parents didn't give them a clear message. Only 8% of teens whose parents said that underage drinking was unacceptable were active drinkers. Nearly 50% of teens whose parents thought that underage drinking was acceptable or somewhat acceptable were active drinkers.

Online survey of 663 high school students by MADD.

Teens Who Dine with Their Families May Be Slimmer Adults

Jerica Berge, PhD, MPH, assistant professor, department of family and community medicine, University of Minnesota Medical School, Minneapolis.

Kristi King, RD, MPH, clinical dietitian, Texas Children's Hospital, and clinical instructor, pediatrics, section of gastroenterology, hepatology and nutrition, Baylor College of Medicine, Houston.

Journal of Pediatrics

For those teens who try to avoid spending time with their parents and siblings, research research suggests that sitting down for family meals might help them stay slim as adults.

Despite everyone's busy schedules, researchers found that just one or two gatherings around the kitchen table each week were well worth the effort.

"There are numerous distractions that could keep families from having family meals. However, this study shows that even trying to have a few family meals a week could be beneficial for guarding against overweight and obesity in adulthood," noted study author Jerica Berge, PhD, MPH, an assistant professor in the department of family and community medicine at the University of Minnesota Medical School, in Minneapolis.

OK on the PB and J !

Young girls who eat peanut butter reduce their risk of developing benign breast disease. Eating peanut butter or nuts three days a week between the ages of nine and 15 lowered the risk for breast disease by 39% 15 years later. Benign breast disease—noncancerous changes in the breast tissue—affects about one-fourth of all women and is considered a risk factor for later development of breast cancer.

Graham Colditz, MD, DrPh, associate director for cancer prevention and control, Alvin J. Siteman Cancer Center and professor of medicine, Washington University School of Medicine, both in St. Louis, and leader of a study of 9,039 schoolgirls, published in *Breast Cancer Research and Treatment*.

THE STUDY

Using data from a 10-year study involving more than 2,000 teenagers, the researchers examined variables that could affect young people's weight, such as diet and physical activity. The teens were asked how often they sat down for family meals. The researchers also recorded each teen's body mass index (BMI)—a measurement that determines whether a person is a healthy weight for their height.

After a decade, 51% of the teens involved in the study were overweight and 22% were obese overall, the study published recently in the *Journal of Pediatrics* found.

The researchers noted that when the study began, 15% of the teens said they never ate family meals. Of those teens, 60% were overweight at the 10-year follow up and 29% were obese.

Meanwhile, among the teens that reported eating between one and five family meals per week, only 47% to 51% were overweight a decade later, and 19% to 22% were obese.

EXPLANATION

So, how do family meals help prevent weight gain? The protective effect is likely due to a combination of factors, according to Dr. Berge. "Although we don't know exactly why having family meals is protective, family meals may provide a combination of activities such as opportunities for healthful eating, connection among family members, creating a supportive environment for emotion regulation and a sense of security that give children the ability to regulate their own eating behaviors in their day-to-day lives," she explained.

Research has shown that American children and teens sit down for an average of about two to four family meals per week, according to Dr. Berge. She noted this includes breakfast and lunch, as well as dinner.

Another study Dr. Berge conducted, which was published in the journal *Pediatrics*, found that calm, positive family meals might help a child avoid becoming overweight or obese.

One expert noted that her clients are really trying to carve out time for family meals.

"The '50s were the epitome of the family meal," explained Kristi King, RD, MPH, a clinical dietitian at Texas Children's Hospital in

Possible ADHD Link

Acetaminophen may be linked to ADHD. Pregnant women who take Tylenol and other medications with acetaminophen are 13% more likely to have children diagnosed with attention-deficit/hyperactivity disorder (ADHD).

Study of more than 64,000 Danish mothers and children by researchers at University of California, Los Angeles, Fielding School of Public Health, published in *JAMA Pediatrics*.

Houston. "As society became more fast-paced, we found ourselves drifting away from the family meal time. Now, in practice, I see families very much wanting to try and slow down and reinstitute the family meal on a regular basis."

King also pointed out that meals at home are typically lower in calories and contain more fruits and vegetables.

RECOMMENDATIONS

For busy families, having just one family meal is a great place to start, Dr. Berge pointed out. "It may not matter which day of the week it occurs or that it is the dinner meal. The important thing is to start making family meals a regular occurrence," she said.

Limiting distractions can also help, advised King.

"Just one meal can give families the opportunity to 'check-in,' but that is assuming technology takes a backseat during meal time," she said. "Kids learn by watching their parents. So parents should set the example they wish their children to follow. Try having the whole family disconnect for 30 minutes during meal time and actually having a conversation."

info For more information on preventing obesity, visit the website of the U.S. National Heart, Lung, and Blood Institute, *www. nhlbi.nih.gov*, and search "How can overweight and obesity be prevented?"

Fitness May Boost Kids' Brainpower

Laura Chaddock-Heyman, PhD, postdoctoral researcher, department of psychology, University of Illinois at Urbana-Champaign.
Bonita Marks, PhD, professor, exercise physiology, and director, Exercise Science Teaching Lab, department of exercise and sport science, University of North Carolina at Chapel Hill.
Megan Herting, PhD, postdoctoral fellow, division of research on children, youth and families, Children's Hospital of Los Angeles.
Frontiers in Human Neuroscience

Exercise and brainpower in children may not seem closely related, but a small recent study hints that fitness may supercharge kids' minds.

The finding doesn't prove that fitness actually makes children smarter, but it provides support for the idea, the researchers said.

"Our work suggests that aerobically fit and physically fit children have improved brain health and superior cognitive [thinking] skills than their less-fit peers," said study author Laura Chaddock-Heyman, PhD, a postdoctoral researcher with the department of psychology at the University of Illinois at Urbana-Champaign. "Hopefully, these findings will reinforce the importance of aerobic fitness during development and lead to additional physical activity opportunities in and out of the school environment."

BACKGROUND

The researchers launched their study to gain more insight into the connections between fitness and the brain in children. Other research has connected higher levels of fitness to better attention, memory and academic skills, Dr. Chaddock-Heyman said.

And two recent studies found that fit kids are more likely to have better language skills and to do better on standardized tests for math and reading.

But there are still mysteries. While moderate exercise boosts brainpower for a few hours—making it a good idea to work out before a test—it's not clear how fitness affects the brain in the long term, said Bonita Marks, PhD, director of the Exercise Science Teaching Lab at the University of North Carolina at Chapel

Hill. "The chronic impact is less certain and, for health, really the key for future research and health management," she added.

STUDY FINDINGS

The recent study didn't examine any thinking skills, but instead looked only at the brain's "white matter," which helps different brain regions communicate with each other. The researchers scanned the brains of 24 kids aged nine and 10, and found that white matter was different in the fitter kids, potentially a sign of better-connected brains.

Higher levels of fitness may boost blood flow, increase the size of certain brain areas and improve the structure of white matter, Dr. Chaddock-Heyman said.

The study was published in the journal *Frontiers in Human Neuroscience*.

IMPLICATIONS

What do the findings mean in the big picture?

It's hard to know for sure. Megan Herting, PhD, a postdoctoral fellow with the division of research on children, youth, and families at Children's Hospital of Los Angeles, pointed out that the kids with lower fitness levels also weighed more, "so it is unclear if it is actually fitness or 'fatness' that may be affecting the brain. "Studies show that individuals with obesity have different brains compared to their healthier-weight peers," she said.

As for the stereotype of the 99-pound weakling nerd, Dr. Herting suggested it may be time for a rethink. "These findings do challenge that if you are aerobically fit, you are likely to be dumb. In fact, from an evolutionary perspective, we were made to move. So rather than fit-

ness being 'good' for the brain and cognition, it is feasible that being sedentary may be 'bad.'"

NEW STUDY IN PROGRESS

The researchers are now working on a study that assigns some kids to take part in exercise programs to see what happens to their brains over time when compared with other kids, Dr. Chaddock-Heyman said.

info For more about fitness, visit the website of the American Academy of Pediatrics, *www.healthychildren.org*, and search "How to get fit."

High Tech Reins In Teen Drivers

Roundup of experts on automotive technology, reported at *CBSNews.com*.

Use technology to set limits on teenage drivers. Ford models equipped with the MyFord Touch system (available with Ford's Sync system, which costs $60/year) let you set maximum speed, give beeper reminders as the vehicle reaches designated speeds and put limits on the volume of the audio system. And the radio will not turn on if seat belts are not fastened. General Motors Family Link, a $3.99/month add-on to the GM OnStar service—which costs $20 to $30 a month—lets you stipulate where a teen can drive, providing text messages if he/she leaves the area.

Heart & Stroke

6 Secrets to Holistic Heart Care

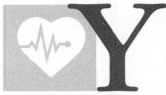

You don't smoke, your cholesterol levels look good and your blood pressure is under control.

This means that you're off the hook when it comes to having a heart attack or developing heart disease, right? Maybe not.

Surprising statistic: About 20% of people with heart disease do not have any of the classic risk factors, such as those described above.

The missing link: While most conventional medical doctors prescribe medications and other treatments to help patients control the "big" risk factors for heart disease, holistic cardiologists also suggest small lifestyle changes that over time make a significant difference in heart

*To find a holistic cardiologist, go to the website of the American Board of Integrative Holistic Medicine, *ABIHM.org*, and search the database of certified integrative physicians.

disease risk.* *My secrets for preventing heart disease...*

SECRET #1: Stand up! You may not think of standing as a form of exercise. However, it's more effective than most people realize.

Think about what you're doing when you're not standing. Unless you're asleep, you're probably sitting. While sitting, your body's metabolism slows...your insulin becomes less effective...and you're likely to experience a gradual drop in HDL "good" cholesterol.

A study that tracked the long-term health of more than 123,000 Americans found that those who sat for six hours or more a day had an overall death rate that was higher—18% higher for men and 37% for women—than those who sat for less than three hours.

What's so great about standing? When you're on your feet, you move more. You pace...fidget...

Joel K. Kahn, MD, clinical professor of medicine at Wayne State University School of Medicine in Detroit and director of Cardiac Wellness at Michigan Healthcare Professionals. He is a founding member of the International Society of Integrative, Metabolic and Functional Cardiovascular Medicine and author of *The Whole Heart Solution. DrJoelKahn.com* move your arms…and walk from room to room. This type of activity improves metabolism and can easily burn hundreds of extra calories a day. Standing also increases your insulin sensitivity to help prevent diabetes. So stand up and move around when talking on the phone, checking e-mail and watching television.

SECRET #2: Count your breaths. Slow, deep breathing is an effective way to help prevent high blood pressure—one of the leading causes of heart disease. For people who already have high blood pressure, doing this technique a few times a day has been shown to lower blood pressure by five to 10 points within five minutes. And the pressure may stay lower for up to 24 hours.

During a breathing exercise, you want to slow your breathing down from the usual 12 to 16 breaths a minute that most people take to about three breaths. I use the "4-7-8 sequence" whenever I feel stressed.

What to do: Inhale through your nose for four seconds…hold the breath in for seven seconds…then exhale through the mouth for eight seconds.

Also helpful: A HeartMath software package, which you can load on your computer or smartphone, includes breathing exercises to help lower your heart rate and levels of stress hormones.

Cost: $129 and up, at *HeartMath.org*. You can also sign up for some free tools on this website.

SECRET #3: Practice "loving kindness." This is an easy form of meditation that reduces stress, thus allowing you to keep your heart rate and blood pressure at healthy levels.

Research has shown that people who meditate regularly are 48% less likely to have a heart attack or stroke than those who don't meditate. "Loving kindness" meditation is particularly effective at promoting relaxation—it lowers levels of the stress hormones adrenaline and cortisol while raising levels of the healing hormone oxytocin.

What to do: Sit quietly, with your eyes closed. For a few minutes, focus on just your breathing. Then imagine one person in your life whom you find exceptionally easy to love. Imagine this person in front of you. Fill your heart with a warm, loving feeling…think about how you both want to be happy and avoid suffering…and imagine that a feeling of peace trav-

---

How Heart Patients Can Lower Risk for Early Death by 55%

When cardiac patients talked with nurses and doctors about their treatment and other concerns…did relaxation exercises…and/or participated in music therapy during their hospitalization or rehabilitation, they were 55% less likely to die or have another cardiovascular event after two years, in a recent study.

How heart patients can get this type of support: Ask health-care providers more questions about their treatment…and seek out activities, such as music or exercise programs, group psychotherapy and meditation.

Zoi Aggelopoulou, PhD, RN, head of continuing education, NIMTS Veterans Hospital of Athens, Greece.

---

els from your heart to that person's heart in the form of white light. Dwell on the image for a few minutes. This meditation will also help you practice small acts of kindness in your daily life—for example, giving a hand to someone who needs help crossing the street.

SECRET #4: Don't neglect sex. Men who have sex at least two times a week have a 50% lower risk for a heart attack than those who abstain. Similar research hasn't been done on women, but it's likely that they get a comparable benefit.

Why does sex help keep your heart healthy? It probably has more to do with intimacy than the physical activity itself. Couples who continue to have sex tend to be the ones with more intimacy in their marriages. Happy people who bond with others have fewer heart attacks—and recover more quickly if they've had one—than those without close relationships.

SECRET #5: Be happy! People who are happy and who feel a sense of purpose and connection with others tend to have lower blood pressure and live longer than those who are isolated. Research shows that two keys to happiness are to help others be happy—for example, by being a volunteer—and to reach out to friends and neighbors. Actually, any shared activity, such as going to church or doing group hobbies, can increase survival among heart patients by about 50%.

SECRET #6: Try Waon (pronounced Wa-own) therapy. With this Japanese form of "warmth therapy," you sit in an infrared (dry) sauna for 15 minutes then retreat to a resting area for half an hour, where you wrap yourself in towels and drink plenty of water. Studies show that vascular function improves after such therapy due to the extra release of nitric oxide, the master molecule in blood vessels that helps them relax.

Some health clubs offer Waon treatments, but the dry saunas at many gyms should offer similar benefits. I do not recommend steam rooms—moist heat places extra demands on the heart and can be dangerous for some people.

Heart Murmur Concern

Michael Miller, MD, professor of cardiovascular medicine, University of Maryland School of Medicine, Baltimore, and author of *Heal Your Heart*.

Do individuals with a heart murmur have a higher risk of heart disease?

Usually not. A heart murmur is an extra sound made during a heartbeat, often caused by a heart valve that doesn't fully close. Most lifelong heart murmurs do not raise risk for heart disease or need treatment.

However, a heart murmur that begins in older age (over age 60) can indicate progressive changes in the heart such as narrowing of a valve due to calcium buildup. If your doctor hears a murmur that was not present before, you may want to have an ultrasound of the heart (echocardiogram) to evaluate your heart valves and function in order to better estimate your risk for heart disease.

Combo Drug Prevents Heart Attacks

Robert M. Califf, MD, vice-chancellor for clinical and translational research and director of the Duke Translational Medicine Institute, Durham, North Carolina. He led a study presented at a recent meeting of the American Heart Association.

Combination drug prevents heart attack and stroke better than a statin alone. Vytorin, which contains the statin *simvastatin* plus *ezetimibe*, a drug that prevents the body from absorbing cholesterol, brought down levels of LDL (bad) cholesterol more than simvastatin did on its own. Vytorin had no more side effects than taking a statin alone. Patients who took Vytorin had 6.4% reduced risk for cardiac events. Vytorin should be considered when a statin alone leaves the patient with LDL greater than 70 mg/dL or when the patient cannot take a full dose of a statin because of a side effect.

The Hidden Heart Disease Even Doctors Miss

Holly S. Andersen, MD, attending cardiologist and director of Education and Outreach at the Ronald O. Perelman Heart Institute of New York-Presbyterian Hospital in New York City and medical adviser to the Women's Heart Alliance. She is an expert in the field of heart disease in women.

It's hard to imagine that with all the technology available today that heart disease could be completely missed. But that's exactly what's frequently occurring with a tricky heart condition known as small vessel disease or coronary microvascular disease (MVD).

Here's what happens: Patients, most often women, have chest pain, other symptoms that suggest heart disease or even heart attacks. But when doctors examine their coronary arteries, they find no evidence of blockage and often rule out heart disease.

Result: Patients go without the vital treatment they need.

Mystery solved: The problem in these cases, researchers have recently discovered, often lies in the tiny blood vessels—which can't be seen with the naked eye or conventional heart disease testing—that branch off the larger coronary arteries in the heart.

Researchers still have much to learn about MVD, but here's what's known now and what you can do to protect yourself…

A DIFFERENT KIND OF HEART DISEASE

The most common variety of coronary heart disease (CHD) is caused by atherosclerotic plaques—cholesterol-containing deposits that pile up and narrow one or more of the large arteries that carry blood to the heart, restricting flow. When the heart gets too little blood to meet its needs—during exertion, for example—people with CHD have chest pain (angina). And if blood flow is restricted even further—usually due to a clot lodged in the narrowed artery—a heart attack and death may occur.

Plaque is often involved in MVD, too. But instead of accumulating in clumps that block off segments of specific coronary arteries, cholesterol is deposited more evenly inside whole areas of microscopic circulation. Additionally, in MVD the walls of the tiny arteries are injured or diseased—instead of opening wider to allow more blood to reach the heart during exercise or at times of emotional stress, they tighten up, constricting blood flow when it's needed most.

The reason for this is unclear, but it seems that at least some of the time, it's due to malfunction of the endothelial cells that line the blood vessels. The resulting symptoms can be indistinguishable from garden-variety CHD—and the risk for heart attack may be just as real.

DO YOU HAVE MICROVASCULAR DISEASE?

Diabetes and high blood pressure raise one's risk for MVD, as does CHD. High cholesterol, obesity, smoking and a lack of physical activity are risk factors, too, and like CHD, MVD becomes more common with advancing age.

Symptoms of MVD can be identical to the classic signs of CHD—pain, a squeezing sensation or pressure in the chest, usually during activity or emotional stress. The discomfort can also occur in the shoulders, arms, neck or jaw.

MVD tip-off: Painful episodes of MVD usually last longer—more than 10 minutes, and sometimes longer than 30 minutes—than those of classic CHD.

Other symptoms of MVD: Fatigue or lack of energy, trouble sleeping and shortness of breath. Women are particularly likely to have these vague manifestations rather than the kind of distinct chest pain that we usually associate with heart disease. Forty percent of women don't have chest pain even while having a heart attack, whether it's caused by CHD or MVD.

Another clue: With MVD, patients often notice symptoms during daily activities and/or during times of mental stress rather than during times of physical exertion as is more often the case with CHD.

GETTING A DIAGNOSIS

The standard tests for heart disease may not uncover MVD. If you suspect you have the condition, be sure to see a cardiologist with significant experience in treating MVD. An academic medical center is the best place to find such a doctor. *He/she may be able to diagnose it from your symptoms, medical history and earlier test results, or he may order additional tests…*

•**Nuclear imaging,** which uses a radioactive compound injected into the bloodstream to reveal a detailed image of the heart and blood flow through the arteries, including microcirculation.

•**Magnetic resonance imaging (MRI)** to produce a picture of the heart and its circulation without subjecting the patient to dye or radiation.

•**Positron emission tomography (PET),** which provides information on metabolism in the heart. This can uncover certain areas that aren't getting enough fuel and oxygen, suggesting MVD.

IF YOU HAVE MVD

If MVD is diagnosed, the goal is to keep it from progressing and to prevent heart attack and stroke. *Key strategies…*

•**Tweak your diet, and punch up your exercise routine.** A healthy eating plan, such as the Mediterranean diet, emphasizes fruits, vegetables, legumes, whole grains and nuts and fish, which contain healthy fats. Weight control and exercise reduce heart disease risk overall and also reduce blood pressure and help prevent diabetes, which are additional MVD risk factors. Beyond its general cardiovascular benefits, regular exercise appears to improve the function of the endothelial cells that line blood vessels and function poorly in MVD.

•**Get help from medication.** Doctors prescribe the same medications to treat MVD as for CHD—to reduce blood pressure and cholesterol. Aspirin or other drugs to reduce clotting risk are recommended as well.

Some evidence suggests that statins may be particularly useful because they not only reduce cholesterol but also improve endothelial function and relax the muscles around tiny blood vessels.

Similarly, calcium channel blockers, such as *amlodipine* (Norvasc), and ACE inhibitors, like *enalapril* (Vasotec), may be good choices for lowering blood pressure because they too help keep arteries open.

•**Get treated for anemia if you have it.** Anemia (low red blood cell count) may slow the growth of cells that help repair artery walls. This condition is treated with iron or B-12 supplements.

Note: If you have CHD and MVD (it's possible to have both) and have had angioplasty, a stent or bypass surgery, be aware that these procedures do not help MVD.

Add Fiber...Help Your Heart: No Fancy Diet Needed

Study of 240 people with metabolic syndrome led by researchers at University of Massachusetts Medical School, Worcester, published in Annals of Internal Medicine.

Overweight adults who ate more fiber lost nearly as much weight as others who followed a more complex diet. The fiber group also lowered their blood pressure and controlled their insulin levels as much as those who followed the more complex diet. Participants were told to increase fiber to 30 grams per day but were not given a diet plan. Weight loss was compared with those who followed the American Heart Association diet.

Underused Stroke Drug

Only about 4% of stroke patients receive a drug that could save their lives. Tissue plasminogen activator (tPA) was shown 20 years ago to dissolve stroke-related clots that can cause brain damage, but most patients don't receive it. The drug must be given within 4.5 hours of a stroke. If you are having possible stroke symptoms, seek medical attention immediately.

Study by researchers at University of Cincinnati, presented at the American Heart Association/American Stroke Association's annual International Stroke Conference 2014 in San Diego.

Artery Inflammation: Six Simple, Lifesaving Tests

Bradley Bale, MD, medical director, Grace Clinic Heart Health Program, Lubbock, Texas, and cofounder, Heart Attack & Stroke Prevention Center, Spokane. He is co-author, with Amy Doneen, ARNP, and Lisa Collier Cool, of Beat the Heart Attack Gene: The Revolutionary Plan to Prevent Heart Disease, Stroke and Diabetes.

A fire could be smoldering inside your arteries...a type of fire that could erupt at any moment, triggering a heart attack or stroke. In fact, the fire could be building right this minute and you wouldn't even know it. That's because the usual things doctors look at when gauging cardiovascular risk—cholesterol, blood pressure, blood sugar, weight—can all appear to be fine even when your arteries are dangerously hot.

What does work to detect hot arteries? A set of six simple, inexpensive and readily available blood and urine tests.

Problem: Few doctors order these tests, and few patients know enough to ask for them. *Here's how to protect yourself...*

THE BODY'S ARMY ON ATTACK

Hot arteries are not actually hot (as in very warm)—instead, in this case "hot" refers to the effects of chronic inflammation. Why call them hot, then? Chronic arterial inflammation can put you on the fast track to developing vascular disease

Surprising Heart Danger

Women who lived within 164 feet of a major roadway were 38% more likely to suffer sudden cardiac death than those who lived farther away, according to a recent study.

Possible reason: Increased air pollution.

Circulation

by speeding up the aging of your arteries. It's so dangerous to the arterial lining that it's worse than having high LDL cholesterol. And if your arteries are already clogged with plaque—which acts as kindling for a heart attack or stroke—inflammation is what lights the match.

Inflammation in the body isn't always bad, of course. In fact, it's an important aspect of healing. When something in your body is under attack, the immune system sends in troops of white blood cells to repair and fight off the attacker, and temporary inflammation results. That's why when you cut yourself, for example, you'll see swelling at the site of the injury—it's a sign that your white blood cells are at work for your benefit.

But: When an attack against your body persists (for instance, as occurs when you have an ongoing infection of the gums), your white blood cells continue to drive inflammation. When it turns chronic, inflammation becomes highly damaging to many tissues, including the arteries.

Normally, the endothelium (lining of the arteries) serves as a protective barrier between blood and the deeper layers of the arterial wall. However, when that lining is inflamed, it can't function well and it gets sticky, almost like flypaper, trapping white blood cells on their way through the body. The inflamed endothelium becomes leaky, too, allowing LDL "bad" cholesterol to penetrate into the wall of the artery. The white blood cells then gobble up the cholesterol, forming fatty streaks that ultimately turn into plaque, a condition called atherosclerosis. Then when the plaque itself becomes inflamed, it can rupture, tearing through the endothelium into the channel of the artery where blood flows. This material triggers the formation of a blood clot—a clot that could end up blocking blood flow to the heart or brain.

THE 6-PART FIRE PANEL

Just as firefighters have ways of determining whether a blaze is hiding within the walls of a building, certain tests can reveal whether inflammation is lurking within the walls of your arteries. I use a set of six tests that I call the "fire panel." Each reveals different risk factors and, for several of the tests, too-high scores can have more than one cause—so it's important to get all six tests, not just one or two.

The fire panel can identify people at risk for developing atherosclerosis…reveal whether patients who already have atherosclerosis have dangerously hot arteries that could lead to a heart attack or stroke…and evaluate patients who have survived a heart attack or stroke to see whether their current treatments are working to reduce the inflammation that threatens their lives. Your individual test results will help determine your most appropriate course of treatment.

I recommend that all adults have this panel of tests done at least every 12 months—or every three to six months for patients at high risk for heart attack or stroke. All of these tests are readily available…are inexpensive and usually covered by insurance…and can be ordered by your regular doctor. *Here are the six tests…*

•**F2 Isoprostanes.** My nickname for this blood test is the "lifestyle lie detector" because it reveals whether or not patients are practicing heart-healthy habits. The test, which measures a biomarker of oxidative stress, helps determine how fast your body's cells are oxidizing, or breaking down. According to one study, people who have the highest levels of F2 isoprostanes are nine times more likely to have blockages in their coronary arteries than people with the lowest levels.

The score you want: A normal score is less than 0.86 ng/L…an optimal score is less than 0.25 ng/L.

•**Fibrinogen.** An abnormally high level of this sticky, fibrous protein in your blood can contribute to the formation of clots…it's also a marker of inflammation. One study divided people into four groups (quartiles) based on their fibrinogen levels and found that stroke risk rose by nearly 50% for each quartile. High fibrinogen is particularly dangerous for people who also have high blood pressure because both conditions damage the blood vessel lining and make it easier for plaque to burrow inside.

Normal range: 440 mg/dL or lower.

•**High-Sensitivity C-Reactive Protein (hs-CRP).** Your liver produces C-reactive protein, and the amount of it in your blood rises when there is inflammation in your body—so an elevated hs-CRP level generally is considered a precursor to cardiovascular disease. The large-scale Harvard Women's Health Study cited this test as being more accurate than cholesterol in predicting risk for cardiovascular disease…while another study of women found that those with high scores were up to four times more likely to have a heart attack or stroke than women with lower scores. A high hs-CRP score is especially worrisome for a person with a large waist. Excess belly fat often is a sign of insulin resistance (in which cells don't readily accept insulin), a condition that further magnifies heart attack and stroke risk.

The score you're aiming for: Under 1.0 mg/L is normal…0.5 mg/L is optimal.

•**Microalbumin/Creatinine Urine Ratio (MACR).** This test looks for albumin in the urine. Albumin is a large protein molecule that circulates in the blood and shouldn't spill from capillaries in the kidneys into the urine, so its presence suggests dysfunction of the endothelium. Though this test provides valuable infor-mation about arterial wall health, doctors rarely use it for this purpose.

Important: New evidence shows that MACR levels that have traditionally been considered "normal" can signal increased risk for cardio-vascular events.

Optimal ratios, according to the latest research: 7.5 or lower for women and 4.0 or lower for men.

•**Lipoprotein-Associated Phospholipase A-2 (Lp-PLA2).** This enzyme in the blood is attached to LDL cholesterol and rises when artery walls become inflamed. Recent research suggests that it plays a key role in the athero-sclerosis disease process, contributing to the formation of plaque as well as to the plaque's vulnerability to rupture. People with periodon-tal (gum) disease are especially likely to have elevated Lp-PLA2 scores—chronic inflammation can start in unhealthy gums and, from there, spread to the arteries.

Normal range: Less than 200 ng/mL.

•**Myeloperoxidase (MPO).** This immune system enzyme normally is found at elevated levels only at the site of an infection. When it is elevated in the bloodstream, it must be assumed that it's due to significant inflammation in the artery walls and leaking through the endothelium. This is a very bad sign. MPO produces numerous oxidants that make all cholesterol compounds, including HDL 'good' cholesterol, more inflam-matory. If your blood levels of MPO are high, HDL goes rogue and joins the gang of inflam-matory thugs. It also interacts with another substance in the bloodstream to produce an acid that can eat holes in blood vessel walls. Smokers are particularly prone to high MPO levels.

Normal range: Less than 420 pmol/L.

HOW TO PUT OUT THE FIRES

While the "fire panel" tests above may seem exotic, the solution to the hot artery problem, for most of us, is not. That's because the best way to combat chronic inflammation is simply to maintain a healthful lifestyle. You just have to do it! Key factors include…

•**Following a heart-healthy Mediterra-nean-style diet.**

•**Managing stress.**

New Heart Disease Test

Recently approved by the FDA, the PLAC blood test measures the activity of Lp-PLA2, an enzyme that is a marker for vascular in-flammation. Elevated levels indicate a greater risk for heart disease and heart attack. The test is recommended for people with heart disease risk factors, such as high blood pres-sure or elevated cholesterol, and may be cov-ered by insurance.

Robert M. Stark, MD, medical director, Cardiovascu-lar Prevention Program, Greenwich Hospital/Yale New Haven Health, Connecticut.

- **Getting plenty of exercise.**
- **Guarding against insulin resistance.**
- **Taking good care of your teeth and gums.**
- **Not smoking.**

In some cases, lifestyle changes alone are enough to quell the flames of chronic inflammation and to put your arteries on the road to recovery. In other cases, patients also need medication such as statins and/or dietary supplements such as niacin and fish oil. Either way, the good news is that once you shut the inflammation off, the body has a chance to heal whatever disease and damage has occurred—so you're no longer on the fast track to a heart attack or stroke.

Puzzling Palpitations?— Here's How to Tell What They Really Mean...

Robert Stark, MD, an internist and a cardiologist who is the medical director of the Cardiovascular Prevention Program at Greenwich Hospital/Yale New Haven Health and a clinical faculty member at New York Medical College in Valhalla. *RobertStarkMD.com*

Chances are, you hardly ever notice the steady rhythm of your heart, even though it beats approximately 100,000 times a day. But there may be times when you can feel your heart beating. Perhaps it's racing, even though you haven't done anything strenuous. Or maybe you notice a fluttering sensation...an abrupt thump...or a flip-flop feeling.

Is this a sign that something is seriously wrong with your heart or just a harmless "glitch" in your normal heartbeat?

LISTENING TO YOUR HEART

Most people think of heart palpitations as a racing or pounding sensation in the heart, but the term actually applies whenever you have any unpleasant awareness of your own heartbeat. Palpitations can be normal—when you exercise, for example, you'll feel your heart pounding.

Heart palpitations also can be caused by arrhythmias, heartbeat irregularities that may (or may not) be harmless. For example, if you're under a lot of stress, drink too much coffee or use a cold medicine with a stimulating ingredient (such as *pseudoephedrine*), you may experience arrhythmias.

When there may be a problem: If palpitations are repetitive or recurrent over the course of a day, this could be a sign of heart damage or disease. So could palpitations that last more than a few seconds or are accompanied by dizziness, shortness of breath or other symptoms. These palpitations should always be checked by a physician (in some cases, on an emergency basis). You might need tests—including blood work and an electrocardiogram (EKG or ECG)—to analyze the heartbeat and identify likely problems. *Unusual heart sensations—and what they could mean...*

- **Sensation—Skipped beats.**

What it could be: Premature atrial contractions (PACs), which occur in the heart's upper chambers, or atria...or premature ventricular contractions (PVCs), which affect the lower chambers, or ventricles. These are the most common types of palpitations—and usually the least serious.

With these palpitations, the heart simply beats earlier than it should. You might feel a "pause"

Roll Up the Windows

Car air-conditioning is better for your heart than driving with the windows open. Heart-rate variability—a measure of cardiovascular health—was 32% better in people who ran air-conditioning during a two-hour commute than in people who drove with open windows.

Possible reason: Air-conditioning filters exhaust particles and pollutants that cause internal inflammation and disrupt the heart's electrical signals.

Study of 60 people by researchers at Taipei Medical University, School of Medicine, Taiwan, published in *Science of the Total Environment*.

in your heartbeat, followed by a strong "thump" as the heart compensates for the delayed beat.

Most individuals have occasional PVCs. PACs are also common. If you don't have a history of heart disease (including atherosclerosis), your doctor will probably tell you not to worry.

Exception: When PVCs are repetitive, with one following right after the other for seconds or minutes. This pattern increases the risk for a more serious arrhythmia called ventricular tachycardia.

Treatment options: For frequent premature heartbeats, you may need an antiarrhythmic medication. There are many such drugs, including *disopyramide* (Norpace), *propranolol* (Inderal) and *sotalol* (Betapace).

Helpful: Cutting back or avoiding alcohol, caffeine, smoking and emotional stress often can reduce the frequency of PVCs and PACs and may prevent the need for medication.

•**Sensation—Racing** (as with a very fast pulse) and/or fluttering.

What it could be: Atrial fibrillation. It's a serious arrhythmia that you may or may not feel—and it might occur with sudden sweating or chest pain that feels like a heart attack. It also can cause dizziness, weakness and/or shortness of breath. With atrial fibrillation, the heart's upper chambers beat too erratically to efficiently pump blood to the lower chambers.

Result: Blood pools in the atria and may form clots. Each year, about 8% of people with untreated atrial fibrillation have a stroke.

If you have racing and/or fluttering sensations in your heart, go to a hospital emergency department. If your heart turns out to be healthy, you might have had lone atrial fibrillation, a onetime event that's unlikely to be dangerous. But if you keep having these sensations, or they last a long time (or never go away), you're going to need treatment.

Treatment options: If you are experiencing atrial fibrillation, your doctor will try to convert the heartbeat back to a normal rhythm. This can sometimes be done with anti-arrhythmic drugs or with electrical cardioversion, in which an electrical shock is delivered to restore the heart's normal rhythm.

Relationships Affect Heart Health

•**Marriage can hurt your heart.** Long-time married couples who have mixed feelings toward each other had the highest rate of coronary artery calcification (a predictor of coronary artery disease), according to a recent study of 136 couples married for an average of 36 years.

Reason: Constant ambivalent feelings create stress, which can raise blood pressure.

Bert Uchino, PhD, professor of psychology, The University of Utah, Salt Lake City.

•**Good neighbors boost heart health.** According to recent research, when more than 5,000 adults were followed for four years, those who rated their neighborhoods as friendly had a 67% lower risk for heart attacks than people who rated their neighborhoods negatively.

Possible explanation: Strong social support has been linked to better health (including heart health) in past studies, so tight-knit, friendly neighborhoods are also believed to confer that benefit.

Eric Kim, MS, researcher, University of Michigan, Ann Arbor.

If this treatment doesn't work, you might be given a prescription for a beta-blocker, a calcium channel blocker or other drugs that prevent the heart from racing or fluttering, along with blood-thinning medications to prevent clots. You'll probably need to take the drugs for life. Another approach, known as radiofrequency ablation, uses electricity to permanently damage (ablate) the cells in the heart that are causing abnormal rhythms. This is usually done only when medications and other approaches haven't helped.

•**Sensation—A sudden burst of rapid beats lasting seconds to hours.**

What it could be: Ventricular tachycardia (V tach). Get to an emergency department! V tach usually occurs in people with a history of heart disease. The lower chambers of the heart can start beating faster than 170 times a minute.

Super Food for a Healthy Heart

● **Apples act like statins.** A British study found that eating one apple a day could prevent 8,500 deaths a year from heart attacks and strokes in people over age 50 in the UK. Apples act like statins to reduce LDL "bad" cholesterol, a risk factor for heart attacks and stroke.

Study by researchers at University of Oxford, England, published in the *BMJ*.

● **Tomatoes keep blood vessels strong.** Getting a daily dose of the antioxidant lycopene improved the inner linings of blood vessels (endothelia) in people with heart disease, a recent study has found. Healthy endothelia help curb the progression of heart disease. The study participants received a lycopene extract (7 mg daily). You can, of course, get lycopene from food—enjoy tomatoes (your body will absorb more of the antioxidant if they're cooked)…watermelon…and apricots.

Joseph Cheriyan, MD, associate lecturer in medicine, University of Cambridge, UK. The research appeared in PLOS ONE.

It can lead to ventricular fibrillation, a dangerous arrhythmia that causes the heart to quiver instead of pump. It's the main cause of sudden cardiac arrest, which is usually fatal.

How can you distinguish a racing heart from V tach? You can't. You must be treated at a hospital emergency department, particularly if you're dizzy or have actually lost consciousness—both symptoms of insufficient blood flow.

Treatment options: People with V tach are often treated in an emergency department with antiarrhythmic medications. They might be given a strong electrical shock to restore the heart's normal rhythm. Once the heart has stabilized, you might need long-term care to prevent future attacks.

Possibilities: An implantable cardioverter defibrillator (ICD), a surgically implanted device that analyzes the heartbeat and administers shocks to prevent ventricular fibrillation…or radiofrequency ablation, which, as mentioned above, purposely damages the parts of the heart that cause abnormal beats.

Aspirin for DVT

Study of 1,224 people by researchers at University of Sydney, Australia, published in *Circulation*.

Aspirin for blood clot prevention may be an alternative to *warfarin* for deep vein thrombosis (DVT) patients. DVT often is treated with the anticoagulant drug warfarin.

But: Long-term use of warfarin to prevent clots may require frequent blood tests and dosage adjustments, and it may cause bleeding in some patients. Newer drugs such as *dabigatran* (Pradaxa) and *rivaroxaban* (Xarelto) are effective, but they can be expensive and some patients cannot tolerate them. An inexpensive daily aspirin reduces risk for clots by 42% without causing excessive bleeding.

Caution: Do not switch from warfarin to aspirin unless you speak to your doctor first.

Could Wine, Chocolate Help Shield Your Heart From Smog?

Jia Zhong, MS, doctoral student, Harvard School of Public Health, Boston.
Andrea Baccarelli, MD, MPH, PhD, associate professor of environmental epigenetics, Harvard School of Public Health, Boston.
Russell Luepker, MD, professor of epidemiology and community health, University of Minnesota School of Public Health presentation, American Heart Association annual meeting, Chicago.

A diet rich in chocolate, wine, fruits and vegetables may help protect people from heart disease caused by air pollution, recent research suggests.

The researchers found that elderly men were less likely to experience changes in heart function during heavy smog days if they ate foods loaded with flavonoids, an antioxidant found in plants.

For example, eating about 100 grams of blueberries (about three-quarters of a cup) every day might protect older men from smog-related heart disease, said lead researcher Jia Zhong, a doctoral student at the Harvard School of Public Health.

"We as individuals have no regular means to protect ourselves from air pollution," said Zhong's mentor, Andrea Baccarelli, MD, MPH, an associate professor of environmental epigenetics at the Harvard School of Public Health. "Here we have a potential avenue where we can protect ourselves."

SMOG'S LINK TO HEART DISEASE

Smoggy air can reduce the heart's ability to vary its rhythm. Reduced heart rate variability has been linked to death from heart attacks and heart disease among older people, Zhong said.

"We were looking if there were any factors that could make the harm less significant," Zhong said.

The researchers landed on flavonoids, which are compounds in plants that provide their color. Flavonoids are well-known antioxidants—substances that may prevent or delay some types of cell damage.

STUDY DETAILS

For their study, the researchers focused on 573 Boston-area elderly men taking part in an aging study. They compared clinical measurements taken of the men against air quality measures for their community, and had the men fill out diet questionnaires.

Over an 11-year period, the men tended to suffer from reduced heart rate variability when smog levels rose for 48 hours, the researchers found.

The effect was even worse for men whose genetics tended to suppress a protein called toll-like receptor 2, which detects foreign substances and passes on signals to the immune system.

But the air pollution and genetics had a far weaker effect in men who consumed high levels of flavonoids in their diets, the researchers found.

EXPLANATION

Flavonoids may help protect against pollution-related heart risk by helping regulate the body's immune system response, the researchers said.

"Diet makes a difference," Dr. Baccarelli said. "The amount of flavonoids found in chocolate or blueberries can reprogram our genes."

The researchers warned that this shouldn't be taken as an indication to gorge on chocolate bars or guzzle wine. "If you eat too many calories, that's not going to be good for your heart," Dr. Baccarelli said.

Dr. Baccarelli added that because the study is observational, it does not prove any cause-and-effect link between flavonoids and heart rate variability. Clinical trials will be required before any dietary changes can be recommended.

The research was presented at the American Heart Association annual meeting in Chicago.

EXPERT REACTION

Russell Luepker, MD, a professor of epidemiology and community health at the University of Minnesota School of Public Health, agreed that these results should not lead anyone to drastically change their diet.

"There are a whole bunch of links here that are speculative, and a study that talks about associations can't fill in these speculative links," Dr. Luepker said. "This is only a first step. We need a lot more before we start telling people to do different things."

info For more on antioxidants, visit the website of the National Institutes of Health, *www. nlm.nih.gov/medlineplus/antioxidants.html.*

A Charley Horse...or a Deadly Blood Clot?

Daniella Kadian-Dodov, MD, assistant professor of medicine in the department of vascular medicine at the Zena and Michael A. Wiener Cardiovascular Institute and the Marie-Josée and Henry R. Kravis Center for Cardiovascular Health at the Icahn School of Medicine at Mount Sinai Hospital in New York City.

If you've ever been stopped cold by a charley horse, you know just how excruciating these muscle spasms can be. But are you sure it's just a muscle spasm? Or is that leg pain due to something far more serious?

What can cause leg pain...

PERIPHERAL ARTERIAL DISEASE (PAD)

This is one to worry about. Even though the pain usually isn't intense, it can triple your risk of dying from a heart attack or stroke.

What it feels like: About 10% of people with PAD suffer leg cramps, leg aching and leg fatigue that occur only during physical activity involving the legs (any type of activity can trigger it—even just walking). When you rest your legs, the discomfort goes away, usually in 10 minutes or less. As PAD becomes more severe and blood circulation worsens, pain can occur during rest and result in leg ulcers and even gangrene.

What to do: See a doctor. PAD is usually caused by atherosclerosis, the same condition that leads to most heart attacks. Your doctor will compare the blood pressure in your arms to the pressure at your ankles. If there's a significant difference, that could mean that you have PAD and you'll need an ultrasound of the legs to determine the extent and location of arterial obstructions.

Next steps: The same practices that protect your heart—such as not smoking, controlling diabetes, maintaining healthy blood pressure and getting plenty of exercise—will help stop PAD from worsening and could even reverse it.

Important: You must walk—even when it hurts. Walking ultimately reduces pain and improves circulation by stimulating the growth of blood vessels that bypass the damaged ones. With your doctor's OK, walk five times a week, for 30 to 45 minutes each time. I usually advise my patients to walk fast for two blocks or until they feel moderate pain, then rest a moment and walk fast for two blocks again, repeating until the end of their workout.

DEEP VEIN THROMBOSIS (DVT)

It doesn't always cause leg pain, but if pain occurs, this warning could save your life. DVT means that you have a blood clot—most often deep in a leg vein. It can be fatal.

What it feels like: You might notice a sudden, pulsating or aching pain deep in your calf or thigh, sometimes accompanied by redness and/or swelling. DVT usually occurs after you've been immobile for a long time—you're

Watch Out for This Heart Drug

Widely prescribed heart drug is dangerous for patients with atrial fibrillation (abnormal heart rhythm). There is increasing evidence that those patients taking *digoxin* are at increased risk for death, compared with patients treated with beta-blockers and calcium channel blockers such as *diltiazem* and *verapamil*. About one-quarter of people with atrial fibrillation still are prescribed digoxin, partly because it has been used for so long. But do not stop taking it until you see your doctor.

Samy Claude Elayi, MD, associate professor of medicine at Gill Heart Institute of University of Kentucky, Lexington.

laid up in bed after surgery, for example, or following a long car or plane trip.

What to do: Get to an emergency department or a physician's office where you can get an immediate ultrasound. The clot could break free, travel to the lungs and cause pulmonary embolism, a clot in the lungs that's fatal in up to 30% of cases.

If you have a DVT, your doctor will probably give intravenous or injectable *heparin*, a blood-thinning drug that prevents the clot from growing. After a day or two, you'll be switched to oral blood-thinning medication, such as *warfarin* (Coumadin) or *dabigatran* (Pradaxa). You'll need to take the medication for about six months. If the clot is not entirely dissolved after treatment, it should be monitored with ultrasound—and if you have had one clot, you might get another one. Prevention is critical.

Everyone—whether you've had a DVT or not—should flex the ankle and calf muscles for about 30 seconds every 20 or 30 minutes when sitting for longer than four hours. Stand up and move around at least every hour or so.

If you have risk factors for blood clots—you're over age 40, obese, have a family history of blood clots or use hormone replacement therapy—ask your doctor about such precautions as taking aspirin before travel and/or wearing compression stockings while you're immobile.

SCIATICA

This back condition is typically caused by a herniated spinal disk. The legs become involved because the disk exerts painful pressure on the sciatic nerve, which runs down the backs of the legs.

What it feels like: Intense, shooting and/or knifelike pains may extend through the buttocks and into one leg. Sciatica also can cause leg and/or ankle weakness.

What to do: See your doctor. If you do have sciatica, you may get better within eight weeks by doing physical therapy and using a nonsteroidal anti-inflammatory medication such as *ibuprofen* (Motrin)—90% of sciatica patients do.

Next steps: Consider surgery for a herniated disk/sciatica only when the pain is too intense to handle…you have responsibilities that don't permit extended downtime…or you're having additional symptoms such as muscle weakness or a loss of bowel/bladder control.

WHEN IT REALLY IS A CHARLEY HORSE

If you're getting muscle spasms with any sort of regularity, see your doctor. Muscle spasms have a variety of causes—for example, you may have overworked your legs by doing yard work…you may be dehydrated (without enough water, muscle cells can spasm)…or a medication you're taking, such as a diuretic, may be the culprit.

Helpful: Because most muscle spasms are caused, in part, by tight hamstrings (the muscles in the backs of your upper legs), I recommend doing a standing hamstring stretch on a regular basis. Start in a standing position with your knees straight…bend at the waist…and reach for your toes or the floor until you feel a stretch in your hamstrings. Hold for a few seconds, and repeat a few times a day.

Lifesaving Vest for Heart Health

A lifesaving vest that delivers electrical shocks to keep the heart beating is more comfortable—and possibly more reliable—than older wearable defibrillators worn by heart patients. The vest, still in development, can be worn under clothes and washed at home.

Johns Hopkins University.

Heart-Device Danger

Jeffrey L. Williams, MD, medical director of electrophysiology at The Good Samaritan Hospital, with a private practice at Lebanon Cardiology Associates, both in Lebanon, Pennsylvania. He is author of *What Is a Pacemaker?*

Too many people are getting heart defibrillators.

Unsettling fact: A large study concluded that more than 20% of people who have an implanted cardioverter defibrillator (ICD) don't meet the expert guidelines for who should have the device.

An ICD is a pacemaker-like device that delivers a brief shock when it detects ventricular fibrillation, a life-threatening arrhythmia that can cause cardiac arrest and sudden death. The device is recommended for patients with ventricular defibrillation…those who have already suffered from cardiac arrest…and those with an ejection fraction (a measure of the heart's pumping ability) below 35% that doesn't improve with other treatments.

Researchers at Duke University examined nationwide data involving nearly 112,000 patients. Those who received ICDs who did not meet the guidelines were more likely to suffer infections and complications. They spent more time in the hospital and were more likely to die in the hospital.

Why don't more doctors follow the guidelines? Some simply don't keep up with the latest recommendations. There also is concern that because Medicare pays $50,000 for the procedure, some hospitals might simply be cashing in. The Department of Justice opened an investigation of ICD overuse in 2010 that is still ongoing.

The guidelines specify a 40-day waiting period after a heart attack before implanting an ICD. If your doctor recommends an ICD sooner than this or if you don't meet the guidelines above, ask him/her why you need the device. In the study, electrophysiologists (who have the most experience with ICDs) were more likely to follow the guidelines than other doctors.

Drug Gives "New Hope" Against Heart Failure

John McMurray, MD, professor, cardiology, British Heart Foundation Cardiovascular Research Center, University of Glasgow, U.K.

Mariell Jessup, MD, professor, medicine, Perelman School of Medicine, University of Pennsylvania, Philadelphia

Gregg Fonarow, MD, professor, cardiology, University of California, Los Angeles.

New England Journal of Medicine

European Society of Cardiology annual meeting, Barcelona.

In a head-to-head comparison, an experimental drug was more effective than standard treatment at preventing deaths and hospitalizations in heart failure patients.

According to the study authors, the trial was stopped early because of the marked benefit of the new drug, dubbed LCZ696.

STUDY DETAILS

In the trial, 26.5% of those getting the standard medication, *enalapril* (Vasotec), either died or were hospitalized due to heart failure, compared with 21.8% of those on the new drug. Enalapril belongs to a class of blood pressure-lowering medications known as ACE inhibitors.

"LCZ696 could become the new gold standard, replacing ACE inhibitors," said lead researcher John McMurray, MD, a professor of cardiology at the British Heart Foundation Cardiovascular Research Center at the University of Glasgow, in Scotland.

Anger Can Kill

Angry outbursts increase risk for heart attack fivefold—and risk for stroke fourfold. The higher risk disappears in about two hours but is significant. Risk is highest among people who often get angry and have existing risk factors, such as prior heart problems.

Probable reason: Anger causes a stress response in the body that raises heart rate and blood pressure.

Analysis of case studies conducted between 1966 and 2013 led by researchers at Harvard Medical School and Beth Israel Deaconess Medical Center, both in Boston, published online in *European Heart Journal*.

LCZ696 combines two blood pressure drugs—an angiotensin II receptor blocker (ARB) and the neprilysin inhibitor known as *sacubitril*.

"We found that LCZ696 was superior to the gold-standard ACE inhibitor for heart failure—an ACE inhibitor being the absolute cornerstone of treatment for this problem," he said.

Not only did LCZ696 beat enalapril, but it did that even when added to other treatments, Dr. McMurray noted.

"The new treatment was very well tolerated, with no significant safety concerns," he added.

The report was published online in the *New England Journal of Medicine*, to coincide with a presentation at the European Society of Cardiology annual meeting in Barcelona. The trial was funded by Novartis, the maker of LCZ696.

EXPERT RESPONSE

Mariell Jessup, MD, a professor of medicine at the University of Pennsylvania's Perelman School of Medicine, said, "There is new hope for heart failure."

She added, "We have not had a new drug for heart failure for many years. LCZ696 is a unique compound that may represent a new approach."

Doctors have relied on ACE inhibitors for over two decades, she said. According to Dr. Jessup, who wrote an accompanying editorial, "Newer drugs that work via alternate pathways may [show] benefit beyond the medical therapy that is used today."

For the study, over 8,400 patients with heart failure were randomly chosen to receive LCZ696 or enalapril.

Over an average of 27 months of follow-up, LCZ696 reduced the risk of hospitalization for heart failure by 21%, compared with enalapril, the findings showed.

Moreover, among the 1,251 people who died from heart disease during the trial, 558 were taking LCZ696 (13.3%) and 693 were taking enalapril (16.5%), the researchers noted.

Gregg Fonarow, MD, a professor of cardiology at the University of California, Los Angeles, commented, "The results of this study are terrific news for patients with heart failure, and represent landmark findings."

If approved by the U.S. Food and Drug Administration, this new medication should help doctors improve outcomes for the millions of men and women with chronic heart failure worldwide, he said.

 Visit the American Heart Association for more on heart failure at *www.heart.org.*

Dangerous Antibiotic

Suzanne Steinbaum, DO, director of Women's Heart Health, Heart and Vascular Institute, Lenox Hill Hospital, New York City, and author of *Dr. Suzanne Steinbaum's Heart Book. SRSHeart.com*

A popular antibiotic can be dangerous for people with heart conditions. Respiratory infections often are treated with the antibiotic *clarithromycin*, but in a recent study, clarithromycin was associated with a 76% greater risk for cardiac death than *penicillin.*

Reason: Clarithromycin can affect the heart's electrical activity.

Among the safest antibiotics for heart patients: Penicillin, *amoxicillin* and related drugs.

Daily Aspirin for Heart Health: Is It Helping or Harming You?

Salim S. Virani, MD, PhD, investigator, Health Policy, Quality & Informatics Program, Michael E. DeBakey Veterans Affairs Medical Center, and associate professor, section of cardiovascular research, Baylor College of Medicine, both in Houston.

If you are taking aspirin every day to ward off heart attack and stroke, just like more than one-third of Americans do, you may actually be putting yourself in harm's way. Some doctors may not even be following long-known guidelines about who should and shouldn't be taking daily aspirin!

"Heartbroken" in the South?

Possible reason: Compared with the rest of the country, there are higher rates of diabetes, obesity, hypertension—and smoking—in southern states.

Southerners are more likely to die from heart attacks than people who live in other regions of the US.

University of Arkansas for Medical Sciences.

WHO NEEDS IT?

Aspirin is a blood thinner that helps prevent artery-blocking clots. But the same anticlotting mechanism that can prevent heart attacks and strokes can cause serious and deadly internal bleeding in the form of stomach ulcers and bleeding in the brain.

While daily aspirin has been shown to reduce risk of heart disease and ischemic stroke in people with heart disease, risk of hemorrhagic stroke is very slightly increased. Meanwhile, studies have shown that people who take daily aspirin but do not have heart disease have a 30% increased risk of internal bleeding (including deadly hemorrhagic stroke) compared with healthy people who do not adopt this regimen.

So, the only people who should be taking daily aspirin are those in whom its cardiovascular benefits outweigh its health risks. These people include those who already have had a heart attack or stroke and those at medium-to-high risk for having one. But researchers from Baylor College of Medicine in Texas discovered that about one in 10 people who take daily aspirin are not in these categories.

They found this out by analyzing five years' of medical records from 119 cardiology practices across America. This allowed them to identify nearly 69,000 patients who were taking daily aspirin even though they never had had a heart attack or stroke. Although most of these patients were at medium-to-high risk for these deadly cardiovascular events, roughly 12% were at low risk and, therefore, should not have been taking daily aspirin. Risk factors for heart attack and stroke can include a family history, older age,

Take Those Extra Steps

Walking 2,000 extra steps a day lowers heart attack risk by 10%. This is the equivalent of a 20-minute walk. Over the course of a six-year study, each time a person increased his/her activity by another 2,000 steps, his risk for heart attack went down by another 8%.

Study of 9,306 adults from 40 countries for six years by researchers at University of Leicester, UK, published in The Lancet.

smoking, and, of course, high blood pressure, high cholesterol, obesity, physical inactivity and diabetes. Level of risk hinges on the number and severity of risk factors a person has.

When the researchers looked into how aspirin was being prescribed to patients, they found a lot of variation. The percentage of inappropriate aspirin prescriptions per cardiology practice ranged from 0% to 72%.

TAKE CHARGE!

This study looked at people who took aspirin who were under the care of cardiologists, but how many of you are taking daily aspirin because your primary care doctor told you to or because you simply read somewhere that it was a good idea? Many more people than those identified in the study are probably risking gut ulcers and deadly brain bleeds by taking aspirin they don't need.

You may be able to know whether the benefits of aspirin outweigh the risks for you personally without first consulting a doctor. If you already know your blood pressure levels and either your cholesterol level or body mass index, you can calculate your cardiovascular disease risk with the same calculator used in the study. After you click on the link, find where it says "Risk Score Calculators" on the Web page and select either the calculate-by-BMI or calculate-by-lipids option. If your 10-year risk of cardiovascular disease is below 6%, then you may be better off avoiding an aspirin-a-day. If higher, then it is best to talk to your doctor about whether the benefits of daily aspirin

to prevent cardiovascular disease outweigh the risks. But be sure your doctor engages with you on the pros and cons and doesn't just push the aspirin right at you.

info The U.S. Department of Health has more on aspirin for preventing cardiovascular disease at *healthfinder.gov* (search "aspirin").

Implanted Device May Improve Hard-to-Treat Chest Pain

Shmuel Banai, MD, director, interventional cardiology, Tel Aviv Sourasky Medical Center, Israel.
Christopher Granger, MD, director, Cardiac Care Unit, Duke University Medical Center, Durham, North Carolina.
New England Journal of Medicine

A stent-like device placed in a heart vein may bring relief to some people with otherwise untreatable cases of angina, a small clinical trial finds.

The study, published in the *New England Journal of Medicine*, included 104 patients with severe angina that had eluded conventional therapies—in what doctors call "refractory" angina.

Angina refers to chronic chest pain, fatigue and breathing problems caused by atherosclerosis—a hardening and narrowing of arteries supplying blood to the heart. Usually, the symptoms can be treated with lifestyle changes, medications, or procedures that open up the narrowed arteries and improve blood flow.

But when the standard treatments don't work, patients are out of options, said Shmuel Banai, MD, the senior researcher on the recent study and director of interventional cardiology at Tel Aviv Sourasky Medical Center in Israel.

The device his team studied, called the Reducer, is already approved in Europe but not yet in the United States. It is similar to a stent, the scaffold-like device that doctors commonly implant to prop open clogged heart arteries. But the Reducer has an hourglass shape, and instead of being placed in an artery, it's implanted in a large heart vein, to alter the flow of blood out of the heart.

That helps keep more oxygen-rich blood circulating in the parts of the heart muscle that need it, according to Neovasc, the company that markets the device and funded the recent research.

STUDY DETAILS

For the study, Dr. Banai's team recruited 104 patients with class 3 or 4 angina who'd failed to improve with medication and could not have the standard invasive procedures—namely, traditional stents or bypass surgery. The classes, on a scale from 1 to 4, rate lower to greater activity limitations due to angina.

His team randomly assigned half of the patients to have the Reducer device implanted, which involves threading a catheter into the heart vein under local anesthesia. The rest of the patients were assigned to a "sham" procedure, in which the catheter was inserted but no device was implanted.

Over the next six months, 35% of patients with the device saw their symptoms improve by at least two "angina classes"—which is considered substantial in real-life terms, according to Dr. Banai. That compared with 15% of the sham-treatment group.

Other patients got relief, too. In all, 71% of those with the device improved by at least one angina class, versus 42% of the sham group.

"For these patients who are very limited in their daily activities, even one class improvement is important, and a two-class improvement is critically important," Dr. Banai said.

One patient who received the implant suffered a heart attack soon after the procedure. But in general, the treatment appears relatively safe, according to Dr. Banai.

EXPERT COMMENTARY

A cardiologist not involved in the study called it "good news for patients."

"This condition is fairly common, and can be debilitating," said Christopher Granger, MD, director of the Cardiac Care Unit at Duke University Medical Center in Durham, North Carolina.

It's been estimated that refractory angina affects up to two million people in the US, according to Granger, who cowrote an editorial published with the study.

Still, larger and longer-term studies are needed, Dr. Granger stressed. "This is a well-done study, and it's an important study," he said. "But it's still a small study."

So far, the device seems "well-tolerated," Dr. Granger noted. But there are, as with any medical implant, safety concerns, he said.

"There can be complications when the device is implanted, such as bleeding or infection," Dr. Granger said. And if the device were to become blocked, that could affect the outflow of blood from the heart muscle.

What about all the patients in the sham group who also saw improvement? Dr. Granger said that could be related to the normal fluctuations in angina symptoms. Patients are enrolled in a trial when their symptoms are at their worst, and then there's a natural wane. He said there could also be a "placebo effect" at work.

For now, he said, the best thing most people can do is to take steps to prevent angina, or keep it from worsening. That includes not smoking, eating a healthy diet, and keeping blood pressure and cholesterol down—with medications, if needed.

info The U.S. National Institutes of Health has more on preventing and treating angina at *http://www.nhlbi.nih.gov.*

Heart Attacks and Depression

Heart attacks are more likely to cause depression in women than in men. Survivors of both genders report more sadness, worry and stress in life. But the gap between feelings before and after the heart attack is greater in women. And significantly more women who had heart attacks (35%) were diagnosed with depression than men who had heart attacks (24%).

Bottom line: Both men and women—but especially women—need extra social support after a heart attack.

Results of 353,492 interviews by Gallup-Healthways Well-Being Index, reported in *USA Today.*

Exercise, Diet May Be Key to Beating a Common Irregular Heartbeat

Rajeev Pathak, a cardiologist and electrophysiology fellow at the University of Adelaide in Australia.
University of Adelaide, news release.

Atrial fibrillation is a potentially danger-ous form of irregular heartbeat for older Americans. However, a recent study sug-gests healthy changes in eating and exercise habits can help ease the condition.

According to the Australian researchers, atrial fibrillation is the most common cause of irregu-lar heartbeat, and it has been linked to a height-ened risk for dementia, stroke and death.

RECENT STUDY

The recent study included more than 149 people who had undergone a procedure called catheter ablation to treat the condition. In this procedure, the tissue surrounding the problem area in the heart is burned.

In addition, 61 of the patients also took part in an aggressive "risk factor management" pro-gram after they underwent catheter ablation. The program was designed to reduce lifestyle risk factors such as being overweight, having high blood pressure, high cholesterol or high blood sugar levels, sleep breathing problems (such as sleep apnea), and smoking and drinking.

After five years, patients who managed these lifestyle factors were five times more likely to be alive and to be free of heart rhythm problems such as atrial fibrillation than those who hadn't gotten healthier—87% versus 18%.

The study was published in the *Journal of the American College of Cardiology*.

IMPLICATIONS

"This is a very important finding because it shows the huge gap between what happens when patients are able to manage the underly-ing risks of their health and those who rely solely on medical intervention," said lead author Rajeev Pathak, MD, a cardiologist and electrophysiology fellow at the University of Adelaide in Australia.

"This study should serve as a wake-up call to physicians to begin prevention programs to reduce disease states rather than focus on their treatment only, and the good news is it is never too late to start," he added.

info For more information about atrial fibril-lation, visit the Website of the U.S. Na-tional Heart, Lung, and Blood Institute, *www. nhlbi.nih.gov*, and search "atrial fibrillation."

Stroke Risk Self-Test

Can you balance on one leg unassisted for 20 seconds? In a study of nearly 1,400 men and women, one-third of those who couldn't do this had mild memory loss and brain MRIs that showed two or more microbleeds (com-mon precursors of serious strokes). These small strokes are caused by narrowing or leakage of tiny blood vessels deep within the brain. If you fail this balancing test, see your doctor to find out why.

Yasuharu Tabara, PhD, associate professor, Cen-ter for Genomic Medicine, Kyoto University Graduate School of Medicine, Japan.

Could a Jolt to the Neck Cause a Stroke?

Rebecca Gottesman, MD, associate professor of neu-rology and epidemiology at The Johns Hopkins Univer-sity School of Medicine and director of clinical research at Johns Hopkins Bayview Neurology, both in Baltimore.

Most strokes occur due to years of high blood pressure…or when the gradual buildup of fatty substances (plaque) in the arteries cuts off blood flow to the brain.

An unusual and little-recognized trigger: Some people get strokes from simply moving the neck in an extreme way or holding it in an odd position. This sort of neck movement might oc-cur during a car accident, for example—but it might also be caused by normal activities such as riding a roller coaster, craning your neck to paint a ceiling or leaning back to have your hair shampooed at a hair salon (the so-called "beauty parlor syndrome").

The culprit in such strokes is a vertebral artery dissection (VAD), a tear in the innermost or middle layer of the three-layered vertebral artery wall, which can disrupt blood flow to the brain. Sometimes, the damage is minor and the artery repairs itself without difficulty. In other cases, however, the arterial injury leads to a stroke.

Recent development: The American Heart Association (AHA) recently issued a warning that neck manipulation (used, for example, during certain chiropractic or physical therapy treatments) has been linked to stroke due to such arterial injuries. While no direct cause-and-effect relationship has been found, the AHA now advises health-care practitioners to inform their patients of the association before performing neck manipulation.

WHEN AN ARTERY SHREDS

The right and left vertebral arteries run up the back of the neck and into the skull, carrying blood to the brain. A stroke-inducing arterial tear can result from virtually any sudden and/or extreme movement that turns or stretches the neck excessively. But in many cases, people with VAD can recall nothing more unusual than a sneeze or vigorous sexual activity in the preceding days, and sometimes there is nothing to blame it on.

Why the cause can be elusive: Some people are apparently more vulnerable to VAD than others. It is more common in those with known connective tissue disorders such as Marfan's syndrome or fibromuscular dysplasia. Also, some studies have found that artery walls in people who have suffered dissections look subtly abnormal under the microscope, suggesting a congenital abnormality.

But practically speaking, there is no way to predict who will get a VAD or what will cause it. There are warning signs, though. And if you've already suffered a VAD, there are steps you can take to help prevent another one.

RED FLAGS FOR VAD

Each year, approximately 4,500 Americans suffer VAD. The condition is a leading cause of

---

Exercise Works Better Than Meds

Exercise may work better than medication after a heart attack or stroke to prevent early death. At least two-and-a-half hours a week of moderate-intensity aerobic activity, such as brisk walking, was as good as drugs for heart attack patients and more effective than medicine for stroke patients who were capable of exercising—although such patients may have been healthier to begin with. Doctors should discuss lifestyle changes as well as medication use with patients who have had strokes or heart attacks—a combination of medicine and exercise may be best for many people.

Huseyin Naci, doctoral candidate in pharmaceutical policy and economics at London School of Economics, fellow at Harvard Medical School, Boston, and leader of an analysis of 305 studies, published in BMJ.

---

stroke in adults under age 45. VAD also can occur, though less commonly, in older adults. Of course, the best course is to spot a VAD early—before it can cause a stroke.

Recent finding: An analysis of 75 studies involving nearly 2,000 people diagnosed with VAD found that dizziness or vertigo was the most common symptom, reported by 58% of sufferers, with headache (51%) and neck pain (46%) close behind.

The trouble is that dizziness, headache and neck pain are extremely common and can be caused by many different conditions. And you can't run to the doctor to check out every headache or dizzy spell.

When to be concerned: If you have a headache that is more severe than usual…suffer extreme dizziness…have neck pain that is unusual for you…or if any of these symptoms occur at the same time or last longer than a day. Call or visit your doctor without delay.

When to be very concerned: If you develop symptoms such as double vision, difficulty walking, speaking or swallowing, and/or weakness on one side of your face or body, particularly if they occur with dizziness, neck pain or headache. These could be signs that a stroke or transient ischemic attack (TIA), a temporary blockage of brain circulation, is occurring.

A sudden and severe "thunderclap" headache (the kind that people describe as "the worst headache of my life") may indicate that a brain hemorrhage is imminent or has happened.

Prompt emergency care in these situations could mean the difference between complete recovery and disability or death.

PREVENTING AN ARTERIAL TEAR

If you have ever had an episode of VAD, you are at increased risk for another. This doesn't mean that you should stop all exercise or keep your neck in a brace, but you may want to pass on activities that could easily lead to a neck injury, such as mountain biking and skydiving.

Also, if you've had a VAD, avoid any situations where your neck is stretched out for prolonged periods—for example, try to avoid hyperextending your neck at an extreme angle backward while getting your hair shampooed or styled. Don't give up yoga, but skip postures that stress your neck. If you receive chiropractic care, it's safest for manipulations to be performed below neck level.

DIAGNOSING AND TREATING AN ARTERIAL TEAR

If your doctor suspects that you've suffered a vertebral artery dissection (VAD), he/she will probably order a CT scan or MRI. Treatment for a VAD usually includes a drug to keep clots from forming, most commonly *warfarin* (Coumadin). If you have a VAD, it's common to take the drug for three to six months. If symptoms persist, your doctor may recommend that a stent or coil be surgically placed in the damaged artery.

Precautions: While VAD is less likely to cause a stroke once you begin taking an anticoagulant, anticlotting drugs themselves carry the risk of bleeding. Your doctor should advise you what activities to avoid during this time—this usually includes anything that could cause head injury. Patients on oral anticoagulants also should have their blood levels checked regularly and need to maintain a regular diet in order to keep their blood thin enough while they are taking this medication.

Delay Surgery After Stroke

In more than 480,000 surgeries, patients who underwent elective, noncardiac procedures following an ischemic stroke had the lowest risk for complications if their surgeries took place more than nine months after their strokes, a recent analysis found. Patients who received surgery within the first three months after their strokes were at highest risk of suffering another stroke or even death. Risk gradually decreased after three months, possibly due to stabilization of blood flow to the brain.

Mads Jorgensen, MB, research assistant, The Cardiovascular Research Center, Gentofte Hospital, Denmark.

Check Heart Rhythm After Surgery

Hooman Kamel, MD, a neurologist at the Brain and Mind Research Institute, Weill Cornell Medical College, New York City, and coauthor of a study of more than 1.7 million people, published in The Journal of the American Medical Association.

Stroke risk doubles after surgery among people who develop irregular heart rhythms during their hospital stays. Heart flutters and fibrillations may result from the short-term stress associated with any surgery and may not be any cause for concern. But they also could be a sign of increased stroke risk and need to be followed up. Be sure to ask your doctor whether you have any heart-rhythm irregularities after surgery.

Certain Painkillers Tied to Raised Risk of Death After Stroke

Morten Schmidt, MD, cardiovascular research coordinator, Aarhus University Hospital, Denmark.
Ralph Sacco, MD, chairman, neurology, University of Miami Miller School of Medicine Neurology, online.

Arthritis pain relievers known as COX-2 inhibitors, including *celecoxib* (Celebrex) and *etodolac* (Lodine), are associated with an increased risk of dying within a month after a stroke, according to a recent study.

"This large study from Denmark adds to the prior concerns about COX-2 inhibitors and stroke risks," said Ralph Sacco, MD, chairman of neurology at the University of Miami Miller School of Medicine.

"Patients at high risk for stroke should be cautious about taking such medications and should consult their physicians as to the best medications to treat inflammation and pain," Dr. Sacco said.

However, while the study found an association between use of these painkillers and death in stroke patients, it did not prove cause-and-effect.

Other types of nonsteroidal anti-inflammatory painkillers (NSAIDs)—including *ibuprofen* (Advil, Motrin) and *naproxen* (Aleve)—weren't linked to an increased risk of death after stroke, the study authors said.

BACKGROUND

COX-2 inhibitors have previously been linked to an increased risk for both heart attack and stroke. In 2004, Merck pulled the popular painkiller Vioxx from the market because of this association.

The next year, the U.S. Food and Drug Administration asked Pfizer to voluntarily stop selling *valdecoxib* (Bextra) because of its link with an increased risk of heart attack and stroke.

Celebrex, however, which is in the same class of drugs and also made by Pfizer, remains on the market.

NEW FINDINGS

In the recent study—based on more than 100,000 people hospitalized for a first stroke between 2004 and 2012—the investigators wanted to see if the painkillers affected recovery from a stroke.

The researchers found that use of Celebrex prior to hospitalization for ischemic stroke was associated with a 19% increase in risk of death within a month, compared with non-use of the drug.

Ischemic stroke, the most common type of stroke, is caused by a clot that blocks blood flow to the brain.

"Much of this result came from new users of the drugs, who were 42% more likely to die from stroke than those who were not taking the drugs," said lead researcher Morten Schmidt, MD, the cardiovascular research coordinator at Aarhus University Hospital.

"The results were also stronger for those taking the older COX-2 inhibitors," he added.

The older drugs—for example, *etodolac* (Lodine)—raised the risk of dying from stroke by 53%, the researchers reported.

Of the more than 100,000 stroke patients the researchers looked at, 11% used painkillers prior to admission and 8% were former users.

The report was published in the journal *Neurology*.

IMPORTANT

"There are several cardiovascular risks to consider when prescribing NSAIDs, in particular COX-2 inhibitors," Dr. Schmidt said.

"Efforts should be made to ensure people with a higher risk of stroke are not prescribed these medications when other options are available," he said.

info For more about stroke, visit the U.S. National Library of Medicine at *www.nlm. nih.gov/medlineplus/stroke.html*.

Better Stroke Follow-Up

Bernd Kallmünzer, MD, stroke unit physician, University of Erlangen-Nuremberg, Germany.

Monitoring a stroke patient's pulse at home may help guard against a second stroke—and you don't have to be a doctor to do it. Pulse can reveal an irregular heartbeat, a major cause of second strokes. When patients and family members were trained to properly take a pulse in a study of 256 stroke survivors, their measurements were almost as accurate as those taken by health-care professionals and correctly identified most arrhythmias, which can be treated with medication.

Bed Position Important for Recovery

Murray Flaster, MD, PhD, a neurologist and stroke specialist at Loyola University Medical Center, Maywood, Illinois. He reported on stroke-care issues in *MedLink Neurology*.

Better stroke recovery depends on bed position, reports Murray Flaster, MD, PhD. Doctors must evaluate the type of stroke and initial progress of the patient to decide what bed position in the first 24 to 48 hours is best for recovery. Sitting upright can harm some patients by decreasing blood flow to the brain.

Faster Stroke Test Coming

A helmet called Strokefinder uses microwaves to examine brain tissue. It can accurately tell within 10 minutes if a stroke is caused by bleeding or clots even before patients arrive at the hospital. Testing is under way.

Chalmers University of Technology.

For those patients, lying flat can improve blood flow. But if a stroke increases brain swelling, sitting upright can improve blood drainage and make damage from the swelling less likely. Ask your doctor which position is best for you.

Infectious Diseases

How to Wreck Your Immune System

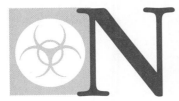obody wants to spend time sick in bed feeling miserable with a cold, the flu or any other illness.

But here's the catch: Even if you stay well rested, exercise and eat healthfully, you still could be sabotaging your immune system. Most people are unknowingly making it harder for their bodies to fight off illnesses. *How to stop hurting your immune system…*

• **Skip the germ-killing soaps.** Studies now show that *triclosan*, the key ingredient in many antibacterial hand soaps (as well as some shaving gels, shampoos, cosmetics, deodorants and other personal-care items), fuels the growth of antibiotic-resistant bugs in the public at large. With frequent use, triclosan also can hurt you personally by setting up your body to

develop a secondary "superinfection" that can occur as a complication of colds, the flu or viral pneumonia.

Among the best ways to prevent colds and the flu: Vigorous, frequent hand-washing with plain soap is all you need, but here's the key—you need to scrub long enough (count to 20).

If you like the reassurance offered by a hand sanitizer, products with at least 60% alcohol, such as Purell or Germ-X, are widely recommended. However, the alcohol in such hand sanitizers can lead to dry, cracked skin, which provides an entry point for bacterial or fungal skin infections. Alcohol-based products are supported by strong research, but if dry skin is a problem, rely on hand-washing and/or a hand sanitizer that contains natural antibacterial plant oils such as citrus, oregano, rosemary and/or thyme.

Good choice: CleanWell, $10.99 for three one-ounce spray bottles, *CleanWellToday.com*.

Robert Rountree, MD, a family physician in private practice and owner of Boulder Wellcare in Boulder, Colorado. He is coauthor of numerous books, including *Immunotics: A Revolutionary Way to Fight Infection, Beat Chronic Illness and Stay Well.*

Faster Blood Test for Infection

Previously, yeast infections in the blood-stream (which most often affect patients with weakened immunity and can lead to severe complications and death if not treated quickly) were diagnosed with blood cultures that took six days or longer for results.

Now: The T2Candida blood test, recently approved by the FDA, provides identification in three to five hours, so antifungal treatment can begin much sooner, reducing risk for complications and death.

Alberto Gutierrez, PhD, director, Office of In-Vitro Diagnostics and Radiological Health, FDA, Silver Spring, Maryland.

•**Take a pass on sugar.** Sugar, refined carbohydrates and high-fructose corn syrup can impair the effectiveness of our immune cells. As soon as you notice cold or flu symptoms, cut these foods out of your diet.

Beware: The caramelized sugar found on cinnamon rolls, donuts or sticky buns is particularly harmful to our immunity. Certain molecular structures in this type of sugar resemble bacteria, and our immune system receptors mistakenly bind to them, interfering with their ability to respond effectively to true infections.

If you need a sweetener: Try raw honey, which has immune-building properties.*

•**Watch out for pesticides.** Most nonorganic produce gets showered with pesticides, which damage your immune system.

What to try instead: Load up on fresh, organic fruits and vegetables to arm your immune system with disease-fighting vitamins and nutrients. Organic berries, citrus fruits, grapes and spinach are especially rich in antioxidants that support immune function. When fresh berries aren't available, try frozen organic berries. You can save money by opting for nonorganic citrus fruits and other peelable items (such as bananas) that are less likely to harbor dangerous pesticides than produce without peels.

*Infants under age one and people who are allergic to pollen or immunocompromised should not consume raw honey.

POWER UP YOUR IMMUNITY

Many people rely on well-known immunity boosters such as vitamin C and/or echinacea, but you're likely to get better results from using the following on a daily basis as a preventive during cold and flu season (or year-round if you work directly with the public)...**

•**Probiotics.** By far, probiotics are the best way to enhance your immunity. These "good" bacteria, including Lactobacillus and Bifidobacterium, reside in your digestive tract, where they keep intestinal microbes in check and elevate your number of infection-fighting T cells.

Fermented foods, such as kefir, yogurt, kimchi, sauerkraut and kombucha, are all naturally rich in probiotics. Aim for two (four- to six-ounce) servings a day.

In general, however, probiotic supplements are more potent and may be more reliable than probiotic-rich foods. If you opt for a supplement, use a combination of Bifidobacterium and/or Lactobacillus species.

A probiotic found in studies to boost immunity: Culturelle, $39.99 for 80 capsules, Amazon.com.

•**N-acetylcysteine (NAC).** The body easily converts this amino acid into a usable form of glutathione, an immunity-protecting antioxidant that itself is poorly absorbed from the gastrointestinal tract.

Scientific evidence: Italian researchers found that taking 1,200 mg daily of NAC throughout flu season reduced the frequency, severity and intensity of flu-like symptoms.

Typical dose: 600 mg to 1,200 mg daily as a preventive...at the first sign of infection, increase the dose to 3,000 mg daily (taken in doses of 600 mg each throughout the day).

• **Elderberry syrup.** When used within the first 48 hours of feeling flu-ish, this syrup (made from naturally antiviral elderberries) has been shown to relieve symptoms four days faster than a placebo.

If you are not taking elderberry syrup as a daily preventive, start using it within the first

**Consult your doctor before trying dietary supplements—especially if you take prescription medication and/or have a chronic medical condition.

two days of developing cold or flu symptoms. Follow label instructions.

Good choice: Sambucol Black Elderberry Immune System Support, $19.99 for 7.8 ounces, *Drugstore.com.*

DON'T GO IT ALONE!

What do close relationships have to do with immunity? A lot, according to research.

When researchers exposed 276 adults to a rhinovirus (a cause of the common cold), subjects with only one to three relationships (such as fulfilling marriages or friendships with colleagues, neighbors and religious community members) were four times more likely to get sick than those who had more than six relationships.

Possible explanation: Social interactions help ease the negative effects of stress—a known threat to immunity.

The Germiest Spots in Public Places

Philip M. Tierno, Jr., PhD, microbiologist and director of clinical microbiology and diagnostic immunology at New York University Langone Medical Center. He is author of *The Secret Life of Germs.*

You're not paranoid—germs really are out to get you. But not from the much publicized diseases such as Ebola. The real risk comes from mundane microbes lurking where you might not expect them. *Here's where they are and what to do about them…*

LYING IN WAIT

About 80% of all infections are caused by touch—either from direct contact or from touching a contaminated surface. And when you're in a public place, just about every surface is contaminated.

When researchers at University of Arizona applied a noninfectious virus to an office door—a virus that was not naturally present in the office—the virus was detected on more than half of the office surfaces (and on the hands of office workers) within just four hours.

Don't count on people washing their hands. Researchers observed the hand-washing habits of nearly 4,000 people in public restrooms. They found that about 10% didn't wash at all. Among those who did, about two-thirds didn't use soap, and only 5% washed long enough to thoroughly remove harmful organisms.

PUBLIC OFFENDERS

Bacteria and viruses can survive on hard surfaces for anywhere from a few hours to several days—and sometimes longer when they're protected by a sheen of hand lotion or residue from a greasy meal. *Watch out for…*

• **Coffee-cup lids.** A University of Arizona professor found that about 17% of disposable coffee-cup lids placed on cups by coffee shop workers were contaminated with fecal bacteria.

Solution: Skip the lid, or pour the coffee into your own thermos cup.

• **Office coffeepot handles.** The pots usually get rinsed out, but the handles are rarely cleaned.

Solution: Wash your hands after pouring your coffee, or use a disposable wipe to wipe down the handle before using.

• **ATM machines.** A British study found that ATM machines were heavily contaminated with bacteria at the same levels as nearby public toilets.

Solution: Bring a disposable wipe to wipe the keypad or touch screen, or clean your hands with a disposable wipe immediately after using the machine.

• **Supermarket checkout conveyor belts.** Juices from raw poultry and beef, which may be contaminated with dangerous bacteria, including salmonella and E. coli, may leak onto the belts. Other food-related bacteria end up there, too. A study by Michigan State University tested 100 belts in 42 grocery stores. All 100 belts were found to have mold, yeast, the disease-causing bacteria Staphylococcus aureus (staph) and other bacteria.

Solution: When you get home, wash your hands before opening cabinets and the refrigerator. Wash them again when you're done unpacking your groceries. Put packaged raw meat and poultry in plastic bags before you refrigerate or freeze it. Wash off the tops of cans before you open them.

•**Public telephones.** Though pay phones have all but disappeared, you still find telephones for public use in office lobbies, conference rooms, hotel lobbies, etc. They're rarely cleaned.

Solution: Use a disposable wipe to clean the mouthpiece…the part that presses against your ear…and the buttons before using public phones.

HOTELS

•**Bathtubs.** Don't be fooled by the gleaming white porcelain and legions of bustling hotel maids. When we took cultures from hundreds of apparently clean bathtubs, about 60% were contaminated with staph.

Rinsing a tub doesn't help because staph survives in biofilm, an invisible coating that forms in tubs and keeps the bacterium moist and viable.

Solution: You need mechanical action to remove biofilm. If you know that you'll want to take a bath in your hotel, bring a small scrub brush and a few ounces of bleach. A solution of one part household bleach to nine parts water and a few drops of soap (such as the shampoo or shower gel at the hotel) will kill most microbes within a few seconds, and the brush will remove them.

•**Pillows.** Pillows are rarely laundered. When I travel, I always bring protective covers (look for antiallergy pillow casings). I wash them each time I return home.

Also: Just about everyone knows (or suspects) that the bedspreads used in most hotels aren't laundered anywhere near as often as the sheets.

Solution: Remove the bedspread and toss it in a corner. To stay warm, request additional blankets, which are laundered more often than bedspreads.

•**Carpets.** The carpets in public places can harbor some 200,000 bacteria per square inch—thousands of times more than live on the average toilet seat. Since carpets aren't deep-cleaned very often, they provide a veritable buffet for bacteria and other organisms.

Solution: Higher-end hotels often provide a pair of disposable scuffs or slippers. Wear them! Or bring your own slippers or flip-flops.

RESTAURANTS

•**Tables.** Does the server wipe your table before you sit down?

Bad news: The damp wiping cloths should be sanitized between uses but often aren't. They can harbor astonishing amounts of bacteria. One study found that 70% of wiped restaurant tables were contaminated with E. coli and other fecal bacteria.

Solution: When you go to a restaurant, wipe the table yourself with a sanitizing wipe.

•**Toilets.** The top of the toilet seat might be sparkling clean, but most germs are underneath. Your fingertips are contaminated when you raise or lower the seat.

Solution: Use a disposable wipe or a thick layer of toilet tissue to lift the seat.

Also important: Close the lid, if the toilet has one, before you flush. Flushing an old-style toilet can spray bacteria-laden droplets up to 20 feet—the newer, low-flush toilets will spray no more than one foot.

Your Church or Synagogue Can Make You Sick

William Schaffner, MD, professor, department of preventive medicine and medicine/infectious diseases, Vanderbilt University School of Medicine, Nashville.

We certainly don't mean to cast aspersions on anyone's religious practices, but there are a number of hazards lurking in our churches and synagogues—toxins, allergens, irritants, germs, etc.—that can undermine the health of unwary worshippers. *Here's what worshippers should watch out for…*

•**Contaminated holy water.** Researchers from the Institute of Hygiene and Applied Immunology at the Medical University of Vienna in Austria tested samples of holy water from

39 churches and shrines in that country. Christian churches use holy water for baptism. In addition, in Catholic churches and certain other denominations, there is a permanent font (basin) at the church entrance. Worshippers dip their fingers into the holy water, then anoint themselves by touching their faces, chests and shoulders to make the sign of the cross.

Study findings: All holy water samples from churches and hospital chapels showed extremely high concentrations of heterotrophic plate counts (used to measure microorganisms such as bacteria, molds and yeasts in water)… frequently visited churches also showed signs of fecal contamination as well as staphylococcus and other bacteria. The likely source was worshippers' hands. (We can't be sure that holy water in this country has the same problem, but there's no reason to assume that it doesn't.)

Self-defense: If you want to anoint yourself with holy water, dip only a fingertip, then when you touch your face, touch only your forehead—your risk is minimized as long as you avoid your lips and eye area. Wash your hands or use a hand sanitizer as soon as possible afterward. Also, ask your priest or church sexton how often the fonts are emptied, cleaned and disinfected—your concern may encourage increased attention to this matter. If you have an infant who is going to be baptized, make certain that the special font used for baptism will be disinfected right before the service. And never drink the water from a holy spring even if you see others doing so.

•Communal communion chalices. Most Christian denominations include the sacrament of communion, in which wine and bread are shared—and often worshippers drink from a single large cup called a chalice. When offering wine using a communal chalice, officiants generally wipe the rim with a cloth before serving the next person. This reduces the chances of spreading colds, flu, oral herpes and other viruses—but it certainly doesn't eliminate the risk.

Safer: Many churches offer the option of receiving communion from tiny individual cups. If your church does not do this, speak to the minister or priest about implementing this practice.

•Shared yarmulkes. Most synagogues have a basket of the traditional head coverings for men who forget to bring their own. But just as schoolchildren are at risk for catching head lice when they share hats, there is a chance of getting lice by wearing a yarmulke from the communal basket.

Lice avoidance: Remember to bring your own yarmulke! If you are the forgetful type, keep a few spares in places like the glove compartment of your car, your briefcase, coat pockets, etc.

•Burning candles and incense. According to a study from Maastricht University in the Netherlands, after candles and/or incense were burned in the usual manner in chapels and churches of various sizes, the concentration of toxic polycyclic aromatic hydrocarbons (PAHs) in the air increased by a factor of four to 10. PAHs and other types of particulate matter that form when certain substances are burned have been linked to increased risk for lung cancer and other pulmonary diseases. The irritants in smoke from candles and incense can also trigger asthma attacks in susceptible people.

Smoke screen: If your place of worship is not well-ventilated and you have any sort of pulmonary condition or extra sensitivity to airborne irritants, sit as far away from the candles or incense source as possible, preferably near an

---

Hugs Fight Colds

Recent study: More than 400 healthy adults were exposed to a cold virus and quarantined.

Finding: Those who reported getting the fewest hugs in their daily lives were more likely to suffer from severe cold symptoms. While greater conflict was also linked to a greater likelihood of infection for those getting few hugs, those who were hugged the most were protected from infection even when they had conflicts.

Theory: Hugs boost immunity by buffering stress.

Sheldon Cohen, PhD, director, Laboratory for the Study of Stress, Immunity and Disease, Carnegie Mellon University, Pittsburgh.

open window or door. If a lit candle or incense thurible is carried around the church, hold a clean handkerchief over your mouth and nose as it passes your pew.

•**Molds.** This hazard isn't limited to houses of worship, of course. But many churches, synagogues and mosques are located in old buildings, and old buildings frequently are contaminated by mold…and even newer buildings aren't immune. Plumbing leaks, poor insulation, large carpets that are shampooed frequently—all of these factors may turn churches and synagogues into "petri dishes" for mold. Some molds can trigger allergic reactions or asthma attacks in sensitive people…others are known to produce potent toxins and/or irritants, Dr. Schaffner noted.

Best: If you find that you often have respiratory symptoms after visiting your house of worship, talk to the trustees about having the premises inspected by mold-remediation experts—so that you and your fellow worshippers can breathe easier.

Bottom line: There's no need to let concerns about getting sick from your church or temple deter you from your religious observances. Your risk is very low if you follow the commonsense precautions above.

Superbug Danger from a Common Procedure

Lawrence F. Muscarella, PhD, a biomedical engineer and health-care safety expert who advises hospitals about gastrointestinal endoscopy and infection control. Based near Philadelphia, he writes the blog "Discussions in Infection Control." *EndoscopeReprocessing.com*

In February 2015 a "superbug" infected seven patients (two of whom died) during a common medical procedure at a California hospital. The bacterium can't reliably be stopped by any antibiotic and is fatal in at least 40% of cases.

The patients were infected by duodenoscopes that are used to diagnose and treat problems of the liver, bile ducts and pancreas. Within the past two years, 135 scope-related infections

were reported to the FDA. The true number is likely higher because many infections, particularly those caused by less virulent organisms, are never reported.

The scopes have an adjustable tip that is controlled by an "elevator wire." This part of the device tends to collect biological material (including bacteria) that's difficult to remove even when the devices are cleaned. *Here's how to protect yourself if you need a procedure involving a duodenoscope…*

•**Request that the scope be tested.** Some hospitals are doing this now. The scopes are cleaned, disinfected, sampled for bacteria and then quarantined in storage until their safety can be assured.

•**Ask about ethylene oxide (EtO) sterilization.** With this method, a gas is used to sterilize scopes. It's a time-consuming step, however, that isn't available in most hospitals. Ask for it.

If your doctor doesn't address your concerns, or if the medical center doesn't have the enhanced testing or sterilization method mentioned above, consider going somewhere else.

Better Bloodstream Infection Treatment

Deverick J. Anderson, MD, MPH, associate professor of medicine, Duke University School of Medicine, Durham, North Carolina.

Follow up to get the best infection treatment. According to a recent study, 38% of patients with a bloodstream infection got the wrong treatment or were initially given an ineffective antibiotic while the cause of the infection was being investigated.

Most common types of infection: Staph and E. coli. If you develop a bloodstream infection, ask your doctor to review your updated blood culture results if symptoms don't improve within 24 hours.

Lyme Disease May Be Sexually Transmitted

Researchers found Lyme bacteria in all of the vaginal secretions from female study participants and in almost half of the semen from male participants with Lyme disease. Identical strains of the bacteria were found in married couples having unprotected sex, suggesting that sexual transmission occurs. If you are concerned about Lyme disease, talk to your doctor about being tested and treated.

Study led by Marianne Middleveen, MD, veterinary microbiologist, Alberta, Canada, published in *Journal of Investigative Medicine*.

Air Travel Myths Debunked

Roundup of travel and health experts, reported in *USA Today*.

Myth: Cabin air is full of germs.

Reality: Aircraft are equipped with HEPA filters to clean the air. The problems lie on chair upholstery, tray tables, armrests and toilet handles where bacteria such as MRSA and E. coli can live for up to one week.

Myth: Bagged pillows and blankets are safe to use.

Reality: Pillowcases on bagged pillows are rarely changed, and blankets should be used only on your lower legs—not near your eyes, nose and mouth.

Myth: The aircraft is cleaned between flights.

Reality: Airplanes typically are wiped down after every 30 days of service or at 100 flying hours, but the FAA doesn't regulate cleaning, so frequency and thoroughness vary.

Myth: There is nothing you can do to protect yourself in an aircraft cabin.

Reality: Use alcohol-based hand sanitizer… wipe the armrest and tray table with disinfectant wipes…stay hydrated…use tissues to open bathroom doorknobs and touch toilet handles… don't touch your eyes because tear ducts are a fast route to the nose and throat.

Traveler's Diarrhea Self-Defense

Anu Kantele, MD, PhD, associate professor in infectious diseases, Helsinki University Central Hospital, Finland. Her study was published in *Clinical Infectious Diseases*.

When you have a serious infection, you want your antibiotic to work fast and thoroughly and to kill the bacteria before they possibly kill you. But if the bacteria causing infection have learned to outsmart the antibiotic, then you're in real trouble. Overuse and inappropriate use of antibiotics are key factors in training bacteria to trump treatment.

When you overuse antibiotics, you are not only setting yourself up for antibiotic resistance, you are also contributing to a looming threat that affects us all. Now, a large Finnish study warns that antibiotic use to prevent or treat traveler's diarrhea may be the perfect storm for contracting superbugs during your travel.

AN UNWELCOME SOUVENIR

Not everything you bring home from a trip abroad fits in your suitcase. Like rats on an old seafaring ship, organisms can stow away in your body. A study involving 430 Finns who were traveling outside of Scandinavia showed how common a transfer of bacteria from one locale to another is. Travel destinations included South Asia (India, Pakistan and nearby locales), Southeast Asia, East Asia, North Africa and the Middle East, sub-Saharan Africa, South and Central America and the Caribbean, and Europe, Australia and North America.

The results: Among those who got traveler's diarrhea, a stunning 46% who took antibiotics for it came home with antibiotic-resistant intestinal bacteria in their bodies (namely strains of E. coli)…compared with only 17% of those who didn't take antibiotics.

The most likely place to pick up these "bugs" was South Asia, where 46% of visiting travelers were affected. Thirty-three percent of travelers visiting either Southeast Asia, East Asia or North Africa and the Middle East were affected, as were 12% of visitors to sub-Saharan Africa.

Meanwhile, all travelers to Europe, Australia and the Americas returned home unscathed.

AVOID HITCHHIKING SUPERBUGS

Although antibiotics are extremely useful in quashing bacterial infections, they can disrupt the microbial ecosystem in our guts, where "good" bacteria keep the less friendly disease-causing bacteria in check. When antibiotic use upsets the balance, it becomes easier for pathogens to invade the gut, thrive and, among travelers, hitch rides back to a traveler's native land where the bugs can spread to others. If they cause an infection, treatment becomes a challenge because these microbes can be resistant to commonly used antibiotics.

Rather than taking an antibiotic to prevent or treat traveler's diarrhea, the study researchers gave recommendations that mirror those of the US Centers for Disease Control and Prevention and noted that travelers to Asia—particularly South Asia—and Africa should be extra vigilant.

Although the CDC affirms that taking an antibiotic is, in fact, effective in preventing traveler's diarrhea, it recommends that travelers, instead, take bismuth subsalicylate (none other than Pepto Bismol) if they want to take prophylactic treatment. Bismuth subsalicylate provides some protection against harmful gut bacteria without promoting antibiotic resistance, according to the CDC. It recommends two tablets or two fluid ounces of bismuth subsalicylate four times per day but not for more than three weeks. But this prophylactic treatment is not for you if you are allergic to aspirin or on blood thinners, *probenecid* or *methotrexate*—and it should not be used by pregnant women.

Better than taking a drug to prevent traveler's diarrhea, though, the CDC and Finnish researchers both urge you to simply be careful about food and hygiene while traveling to countries known to be hot spots for traveler's diarrhea. *Avoid...*

•**Tap water unless it has been boiled.** Use bottled water for drinking and teeth-brushing—and don't let ice cubes land in your libations.

•**Food and beverages sold by street vendors** and at locales that appear to be off-the-beaten-path or unsanitary.

•**Raw or undercooked meat and seafood as well as uncooked vegetables.** In fact,

make sure that all your meals are served well-cooked and warm.

•**All raw fruit unless the fruit has a thick peel** (examples include bananas, oranges and avocados) that you can wash with bottled water before peeling.

If you get hit with traveler's diarrhea...sure, it's inconvenient, but it is usually a mild illness that resolves within a few days without treatment and is rarely life-threatening, said lead author of the study, Anu Kantele, MD, PhD, associate professor in infectious diseases at Helsinki University Central Hospital. She recommends *loperamide* (Imodium) for people with traveler's diarrhea without fever who need symptom relief—for example, relief from symptoms in order to sit through a long plane flight home.

The recommendation given by the CDC is very basic and what we all know to do—drink lots of clear fluids to stay hydrated. However, the CDC and Dr. Kantele recommend that if symptoms are severe, especially if you are running a high fever or if your stools are bloody, then, taking an antibiotic may be a wise choice despite the risk of contracting antibiotic-resistant bacteria.

Ebola Myths: Cutting Through the Hype

William Schaffner, MD, professor of preventive medicine and infectious diseases, Vanderbilt University School of Medicine, Nashville, and a past president of the National Foundation for Infectious Diseases.

From the public's perspective, the outbreak of Ebola in West Africa is very frightening and tragic. However, the reality for people living in the US is far less dramatic than what has been portrayed in books and movies. Unfortunately, some fundamental misunderstandings about the current outbreak of this illness still persist. *Here are the main myths that are causing so much confusion...*

MYTH: Ebola can't be controlled. Even though the Ebola outbreak in West Africa is indeed unprecedented, the virus typically comes and goes in rural African villages in small outbreaks that are quickly curtailed by diagnosing and treating the condition while also tracing the original source of transmission.

Many people don't realize that the disease, which was first documented in Africa in 1976, usually disappears for three to five years before reemerging. This time, Ebola spread to African cities when doctors brought in sick patients from remote villages, hoping to provide better care.

Even in these cities, proper infection-control systems, such as the use of biohazard suits, are difficult to maintain because of the sweltering heat (it's often very humid and temperatures can reach 100°F). Those bulky, cumbersome, spacesuit-looking forms of protection are like ovens and exhausting to work in. There's also a shortage of necessary medical supplies, such as latex gloves and disinfectant, in underdeveloped parts of Africa.

No one really knows why each Ebola outbreak begins. But experts suspect that the virus is carried by bats or small mammals—monkeys, in particular.

A new round of the disease probably starts when a person is bitten by or exposed to the blood of an infected animal or eats or handles raw or undercooked meat of an infected animal. Authorities suspect that the most recent outbreak began when a two-year-old boy in Guinea became infected.

MYTH: Ebola cannot be treated. The initial symptoms, which develop two to 21 days after exposure to the virus, are not that different from those of the flu and are likely to include fever, aches, sore throat, weakness, nausea, vomiting and diarrhea.

Although there's currently no specific treatment available for the disease, the supportive care that's required is not that specialized. Any decent regional hospital in the US, not just those in major cities, is capable of providing this care safely.

What's most important when treating Ebola is to stabilize the patient's fluids and electrolytes while maintaining his/her blood pressure and oxygenation. As the virus takes hold, however, there may be uncontrollable bleeding from the nose, gums and bowels, and into the whites of the eyes. In severe cases of the illness, general organ failure leads to death.

It's not fully understood why so many people die of Ebola and others survive—scientists suspect that it has to do with the immune system's

Germs in Your Contact Lens Holder

Bacteria can survive in contact lens solution for hours. Pseudomonas aeruginosa bacteria can cause corneal ulceration that can result in vision loss. In a test of nine strains, most were killed within 10 minutes of being placed in contact lens solution. But strain 39016 survived for more than four hours.

Craig Winstanley, PhD, professor, department of clinical infection, microbiology and immunology, University of Liverpool, UK, and leader of a study presented at a recent meeting of the Society for General Microbiology.

ability to withstand the initial viral attack. In the current outbreak, about 40% of people sickened with the virus have survived so far.

MYTH: Ebola is highly contagious. Ebola is not easy to catch—it spreads only by intimate contact with body fluids during the time when a person is actively sick.

It's a particular problem in Africa because funeral rites require that families perform ablutions. This involves washing the entire body of the deceased loved one, including inside the mouth and anus.

Villages actually shun families that don't perform ablutions. Even though village leaders can influence tribal practices in remote villages, it's much harder to contain the disease in teeming urban areas, where the current outbreak is located.

Traveler Warning: New Mosquito-Borne Virus

Phyllis Kozarsky, MD, medical consultant for the Traveler's Health Team, Centers for Disease Control and Prevention, Atlanta.

William Schaffner, MD, professor of preventive medicine and infectious diseases, Vanderbilt University School of Medicine, Nashville, and a past president of the National Foundation for Infectious Diseases.

The disease chikungunya has been reported in the US and the Caribbean as well as in Africa, Asia and islands in the Indian Ocean and Western Pacific. Symptoms of chikungunya, which include fever and severe joint

Germy Gyms

In a study in the *Clinical Journal of Sports Medicine*, cold viruses were found on 63% of equipment in fitness centers. And 80% of infectious diseases are transmitted by contact—either direct (such as kissing, coughing or sneezing) or indirect (for example, touching a contaminated surface, such as gym equipment, and then touching your eyes, nose, mouth or a wound, which are considered portals of entry for germs).

Always make sure to wash your hands with soap and water for at least 20 seconds before eating or drinking anything or before touching those portals of entry. If you're not near a sink, use a hand sanitizer that contains at least 60% alcohol.

Philip M. Tierno, PhD, clinical professor of microbiology and pathology, New York University School of Medicine, New York City.

pain, often in the hands and feet, usually appear three to seven days after a bite from an infected mosquito. Other symptoms sometimes include a reddish rash with slight bumps that may occur on the face, trunk, arms and legs. For most people, CHIKV lasts one to two weeks. But 10% of sufferers may have painful joints for up to a year.

There is no treatment, and the only defense is avoiding mosquito bites.

According to the CDC, as of February 10, 2015, a total of 2,492 chikungunya virus disease cases were reported from US states for 2014. Eleven locally transmitted cases were reported from Florida. All other cases occurred in travelers returning from affected areas.

Better C. diff Cure

Ilan Youngster, MD, clinical fellow, Division of Infectious Diseases, Boston Children's Hospital.

Clostridium difficile (C. diff) infections, which cause severe, sometimes deadly diarrhea, have been treated with fecal transplants—inserting feces from a healthy donor into the patient's gastrointestinal tract to rebalance the gut.

Problem: Fresh donor feces may not be available.

Solution: When frozen feces were given (through colonoscopy or a nasogastric tube), 70% of C. diff patients got better after just one treatment and 90% recovered after a second dose. Currently available at some major medical centers, a frozen fecal capsule is now being developed for widespread use.

The Truth About Flu Shots

Fiona Havers, MD, a medical epidemiologist at the influenza division, National Center for Immunization and Respiratory Diseases, Centers for Disease Control and Prevention in Atlanta, Georgia.

What's your take on flu shots? Are you dutiful about it, or do you take your chances and tough it out? Is it all about you, or do you consider the impact of viral illnesses and vaccination on the world at large? Are you afraid that you'll have a serious adverse reaction to the vaccine? Here, Fiona Havers, MD, a medical epidemiologist at the National Center for Immunization and Respiratory Diseases at the Centers for Disease Control and Prevention (CDC) in Atlanta, fleshes out these concerns about the flu and the vaccine to see who should and who shouldn't get vaccinated…

MYTH-BUSTING THE FLU VACCINE

Commonly held misconceptions, according to research from the CDC, are that the vaccine is not safe, has dangerous side effects and gives you the flu. Other people believe that the vaccine doesn't work or that an annual flu shot is just not necessary.

The truth is, serious allergic reactions to flu vaccine can occur—but the truth also is that these reactions are extremely rare. What causes these rare reactions is not always known. The cause can be an allergic reaction to a preservative added to the vaccine to extend its shelf life, an antibiotic added to inhibit bacterial contamination or the material (eggs for most flu vaccines) that the virus for the vaccine is grown in. To help prevent severe allergic reactions, doctors are trained to examine and question patients to decide whether they may react badly to the vaccine and to have antidotes on hand should a bad reaction occur.

Another truth: Despite what many people think, an association between an uncommon neurologic disease called Guillain-Barré syndrome and currently available flu vaccines is unlikely. In Guillain-Barré syndrome, the immune system attacks the neuromuscular system, causing muscle weakness. The syndrome tends to develop after a person has had a respiratory infection or the flu. Most people recover, but some can have permanent nerve damage or even die, usually from breathing difficulties.

Although a bona-fide association was seen between Guillain-Barré syndrome and the swine flu vaccine of 1976, scientists are now questioning whether a link exists beyond that one year's vaccine. The latest research shows that a person is 17 times more likely to acquire Guillain-Barré syndrome after having the flu than after getting the flu vaccine.

As for whether the flu vaccine can give you the flu, the evidence strongly says no. Although it's true that people who get vaccinated can still get the flu—no one ever claimed that the vaccine is 100% effective—it isn't the vaccine that makes these people sick. Their immune systems might not be strong enough (even after vaccination) to fight off a flu virus they become exposed to—in which case they come down with a milder version of the flu than they would otherwise. Or else they may become infected with a flu strain that differs from that in the vaccine they received. With the introduction of a quadrivalent vaccine (which protects against four different flu strains) and a new high-dose trivalent vaccine (which packs stronger protection against three different flu strains), getting the flu after vaccination is becoming less and less likely.

Yes, you might have a sore arm after getting the flu shot, but what is that compared with days or weeks of being sick and possibly being hospitalized if you catch the flu?

As for fears about mercury-laced vaccines, most currently available vaccines either do not contain the mercury-containing preservative thimerosal or are available in two versions—one with and one without thimerosal.

The amount of thimerosal used in vaccines has been proved to be safe in people of all ages—including people with thimerosal allergies, who are simply more likely to have a sore arm after vaccination. Despite what many people think (and despite many heartbreaking personal anecdotes from parents whose children are autistic), there is no scientific evidence of a correlation between thimerosal in vaccines and autism or any health problem besides injection-site soreness. In any case, thimerosal-free vaccines have been made available to ease public concerns. You can request one from your doctor.

Because a shot in the arm might be traumatic, a nasal-spray vaccine, called FluMist, is also available, but it's not for everyone. You have to be healthy, not pregnant, have no respiratory problems (or allergies) and be between two and 49 years old. It's particularly effective in children and is mainly being made for them. Eligibility is limited because FluMist is the last-standing activated flu vaccine out there. Activated vaccines are made from live virus strains and are associated with more side effects—both mild (sore arms and mild, short-term flu-like symptoms) and severe (allergy-associated anaphylaxis, with estimated incidence of one in 500,000 vaccinations)—than inactivated vaccines.

FLU VACCINE PRECAUTIONS

The CDC recommend that virtually everyone older than six months get the flu vaccine. Still, if you've had a bad allergic response to the flu vaccine in the past, discuss with your doctor whether any of the current vaccines would be safe for you—or if you need to avoid the vaccine altogether.

Also, because nearly all flu vaccines contain a small amount of egg as an ingredient, people with egg allergies need to proceed with caution when it comes to flu vaccines. They can't just walk into a local pharmacy for any free flu shot—but they may be able to be safely vaccinated depending on the severity of the allergy. Vaccination is, therefore, something that a person with an egg allergy needs to carefully discuss with his or her physician.

There is good news for some people with egg allergies, though. An egg-free vaccine called Flublok was recently approved by the FDA for people with egg allergies who are between the ages of 18 and 49. If you have an egg allergy, this is the vaccine to ask your doctor about. If it is right for you, the doctor may have it on hand or may have to order it for you.

Finally, if you come down with bronchitis or a "stomach flu" (which is usually not caused by the seasonal flu but another cause) just when you've decided to run out to get your flu shot, you should postpone getting vaccinated until you feel better. Mild head cold or sore throat is not a deterrent to vaccination.

Many different types of flu vaccines are now available. You can view a list of those approved for this year's flu season at the CDC website, *www.cdc.gov/*. The list includes information on precautions and whether and how much mercury and egg are in each vaccine.

If you are on the fence about getting a flu shot because of safety concerns about mercury content in a vaccine, an egg allergy or other personal medical condition or anything else, print out the CDC list and talk to your doctor about which flu vaccine is best for you.

FDA Approves New Vaccine to Protect Against Meningitis

U.S. Food and Drug Administration, news release.

A new vaccine that could help prevent some cases of life-threatening meningococcal disease was recently approved by the U.S. Food and Drug Administration.

Trumenba is approved to protect people between the ages of 10 and 25 from invasive meningococcal disease caused by Neisseria meningitidis serogroup B bacteria.

The bacteria can infect the bloodstream (sepsis) and the lining that surrounds the spinal cord and brain. It is a leading cause of bacterial meningitis, and infection can occur through coughing, kissing or sharing eating utensils.

Of the 500 cases of meningococcal disease reported in the United States in 2012, 160 were caused by serogroup B, according to the U.S. Centers for Disease Control and Prevention.

Antibiotics can reduce the risk of death or serious long-term problems in patients with meningococcal disease, but immediate medical treatment is crucial. Until now, vaccines in the United States covered four—A, C, Y and W—of the five main N. meningitidis serogroups that cause meningococcal disease.

"Recent outbreaks of serogroup B meningococcal disease on a few college campuses have heightened concerns for this potentially deadly disease," Karen Midthun, MD, director of the FDA's Center for Biologics Evaluation and Research, said in an agency news release.

In 2013, outbreaks of meningitis at the University of California-Santa Barbara (UCSB) and Princeton University prompted those institutions to get special permission from the FDA to use a vaccine that had been sanctioned in Europe but not in the United States.

According to *USA Today*, a total of 12 cases occurred in those two outbreaks. A UCSB lacrosse player had to have his feet amputated due to the meningitis infection, the paper reported. Amputations occur because the bacteria can trigger blood clots that reduce blood flow and can cause gangrene.

However, Dr. Midthun said that "the FDA's approval of Trumenba provides a safe and effective way to help prevent this disease in the United States."

Probiotics Help Cure H. Pylori

Standard "triple therapy" (proton pump inhibitor, *amoxicillin* and *clarithromycin*) for Helicobacter pylori (H. pylori) infection (which can cause ulcers) worked better when a probiotic was added in a study of 804 adults with the infection. After taking a probiotic that contains Lactobacillus and Bifidobacterium, twice daily for six weeks, 88% had no H. pylori infection versus 73% who didn't take probiotics.

Goran Hauser, MD, PhD, gastroenterologist, Clinical Hospital Centre, Rijeka, Croatia.

The FDA's accelerated approval of the new vaccine from Wyeth Pharmaceuticals Inc. was based on three studies in the United States and Europe that included about 2,800 teens. After vaccination with Trumenba, 82% of the teens had antibodies in their blood that killed four different N. meningitidis serogroup B strains, compared with less than 1% of teens before vaccination.

The four strains targeted by the vaccine are the same ones that cause serogroup B meningococcal disease in the United States, according to the FDA.

The safety of Trumenba was assessed in 4,500 participants in studies in the United States, Europe and Australia. The most common side effects were pain and swelling at the injection site, headache, diarrhea, muscle and joint pain, fatigue and chills.

info The U.S. Centers for Disease Control and Prevention has more about meningococcal disease at *http://www.cdc.gov/meningococcal/*.

Hidden Horror in Your Food

Leigh Broadhurst, PhD, a research geochemist in the USDA's Beltsville Agricultural Research Services, Beltsville, Maryland.

We humans aren't the only ones who relish lush, juicy summertime produce—mold, too, thrives happily on the sugar and moisture so readily available in ripe fruits and vegetables. It even can grow deep into these foods where you can't see it…ick! According to Leigh Broadhurst, PhD, research geochemist in the USDA's Beltsville Agricultural Research Services, even invisible mold in your food can make you sick. Just sniffing mold in food can make you very ill with symptoms that can range from slightly nauseous to a life-threatening toxic shock reaction. *Here is her advice…*

•**Citrus fruits.** When you get home from the market, do an immediate and thorough check of citrus fruits in bags and boxes—if you find one or two with even a bit of visible mold, there are likely to be more—return them all to

the store or toss them all into the trash. Mold spreads easily and fast with these fruits, and eating citrus with mold can make you quite ill. And, since it's sometimes hard to see, if a fruit tastes moldy when you bite into it, spit it out.

•**Soft fruits and vegetables.** This category includes peaches, nectarines, plums, grapes, melons, cucumbers, zucchini and the like, all of which are prone to announce mold by developing soft spots. For these, it's OK to cut small moldy spots away (meaning those that are less than a quarter of the total piece), taking one-half inch around the spot. To avoid cross-contamination, don't let the knife touch the mold. Larger soft areas, though, mean mold has invaded the whole fruit or vegetable even though you don't see it…throw the food away.

•**Firm vegetables.** Hard vegetables, like cabbage, cauliflower, carrots, peppers and others, have little moisture, making them less vulnerable to mold. It is fine to cut off any small patches of mold you see, in this case at least one inch around the mold.

•**Tomatoes.** Brown spots on the outside and dark seeds inside mean you should throw the entire tomato away.

•**Berries.** The ones with hollow centers (like raspberries) may grow mold from the inside out, so cut these in half and look before eating.

BLOCK THAT MOLD!

The safest produce, of course, is that which hasn't had a chance to grow mold. *Dr. Broadhurst has a few tips for that as well…*

• **Shop at local farmer's markets,** where produce is more likely to be just picked.

• **Wash produce only when you are ready to eat,** cook or freeze it. Fruits and vegetables naturally have protective microorganisms on their surfaces that are harmless—washing strips these off and opens the way for mold to settle in.

• **Use "freshness preserving" containers and/or bags.** These are designed to release the ethylene gas produced as fruits and vegetables mature, which if allowed to accumulate increases the speed of ripening and thus spoilage.

• **Use the freezer,** in particular for fresh berries you want to save. Place the entire package (washed first) into a sealed plastic bag and put it in the freezer, then use the fruit as you need it. (It won't have the same consistency as fresh fruit, but it's delicious...nutritious, too.)

Also a good choice: Frozen berries from the supermarket—they do not mold and are good year-round.

Fight Off Food Poisoning Naturally

Jamison Starbuck, ND, naturopathic physician in family practice and guest lecturer at the University of Montana, both in Missoula. She is past president of the American Association of Naturopathic Physicians and a columnist for *Bottom Line/Health.*

I s there a way to ward off food poisoning if you think you may have eaten something bad?

Activated charcoal—available at drugstores, natural-food stores and stores such as Target and Walmart—traps toxins and other substances and removes them from the body. To prevent food poisoning or lessen its severity, take two capsules of activated charcoal as soon as possible. Repeat every 30 minutes for several hours.

Also helpful: Probiotics. Take a standard dose—read the label for the correct dosage—every hour for several hours as soon as possible. Don't take probiotics at the same time as activated charcoal. Schedule the doses for in between the charcoal doses.

Important: Consult a health-care provider if you have pain or fever for more than 24 hours after eating contaminated food.

The Handshake—Could Banning It Prevent Infections?

Mark Sklansky, MD, chief of pediatric cardiology, David Geffen School of Medicine at UCLA, University of California, Los Angeles. Dr. Sklansky's article on banning the handshake appeared in *JAMA.*

S hould hospitals ban handshaking? And should you refuse to shake your doctor's hand for your own health?

A handshake can be a sign of welcome, respect, thanks or civility...or it can be something unwittingly sinister because, as you know, it's a great way to spread germs. And yet, ironically, the people who are among those most likely to spread germs via their hands are the ones tasked with fighting infections—health-care workers. This has got one doctor on a campaign to ban the handshake in certain medical settings.

KEEP YOUR HANDS TO YOURSELF

Although there certainly are policies for hospital workers about hand washing and infection control, such policies are not always

The Mumps Is Back

There were 1,078 cases of mumps reported in the first 11 months of 2014, compared with 438 in 2013. Most people born before 1967 have lifetime immunity because they contracted the virus. And most who got the MMR (measles/mumps/rubella) vaccine are immune. But the vaccine's protection declines after a decade or two. Teens and young adults may need a booster if mumps appears in the community.

William Schaffner, MD, professor of preventive medicine and infectious diseases at Vanderbilt University School of Medicine, Nashville.

followed despite numerous studies that have been published over the years about the importance of—but lapses in—hand washing in the hospital setting. According to one recent study, only 40% of health-care workers in the US regularly wash their hands before or after examining patients—that's right, 40%.

As a way to get around this rather longstanding and stubborn problem, Mark Sklansky, MD, chief of pediatric cardiology at the David Geffen School of Medicine at UCLA, argues that it's time to institute handshake-free zones, particularly in intensive- and critical-care units, emergency rooms and patient rooms. That is, doctors, patients and the friends and relatives of patients will all be expected to keep their hands to themselves.

So no more "Nice to meet you, doc"—at least, not with a shake.

Would patients and visitors comply with such a rule? This is doubtful, based on how automatic and reflexive it is for Americans to shake hands. Dr. Sklansky believes people would comply.

"We already have signs in hospitals telling visitors not to enter if they have coughs or rashes. Hospital workers and visitors to the hospital know that the hospital and its grounds are no-smoking zones. If these kinds of rules can be enforced, there is a very good chance that handshake-free zones will also be the norm in the future," said Dr. Sklansky.

In his view, germy hand-to-hand contact doesn't put only hospitalized patients with weakened immune systems at risk—it also has a much broader impact by contributing to the growth and spread of "superbugs," bacteria that are resistant to antibiotics. In other words, the more bacteria that gets passed around, the more antibiotics get used to fight infections, which leads to the development of bacteria that can't be treated with conventional antibiotics, Dr. Sklansky explained.

But as a physician, Dr. Sklansky told me that he understands the value of human touch and is not proposing that doctors and nurses stop touching their patients. He, however, feels strongly that limiting handshakes in certain health-care settings "makes absolute sense and most people in the medical community know it."

Measles Alert

Adults born in 1957 (about the time the measles vaccine began to be widely used) or later who have no record of vaccination or memory of having measles as a child should get a blood test to determine measles immunity. If none is found, they should have at least one dose of the MMR (measles-mumps-rubella) vaccine, according to the CDC. (Those born before 1957 are presumed to have had measles.) Measles is highly contagious, so anyone without immunity is at risk of contracting the disease. Complications from measles can include pneumonia and encephalitis.

Aaron E. Glatt, MD, executive vice president, Mercy Medical Center, Rockville Centre, New York.

But Dr. Sklansky doesn't realistically see banning the handshake or even setting up handshake-free zones coming too soon. "The true value of banning the handshake from the health-care environment will require study," he said. Because of the way science (and bureaucracy) works, "we may first need to find out just how many infections might be prevented by having such a rule in place."

ALTERNATIVES TO THE HANDSHAKE

Now, nothing's going to change the fact that humans need to acknowledge each other, and perhaps no more so than in an intimate, emotionally charged setting like a hospital. We're not going to all walk around greeting each other like robots, no matter what rule a hospital passes, right?

So let's look at some alternatives to the germ-passing handshake. In some places and circumstances, it's already the case that handshakes are not permitted, of course. "There are certain cultural and religious traditions in which handshakes are forbidden between members of the opposite sex, so it is not unusual for the physician or another caregiver to give a nod of the head or place the palm of the hand over one's own heart to acknowledge or greet the patient or his or her family," Dr. Sklansky said.

Other forms of noncontact greeting that can be used include a hand wave with a slight bow, holding up a hand with the palm forward or placing the palms together, as if in prayer, and lightly touching them to one's own the chest. "Meaningful eye contact and a smile works well, too," Dr. Sklansky remarked.

When you think about all those sincere, unmistakable and safe alternatives to convey greetings, and respect, it kind of makes you wonder, what's so great about a handshake, anyway?

You might be fastidious about hand washing and use of hand sanitizers, and some health-care workers and hospitals do keep very strict hygiene practices, but how can you really know if the person or professional extending a hand to you is careful about cleanliness? Even though Dr. Sklansky thinks it may be a while before his suggestion to ban the handshake could take hold in health-care settings, you may want to protect yourself and do your part for public health even more than you already are by adopting new ways to cordially greet other people—especially doctors and other health-care workers—that skip skin-to-skin contact.

Restroom Hand Dryers

Study by researchers at University of Leeds, UK, published in *Journal of Hospital Infection*.

Restroom hand dryers spread more germs than paper towels do. Researchers placed a harmless type of bacteria on the hands of study subjects to imitate poorly washed hands and found bacteria levels around high-powered "jet air" dryers were 27 times higher than levels near paper-towel dispensers...and 4.5 times higher than levels around warm-air dryers. Nearly half the bacteria around dryers remained for five minutes after the units were used—and some bacteria still could be detected after 15 minutes.

Better Antibiotic for Deadly Skin Infections

William Schaffner, MD, professor of preventive medicine and professor of medicine in infectious diseases at Vanderbilt University School of Medicine, Nashville. *NFID.org*

New antibiotic treats serious skin infections in just one dose, says William Schaffner, MD. Potentially dangerous skin and soft-tissue infections, such as MRSA (methicillin-resistant Staphylococcus aureus), often require a week or more of twice-daily antibiotic infusions at a health-care facility. The new IV drug *oritavancin* (Orbactiv) is equally effective—but it is so fast-acting, potent and long-lasting that it needs to be given only once.

Diagnosed with Hepatitis C! Now What?

Sammy Saab, MD, MPH, professor of medicine and surgery, and head of Outcomes Research in Hepatology, Pfleger Liver Institute, all at University of California, Los Angeles.

For the past year or so, many people diagnosed with the potentially deadly hepatitis C virus have been playing a waiting game—hoping that promising new treatments would become available before their livers suffered irreparable damage.

Now the wait is ending, at least for some patients, thanks to the recent approval of a breakthrough drug.

Why does this matter so much? Because more than 3.2 million Americans, mostly in the baby boomer generation, have hepatitis C—and the majority of them do not even know it. *Here's what you need to know about this deadly disease and the exciting new advances in its treatment...*

LIVER AT RISK...OR NOT?

In many patients, chronic hepatitis C infection is present for several decades before it is detected, either through a screening blood test or because liver damage develops. Symptoms of liver damage include fatigue, joint pain, jaundice, nausea and abdominal pain. Cirrhosis (scarring of the liver), liver cancer or liver failure eventually develops in about 30% of cases of chronic hepatitis C. However, the other 70% of patients never develop any significant liver damage—so when patients show no clear signs of advancing disease, doctors have often recommended a wait-and-see approach rather than jumping into treatment.

That's because, until now, the standard treatment for hepatitis C involved a grueling 48-week regimen. Patients had to take as many as 18 pills every day—typically *ribavirin* plus *boceprevir* or *telaprevir* (both FDA-approved in 2011) or the newer *simeprevir* (approved in November 2013)—and also get weekly injections of interferon, which can cause horrid side effects such as extreme fatigue, muscle aches, rashes, flulike symptoms, gastrointestinal problems, anemia, anxiety and depression. These regimens are painful, expensive and fail to cure more than three in 10 patients.

There is no way to accurately predict who will suffer life-threatening complications from the infection and who will remain symptom-free. So once doctors learned about new drugs on the verge of winning FDA approval, many stopped recommending treatment with the older hepatitis C drugs for patients who were not in imminent danger, said Sammy Saab, MD, head of Outcomes Research in Hepatology at the Pfleger Liver Institute at University of California, Los Angeles.

Game changer: In December 2013, the FDA approved the new one-dose-daily oral drug *sofosbuvir* (Sovaldi), which works by inhibiting a particular enzyme that the hepatitis C virus uses to replicate. The FDA even awarded the drug a "breakthrough therapy" designation, reserved for therapies that represent substantial improvement over previously available therapies for treating serious or life-threatening diseases.

Though it's not perfect, sofosbuvir offers significant advantages over the earlier treatment options. For one thing, many (though not all) hepatitis C patients being treated with sofosbuvir do not need to get interferon injections at all…and those who do also need the injections are cured four times more quickly than patients using the older drugs along with interferon. Also, the overall cure rate is substantially higher with sofosbuvir, topping 90%, compared with about 65% to 70% for the older drugs—and studies showed that patients who did not respond to the older drugs were among those who benefited from sofosbuvir.

In clinical trials, sofosbuvir caused only mild side effects, such as slight fatigue and headache. Of course, as with any new medication, only time will tell whether the drug has additional risks or side effects.

All in all, Dr. Saab said, sofosbuvir will make it easier and more logical to treat hepatitis C without waiting to see whether liver damage will develop.

EXPENSIVE DRUG

The biggest problem with sofosbuvir may be the expense—the drug costs about $80,000 to $90,000 for a course of treatment. Dr. Saab noted that this is similar to the full cost of the longer course of treatment needed with the older drugs. Advocacy groups are gearing up to fight for full insurance coverage—but for now, patients have to check with their own insurance companies to see where things stand. Gilead Sciences, the pharmaceutical company behind sofosbuvir, has set up a program called Support Path to offer financial assistance to certain patients.

Salmonella from Frozen Entrees

Frozen meals need standing time to finish cooking. When researchers investigated a salmonella outbreak that was caused by frozen entrées, they found that 12% of the people infected did not follow the package directions and skipped the standing time before eating. Letting the meal rest after taking it out of a conventional oven or a microwave allows it to finish cooking properly.

Morbidity and Mortality Weekly Report by the Centers for Disease Control and Prevention.

On the horizon: Dr. Saab said that he is excited about what's still coming down the pike for hepatitis C patients. Within about another year, he anticipates that several other new drugs will be approved. The upcoming drugs are expected to cure hepatitis C in as little as eight weeks...in some cases, with just a one-pill-per day regimen...and with only minimal side effects.

WHAT'S NEXT FOR YOU

If you have never been screened for hepatitis C: The CDC recommends that everyone born between 1945 and 1965 get the hepatitis C blood test because 75% of infected Americans were born during those years—so talk with your doctor about being tested. Remember, most people who have hepatitis C do not realize it until symptoms of liver damage develop.

If you already have a hepatitis C diagnosis: See your doctor to check your liver function and discuss updating your individual treatment plan. For instance...

•**If you were previously treated but the older drugs failed to cure you,** there's a good chance that you could benefit from sofosbuvir.

•**If you have one of the rare genotypes,** ask your doctor about the evidence suggesting that sofosbuvir is effective for your particular genotype.

•**If you are currently undergoing a 48-week course of treatment with interferon plus the older drugs,** your situation is trickier—because there are no guidelines on this, Dr. Saab said. Your best bet, he advised, is to talk with your doctor about your individual circumstances to determine whether to continue with your current therapy or to switch gears and try the newer treatment.

Bottom line: Hepatitis C is a dangerous disease...but the tools for fighting it are better than they've ever been.

Gene Therapy for Controlling HIV Shows Early Promise

Bruce Levine, PhD, associate professor, cancer gene therapy, University of Pennsylvania Perelman School of Medicine, Philadelphia.

Rowena Johnston, PhD, vice president and director, research, amfAR, the Foundation for AIDS Research, New York City.

New England Journal of Medicine

In an early step toward drug-free HIV therapy, researchers are reporting the first success in genetically "editing" T-cells in patients' immune systems to become resistant to the virus.

The findings, published in a March 2014 issue of the *New England Journal of Medicine*, are based on only 12 patients. But experts were cautiously optimistic about what the study accomplished.

Specifically, researchers were able to take T-cells from the HIV patients' blood, then "knock out" a gene known as CCR5, which controls a protein that allows HIV to enter a cell.

The scientists then infused the genetically altered T-cells back into patients' blood, where they expanded in number. What's more, a few patients were taken off their HIV drugs temporarily and saw their virus levels decrease.

"This is impressive," said Rowena Johnston, PhD, director of research for amfAR, the Foundation for AIDS Research.

Still, she said, there are plenty of questions left and much research ahead. The investigators on the study agreed.

"This was a first-in-human study," said researcher Bruce Levine, PhD, an associate professor of cancer gene therapy at the University of Pennsylvania School of Medicine, in Philadelphia.

That means the trial was designed to see whether it's even safe to use this approach in people with HIV—and not whether it's an effective therapy.

The T-cell infusions did appear safe in the short term: Of the 12 patients, only one had a temporary reaction—developing fever, chills and joint pain within 24 hours of the infusion.

Wash That Stethoscope!

Stethoscopes can transfer bacteria from one patient to another. Bacteria were found on the part of the stethoscope that touches patients' skin. Some were contaminated with the deadly methicillin-resistant Staphylococcus aureus (MRSA).

Self-defense: Ask the doctor to clean the stethoscope with alcohol before using it to examine you.

Study by researchers at University of Geneva Hospitals, Switzerland, published in *Mayo Clinic Proceedings*.

"Right now, we're at the point where we've demonstrated safety and feasibility," Dr. Levine said.

Ultimately, scientists want to develop a "functional" cure for HIV—where people's immune system cells are resistant to the virus, and they can stop taking the lifelong, daily drug regimens currently used to suppress the infection.

Those drugs have turned HIV into a manageable chronic disease for many. But, Levine said, they are costly, cause side effects, and for some people, eventually lose their effectiveness.

No one knows whether the technology used in this study will eventually offer a functional cure. But Levine said there were "hints" that, with further refinement, it could.

One month after the T-cell infusion, half of the study patients stopped their regular HIV drug regimen for up to 12 weeks. Initially, the patients' "viral load" increased, but for the four who were able to stay off their medication for the full 12 weeks, the viral load declined toward the end.

HIV researchers have been studying the CCR5 protein for years. It's long been known, Dr. Levine said, that the protein allows HIV to gain entry into cells. And people who have a particular mutation in both copies of their CCR5 gene (inherited from both parents) are protected from HIV infection.

CCR5 research has gained momentum in the past several years—particularly after the famous case of the "Berlin patient," who is considered the first person to be cured of HIV.

That patient, whose real name is Timothy Ray Brown, was HIV-positive back in 2007, when he underwent a bone marrow transplant to treat leukemia. His bone marrow donor carried two copies of the CCR5 mutation, and the transplant not only cured his cancer, but also knocked his HIV levels below the threshold of detection. He has been off of HIV drugs since 2008.

According to the World Health Organization, most people living with the disease globally do not have access to the current treatments.

But Dr. Johnston said she believes that if scientists can develop an effective gene therapy, others would find a way to get it to people living with HIV.

"I'm optimistic," she said. "For many years, people didn't think it would ever be possible to cure HIV. Now the question is no longer, 'Is it possible?' It's 'How are we going to do it?'"

The study was partly funded by Richmond, California based Sangamo BioSciences. Several co-researchers on the work are employees of the company.

info The Centers for Disease Control and Prevention has more on HIV/AIDS at *www.cdc.gov/hiv*.

"Kissing Bug" Spreading Tropical Disease in U.S.

Melissa Nolan Garcia, MPH, research associate, Baylor College of Medicine, Houston.

Susan Montgomery, DVM, MPH, epidemiology team leader, parasitic diseases branch, U.S. Centers for Disease Control and Prevention.

Presentation, American Society of Tropical Medicine and Hygiene annual meeting, New Orleans.

American Journal of Tropical Medicine and Hygiene, online

Residents of the southern United States may be at risk for a parasitic infection that can lead to severe heart disease and death, three recent studies suggest.

Chagas disease, which is transmitted by "kissing bugs" that feed on the faces of humans at night, was once thought limited to Mexico, Central America and South America.

That's no longer the case, the recent research shows.

"We are finding new evidence that locally acquired human transmission is occurring in Texas," said Melissa Nolan Garcia, MPH, a research associate at Baylor College of Medicine in Houston and the lead author of two of the three studies.

STUDY #1

In one pilot study, her team looked at 17 blood donors in Texas who tested positive for the parasite that causes Chagas disease.

"We were surprised to find that 36% had evidence of being a locally acquired case," she said. "Additionally, 41% of this presumably healthy blood donor population had heart abnormalities consistent with Chagas cardiac disease."

The CDC, however, still believes most people with the disease in the United States were infected in Mexico, Central and South America, said Susan Montgomery, DVM, MPH, of the agency's parasitic diseases branch.

"We don't know how often that is happening because there may be cases that are undiagnosed, since many doctors would not think to test their patients for this disease" she said. "However, we believe the risk of infection is very low."

Maybe so, but kissing bugs—blood-sucking insects called triatomine bugs—are found across the lower half of the United States, according to the CDC. The insects feed on animals and people at night.

The feces of infected bugs contains the parasite Trypanosoma cruzi, which can enter the body through breaks in the skin. Chagas disease can also be transmitted through blood.

It's a silent killer, Garcia said. People don't feel sick, so they don't seek care, but it causes heart disease in about 30% of those who get infected, she said.

ADDITIONAL STUDIES

In another study, Garcia's team collected 40 insects in 11 Texas counties. They found that 73% carried the parasite and half of those had bitten humans as well as other animals, such as dogs, rabbits and raccoons.

A third study found that most people infected with Chagas aren't treated.

For that project, Jennifer Manne-Goehler, MD, a clinical fellow at Harvard Medical School

Hidden Chlamydia

Nearly 400,000 Americans have chlamydia and don't know it. A recent government report estimates that 1.8 million people in the US have the symptomless sexually transmitted disease, but only 1.4 million infections have been reported.

Study by researchers at US National Center for HIV/AIDS, Viral Hepatitis, STD and TB Prevention, a division of the Centers for Disease Control and Prevention, presented at the STD Prevention Conference in Atlanta.

and Beth Israel Deaconess Medical Center in Boston, collected data on nearly 2,000 people whose blood tested positive for Chagas.

Her team found that only 422 doses of medication for the infection were given by the CDC from 2007 to 2013. "This highlights an enormous treatment gap," Dr. Manne-Goehler said in a news release.

The findings of all three studies were published recently in the *American Journal of Tropical Medicine and Hygiene.*

SYMPTOMS

Symptoms of Chagas can range from none to severe with fever, fatigue, body aches and serious cardiac and intestinal complications.

"Physicians should consider Chagas when patients have swelling and enlargement of the heart not caused by high blood pressure, diabetes or other causes, even if they do not have a history of travel," Garcia said.

However, the two treatments for this disease are "only available [in the United States] via an investigative drug protocol regulated by the CDC," Garcia said. They are not yet approved by the Food and Drug Administration.

Efforts are under way to develop other treatments for Chagas disease, Dr. Montgomery said.

"Several groups have made some exciting progress in drug development," she said, "but none have reached the point where they can be used to treat patients in regular clinical practice."

info The U.S. Centers for Disease Control and Prevention has more about Chagas disease at *http://www.cdc.gov/parasites/chagas./*

Longevity and Optimum Aging

What You Know About Aging Is Wrong!

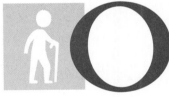ld age is often portrayed as a time of loneliness, depression and significant cognitive decline. But most research shows that the opposite is true for most people.

Among the common myths about getting older…

MYTH #1: Depression hits.

No one loves the physical changes of age, let alone the likelihood of dealing with age-related illnesses. But the emotional prospects are better than you think. The rates of major depression, for example, actually go down with age. A recent study that tracked participants for about 10 years found that their feelings of well-being increased until they reached their 70s. The feelings plateaued at that point but still didn't fall.

People who develop serious medical problems or experience traumatic life events (such as the death of a spouse) obviously will be more likely to suffer from depression than those who have an easier path. But even in the face of adversity, older people are resilient—they've accumulated enough wisdom to help them through hard times.

MYTH #2: You'll be lonely.

One of the inevitabilities of aging is the loss of friends and family members. Older people do spend more time alone. But that's not the same as feeling lonely or isolated.

A number of studies have shown that the quality of relationships improves with age. You may have fewer close friends in your 70s than you did in your 50s, but you'll probably find

Marc E. Agronin, MD, an adult and geriatric psychiatrist who is medical director for mental health and clinical research at Miami Jewish Health Systems and affiliate associate professor of psychiatry and neurology at University of Miami Miller School of Medicine, both in Florida. He is a contributor to *The Wall Street Journal* experts blog at *Blogs.WSJ.com/experts*.

that the connections have matured and become richer and more fulfilling.

Remember your earlier relationships—how often were they tumultuous and emotionally fraught? Studies have shown that older adults tend to be more positive about their relationships and less likely to experience social tensions.

MYTH #3: Your mind slips.

Yes, it will, in some ways—but the typical "slips" that most people experience will be offset by improvements in other mental areas.

Take memory and the ability to concentrate. Both start to decline by middle age. You won't be as quick at math, and your verbal skills won't be quite as sharp. You'll retain the ability to learn, but new information will take longer to sink in.

At the same time, you'll notice improvements in other mental abilities. You'll have a lot of accrued knowledge, along with an edge in reasoning and creative thinking. You won't keep up with the youngsters on cognitive tests, but you may perform better in real-world situations.

To keep your mind active, take up painting or other hobbies. Read challenging novels. Learn another language, or learn to play a musical instrument. People who stretch themselves mentally can improve memory and cognitive skills and possibly slow the rate of subsequent declines.

MYTH#4: There will be no more sex.

In surveys, older adults often report more sexual satisfaction than is reported by their younger counterparts. They might have sex less often, but they tend to enjoy it more.

A national survey of sexual attitudes, published in *The New England Journal of Medicine*, found that, on average, the frequency of sexual activity declines only slightly from the 50s to the 70s.

And the sexual attitudes among seniors are sufficiently frisky to make their grandchildren blush. About 50% of people ages 57 to 75 reported engaging in oral sex. More than half of men and about 25% of women masturbated.

Good health (and an available partner) are among the best predictors of a robust sex life. Sex-specific disorders—such as erectile dysfunction in men and vaginal dryness in women—now can be overcome with a variety of aids and treatments. Even when sexual activity does decline (or disappear), older adults enjoy cuddling and other intimacies.

MYTH #5: Falls are normal.

Falls are never a normal part of aging...and they're not merely accidents. Anyone who is unsteady on his/her feet has a health problem that needs to be addressed. It could be osteoporosis, reduced muscle strength, impaired vision, disturbed sleep or side effects from medications.

Warning: Falls are the main cause of more than 90% of hip fractures and a leading cause of emergency room visits and deaths.

People who get any kind of exercise—a daily walk, working around the house, digging in the garden—are much less likely to fall or to suffer serious injuries should they have a misstep.

Important: A good night's sleep. We've found that people who don't sleep well tend to have more disorientation and balance problems, particularly if they happen to be taking sleep medications that contain the antihistamine *diphenhydramine*.

Practice good sleep hygiene—go to bed and get up at the same times each day...avoid sleep distractions (such as watching TV in bed)... don't drink caffeinated beverages late in the day...and drink a soothing cup of warm milk or chamomile tea at bedtime.

---

5 DIY Tests That Could Save Your Life

David L. Katz, MD, MPH, an internist and preventive medicine specialist. He is also president of the American College of Lifestyle Medicine and author of *Disease-Proof: The Remarkable Truth About What Makes Us Well* (Hudson Street).

If you're conscientious about your health, you probably see your doctor for an annual physical...or perhaps even more often if you have a chronic condition or get sick.

But if you'd like to keep tabs on your health between your doctor visits, there are some easy, do-it-yourself tests that can give you valuable information about your body. These tests can sometimes tip you off that you may have a serious medical condition even though you don't have any symptoms.

Here are self-tests that you can do at home—repeat them once every few months, and keep track of results. See your doctor if you don't "pass" one or more of the tests...*

TEST #1: Stairs Test

Why this test? It helps assess basic lung and heart function.

The prop you'll need: A single flight of stairs (about eight to 12 steps).

What to do: Walk up the steps at a normal pace while continuously reciting "Mary had a little lamb" or some other simple verse.

Watch out: You should be able to talk easily while climbing the stairs and when at the top—without feeling winded. If you cannot continue to talk, or if you feel discomfort or tightness in your chest at any time during this test, see your doctor as soon as possible.

Beware: If the small stress of climbing one flight of stairs causes physical problems, it could be a sign of hardening of the arteries (arteriosclerosis) or heart disease.

For some individuals, being out of breath could mean that they have asthma or bronchitis...chronic obstructive pulmonary disease (COPD), including emphysema...or even lung cancer.

TEST #2: Gravity Test

Why this test? It measures how well your body adapts to changes in position, which can signal a variety of health problems, ranging from anemia to medication side effects.

The prop you'll need: Either a stopwatch or clock that measures seconds.

What to do: Lie down on a bed or the floor, and rest there for a minute or two. Then, start the stopwatch and stand up at a normal pace with no pauses (it's OK to use your hands).

Watch out: If you feel dizzy, make note of this. Most people can go from lying down to standing up within five seconds—and feel perfectly normal. In a healthy person, the body responds to the change in posture by pumping blood more strongly to the head.

*These self-tests are not a substitute for a thorough physical exam from your doctor. Use them only as a way to identify potential problem areas to discuss with your physician.

Beware: Dizziness can signal any of the following...

• **Low blood pressure.** With orthostatic hypotension, your body doesn't pump enough blood to counteract the effects of gravity when you stand up.

• **Medication side effects,** especially from diuretics, such as *furosemide* (Lasix)...beta-blockers, such as *atenolol* (Tenormin) or *propranolol* (Inderal)...drugs for Parkinson's disease, such as *pramipexole* (Mirapex) or *levodopa* (Sinemet)...tricyclic antidepressants, such as *imipramine* (Tofranil) or *amitriptyline* (Elavil)...or drugs to treat erectile dysfunction, such as *sildenafil* (Viagra) or *tadalafil* (Cialis).

• **Dehydration.**

• **Anemia.**

• **Atherosclerosis,** in which blood flow is partially blocked by fatty deposits in blood vessels, or other vascular problems.

TEST #3: Pencil Test

Why this test? It checks the nerve function in your feet—if abnormal, this could indicate diabetes, certain types of infections or autoimmune disease.

The prop you'll need: A pencil that is freshly sharpened at one end with a flat eraser on the other end...and a friend to help.

What to do: Sit down so that all sides of your bare feet are accessible. Close your eyes, and keep them closed throughout the test.

Have your friend lightly touch your foot with either the sharp end or the eraser end of the pencil. With each touch, say which end of the pencil you think was used.

Ask your friend to repeat the test in at least three different locations on the tops and bottoms of both feet (12 locations total). Have your friend keep track of your right and wrong answers.

Watch out: Most people can easily tell the difference between "sharp" and "dull" sensations on their sensitive feet. If you give the wrong answer for more than two or three locations on your feet, have your doctor repeat the test to determine whether you have nerve damage (neuropathy).

Beware: Neuropathy is a common sign of diabetes...certain autoimmune disorders, including lupus and Sjögren's syndrome…infection, such as Lyme disease, shingles or hepatitis C…or excessive exposure to toxins, such as pesticides or heavy metals (mercury or lead).

TEST #4: Urine Test

Why this test? It helps evaluate the functioning of your kidneys.

The prop you'll need: A clear plastic cup or clean, disposable clear jar.

What to do: In the middle of the day (urine will be too concentrated if you do this first thing in the morning), urinate into the cup or jar until you have caught at least an inch of urine. Throughout the day, note how often you urinate (about once every three waking hours is typical).

Watch out: The urine should be a pale, straw color—not deep yellow, brown or pinkish. Urine that's discolored could indicate dehydration, abnormal kidney function or another health problem.

Next, smell the urine. It should have nothing more than a very faint urine odor (unless you recently ate asparagus).

Beware: While dark-colored or smelly urine could simply mean that you are dehydrated, there are too many other potentially serious causes to ignore the signs.

Some of the disorders that can affect urine include…

•**Kidney or bladder infection,** which can cause discolored urine and frequent urination.

•**Kidney disease,** which can cause smelly, discolored urine. Interestingly, both too frequent urination and infrequent urination are signs of kidney disease.

•**Diabetes or enlarged prostate,** which can cause frequent urination.

TEST #5: "Rule of Thumb" Test

Why this test? It can help identify hearing loss.

The prop you'll need: A perfectly quiet room.

What to do: Rub your right thumb and index finger together continuously to create a kind of "whisper" sound. Raise your right arm so that it's level with your ear and your arm is roughly forming a right angle. Continue rubbing your thumb and index finger together. Can you still

hear the sound? If not, move your hand toward your right ear, stopping when you can just hear the sound. Repeat on the left side.

Watch out: You should be able to hear this "finger rub" when your hand is six inches or more away from your ear.

Beware: If you need to be closer than six inches to hear the sound in either ear, you may have hearing loss. See an audiologist or otolaryngologist (ear, nose and throat specialist) for an evaluation.

While many people dismiss hearing loss as a mere inconvenience, it can have serious repercussions, such as getting into a car wreck because you can't hear the sound of a car approaching from the side.

Grow Young with Powerful Mental Techniques

Ellen Langer, PhD, professor of psychology, Harvard University, Cambridge, Massachusetts and head of the Langer Mindfulness Institute at Harvard. *LangerMindfulnessInstitute.com*

Did you know that you can turn back the clock and regain the vigor of your youth by putting yourself in a "time capsule" for a few days? Sounds crazy, but it's actually fun, festive and easy to do. And it's based on ongoing research from Ellen Langer, PhD, a professor of psychology at Harvard University and head of the Langer Mindfulness Institute. Learning more about this unique exercise and four more mind-bending tricks from Dr. Langer's research will prove to you that mind over matter is for real when it comes to staying healthy and fit.

THE MIND-BODY CONNECTION

"Our culture operates on the assumption that the mind and body are separate," said Dr. Langer. "What we're learning is that you can't separate them…the mind and body are one." And prioritizing the mind-body connection is fast becoming the best approach to not only physical health, but all-around well-being.

Take, for instance, that time-machine study on ageless aging—a program you can easily do with a group of friends in your age bracket. The study involved a group of 80-year-olds who were basically put in a time machine for a week. Yes—a time machine. They were first tested on vision and hearing, grip strength, memory and dexterity before being taken to a monastery that was decorated to replicate life in 1959. The décor included photos of their younger selves. The participants wore 1950s fashions during their stay, and entertainment consisted of TV shows, movies, books, newspapers and music of the 1950s. The participants also were instructed to discuss sports and events that occurred during that era in the present tense. Most importantly, the participants were told to not reminisce about the old days, but, instead, to think of themselves as actually being younger.

Five days later, the participants did, in fact, look younger and their scores on grip strength, dexterity, memory and even eyesight had improved. Dr. Langer showed that thinking you're in your prime (even if you are way past it) can trigger the body to become healthier. Britain, South Korea and The Netherlands have since created TV shows based on Dr. Langer's study—and have gotten similar results.

THINK YOURSELF WELL

Here's more on how you can be inspired by Dr. Langer's provocative research for a healthier and younger you.

•**Believe you're in control of your health.** But you really have to believe.

Real-life results from Dr. Langer: A group of college students hoping to enter the military were divided into two subgroups. All participants had 20/20 vision or better. One group was given flight suits to wear and told to think of themselves as Air Force pilots doing flight simulation exercises while they used flight simulators. The other group was just seated at the flight simulators and told that the simulator was broken and that they should just pretend to fly the plane. After the exercise, the participants' were given vision tests. The eyesight of the group members who believed they were actually enacting a flight simulation—a skill that requires precise vision—was 40% better than those in the group that was just pretending.

•**Transform the mundane into a vital health routine.** For example, recognize that any kind of physical activity—not just sweating through a Zumba workout—can be a calorie-burning exercise. Be like a group of maids who were told that cleaning is good exercise. They lost weight and had improved body mass indices and hip-to-waist ratios compared with maids who weren't told this. When questioned, those other maids said that they didn't think of housecleaning as exercise. They didn't lose any weight at all.

•**Describe your health in the most positive terms possible.** Although doing so won't necessarily miraculously cure you of whatever you've got, it can make living with a chronic disease or health risk a lot easier by relieving pain and stress. For example, don't be like a group of breast-cancer survivors who said they were "in remission." They were less functional, in more pain and in poorer health than another group who thought of themselves as "cured."

•**Act how you want to feel.** Surely, you have had experiences when you've "thought yourself well"—or "made yourself sick." Dr. Langer proved how easy it is to do.

This "don't try this at home" experiment makes a strong point: Healthy volunteers were given tissues and asked to act as if they had a cold while watching a film of people coughing and sneezing. Forty percent of the volunteers reported cold symptoms afterward, and blood tests taken at that time showed that all of those reporting symptoms had high levels of IgA antibody, which means that their bodies were launching an immune response against a cold they were imagining that they had!

Practice thinking of yourself as healthy, vibrant, young and resilient, and engage your imagination to cause change in accordance with will.

It Takes a Virtual Village

Karen Larson, editor, *Bottom Line Personal.*

My mother-in-law, a widow, would have liked to "age in place" in her house in New Jersey, but she was feeling isolated and moved to a senior living facility.

Back in 1999, Susan McWhinney-Morse faced a similar dilemma. She loved her Boston town house but was worried that she'd have to struggle to obtain needed support.

Her solution: She helped launch a nonprofit group that would provide her—and other retirees in her area who wished to remain in their homes—with help and social activities. Today that nonprofit group, Beacon Hill Village, has nearly 400 members. What's more, it has inspired approximately 150 similar "virtual villages" around the country, with roughly 120 more in the planning stages.

These virtual villages do not typically provide actual day-to-day support to members, just guidance about where and how to obtain support. They vet local service providers—from plumbers to home health aids. (Some of these providers offer discounts to group members.) They connect members in need of assistance with fellow members or local volunteers who are willing to help. And they typically have someone on staff who can advise members about the ins and outs of senior services. Virtual villages also sponsor get-togethers and outings, says McWhinney-Morse, who still is in her town house as she enters her 80s. Membership fees typically are $300 to $500 a year, though a few villages charge as much as $1,000.

The Village to Village Network website (*VT VNetwork.org*) can help you locate groups in your area. If there is no group nearby, click the "Start a Village" link on the site to learn more.

High-Tech Ways to Age at Home

Majd Alwan, PhD, senior vice president of technology and executive director of the LeadingAge Center for Aging Services Technologies, a nonprofit for aging advocacy in Washington, DC. *LeadingAge.org/CAST*

W here do you plan to live during your retirement years—including your latest years? If you're like most people, you want to stay right at home.

But that doesn't work for everyone. People with chronic illnesses and/or physical disabili-

ties may end up moving into assisted-living facilities or nursing homes—and often sooner than they had hoped.

Now: High-tech devices can help you stay in your home much longer than before (even if you live alone) while also giving loved ones the assurance that you are safe.

To stay at home as long as possible, people have traditionally installed ramps, grab bars, brighter lighting and other such products to accommodate their changing needs. But that doesn't scratch the surface of what's available today.

Impressive high-tech devices to help you stay at home as you age…

"CHECKUPS" AT HOME

There's now an easy way to quickly alert your doctor of important changes in your health that may be occurring between office visits.

What's new: Remote patient monitoring. You can use an at-home glucose monitor, weight scale, pulse oximeter (to measure oxygen in the blood) and other devices that store readings, which you can then easily share with your doctor—on a daily, weekly or monthly basis, depending on your condition and how well you're responding to treatments.

Example: A wireless glucose monitor, such as the iHealth Align ($16.95, without test strips), available at *iHealthLabs.com*. It works with a smartphone to take glucose readings and automatically log/track measurements over time and send them to the doctor.

In development: Systems with wearable sensors that automatically take and transmit important readings. A steering wheel that measures blood glucose? Watch for that too in the next few years!

FALL MONITORS GO HIGH-TECH

We're all familiar with the older fall-monitor systems that require users to press a button on a pendant to initiate communication with a call center. Staffers then contact you (via an intercom-like device) to ask if you need help.

What's new: Devices that don't require the push of a button, so fall victims who are immobilized or unconscious also can be helped.

New-generation fall monitors are equipped with accelerometers that can tell when you've fallen. The units, worn around the neck, on the wrist or clipped to a belt, contact a call center or a designated caregiver. If you don't answer a follow-up call, emergency responders will be sent to your address.

Why the new technology is important: Fall victims who receive help within one hour of a fall are six times more likely to survive than those who wait longer.

Examples: Philips Lifeline HomeSafe with AutoAlert (automatic fall detection with push-button backup, 24-hour call center/emergency response) starts at $44.95/month. GoSafe is a wireless version that starts at $54.95/month, plus a onetime GoSafe mobile button purchase of $149. Both are available at *LifelineSys.com*.

Traditional-style fall monitor: Walgreens Ready Response Vi Alert System (390-foot range, 24-hour call center/emergency response) requires the fall victim to push a button. Available at *WalgreensReadyResponse.com* for $29.99/month.

ACTIVITY MONITORS

By tracking activity—and noting changes in routines—an off-site loved one or caregiver can tell when you've become more or less active or when you're spending more time in certain parts of the house. A sudden increase in bathroom visits, for example, could indicate a urinary tract infection that hasn't yet been diagnosed.

What's new: Sensors that track daily activity—for example, how often refrigerator doors are opened, when the stove is turned on and how often the bathroom is used.

Examples: GrandCare Activity Monitoring Package. A caregiver can log in to the system to view activity reports and/or set up "alert parameters" that will trigger a text if there's no movement at expected times. Available at *www. us.GrandCare.com*, $499.99, plus $49/month.

A less expensive option is Lively Activity Sensors for Living Independently. Small, disk-shaped sensors are attached to household objects such as the refrigerator and a pillbox. The sensors detect and send text/e-mail notifications when there's a movement, such as the opening of a refrigerator door. A package of six is available at *Amazon. com* for $9.99, plus $24.95/month.

HOW'S YOUR WALKING

A change in walking speed could indicate that someone has balance problems, muscle weakness or other issues that can interfere with daily living.

What's new: Wearable devices (available from your doctor or physical therapist) that monitor gait, balance and walking speed. The devices store information that can be electronically transmitted to a doctor or physical therapist.

If walking speed has declined, it could mean that an underlying health problem—such as congestive heart failure—isn't well-controlled by medication…or that you need physical therapy to increase muscle strength and stamina. Detecting such changes in gait in high-risk patients can allow treatment adjustments that help prevent falls and improve mobility—critical for staying (and thriving) at home.

Examples: StepWatch from Modus Health straps onto your ankle and has 27 different metrics to measure gait and speed. Available at *ModusHealth.com*. LEGSys from Biosensics includes portable, wireless sensors that analyze gait and generate easy-to-read reports. It's easy to put on with a Velcro strap. Available at *Biosensics.com/LEGSys-overview*.

Make Your Bathroom Safer

Highly glazed ceramic floor tile can be slippery. Consider replacing it with slip-resistant tiles or tiles with a surface that mimics natural stone. Also, opt for smaller tiles because smaller tiles mean more grout, and grout is less slippery.

Alternative: Rubber or vinyl flooring.

Also: Install screw-mounted grab bars—suction cups can come away from the wall. Attach to the wall studs, not just drywall. And it's best if the bars run horizontally, not vertically or at an angle, as your hand could slip.

Sheila Barton, LCSW, social worker at Mount Sinai School of Medicine, New York City, writing in *Focus on Healthy Aging*.

Urgent: How Good Is Your Sense of Smell?

Jayant Pinto, MD, associate professor of otolaryngology–head and neck surgery in the department of surgery at The University of Chicago Medicine. He is lead author of *"Olfactory Dysfunction Predicts 5-Year Mortality in Older Adults,"* a study published in the online journal *PLOS ONE.*

Can you smell the rose that's under your nose? What about the odor of burning toast? Or the foul smell of spoiled food?

Just as it's common to have fading vision or diminished hearing as you age, many people lose at least some of their ability to smell. In fact, about 25% of adults over the age of 53 have a reduced sense of smell, and the percentage rises to more than 60% in those age 80 and older.

AN EARLY ALERT

You're probably well aware that a decreased sense of smell can affect appetite. People who can't smell and/or taste their food tend to eat less and may suffer from weight loss or nutritional deficiencies. But you might not know that a diminished sense of smell could also be an early indicator of a serious health problem…

Surprising finding: In a recent study, people ranging from ages 57 to 85 who lost their ability to smell were more than three times more likely to die within five years than those with a normal sense of smell—the risk of dying was even higher than for individuals diagnosed with lung disease, heart failure or cancer.

This study didn't uncover the exact link between smelling loss and earlier-than-expected deaths. But the risk for neurodegenerative diseases could be a factor. For example, people who eventually develop Parkinson's or Alzheimer's disease may notice a diminished sense of smell long before they have neurological symptoms.

It's also possible that cellular senescence, the age-related reduction in cell regeneration, affects the olfactory bulb or other parts of the olfactory system before it becomes apparent in other parts of the body.

TEST YOURSELF

Even if you think your sense of smell is fine, some basic testing might show otherwise. In the study mentioned earlier, some individuals who thought they had a good sense of smell actually didn't, while some people who thought they had a problem with their sense of smell actually did well on the smell tests.

How to test yourself…

•**The alcohol test.** Hold an alcohol-swab packet near your belly button and open it up. If your sense of smell is perfect, you will detect the odor. If you can't smell it, raise it higher until you can. Some people won't detect the odor until it's just a few inches from the nose—or not even then. You can do the same test with anything that's strongly scented. The closer the item needs to be for you to smell it, the worse your sense of smell is.

•**Compare yourself to others.** Suspect that you have a problem if you're the only one in the family who doesn't notice the wonderful smell of brownies in the oven. Or if you say "Huh?" when your spouse mentions that the fireplace is smoking or that there's a nasty smell in the refrigerator.

If you think you have a diminished sense of smell: Get evaluated by an otolaryngologist or a neurologist. He/she can determine if your impairment is due to aging or a more serious problem that may have a better outcome if it is detected early.

WHAT YOU CAN DO

So far, a reduced sense of smell can't be restored.* *What can help…*

•**Practice smelling.** German scientists report that it may be possible to improve your sense of smell by smelling more. Spend a few minutes every day sniffing a variety of scents—spices, perfumes, aromatic foods, etc. This approach hasn't been proven, but it could be helpful for some people.

•**Eat a well-balanced diet and take a multivitamin,** which will provide the necessary micronutrients that help slow aging of the olfactory system and promote regeneration.

If you have appetite loss due to a reduced sense of smell…

*Exception: If your loss of smell is due to nasal inflammation—from allergies, chronic sinusitis, etc.—intranasal steroid sprays and antihistamines may restore it.

•**Kick up the seasoning.** Food will not be very appealing if you can't smell or taste it. To make your dishes as flavorful and aromatic as possible, use plenty of strong spices, such as pepper, garlic, cilantro, ginger, etc., in your cooking.

•**Focus on preparation and presentation.** Chefs have a saying: "The eyes eat first." Use brightly colored fruits and vegetables and other colorful ingredients, and add garnishes to your plate. Also, vary the textures of the foods you eat.

"Long Life" Gene Might Make Some Smarter, Too

Jennifer Yokoyama, PhD, assistant professor, neurology, University of California, San Francisco.

Dena Dubal, MD, PhD, assistant professor, neurology, and David A. Coulter Endowed Chair in Aging and Neurodegenerative Disease, UCSF.

Gayatri Devi, MD, neurologist, Lenox Hill Hospital, New York City.

Annals of Clinical and Translational Neurology

A gene variant believed to "wire" people to live longer might also ensure that they keep their wits about them as they age, a recent study reports.

People who carry this gene variant have larger volumes in a front part of the brain involved in planning and decision-making. They performed better on tests of working memory and the brain's processing speed, both considered good measures of the planning and decision-making functions controlled by the brain region in question.

"The thing that is most exciting about this is this is one of the first genetic variants we've identified that helps promote healthy brain aging," said study lead author Jennifer Yokoyama, PhD, an assistant professor of neurology at the University of California, San Francisco (UCSF). She noted that genetic research has mainly focused on abnormalities that cause diseases such as Alzheimer's and Parkinson's.

BACKGROUND ON THE GENE

The gene involved, KLOTHO, provides the coding for a protein called klotho that is produced in the kidney and brain and regulates many processes in the body, the researchers said.

Previous research has found that a genetic variation of KLOTHO called KL-VS is associated with increased klotho levels, longer lifespan and better heart and kidney function, the study authors said in background information. About one in five people carries a single copy of KL-VS, and enjoys these benefits.

STUDY DETAILS

For this study, the researchers scanned the healthy brains of 422 men and women aged 53 and older to see if having a single copy of KL-VS affected the size of any brain area.

They found that people with this genetic variation had about 10% more volume in a brain region called the right dorsolateral prefrontal cortex, Dr. Yokoyama said.

This region is especially vulnerable to atrophy as people age, and its age-related decline may be one reason why older people can be easily distracted and have difficulty juggling tasks, she said.

Referring to the region as the "conductor of the brain's orchestra," Dr. Yokoyama said that it helps people "pay attention to certain types of things, to appropriately shift your attention and to engage working memory," which is the ability to keep a small amount of newly acquired information in mind.

The brain region shrank for everyone, but those with one copy of KL-VS had larger volumes than either people without the genetic variant or those with two copies, the researchers said.

Subsequent "brain game" testing found that the size of this brain region predicted how well people performed on memory and problem-solving tests.

Following up on this finding, researchers genetically engineered mice to have higher levels of klotho, said study senior author Dena Dubal, MD, PhD, an assistant professor of neurology at UCSF.

"Not only did the mice live longer, but they were smarter at baseline," she said.

In essence, the one in five people with a single copy of this genetic variation will undergo natural aging of brain function slower than everyone else, Dr. Dubal said.

"Our data show that carrying one copy of that variant really confers a decade of deferred decline that you see in aging of that brain region," she said.

The study was reported in the *Annals of Clinical and Translational Neurology*.

EXPERT COMMENT

The findings provide some insight into how medical science may have created a disconnect between the aging of the body and the mind, said Gayatri Devi, MD, a neurologist at Lenox Hill Hospital in New York City.

"Because of modern advances in medicine we are living longer," even if our genetics would otherwise condemn us to an earlier death, Dr. Devi said. "But as we live longer and longer lifespans, we come into contact with more illnesses that are brain-related." In other words, medicine to help the brain age gracefully has not kept pace with medicine that helps the body live longer.

While these findings are very preliminary, they could one day lead to treatments that slow brain aging and help people suffering from dementia, Dr. Dubal said.

"If one can boost brain structure and function, maybe that could counter the effects of devastating diseases like Alzheimer's and Parkinson's," she said.

info For more on the aging brain, visit the U.S. National Institutes of Health at *www.nia.nih.gov* (search "the changing brain").

Don't Let Dementia and Age-Related Diseases Catch You Off-Guard

Jullie Gray, MSW, LICSW, CMC, co-owner of Aging Wisdom, a life-care management firm in Seattle. Gray is the president of the National Academy of Certified Care Managers and past president of the National Association of Professional Geriatric Care Managers.

Few situations could be more tragic for older adults than being treated as if they have Alzheimer's disease when they really have a treatable health issue, such as a drug side effect or depression. Equally pathetic is not knowing what is happening or where to turn if Alzheimer's or a movement disorder, such

as Parkinson's disease, is setting in. This is especially true for older people who live alone and away from family. It happens every day to thousands of mature adults. They end up malnourished and living in squalor, forgotten in suboptimal nursing facilities—or on the street.

Don't let any of this happen to you.

Help is available—help that can ensure you get the right diagnosis and treatment. And, just like estate planning, it can assist you in making arrangements in advance for health and physical needs if you have the beginnings of an incurable and progressive age-related disease.

WHEN DAILY LIVING BECOMES A CHALLENGE

The doorway to help is through a process called a geriatric assessment. Besides physical and psychological health, a geriatric assessment evaluates whether activities of daily living are becoming challenging. Activities include ordinary tasks such as eating, bathing and dressing as well as taking medications, keeping appointments, paying bills and getting around.

The first step is to make an appointment with your primary care physician for a geriatric assessment. The doctor will give you a physical exam and interview you to assess activities of daily living. If an age-related health issue is found, the doctor may act as the point person for a team of specialists who will take care of your health needs and help you plan for the future, whether that be making arrangements for physical therapy, optimizing your home to help you live there safely, getting transportation or a visiting nurse service or home-delivered meals, or arranging for nursing home care. Or the doctor may refer you to a geriatric specialist to assess your health and act as the point person for multispecialty care.

KNOW WHEN TO GO

A recent health alert by the division of geriatrics and palliative medicine at University at Buffalo, The State University of New York, gave guidance about when to arrange for a geriatric assessment of a parent, spouse or sibling by observing how that person manages the activities of daily living. It's easy to see when someone close to you is becoming frail and physically or mentally challenged—but what about when you have to make that decision about yourself? Geriatric specialist Jullie Gray, principal at Aging Wisdom, a life-care-management firm in Seattle, says that a geriatric assessment may be wise if you answer yes to even one of these questions...

•**Are you more forgetful,** distracted and irritable than usual, and are you worried that your memory is failing?

•**Do you feel not as steady on your feet,** resulting in having a fall?

•**Is taking care of your house,** paying your bills and taking care of your health becoming more challenging?

•**Do you have more than one chronic health problem?**

•**Are you worried about changes in your health** and feel confused about what to do or who to turn to for help?

PREPARING FOR AGING

Whether or not you decide to have a geriatric assessment, there are ways to ease age-related challenges that you can do on your own. For one, you can optimize your living space with better lighting, grab rails, easy-to-reach cabinets and drawers, elevated toilets and open showers.

Catch Your Balance Before It's Too Late

Jason Jackson, MSPT, a physical therapist in the outpatient rehabilitation department at Mount Sinai Hospital in New York City, where he specializes in balance training, along with prosthetic training, manual therapy and neuromuscular disease.

No one expects to get seriously injured—or even die—from a fall. But it happens all the time. And while older adults are at greatest risk for falls, there are no age requirements for taking a tumble.

Surprising statistic: Even among adults in their 30s, 40s and 50s, falls are the leading cause of nonfatal injuries (more than three million each year) that are treated in US hospital emergency departments. For adults age 65 and older, falls are the leading cause of fatal injuries.

Certain "fall hazards" are well known—electrical cords and area rugs...slippery floors...medications such as sleeping pills and blood pressure drugs...vision problems...and even poorly fitting shoes.

What often gets overlooked: Subtle changes in the neuromuscular system (the nervous system and muscles working together), which helps keep us upright. Regardless of your age, exercising and strengthening this system before you get unsteady (or fall) is one of the best steps you can take to protect your health. *Here's how...*

WHY OUR BALANCE SLIPS

Does your foot or ankle feel a little wobbly when you stand on one leg? Some of that is probably due to diminished strength and flexibility. After about age 40, we begin to lose roughly 1% of our muscle mass every year. As we age, we also become more sedentary and less flexible. These factors make the body less able to adapt to and correct a loss of balance.

The nervous system also gets less sensitive with age.

Example: Sensory receptors known as proprioceptors are found in the nerve endings of muscles, tendons, joints and the inner ear. These receptors make us aware of our bodies in space (proprioception) and can detect even the slightest variations in body positions and movements. But they don't work well in people who don't exercise them (see suggestions below)—and these people find it harder to keep their balance.

The other danger: Muscle weakness, even when it's slight, can lead to apprehension about losing your balance. You might then start to avoid physical activities that you feel are risky—walking on uneven pavement, for example. But avoiding such challenges to your balance actually accelerates both muscle and nervous system declines.

ARE YOU STEADY?

If you're afraid of falling or have a history of falls, a professional balance assessment, done by your doctor or a physical therapist, is the best way to find out how steady you are on your feet. The assessment usually includes tests such as the following (don't try these tests on your own if you feel unsteady)…

•**Sit-to-stand.** Sit in a straight-backed chair. If your balance and leg strength are good, you'll be able to stand up without pushing off with your hands.

•**Stand with your feet touching.** You should be able to hold this position for 15 seconds without any wobbling.

•**The nudge test.** Ask someone to gently push on your hip while you're in a normal stance. If you stagger or throw out your hands to catch yourself, your balance is questionable. If you start to fall, your balance needs improvement.

BOOST YOUR BALANCE

Balance, like strength and endurance, can be improved with simple workouts. Incorporate the exercises below into your daily routine—while at the grocery store, in the office, while watching TV, etc. Do them for about 15 minutes to 30 minutes a day, three to four days a week (daily if you have the time). *What to do…**

•**One-legged stands.** You don't have to set aside time to do this exercise. You simply stand on one leg as you go about your daily activities—while waiting in line, for example. Lift your foot about six inches to 12 inches off the floor to the front, side and back. Try to hold each position for about 15 seconds, then switch legs. This strengthens the muscles in the ankles, hips and knees—all of which play a key role in one's balance.

•**Heel raises.** This move is good for balance and strength. While standing, rise up on your toes as far as you can. Drop back to the starting position, then do it again. Try for 10 repetitions. You can make this exercise more difficult by holding weights. Start with three-pound weights, gradually increasing weight as you build tolerance.

*Do these exercises next to a stable object, such as a countertop, if you feel unsteady. Also, they are more easily done while wearing shoes. When you feel comfortable doing these moves, you can perform them barefoot to add difficulty.

FOR MORE BENEFITS

Once you have become comfortable with the exercises described earlier, you can up your game with the following to keep you even safer from falling…

•**Balance on a Bosu ball.** It's a rubberlike half-ball (about two feet in diameter) that you can use for dozens of at-home workouts, including balance and abdominal exercises.

Cost: About $100, on *Amazon.com* and in some sporting-goods stores.

Example: With the flat side on the floor, start by standing with both feet on the ball. Your muscles and joints will make hundreds of small adjustments to keep you balanced. When you get better at it, try to stand on one leg on the ball. When you're really comfortable, have someone toss you a basketball or tennis ball while you maintain your balance.

JUST FOR FUN

You don't always need formal balance exercises. *Try this…*

•**Walk barefoot.** Most of us spend our days in well-padded shoes that minimize the "feedback" between our feet and the ground. Walking without shoes for at least a few minutes each day strengthens the intrinsic muscles in the feet and improves stability. If you prefer to wear socks, be sure to use nonslip varieties that have treads to avoid slipping on wood or tiled floors.

Also helpful: Minimalist walking/running shoes. They're made by most major footwear companies, such as New Balance, Adidas and Nike, as well as by Vivobarefoot. Because they have a minimal amount of heel cushioning and arch support, they give the same benefits as barefoot walking but with a little extra protection.

Hidden Bone Loss Danger

Angelico Mendy, MD, MPH, researcher in epidemiology, The University of Iowa College of Public Health, Iowa City.

Low bone density is known to boost fracture risk, but a recent study shows that it also impairs balance and hearing. Participants age 65 and older with low bone density were almost four times more likely (and those 40 and older twice as likely) to fail a balance test than those with normal density.

Explanation: Bone loss affects the entire body, including bones in the skull that house the organs for balance and hearing.

Keep Your Hips Forever!

Mitchell Yass, DPT, a physical therapist and founder/owner of PT2 Physical Therapy and Personal Training in Farmingdale, New York. He is author of *Overpower Pain: The Strength-Training Program That Stops Pain Without Drugs or Surgery. MitchellYass.com*

If you're tired of hobbling around on an aching hip, surgery to replace that failing joint might sound pretty good.

Every year, more than 330,000 Americans get this operation. For those who have severe joint damage (for example, bone-on-bone damage that prevents full range of motion), hip replacement can be an excellent choice.

Here's the rub: Many people who receive a hip replacement aren't in this category. They undergo hip replacement but don't realize that the cause of their pain could be in hip muscles, not joints.

IDENTIFY THE PROBLEM

If you complain about persistent groin pain (one of the most common symptoms of hip dysfunction), your doctor will probably order an imaging test (such as an X-ray and/or MRI scan).

What you need to know: Even though imaging tests can give doctors a great deal of information about the condition of a joint, they aren't as conclusive as you might think. For example, an X-ray can show a decrease in cartilage and less space between the thighbone and hip socket, but doctors differ in deciding at what point surgery becomes necessary. Virtually everyone who's age 50 or older will show some degree of joint damage just from normal wear and tear. A decrease in range of motion at the hip joint is key to the need for surgery.

Does a diagnosis of arthritis at the hip joint mean that you need surgery? Not necessarily. Most hip and groin pain is caused by muscle weakness or a muscle imbalance. People who correctly exercise these muscles can often eliminate—or at least greatly reduce—their discomfort. Strengthening these muscles also can help ease pain in those who have already had hip replacements...and improve balance.

THE BEST WORKOUTS

The following exercises are ideal for hip or groin pain. After getting your doctor's OK, start by trying to repeat each one 10 times. Take a one-minute break, then repeat two more sets. The whole routine, which should be done two or three times a week, takes about 20 minutes.

●**Hamstring curl.** The hamstrings (in the back of the thigh) play a key role in the functioning of the hip joints. However, the hamstrings are weak in most people—mainly because these muscles aren't used much in normal daily movements.

How this exercise helps: It strengthens hamstrings and helps prevent the opposing muscles (the quadriceps, in the front of the thigh) from shortening and causing muscle strain and/or spasms.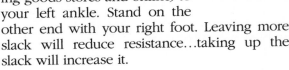

How to do it: Attach one end of a piece of elastic exercise tubing (available in sporting-goods stores and online) to your left ankle. Stand on the other end with your right foot. Leaving more slack will reduce resistance...taking up the slack will increase it.

With your feet a few inches apart and knees slightly bent, raise your left foot and curl it backward toward your buttocks as far as you comfortably can. Then return to the starting position. If you feel unsteady, put one hand (on the side opposite the leg you're working) on a wall. Switch legs and repeat.

●**Hip abduction.** This is great for hip or groin pain because the abductor muscles (on the outer thighs) tend to be much weaker than the opposing adductor muscles.

How this exercise helps: Weakness in the abductors can allow the pelvis to drop on one side, which can cause groin muscles to tighten and become painful.

How to do it: Lie on the side that's not painful (or less painful) on a mat or a carpeted floor. Your painful side will be on top. Place your arm under your head, and

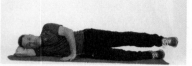

bend your other leg's knee for better support and balance.

Slowly raise your affected leg, keeping it in line with your torso. Keep the knee straight, and don't roll forward or backward. Raise your leg only to hip height (a few inches). Then slowly lower your leg back to the starting position. After performing a set, roll over and repeat the exercise with the other leg, only after pain has eased in the affected leg. Otherwise, focus only on strengthening the painful side.

• **Hip flexor stretch.** This exercise is vital. Most of us spend a lot of time sitting, causing these muscles to shorten and tighten.

How this exercise helps: It stretches tight hip flexors, which can stress the low back.

How to do it: Kneel on your right knee on a mat or a carpeted area. (If you need more padding, you can put a folded towel under the knee.) Place your left foot flat on the floor in front of you, with the knee bent. Rest your left hand on your left thigh and your right hand on

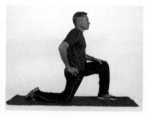

your right hip. Keeping your back straight and abdominal muscles tight, lean forward so that more of your weight is on the front leg. You'll feel a stretch in your right upper thigh. Hold for 20 to 30 seconds. Switch sides.

• **Quad stretch.** Overly tight quad muscles can pull the pelvis downward—a common cause of low-back and hip pain.

How this exercise helps: Stretching the quads helps distribute weight evenly through the pelvis.

How to do it: Stand near a wall for support. Rest your right hand on the wall, then reach

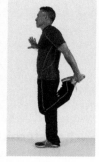

back with your left hand to grip your left foot/ankle. Pull your heel upward toward your buttocks—and eventually behind the hip. Keep pulling, gently, until you feel a stretch in the front of your thigh. Tighten your abdominal muscles. Hold for about 20 to 30 seconds. Repeat on the other side.

If your pain doesn't improve after a month of performing these exercises, consult your doctor.

Surprising Ways to Improve Your Hearing

Michael Seidman, MD, director of the Otolaryngology Research Laboratory and the Division of Otologic/Neurotologic Surgery and chair of the Center for Integrative Medicine at the Henry Ford Health System in Detroit. Dr. Seidman is coauthor, with Marie Moneysmith, of *Save Your Hearing Now. BodyLanguageVitamins.com.*

Aside from protecting your ears from blasting stereos and jackhammers, there's not much you can do to control what happens to your hearing, right? Wrong!

It's true that genetic and environmental factors (such as loud noises) are usually what cause hearing loss. But most people have far more ability to prevent hearing loss—or even improve their hearing—than they realize.

Here's why: Most problems with hearing begin when the hair cells located in the cochlea, or inner ear, don't work well or stop functioning and die. Improving blood supply to the inner ear and tamping down inflammation within the body are among the strategies that may help keep your hearing sharp.

At first glance, you wouldn't think that the steps below would have anything to do with your hearing. But they have a lot to do with it.

Here's my advice for improving your hearing or keeping it intact...

CHECK YOUR MEDS

If you're having trouble hearing, see an otolaryngologist (ear, nose and throat specialist) or audiologist for an evaluation—and ask your doctor about the medications you take. Among the many medications that are "ototoxic"—that is, they can lead to hearing loss…

•**Antidepressants** such as *fluoxetine* (Prozac) and *amitriptyline* (Elavil).

•**Antibiotics,** such as *erythromycin, gentamicin* and *tetracycline.*

•**Nonsteroidal anti-inflammatory drugs (NSAIDs),** such as aspirin and *ibuprofen* (Motrin).

If medication is causing your hearing loss, stopping the drug or switching to a new one, under your doctor's supervision, may improve your hearing.

For a list of drugs that can cause hearing loss: Go to the American Tinnitus Association's website, *ATA.org*, and click on "Ototoxic Drug Information."

GET THE RIGHT NUTRIENTS

Certain nutrients are known to promote blood flow and help fight inflammation throughout the body—including in the ears.

To ensure that you have adequate levels of such nutrients, consider taking targeted supplements to protect your hearing. Among those that are beneficial are alpha lipoic acid, acetyl-L-carnitine, L-glutathione and CoQ10. Taking these supplements may help slow hearing loss and protect against damage from loud noises.

What to do: To determine which supplements (including doses) are best for you, consult an integrative physician. To find one near you, contact the American Holistic Medical Association at *HolisticMedicine.org.*

LOOK AT YOUR LIFESTYLE

Other ways to increase your odds of keeping your hearing sharp as long as possible…

•**Chill out.** If you're late for a meeting and stuck in traffic, your stress levels will probably climb. But what's that got to do with your hearing? Quite a lot, actually.

Research has now shown that brain chemicals called dynorphins respond to stress by triggering inflammation in the brain—and in the inner ear. Inflammation not only exacerbates hearing loss but also hearing-related problems such as tinnitus.

What to do: Setting aside time each day for anything that alleviates tension—be it daily meditation, yoga or listening to restful music—may reduce your stress levels…and improve your hearing or help prevent hearing loss.

Surprising recent research: Chewing gum may curb hearing loss in some cases—perhaps by distracting the brain from stress that may be interfering with the brain's processing of sound.

•**Keep off the pounds.** Evidence is continuing to mount that the more a person is overweight, the greater his/her risk for hearing loss. What's the link? Factors closely related to obesity, such as high blood pressure, are believed to restrict blood flow to the inner ear.

What to do: Both men and women should aim for a body mass index (BMI) of 18.5 to 24.9.

•**Get enough exercise.** In recent research, women who walked at least two hours a week had a 15% lower risk for hearing loss, compared with those who walked less than one hour a week. The hearing protection conferred by exercise is also believed to apply to men.

What to do: To protect your hearing—and perhaps even improve it—spend at least two hours a week doing exercise, such as brisk walking.

•**Avoid cigarette smoke.** Smoking is bad for the lungs, the heart and many other parts of the body. But the ears? Absolutely! In a study of adults ages 48 to 92, smokers were more likely than nonsmokers to have hearing impairment. And though it's not well-known, even nonsmokers who live with smokers (this includes cigar and pipe smokers, too) are more likely to have hearing loss, suggesting that secondhand smoke can cause damage that impairs hearing.

What to do: Kick the tobacco habit—and encourage family members to do the same.

GETTING ENOUGH ZZZs

Sleep apnea, a disorder marked by chronic breathing pauses during sleep, has been recently linked to a 90% increased risk for low-frequency hearing loss (difficulty hearing conversation on the phone is a hallmark) and a 31% increased risk for high-frequency hearing loss (this often makes it hard to understand higher-pitched sounds, such as a woman's voice).

The results are preliminary, but some researchers believe that sleep apnea may trigger hearing loss due to poor blood flow to the cochlea, or inner ear.

What to do: If you snore (a common symptom of sleep apnea), see a doctor to determine whether you have sleep apnea and ask whether you should also have your hearing tested. If you have sleep apnea, it's possible that treating it will improve your hearing.

What's Going on with My Fingernails?

Jeffrey Benabio, MD, physician director of health-care transformation, Kaiser Permanente, San Diego. *Benabio. com*

L ike wrinkles on your face, ridges and discoloration in fingernails are a normal sign of aging. One of my patients humorously refers to them as a "sign of maturity."

Fingernail ridges (which run from cuticle to nail tip) can appear as early as one's 30s but are most common after age 60.

Although fingernail ridges are usually on just one or two nails, they may eventually develop on all of your fingernails. Nails also become drier as you age and tend to split more easily.

In some people as they age, the lunula (the white half moon at the base of the fingernail) can even disappear.

Even though fingernails also can become yellowed or grayish over time, discoloration could indicate a fungal infection or even a health condition such as diabetes.

At your next checkup, be sure to show your doctor your fingernails so that he/she can examine them. You may need blood tests to check for diabetes or a scraping of the nail to determine whether you have a fungal infection.

Nothing can reverse age-related changes in the fingernails. But your fingernails will look and feel better if you moisturize frequently with hand cream. Also, since removing and reapply-

ing nail polish dries the nails, try to do this no more than once a week.

Prevent Glaucoma with a Folate Supplement

Study titled "A Prospective Study of Folate, Vitamin B-6, and Vitamin B-12 Intake in Relation to Exfoliation Glaucoma or Suspected Exfoliation Glaucoma," published in *JAMA Ophthalmology*.

G laucoma is an insidious disease—literally happening before your very eyes undetected, having virtually no symptoms until, in a blink, you've got eye surgery on your plate and you may even be going blind. You may think that, nowadays, glaucoma is easily treatable, but one form of glaucoma, pseudoexfoliation glaucoma (called "PEX" or sometimes just exfoliation glaucoma) is much harder to fix than others. Research from Harvard Medical School, though, is showing that the more folate you get each day, the less likely PEX will develop.

ARE YOU AT RISK?

PEX is caused by pressurized buildup of debris that clogs the eye's ability to drain, and it can lead to cataract formation, destruction of the optic nerve and blindness. PEX can happen because it's in your genes or because your eyes have been exposed to too much of the sun's ultraviolet (UV) light. People who live in some northern parts of the world, such as Scandinavia (possibly because of genes) and higher altitudes (where the thin air encourages more UV-radiation exposure) are also more at risk for this eye disease. People with PEX also have high levels of an amino acid called homocysteine in their blood, tears and eye fluid. Because B vitamins can help keep homocysteine levels in check, some researchers thought that getting enough B vitamins was the key, but the team from Harvard Medical School discovered that it's not quite that simple—it appears that you must get a certain B vitamin in a certain specific way.

UNCOVERING THE PRECISE NUTRITIONAL LINK

To get a clearer picture, the Harvard researchers analyzed information from about 120,000 people from two very large, long-term health study databases, the Nurses' Health Study and the Health Professionals Follow-up Study, with a specific focus on people who were 40 years old or older, were free of glaucoma at the start of the study, had had eye exams within a certain two-year period and had provided information about their dietary habits. They discovered that people who ultimately got PEX were deficient in one particular B vitamin, folate. They also found that, although the amount of folate gotten only from food had little impact on prevention of PEX, getting enough from a supplement made a big difference.

FOLATE IS AN EYE-SAVER

People with the highest intake of folate—at least 335 micrograms (mcg) per day for women and 434 mcg for men—from vitamin supplements had an 83% reduced risk of PEX compared with people who did not take such supplements. The good news is that any high-quality B complex vitamin supplement, which will generally contain 400 mcg of folate, together with a diet rich in green leafy vegetables, fortified whole grains, beans and peas and especially beef liver (if you have a taste for it) will supply you with enough folate to protect you from PEX. You can even find folate supplements that contain 800 mcg or more, but be aware that the daily tolerable upper limit of supplemental folate for adults, according to the Institute of Medicine, is 1,000 mcg. Also, be aware that folate supplements can interfere with the anticancer effectiveness of the drug *methotrexate*. Speak with your doctor if you take that drug. Folate supplements also aren't well absorbed in people taking antiepileptic drugs or *sulfasalazine* (Azulfidine, used to treat ulcerative colitis), so guidance about folate supplement dosage, in these instances, also should be discussed with a doctor.

We're increasingly being told by medical experts to ditch vitamin supplements and get our nutrients from whole foods. Although this is generally sound advice over pill-popping, even if those pills are vitamins, it's important to pay heed to studies like this one that show that a supplement is exactly what's needed to stave off a serious condition. And sight-robbing glaucoma is serious enough in anyone's book!

Save Your Sight from Macular Degeneration While Avoiding an Eye-Vitamin "Rip-Off"

Paul B. Greenberg, MD, clinical professor of surgery (ophthalmology), Warren Alpert Medical School, Brown University, Providence. His study was published in *Ophthalmology*.

You already know that serious vision problems—problems that can result in blindness—can creep up with aging. Age-related macular degeneration (AMD) is one of the most common. It strikes millions of Americans and involves the gradual deterioration of the part of the eye that detects light, fine detail and color. There are certain "eye vitamins" that could help your vision. In fact, major research has spelled out the exact mix of vitamins and other nutrients that do the trick. The problem is…you may be throwing away good money on bad "medicine" when you're choosing a vision supplement in your pharmacy or health-food store—unless you know which vitamin supplement really will help your vision.

THE MAGIC FORMULA

We know what works to reduce progression to advanced AMD in people who already have it. It's been clearly spelled out in two clinical studies that are, together, called the Age-Related Eye Disease Studies (AREDS). The second study of the two is an update (with important revisions) of the first.

The first AREDS formula was 500 mg of vitamin C, 400 IU of vitamin E, 15 mg of beta-carotene, 80 mg of zinc and 2 mg of copper per day. The second, updated study nixed beta-carotene, though, because it's been associated with a higher risk of lung cancer in smokers. It

Don't Catch Pneumonia from Your Dentures

According to a recent study, adults who wore dentures during sleep were twice as likely to develop pneumonia as those who removed their dentures before bedtime.

Why: Bacteria grow more rapidly on dentures that are worn constantly and can spread to the lungs. The denture-wearers were also more likely to have dental plaque, gum inflammation and oral fungus.

What to do: Remove dentures at night and clean them thoroughly.

Toshimitsu Iinuma, DDS, PhD, assistant professor of complete denture prosthodontics, Nihon University School of Dentistry, Tokyo, Japan.

was replaced with two antioxidants—lutein (10 mg) and zeaxanthin (2 mg).

So that does it. You would think that any reputable eye vitamin for AMD would have this mix of nutrients in it. But that is not so, according to a team of researchers from Yale, Penn State and Brown University. The team examined 11 eye vitamins from the five top-selling ocular nutritional supplement brands. Their goal—to compare how well the ingredients matched the winning formula. The results confirm that you should keep up with health news and scrutinize products you buy.

THE RIGHT STUFF

Although it turned out that all of the eye vitamins evaluated did contain the ingredients known to help protect against AMD progression, only four out of the 11 products—various formulations of PreserVision Eye Vitamins manufactured by Bausch & Lomb and Alcon's ICaps Eye Vitamin AREDS Formula—provided the ingredients in all the proper doses. The remaining seven products left something to be desired. For example, Alcon's ICaps Eye Vitamin Lutein & Omega-3 Formula had only 3% of the recommended dose of vitamin E and 9% of the recommended doses of vitamin C and zinc, while several other brands skimped on the lutein and zeaxanthin and, overall, provided

lower doses of most of the ingredients in the proven formula.

What's more, the study researchers felt that some of the information found on manufacturers' websites might be misleading or provide false hope about eye health and AMD. They found that, although many of the products did not contain the proper proportions of the formula established by the Age-Related Eye Disease Studies, the websites claimed that their products were based on the formula. Also, none of the websites specifically stated that, while their products may protect against progression of AMD, they have not been proven to prevent AMD. (They might have a preventive effect, but as a consumer, you have a right to know that this effect has not been proven.)

SMART SELECTION

Now that you know about the scientifically studied vitamin mix for reducing AMD symptoms, make sure to read eye vitamin labels to ensure that yours has the right stuff in the right proportion. Also, don't rely on the manufacturer's website and promotional materials for the real skinny on what the supplement can and can't do. For more information on AMD and the studies that discovered what nutrients are needed to protect your vision, visit the website of the National Eye Institute at *nei.nih.gov.*

Longer-Lasting Relief for Dry Eyes

Study titled "Clinical and Biochemical Tear Lipid Parameters in Contact Lens Wearers," from the School of Optometry and Vision Science at the University of New South Wales in Australia, published in *Optometry and Vision Science.*

Many of us assume that replenishing tears is all that's needed to moisten eyes and that tears are simply salt water—saline. But that isn't so. Your eyes need more than a little watering to keep them moist—but it's not hard to get the eye relief you long for.

PROTECT YOUR TEARS

If dry eyes are a problem for you, your best move may be to stop using the ineffective artificial-tear products you've been toting around. Eyes actually have a multipoint moisture defense system called the tear film. The outermost part of this film is a layer of lipids—an oily, fatty coating that lies over tears that coat the eye and keeps them from evaporating. And that, in part, is why saline-based eye moisteners and especially plain water often don't bring lasting relief. Eye moisture is about the integrity of that lipid layer (a complex mix of lipids and other compounds)—not how much you try to replace tears.

A team of ophthalmologists from the University of South Wales School of Optometry and Vision Science in Sydney, Australia, illustrated this in a study that investigated the relationship between contact lens discomfort and damage to the lipid layer of the eye. They theorized that tears dry too quickly in people whose lipid layer has worn down and become imbalanced—a common problem in contact lens wearers. They compared two groups of contact wearers—those who reported that their lenses were comfortable and those who reported they weren't.

All of the study participants were asked to wear soft hydrogel lenses for six hours. Then, the surface dryness of their eyes was measured and tear samples collected. Surface dryness was defined as how many seconds it took for a dry spot to appear on the eye before blinking.

The result: The eyes of the group who said that their contact lenses were uncomfortable went dry in half the time of the eyes of the group who reported no discomfort. Time for the first dry spot to appear after blinking was 4.5 seconds for the contact lens discomfort group versus 10 seconds for the no-discomfort group—a big difference when multiplied by a full day of comfort or discomfort.

Next, the team took those participants with dry-eye problems and treated the eyes of half with a liposomal spray, made of lipids found naturally in tear film, and the other half with a saline spray. The same experiment was repeated two days later, but the group that first received the liposomal spray received the saline spray

this time and vice versa. As predicted, when eyes were treated with the liposomal spray, they stayed moist and comfortable longer. Even two hours after treatment, the liposomal spray kept eyes moist between blinks an average of 13% longer than the saline spray.

PROTECT YOUR EYES

Eyes have to be moist to retain comfort, maintain clear vision and be protected from infection. One of the simplest defenses against dry

---

Vision Problems Can Be Deadly...

•**Better eyeglass safety.** Adults over age 65 whose prescription changed substantially fell more often than those who had small changes in their eyeglasses, according to a recent study. Other research found an increased risk for falls in older people who got new prescriptions for progressive lenses or bifocals.

Why: A big change in lenses can make objects appear closer or farther than they are.

If you are vulnerable to falls: Give yourself extra time to adapt to new lenses by asking your optometrist to make small and gradual changes to your prescription

David Elliott, PhD, professor of clinical vision science, University of Bradford, West Yorkshire, UK.

•**Protect your eyes.** In a study of 2,520 adults (ages 65 to 84), vision decline—as measured by the mistaken identification of one additional letter per year on a visual acuity chart—was associated with a 16% increased risk for death from any cause over eight years.

Possible reason: Visual acuity is closely associated with a person's ability to perform daily activities such as shopping and doing housework—and risk for death increases with the inability to perform daily tasks.

What to do: As you age, be sure to get an eye exam every year or two and corrective lenses if needed.

Sharon Christ, PhD, assistant professor of human development & family studies, Purdue University, West Lafayette, Indiana.

---

eyes is blinking. Every time you blink, you wash your eyes with a fresh layer of tears and lipids and clear away debris. So be sure to consciously blink and rest your eyes from time to time by looking away from the computer screen or whatever you've been focusing on—even if you have to set a timer to do so. Also keep your eyes moist with lipids from the inside out by eating foods containing healthful fats, such as fish, or consider a fish oil supplement. And, as suggested by the study findings, instead of plain saline, it may help to opt for eye-moistening products labeled "liposomal." The liposomal spray used in the Australian study was Tears Again, manufactured by BioRevive. That particular product is not available in the US, but you can find similar liposomal eye sprays here. (The researchers had no relationship with BioRevive and did not receive financial support from it for the study.)

Age-Related Macular Degeneration: Let These Strategies Keep You Active and Happy

Barry W. Rovner, MD, professor of psychiatry and neurology, Thomas Jefferson University, Philadelphia. His study was published in *Ophthalmology*.

Doctors have known that AMD and depression are linked, but it is only now that they are figuring out what to do about it. A team from Thomas Jefferson University in Philadelphia is the first to look into it through a study of a program that purred elderly folks with AMD to be proactive about problem-solving and staying active. The program, called Behavior Activation, was shown to be nearly 50% better than basic mental health counseling in the study, which compared the two techniques.

A KILL-JOY DISEASE

In AMD, the macula, a small spot toward the back of the eyeball near the optic nerve that allows us to see what is directly in front of us in detail, starts to deteriorate. This causes blurring smack-dab in the middle of a person's visual field. It can worsen, leading to vision that is peppered with blank spots as the disease progresses.

SOLUTION SEEKING

To see whether their Behavior Activation program could prevent full-blown depression in folks with AMD, researchers at Thomas Jefferson University recruited 188 people who were mostly in their mid-80s, had AMD in both eyes and also were slightly depressed. All of the people were evaluated by optometrists and received $350 to purchase basic low-vision aids. Low-vision aids generally are large magnifying lenses or magnifying glasses but can also be electronic magnifiers that use video technology to enlarge type and also extra-large–type gadgets, such as clocks, watches, phones and calculators.

Half of the study participants did not receive the Behavior Activation intervention. They were, however, visited six times over eight weeks by a social worker for one-hour counseling sessions. The other group received six one-hour sessions of Behavioral Activation with a specially trained occupational therapist over the course of eight weeks.

Behavioral Activation included low-vision rehabilitation, which teaches people with AMD

Less Costly Drug to Prevent Blindness Available

Avastin, a medicine approved only for use in cancer treatment, is as effective as Lucentis in treating the wet form of age-related macular degeneration (wet AMD), the leading cause of blindness in the elderly. Avastin costs about $50 per injection...Lucentis, about $2,000. The same company makes both—but Avastin is not approved for use in the eye, and the manufacturer says it may have a greater danger of severe side effects.

But: Doctors have been prescribing Avastin as an off-label treatment for AMD.

The Washington Post

how to best use their low-vision aids. It also teaches eye exercise tricks and techniques to compensate for vision problems and provides suggestions about how to use voice-activated technology and make living spaces as organized and accommodating as possible. And instead of psychotherapeutically talking about having AMD, people in the Behavior Activation group learned from their occupational therapists how to increase self-sufficiency by discussing how moods affect actions instead of just talking about their moods, which is what people in the basic mental health counseling sessions did. They also received advice about how to be as self-sufficient as possible, keep up with hobbies and interests and keep socially active.

At the end of the study, depression worsened to full-blown depression in 23% of people in the talk-therapy group (basically no change from the percent otherwise seen among people with AMD) compared with 13% of the people in the Behavior Activation group. This implies that practical rehabilitation focused on how to compensate for physical disabilities and stay active instead of pity-partying can make a significant difference for older people dealing with vision loss.

But, AMD is not just a disease of elderly people. It can begin to strike in middle age, and Behavioral Activation could very well help younger patients with AMD as well as elderly patients. There is no surefire cure for AMD, although drug treatment, laser surgery and vitamin supplementation can relieve or slow it down in some people, according to the Foundation of the American Academy of Ophthalmology. Its Eye Care America website (*eyecareamerica.org*) is an excellent resource to learn more about preventing and living with AMD and other eye diseases. It even includes an invitation to get free eye care for people age 65 and older that qualify.

How can you stave off depression if AMD is setting in? Take advantage of the resources provided by the American Academy of Ophthalmology, and get a referral from your ophthalmologist to an occupational therapist or certified vision rehabilitation specialist and a mental health professional (psychologist or psychiatric social worker) skilled in behav-ioral therapy. The occupational therapist or rehab specialist can provide low-vision rehabilitation and the mental health professional will help you stay emotionally healthy and resilient, keep up with hobbies and stay socially active.

Seniors Get Too Many Tests Before Cataract Surgery

Catherine Chen, MD, MPH, resident physician, anesthesia and perioperative care, University of California, San Francisco
New England Journal of Medicine

Older Americans get a lot of unnecessary tests before they undergo cataract surgery, a new study suggests.

Experts said the findings highlight an area of wasteful health care spending. Plus, they said, there is a risk for harm if the tests pick up a mild abnormality that prompts further tests, then turns out to be nothing.

Cataracts are protein clumps that cloud the eye's lens. They are exceedingly common among older adults, and cataract surgery is considered one of the most routine and safe procedures performed in the United States.

"It's the prototypical low-risk surgery," said Catherine Chen, MD, the lead researcher on the new study and a resident physician in perioperative care at the University of California, San Francisco. It involves replacing the eye's cloudy lens with an artificial one.

"It takes 10 to 15 minutes for one eye," Chen said, "and it uses local anesthesia."

Because of that simplicity, guidelines from the American Academy of Ophthalmology and other groups say there is no need to routinely do tests ahead of cataract surgery.

Yet, Dr. Chen's study—reported in the *New England Journal of Medicine*—found that more than half of Medicare patients who had cataract surgery in 2011 underwent at least one test beforehand.

That included blood work, urine tests to measure kidney function, and tests of heart and lung function—such as exercise stress tests and electrocardiograms.

Dr. Chen stressed, however, that "this doesn't mean doctors are doing it for the money."

For years, it was simply standard practice to do preoperative testing, she said. Cataract patients are usually elderly and often have chronic health conditions, so it was considered prudent to "be thorough," Dr. Chen explained.

And years ago, cataract surgery took longer and was more extensive than it is today, she added.

But Americans undergo close to 2 million cataract surgeries each year. "So the costs add up," Dr. Chen said. "And those are health care resources that might be better used elsewhere."

Guidelines advising against routine testing came out in 2002. Dr. Chen said research shows that it takes an average of 17 years for new guidelines to become pervasive in everyday medical practice.

"So we weren't actually surprised by our findings," she said.

People can often deal with cataracts by getting a new eyeglass prescription or using brighter lighting. But once their vision problems get in the way of daily life, surgery is the only effective treatment, the U.S. National Eye Institute suggests.

Roughly one-third of ophthalmologists ordered tests for nearly all of their patients, the study found.

It's not that older patients should never undergo tests ahead of cataract surgery. If you have a newly diagnosed medical condition, for example, your doctor might order a test to make sure you are up for the procedure, Dr. Chen noted.

"If your doctor does recommend a test," Dr. Chen said, "you should feel free to ask why. What is the doctor looking for? Is this necessary?"

info For more about cataracts, visit the U.S. National Eye Institute at *https://nei.nih.gov/*

Weight Training Key to Battling Belly Fat As You Age

Harvard School of Public Health, news release.

If you want to battle belly fat as you age, recent research suggests you need to add weight training to your exercise regimen.

Researchers from the Harvard School of Public Health found that combining aerobic activities with weight, or resistance, training is key to preserving muscle and avoiding weight gain, particularly age-related belly fat.

"Because aging is associated with sarcopenia, the loss of skeletal muscle mass, relying on body weight alone is insufficient for the study of healthy aging," study author Rania Mekary, PhD, a researcher at Harvard's department of nutrition, said in a university news release.

The long-term study was conducted between 1996 and 2008. It included more than 10,000 healthy men aged 40 or older whose body mass indexes (BMI) varied widely. BMI measures body fat by looking at weight and height.

The researchers analyzed the men's physical activity, weight and waist circumference to determine which activities had the most significant effect on the men's waistlines, or the amount of belly fat they had.

The men who did 20 minutes of weight training daily had a smaller increase in belly fat than the men who spent the same amount of time engaging in moderate to vigorous aerobic activities, such as stair climbing and yard work, the study, published online in the journal *Obesity*, found.

"This study underscores the importance of weight training in reducing abdominal obesity, especially among the elderly," said study senior author Frank Hu, MD, MPH, PhD, a professor of nutrition and epidemiology, said in the Harvard news release.

info The U.S. Centers for Disease Control and Prevention provides more information on strength training for older adults at *http://www.cdc.gov/physicalactivity/growingstronger.*

Medical Newsmakers

Why Vegetarians Have It All Wrong

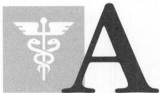

Adiet rich in fruits and vegetables and whole grains, but with little or no meat, has long been touted as the best way to lower your risk for heart disease, prevent weight gain and reduce risk for certain cancers.

But as a medical doctor with progressive multiple sclerosis (MS), I believe that meat (grass-fed beef...organic chicken, pork and lamb...and wild game and fish) has played a critical role in my recovery—and that meat can help protect against other autoimmune diseases, Parkinson's disease, Alzheimer's disease and early cognitive impairment.

HOW MEAT BENEFITS THE BRAIN

•**Meat provides vitamin B-12.** A diet without meat raises your risk for vitamin B-12 deficiency. If your body doesn't get enough B-12,

you can develop neurological symptoms such as problems with balance and coordination, difficulties with decision-making and cognitive decline. Vitamin B-12 is found naturally only in animal foods such as clams, liver, salmon and beef. A synthetic form is often added to cereals and nutritional yeast, but I recommend avoiding gluten because many people are sensitive to it. Alternatively, you could take a B-12 supplement, but I prefer natural food sources, which supply additional vitamins and nutrients.

•**Meat is the best source of complete proteins.** Protein is essential to make, repair and maintain the structure of all the cells in our bodies, including cells in the brain. The amino acids found in protein help the brain produce crucial neurotransmitters that regulate mood and maintain and repair brain cells. If you don't have enough protein to do this, brain function deteriorates.

Terry Wahls, MD, an internist and a clinical professor of medicine at the University of Iowa Carver College of Medicine in Iowa City. She is author of *The Wahls Protocol: A Radical New Way to Treat All Chronic Autoimmune Conditions Using Paleo Principles.*

Meat contains all of the essential amino acids your body needs to manufacture protein. To get a complete protein from a nonmeat source, you would have to combine a grain and a legume, for example.

•**Certain meats provide omega-3 fatty acids.** Cell membranes throughout the body, including in the brain, rely on essential fatty acids to stay healthy. The brain is especially dependent on the omega-3 fatty acids *docosa-hexaenoic acid* (DHA) and *eicosapentaenoic acid* (EPA) that are found in fish such as sardines, herring and anchovies (which have less risk for heavy metal and plastic contamination) as well as organic chicken and grass-fed beef.

While you can get *alpha linolenic acid* (ALA), another omega-3, from plant sources, your body can convert only small amounts of ALA into DHA and EPA. DHA and EPA supplements are available, but numerous studies have shown that foods high in omega-3s are more beneficial to brain health than supplements.

THE BEST MEAT FOR YOUR BRAIN

Most grass-fed meats, game and fish are beneficial for brain health, but organ meats (particularly heart, liver and tongue) provide the most nutrition. Organ meats are chock-full of vitamins A and B and essential nutrients such as creatine, carnitine and coenzyme Q10 (CoQ10). There are a variety of ways to add organ meats to your meals and make them more palatable. *To get the most nutrition from meat…*

•**Start with heart.** Beef and bison heart taste a lot like steak, especially if you serve them up with mushrooms. Just don't overcook organ meat, or it will be dry and tough. Cooking it to medium rare also helps the meat retain vitamins.

•**Try sausage or liver pâté.** Your local butcher can make a sausage out of ground liver and some other ground meat, such as pork or chicken. Start with a ratio of one part liver to six parts ground meat, and work up to a ratio of one to three. If you don't like the taste of liver, ask the butcher to add spices to conceal it.

•**Make a bone broth.** Put the carcass of a chicken or beef or pork knuckle bones into a pot. Add one tablespoon of vinegar per one quart of water, and toss in one whole onion and carrot and a few cloves of garlic. Let the broth simmer for at least six hours, then strain out the bone, vegetables and foam. Use the broth as a stock for soup or drink it.

•**Consider an organ meat supplement.** If you just can't stomach the idea of eating organ meat, consider taking a supplement.

Good choice: Organ Delight from Dr. Ron's Ultra-Pure (*DrRons.com*).

THE WAHLS PROTOCOL

Keep in mind that I'm not advocating a meat-only diet. In fact, the Wahls Protocol diet (the eating plan I developed to combat my own MS) starts by recommending six to nine cups a day (depending on your size and gender) of vegetables, fruits and berries (get twice as many veggies as fruits and berries).

In particular, I prefer green, leafy vegetables…sulfur-rich vegetables in the cabbage and onion families…deeply colored vegetables such as yams, beets, peppers and tomatoes…and brightly colored berries such as raspberries, strawberries and cranberries.

For meat, I recommend six to 12 ounces a day (depending on your size and gender) for disease treatment and prevention.

My regimen also incorporates a CoQ10 supplement, a spirulina or chlorella algae supplement and green tea—which is high in quercetin, an antioxidant with anti-inflammatory properties.

New Thinking on MS

Rob Motl, PhD, associate professor in the department of kinesiology and community health, College of Applied Health Sciences at the University of Illinois at Urbana-Champaign.

Until recently, if you were diagnosed with multiple sclerosis (MS), treatment options were extremely limited. Doctors prescribed powerful drugs to reduce the number of new harmful brain lesions that characterize MS…to help control relapses…and to perhaps even slow progression of the disease.

Unfortunately, these medications, available only by injection, were often inconvenient to use and not always effective. Newer medications (such as Gilenya, Aubagio and Tecfidera) are now available in pill form. But is that enough?

New thinking: Even though medication is still believed to be important for most people with MS and should begin soon after diagnosis (when it is likely to be most effective), researchers are now identifying nondrug therapies that can also help.

BEYOND THE RX

With MS, the immune system mistakenly attacks the myelin sheaths that insulate the nerves, resulting in weakness, tingling, spasticity (marked by stiff or rigid muscles), balance problems and dizziness.

The nondrug therapies below have been shown to help people with MS have the best possible outcomes. Try as many as possible.

•**Walking.** Inactivity is dangerous for a person with MS—it can lead to muscle weakness, shallow breathing and other problems that can be exacerbated by the illness.

In studies of people with MS, walking (a great exercise because it can be adapted to various fitness levels) has been shown to reduce symptoms of fatigue, depression and pain…and improve sleep quality. Walking also may improve cognitive functioning, which can decline with MS, and improve balance, reducing one's risk of falling.

My advice: Walk for at least 15 to 30 minutes three to five times per week. Use a cane or walker if MS symptoms include leg weakness or numbness, spasticity and/or balance problems.

•**Strength training.** Research shows that muscle-strengthening exercises increase bone health and improve bladder and bowel control—all of which can be compromised with MS.

My advice: Twice a week, use weights that target the major muscle groups (such as quads, hamstrings, calves, biceps, triceps, shoulders and core). Do 15 of these exercises for each muscle group per session, and slowly add more repetitions and/or heavier weights.

Important: Speak with your physician before starting an exercise regimen. If you have problems with balance, consider working out with a physical therapist, friend or personal trainer for extra support.

•**Cooling strategies.** Increased activity and warmer temperatures can raise the core body temperature in people with MS. Even a slight increase may temporarily worsen their symptoms. With regular exercise, however, the body becomes more efficient in regulating its temperature, and heat sensitivity decreases.

My advice: While your body is becoming conditioned to respond efficiently to heat during your exercise program, take steps to prevent overheating. For example, exercise in an air-conditioned environment…use fans…wear loose-fitting clothing…and stay well hydrated. Cooling products such as vests, headbands, shirts and hats can help keep your core temperature stable.

Good cooling products include: Vests from GlacierTek (*GlacierTek.com*) or Coolture (*Coolture.net*), which range in price from $100 to $400. The cost may be covered by insurance. Cooling vests and neck, ankle and wrist wraps are also available from the Multiple Sclerosis Association of America (*MyMSAA.org*)—free to those who meet income limits.

•**Salsa dancing.** In a pilot study, people with MS who did salsa dancing for 40 minutes twice a week for four weeks improved their balance and gait and increased their activity levels. The front-to-back and side-to-side movements used in salsa dancing are believed to be especially helpful for those with MS.

My advice: If salsa dancing sounds appealing, ask your doctor whether he/she thinks lessons and regular practice sessions would be appropriate for you. Ballroom dancing and the video game Dance Dance Revolution have also been shown to help MS patients.

•**Acupuncture.** Acupuncture has been found to help with MS symptoms such as bladder problems, sleep disorders and tingling.

My advice: If you want to try acupuncture, look for a licensed acupuncturist. To find one near you, consult the National Certification Commission for Acupuncture and Oriental Medicine, *NCCAOM.org*.

•**Massage.** In a recent study, MS patients who received a 45-minute massage twice a week for

241

five weeks improved their physical and social functioning and suffered less depression. By relaxing the muscles and increasing blood flow, massage may also alleviate spasticity, cramping and pain.

My advice: Consider trying Swedish massage, which uses long strokes and a light touch. Avoid using a table warmer or hot packs during the session, since people with MS tend to get overheated.

Caution: Some people with MS take corticosteroids, which may increase their risk for osteoporosis. If you have osteoporosis, massage may not be advisable unless your physician recommends it.

Scientists Watch Imagination at Work in the Brain

Brigham Young University, news release

Researchers say they've tracked specific activity in the human brain linked to imagining.

It hasn't been clear whether imagination and memory were distinct processes, so a team from Brigham Young University in Provo, Utah, decided to explore the issue.

"I was thinking a lot about planning for my own future and imagining myself in the future, and I started wondering how memory and imagination work together," study coauthor Stefania Ashby said in a university news release.

"I wondered if they were separate, or if imagination is just taking past memories and combining them in different ways to form something I've never experienced before," she explained.

The researchers used MRI scans to monitor brain activity in volunteers while they did tasks that required either memory or imagination.

The results showed that there were distinctive brain patterns for the two processes within an area of the brain that's long been tied to memory, the hippocampus.

"We were able to see the distinctions even in those small regions of the hippocampus," said Ashby. "It's really neat that we can see the difference between those two tasks in that small of a brain region."

The study was published recently in the journal *Cognitive Neuroscience*.

Ashby was a student at Brigham Young University when she conducted the study with Brock Kirwan, an assistant professor of psychology and neuroscience. Ashby is now a research associate at the University of California, Davis.

info The Stanford Encyclopedia of Philosophy has more about imagination at *http://plato. stanford.edu/entries/imagination/*.

When to Try "Keyhole" Surgery

David F. Jimenez, MD, FACS, chairman and professor in the department of neurosurgery at The University of Texas Health Science Center at San Antonio. He is editor and coauthor of *Intracranial Endoscopic Neurosurgery*, a textbook published by the American Association of Neurological Surgeons.

No one likes the thought of undergoing brain or spine surgery. Traditionally, a neurosurgeon would create a four- to six-inch incision and peel back the scalp before drilling through the skull to expose the brain...or make a similar-sized incision in your back, where muscles are then moved to expose the spine.

Recent development: Endoscopic, or minimally invasive, surgery, which has long been offered for such common procedures as gallbladder removal and knee surgery, is now widely available at major US medical centers for neurosurgical operations that involve the brain, spine and peripheral nerves.

Whether it's the removal of a brain tumor or the repair of herniated disks, spinal stenosis or carpal tunnel syndrome, neurosurgeons can now use sophisticated instruments to operate through an incision that's smaller than a dime or even through a natural opening such as a nostril.

This approach allows for a faster recovery and less pain and swelling than the traditional "open" procedures. Older patients frequently respond better to surgery that has minimal blood loss and requires less time under general anesthesia.

Why this matters: Even though endoscopic (sometimes known as "keyhole") neurosurgery is now available, not all surgeons have the training and experience to perform it. This means that you may not be offered endoscopic neurosurgery when it would be a better option than a traditional procedure—or a surgeon may attempt the endoscopic operation without adequate training and/or experience. *What you need to know...*

A NEW GENERATION OF NEUROSURGERY

What makes most types of surgery so challenging has less to do with repairing a problem—whether it's replacing a joint or removing an appendix—than simply getting access to the specific body part.

With endoscopic neurosurgery of the brain, the surgeon makes one or two incisions ranging from one-third to three-quarters of an inch and drills into the skull. A tube (endoscope) is passed through the narrow opening. Everything that's needed to complete the procedure, such as a lighted camera and cutting and scraping tools, is guided into place through the endoscope. Surgeons enter through the nostrils or above the eyebrow to operate on pituitary adenomas and tumors in the front of the brain.

The benefits of endoscopic surgery are largely due to the smaller incision, which is obviously less painful than a large one and has less risk for infection. Since there is less blood loss, there is less need for blood transfusion—another benefit.

Because endoscopic procedures can usually be done faster than traditional surgeries, patients also spend less time under general anesthesia, which reduces postoperative complications, such as cognitive dysfunction and nausea, and improves recovery.

In my practice, at least 30% of brain surgeries (including treatment for hydrocephalus—buildup of fluid in the brain that is drained via a shunt...and removal of skull-base tumors) are minimally invasive. Deep areas of the brain cannot be accessed with endoscopic neurosurgery.

Most of our spine surgeries and virtually all carpal tunnel procedures are done this way.

Examples of when endoscopic neurosurgery can be used...

•**Herniated disk.** Computerized image guidance creates a three-dimensional image of the spine so surgeons can achieve a superb view of the operating field with an endoscopic incision that's barely more than a half-inch long. They use microinstruments to remove the damaged part of the disk.

•**Spinal stenosis.** This narrowing inside the spinal canal (usually due to arthritis) often causes leg pain or other symptoms. It's relatively easy to "open up" the spinal space with endoscopic surgery. Patients often make a full recovery within a month—and may be symptom-free almost immediately—while traditional surgery usually requires a recovery period of at least three months.

IS IT FOR EVERYONE?

In general, endoscopic surgery is a good option for most patients, especially those who are too old, ill or frail to have traditional surgeries.

One patient's story: My oldest patient was a 96-year-old woman whose spinal stenosis was so bad she could barely walk. She might not have done well with a lengthy open procedure, but I knew that I could complete the operation in about 90 minutes—half the usual time. Her pain was gone almost instantly—and a month later, she was bowling and dancing with her boyfriend.

The complication rate (infections and/or bleeding) for endoscopic surgery is at least as good as—and sometimes better than—that of traditional procedures. The numbers will only get better as surgeons gain experience and new approaches and technologies are developed.

FIND THE RIGHT SURGEON

Before agreeing to any type of neurosurgery, ask the surgeon whether the procedure will be open or minimally invasive. While some operations, such as certain brain tumors, still require a traditional approach, most do not.

Chances are that you'll recover much more quickly—and experience less postoperative pain—if you go with endoscopy. If your surgeon doesn't do endoscopic surgery, get a second opinion. You can find a surgeon at the American Association of Neurological Surgeons, *aans.org*.

Experience and training are crucial for surgeons who perform endoscopic surgeries. Compared with traditional operations, endoscopic surgeries require the surgeon to overcome such issues as poor depth perception (from the endoscopic camera) and limited range of motion to manipulate surgical instruments. Make sure your surgeon has several years of experience in performing the procedure you'll be getting and has received endoscopic neurosurgical training.

Tingling in Your Hands and Feet May Be a Sign of Celiac Disease

Study titled "Risk of Neuropathy Among 28,232 Patients With Biopsy-Verified Celiac Disease" by researchers in the department of medical epidemiology and biostatistics, Karolinska Institutet, Stockholm, Sweden, published in *JAMA Neurology*.

If you have peripheral neuropathy, a form of nerve damage that affects your extremities, your doctor may test you for diabetes. It's a common cause. But now research suggests something else to look for as well—celiac disease, the autoimmune disease marked by the body's inability to digest gluten, the protein found in wheat, barley and rye.

If the new finding leads more doctors to test their neuropathy patients for celiac disease, that's a good thing, since 80% of the 2.4 million Americans with celiac disease don't even know they have the disease, according to population studies.

Here's what you need to know about the neuropathy/celiac connection.

A NEW SYMPTOM OF
CELIAC DISEASE

Swedish researchers identified 28,000 people who were diagnosed with celiac disease and compared them with 140,000 subjects who didn't have celiac disease. At the beginning of the study, which lasted about 10 years, none of the subjects had been diagnosed with peripheral neuropathy.

Here's what the researchers found…

•**People with celiac disease were five times more likely to be diagnosed with peripheral neuropathy over the course of the study, compared to people without celiac.** The percentages were small—less than a 1% chance of being diagnosed with neuropathy if you have celiac, but it translates into tens of thousands of Americans.

•**In a separate analysis, the researchers followed people who were diagnosed with peripheral neuropathy over the course of the study but weren't originally known to have celiac disease.** It turns out that they were 80% more likely to end up being diagnosed with celiac than people who didn't have neuropathy.

The new finding suggests that peripheral neuropathy may be an early warning signal for celiac disease. Researchers aren't sure exactly how the two diseases are connected, but they note that celiac is an autoimmune disease, and many autoimmune diseases are linked to nerve damage. That damage may be related to the systemic inflammation that the autoimmune response evokes. (This study doesn't say anything at all about nonceliac gluten sensitivity.)

The good news is that diagnosing and treating celiac disease may help forestall peripheral neuropathy. There is evidence that when people with celiac and peripheral neuropathy go on a gluten-free diet—the only effective treatment for celiac—the neuropathy may stop getting worse.

The bigger picture is that anything that helps diagnose people with celiac disease earlier is incredibly important. Undiagnosed, the disease can cause malnourishment, anemia, infertility, osteoporosis, heart problems and more.

WHAT YOU SHOULD DO NOW

The new finding means that anyone with either condition—or suspicious symptoms—should get tested…

•**If you have peripheral neuropathy, ask your doctor to test you for celiac disease.**

That's the recommendation of the authors of the study.

• **If you suspect you have celiac disease**—common symptoms include bloating and gastrointestinal distress after eating bread or pasta—don't just stop eating foods containing gluten, because you can't be properly diagnosed unless you have been eating gluten. Do go to your doctor for a proper diagnosis.

The Surprising Cause of a Chronic Runny Nose and Cough

Andrew L. Rubman, ND, a naturopathic doctor who specializes in gastroenterology. Dr. Rubman is founder and director of the Southbury Clinic for Traditional Medicines in Southbury, Connecticut. *SouthburyClinic.com*

If you have chronic postnasal drip, a frequent cough and/or a sore throat that won't quit, you might quickly blame it on a persistent cold or allergies.

What you may not know: These same symptoms can be caused by a little-known digestive condition known as airway reflux.

ACID IN THE AIRWAYS

Unless you're among the lucky few, you've probably experienced the burning pain of heartburn, also known as gastroesophageal reflux. This discomfort occurs when harsh digestive fluids surge out of the stomach and into the more vulnerable esophagus.

But another kind of reflux, airway reflux, occurs when irritating acid droplets and vapors escape from the stomach and reach further—as far as the throat, the larynx (voice box) or the back of the nasal airway.

Sometimes called "silent reflux" because many people don't experience telltale heartburn symptoms, common signs of airway reflux include postnasal drip, cough, sore throat and hoarseness. Many people with airway reflux suffer for years because their symptoms are mistakenly attributed to hay fever, a cold, sinusitis or other airway-related problems.

GETTING DIAGNOSED

Doctors who are familiar with airway reflux can usually diagnose it from a description of the symptoms (see above)—particularly if the patient gets worse after meals and/or when he/she lies down.

Another tip-off: A slight feeling of heat in the chest, usually after meals. The sensation isn't as painful as heartburn, and it's likely to occur around the upper part of the breastbone. Heartburn, on the other hand, is felt lower in the chest, somewhere between the nipples and the indentation at the bottom of the sternum.

Important: Many doctors aren't familiar with airway reflux. Even gastroenterologists sometimes miss it. If you suspect you might have airway reflux, your best bet is to see an ear, nose and throat specialist (otolaryngologist).

DRUGS DON'T HELP

Widely used for heartburn, acid-suppressing drugs, such as *cimetidine* (Tagamet) and *omeprazole* (Prilosec), rarely work for airway reflux.*

Why: You actually need some stomach acid to prevent airway reflux.

The stomach's pH (a measure of acidity) is normally between about 1.5 and 3.5. That's strong enough to dissolve most metals! Yet you need this highly acidic environment to kill microorganisms and for efficient digestion.

People who do not produce enough stomach acid—this is common in those age 45 and older and in those who internalize stress or have poor diets—digest their food more slowly.

The stomach compensates with increased muscular contractions (peristaltic action), which help accelerate digestion, but these contractions also increase pressure that can force acid vapors and droplets into the airways.

A clue: If you find yourself burping excessively after eating meals, it's probably because of the carbon dioxide that is released by stomach yeasts—organisms that survive only when stomach acid is low.

*Acid-suppressing drugs can help if you also have an ulcer but should be taken for only a few weeks. Used long-term, they can weaken immunity, decrease your ability to digest food and absorb nutrients and may increase risk for osteoporosis-related fractures and depression.

BEST APPROACH: MORE ACID

For airway reflux, I recommend taking a digestive-enzyme supplement that contains betaine hydrochloric acid (HCl) and pepsin. The two work together to digest food more efficiently. Pepsin, an enzyme that breaks down proteins, is activated by hydrochloric acid.

What I prescribe for my patients: A product called DuoZyme, which contains HCl and pepsin. It should be taken as directed on the label and with meals. This supplement generally improves airway reflux symptoms within a week or even sooner. It's available at health-food stores and online.

Most people do not notice any side effects, although some may experience a little stomach upset when they first start taking the supplement. The stomach discomfort usually goes away within a few days.

Important: Check first with your doctor if you have a peptic ulcer, since this product could worsen symptoms.

Also helpful: A fish oil supplement. It will reduce levels of arachidonic acid, an inflammatory substance in the body that can irritate airway mucous membranes and make you more susceptible to acid vapors.

Nordic Naturals makes high-quality fish oil products. I recommend that patients take fish oil with their evening meals. Check with your doctor before taking it because it may increase bleeding risk.

OTHER EFFECTIVE TREATMENTS

In addition to the steps described earlier, the following strategies can help airway reflux...

• **Fletcherize your food.** "Fletcher chewing," which is named after the Victorian-era health-food enthusiast Horace Fletcher, means chewing each bite of food until it's about the consistency of applesauce. That's a lot more than most people chew.

How it helps: Lengthy chewing will saturate the food with saliva, which jump-starts digestion. That's because food that reaches the stomach in a partially digested form requires less peristaltic action, the vigorous stomach churning that can trigger airway reflux and heartburn.

• **Know your trigger foods.** Most people discover that their symptoms increase when they eat certain foods.

Common offenders include: Tomatoes, onions, chocolate, coffee, peppermint candy and alcohol. Some of these foods weaken the lower esophageal sphincter, the muscle that keeps stomach acids where they belong. Other foods are simply irritating for some people for unknown reasons.

• **Sip—don't gulp—during meals.** If you drink a lot of water during meals, you are adding volume to the *chyme*, the slurry of foods and digestive juices in the stomach. The extra volume can cause a high-velocity spray of acid vapors and droplets.

• **Eat dinner earlier in the evening.** It takes a few hours for the stomach to empty after meals. When you lie down soon after eating, stomach acid is more likely to leak out. Let gravity work in your favor by staying upright for a while after eating.

My advice: Don't eat for at least three hours before bedtime. This is particularly important if you favor desserts or other rich nighttime snacks. High-fat foods take longer to digest.

• **Relax for a few hours after eating.** A leisurely stroll after eating is good for digestion, but a vigorous jog is not. Anything that increases intra-abdominal pressure—vigorous exercise or lots of bending—can increase reflux.

FAST REFLUX RELIEF

An over-the-counter product such as Tums will quickly neutralize that acid-in-the-throat sensation, along with any other reflux symptoms.

But here's an all-natural way to get on-the-spot relief for heartburn and airway reflux...

What to do: Mix one-quarter teaspoon of baking soda and a pinch of Epsom salts in four ounces of spring water, which is free of the contaminants that can sometimes be found in tap water.

When your symptoms flare, sip slowly. You'll typically get relief within a few minutes.

Note: This remedy can be taken up to one-half hour before eating and no sooner than one hour after eating—otherwise, it can dilute the stomach acid needed for digestion.

Surprising Conditions That Can Steal Your Sight

Robert Abel, Jr., MD, an ophthalmologist in private practice in Wilmington, Delaware. He has performed more than 17,000 eye surgeries and helped found three eye banks, which store eye tissue for research and corneal transplantation. Dr. Abel is also author of *The Eye Care Revolution* and cofounder of the American Academy of Ophthalmology's Committee for International Ophthalmology.

You probably know that people with diabetes are at greater risk for eye disease. What you may not realize is that a number of other common physical ailments are hidden risk factors for eye problems, too—and some of them are quite serious.

If you have one of these common medical conditions, you're at increased risk for the following serious vision problems...

HIGH BLOOD PRESSURE

People who have high blood pressure and/or cardiovascular disease are at increased risk for ischemic optic neuropathy (ION).

Sometimes called an "eye stroke," ION is a sudden, painless loss of vision resulting from decreased blood flow to the optic nerve. Untreated high blood pressure can cause blood vessels in the eye to narrow, similar to what happens in the heart. Unlike an ischemic stroke, which affects the brain and typically both eyes when vision loss occurs, the type of ION associated with high blood pressure usually affects only one eye and tends to happen at night when blood pressure naturally drops.

If you awaken to a sudden loss of vision in one eye and are experiencing ION, it may help to breathe into a brown paper bag for about 10 minutes to build up the levels of carbon dioxide in your blood and increase the size of your blood vessels. This technique helps unblock blood flow to the eye. Also, taking an 81-mg aspirin tablet may help protect the other eye.

However, any vision loss could signal a different serious condition, including ischemic stroke. For that reason, the safest approach for anyone experiencing vision loss is to get to an emergency room to be evaluated. Immediate treatment for ischemic stroke is crucial. An eye

New Use for Good Vibrations

A small capsule that vibrates after it's swallowed is being developed as an alternative to laxatives. The experimental capsule stimulates intestinal contractions and doubles the number of bowel movements—without side effects.

The Tel Aviv Sourasky Medical Center.

stroke must also be promptly treated to prevent permanent vision loss from occurring.

Caution: Taking blood pressure medication at night can sometimes increase risk for ION by lowering blood pressure even more than naturally occurs during sleep, further depriving the optic nerve of blood. If you're on blood pressure medication, ask your doctor whether you would benefit from taking it in the morning to avoid this vision-threatening dip. Some blood pressure drugs need to be taken at night, so do not make any changes without talking to your doctor.

ARTHRITIS

If you have arthritis, you're at increased risk for dry eyes. What's the link? Dry eyes and arthritis (osteoarthritis and rheumatoid arthritis) are inflammatory conditions in which antibodies attack tissue linings throughout the body, including in the eyes.

If you have chronic dry eyes: Try an omega-3 fatty acid supplement—1,000 mg of *docosahexaenoic acid* (DHA) and 200 mg of *eicosapentaenoic acid* (EPA) daily.

Good product: Carlson's Super DHA Norwegian Fish Oil Concentrate.

Both DHA and EPA will enhance the quality and quantity of your tears while also improving arthritis symptoms.

Warning: If you take a blood thinner, aspirin or other nonsteroidal anti-inflammatory drug (NSAID), consult your doctor before trying an omega-3 supplement—like these drugs, it can have blood-thinning effects.

If your dry-eye symptoms don't improve within two weeks of taking this supplement, see your eye doctor. An artificial tears product may be prescribed.

Caution: Many brands have ammonia-based preservatives that can worsen dryness. Look for a preservative-free product, such as Systane or GenTeal.

SLEEP APNEA

People with sleep apnea, which interrupts breathing during sleep, are at increased risk for glaucoma.

Here's why: The liver, which metabolizes nutrients and transfers them to the eyes, is most active at night. Because sleep apnea compromises sleep quality and lowers oxygen levels to the retina, it is a little-known but major cause of glaucoma. Sleep apnea sufferers are 1.7 times more likely to develop glaucoma within five years of diagnosis of their sleep disorder than those without sleep apnea.

If you have been diagnosed with sleep apnea: Get treatment. The gold standard is a continuous positive airway pressure (CPAP) machine that helps people with sleep apnea breathe more easily at night. However, if you are waking up with red, irritated eyes, check the fit of your CPAP mask—it may be leaking air and drying out your eyes.

Important: People with sleep apnea should also be sure to get eye exams once a year.

COLD SORES

If you develop cold sores from time to time, you're at increased risk for corneal infection. By age 50, about 90% of American adults are carriers of Herpes Simplex Virus-1 (HSV-1), which can cause cold sores on the lips and inside the mouth. (A different herpes virus, HSV-2, causes most genital herpes.)

More than half of those who are carriers of HSV-1 may develop occasional cold sores that typically last for a week or so. For a small percentage of people who carry HSV-1, an infection may show up in the eye (ocular herpes), beginning with severe irritation and redness, tearing and light sensitivity. The infection can progress to a painful corneal ulcer. When the ulcer heals, scar tissue can form, clouding vision. In severe cases, the scarring can lead to blindness.

If you get cold sores: An HSV-1 outbreak is often triggered by the amino acid arginine, so limit high-arginine foods such as nuts (no more than a handful daily) and chocolate (up to two pieces a day). Also, use UV-protective sunglasses (sunlight is a trigger, too). Taking 500 mg daily of L-lysine, an essential amino acid, can help limit herpes outbreaks as well. It can be used indefinitely for this purpose, but check first with your doctor if you take medication or have a chronic health condition.

Important: Because ocular herpes is a serious complication of HSV-1, anyone diagnosed with this viral infection should keep a prescription for antiviral eyedrops, such as *ganciclovir* (Zirgan) or *trifluridine* (Viroptic), on hand. Begin using the drops as soon as eye symptoms occur, and see an ophthalmologist promptly.

Scientists Set Their Sights on First Whole-Eye Transplant

Jeffrey Goldberg, MD, PhD, professor, director of research, Shiley Eye Center, University of California, San Diego.

Vijay Gorantla, MD, PhD, associate professor of surgery, department of plastic surgery, University of Pittsburgh, and administrative medical director, Pittsburgh Reconstructive Transplant Program at University of Pittsburgh Medical Center.

I n the world of 21st-century medicine, organ transplantation is nothing new.

One major organ still eludes the transplant surgeon, however—the entire human eye. But if one team of U.S. scientists has its way, that dream may become reality, too.

"Until recently, eye transplants have been considered science fiction," said Vijay Gorantla, MD,

---

Help for "Incurable" Hair Loss

For the first time, a patient with alopecia universalis regained a full head of hair, including eyebrows and eyelashes. The disease, thought to be incurable, responded quickly to *tofacitinib* (Xeljanz), an arthritis drug.

Journal of Investigative Dermatology

PhD, an associate professor of surgery in the department of plastic surgery at the University of Pittsburgh. "People said it was crazy, bonkers."

However, "with what we now know about transplantation and, more importantly, nerve regeneration, we are finally at the point where we can have real confidence that this is something that actually can be pursued and eventually achieved," he said.

WHO BENEFITS FROM EYE TRANSPLANTS

Whole-eye transplants would be of enormous benefit for many of the 180 million blind or severely visually disabled people around the world, including nearly 3.5 million Americans, experts say.

"Macular degeneration and glaucoma are the root cause of much of the world's visual impairment," explained Jeffrey Goldberg, MD, PhD, director of research at the Shiley Eye Center at University of California, San Diego.

There are therapies that often help restore sight in these cases, or in people who've lost sight through injury. "But for some people the eye is too damaged or too far gone," Dr. Goldberg said. "For patients with a devastating eye injury where there's no remaining connective optic nerve—or perhaps not even an eyeball in their eye socket—restorative approaches are simply not enough."

In these cases, transplantation of a healthy donor eye would be a solution. "It's a scientific long shot," Dr. Goldberg said. "But it's a very attractive long shot."

RESEARCH BEGINS

So, Drs. Gorantla and Goldberg—and their two universities—have teamed up to push whole-eye transplantation from theory into practice. The effort is funded by the U.S. Department of Defense.

One of the biggest challenges is how to regenerate and regrow delicate optical nerves.

"The chief problem," Dr. Goldberg explained, "is that when you switch out an eyeball you have to completely cut all connections between the optic nerve and the eye. So then you need to reconnect the donor eye's nerve fibers back to the recipient's brain in order to achieve vision restoration. But we know that once you make

Your Own Blood Is Better

A recent study of 32 heart patients has found that recycling a patient's own blood during surgery provides better outcomes than using blood from a blood bank.

Why: Fresh blood from the patient more efficiently delivers oxygen throughout the body than stored blood—even one's own. Using the patient's own blood also reduces risk for harmful transfusion-related reactions. This process is mainly used in orthopedic, heart and vascular operations but can be used in other procedures as well.

Steven Frank, MD, associate professor of anesthesiology, The Johns Hopkins School of Medicine, Baltimore.

that cut, the nerve fibers just do not regrow on their own. That doesn't happen automatically."

"That's what distinguishes an eye transplant from most other types of transplants," Dr. Gorantla added. In other organ transplants, the chief hurdle is simply reconnecting a proper blood supply. "For example, if you get the plumbing connected and the blood going, then a transplanted heart will beat in the recipient patient immediately," Dr. Gorantla said.

"But an eye transplant actually has more parallels with a hand or face transplant," he said. The eye may appear healthy because of a renewed blood supply, but without reconnecting the optic nerve, "there's no motor activity and no sensation or eyesight," Dr. Gorantla said. "The result is functionless and lifeless."

Luckily, various laboratories "have made significant progress" in fostering the long distance regrowth of nerve fibers, Dr. Goldberg said. "In animals with optic nerve injury or degeneration we've even started to see fibers regrow all the way back to the brain," he noted.

The regeneration of cells called retinal ganglia cells—key to achieving discernible vision—has also met with recent success in a lab setting. "The recent indications that such nerve generation is actually possible raises optimism that eye transplantation can really be viable," said Dr. Gorantla, who is also administrative medical director of the Pittsburgh Reconstructive Transplant Program at the University of Pittsburgh Medical Center.

Still, any first attempt at a whole-eye transplant in humans remains years away, the experts cautioned.

"There's a significant amount of work to be done before anything like this can be tried on patients," Dr. Goldberg said. "But when you survey people, losing one's vision comes in just a smidge below death as a thing we fear. There are few things people value more than their vision, so while it may be audacious, it's worth the effort."

info For more information on eye disease and blindness, visit the American Academy of Ophthalmology at *www.aao.org.*

FDA OKs Once-a-Day Drug for Chronic Hepatitis C

Douglas Dieterich, MD, professor, medicine, division of liver diseases, The Mount Sinai Hospital, New York City.
U.S. Food and Drug Administration, news release.
Associated Press

Harvoni, a daily pill that treats the most common form of hepatitis C, has been approved by the U.S. Food and Drug Administration.

It's the first combination pill (*ledipasvir* and *sofosbuvir*) approved to treat the chronic infection, and the first medication that doesn't require that the antiviral drugs *interferon* or *ribavirin* be taken at the same time, the FDA said in a news release.

Both drugs in the combination pill interfere with the hepatitis C virus' ability to multiply. One of the drugs, sofosbuvir (Sovaldi) was approved in December 2013, while ledipasvir is a new antiviral, the agency said.

"With the development and approval of new treatments for hepatitis C virus, we are changing the treatment paradigm for Americans living with the disease," Dr. Edward Cox, director of the Office of Antimicrobial Products in the

FDA's Center for Drug Evaluation and Research, said in the news release. "Until last year, the only available treatments for hepatitis C virus required administration with interferon and ribavirin. Now, patients and health care professionals have multiple treatment options, including a combination pill to help simplify treatment regimens."

One expert applauded Harvoni's approval.

"This is a giant step forward for people with [hepatitis C]. One pill, once daily, no interferon, no ribavirin and 94% to 99% cure! It moves the risk-benefit ratio needle way over toward benefit," said Douglas Dieterich, MD, a professor of medicine in the division of liver diseases at The Mount Sinai Hospital in New York City.

However, price has been an issue with some of the new treatments for hepatitis C. For example, Sovaldi alone costs $1,000 a day and not all insurance companies cover the cost of treatment, experts have noted. Harvoni costs $1,125 a pill, the Associated Press reported. Treatment length varies from 12 to 24 weeks.

Hepatitis C causes inflammation of the liver, which could spark other problems including diminished liver function (cirrhosis), scarring, liver cancer or liver failure. Most infected people aren't aware that they carry the virus until liver damage has occurred, the agency said.

Some 3.2 million Americans are believed to be infected with hepatitis C, the FDA said.

Harvoni was evaluated in three clinical studies involving more than 1,500 people who either hadn't been treated previously or hadn't responded to prior treatment. The most common side effects were fatigue and headache with less common side effects including nausea, diarrhea and insomnia.

Sticky Sea Creatures Might Aid Surgery

Glue made from mussels might be the next big thing.

Reason: Mussels can cling to just about any surface underwater—a quality that could lead to better adhesives, including surgical glues.

American Chemical Society.

The drug is marketed by Gilead, based in Foster City, California.

info The U.S. Food and Drug Administration has more about this approval at *http://www.fda.gov/NewsEvents/Newsroom/PressAnnouncements/ucm418365.htm*.

Experimental Eyewear Helps Surgeons "See" Cancer, Study Says

Washington University School of Medicine, news release.

Experimental glasses that seem to improve a doctor's ability to see cancer cells during surgery may help reduce cancer patients' need for follow-up operations, according to a recent study.

The researchers said that cancer cells can be extremely hard to see, even under high-powered magnification. When viewed through this new high-tech eyewear, cancer cells glow blue and are apparently easier to distinguish from healthy cells. This means stray tumors are less likely to be left behind after surgery, the researchers said.

The new system was developed by a team at Washington University School of Medicine in St. Louis that was led by Samuel Achilefu, PhD, a professor of radiology and biomedical engineering. Julie Margenthaler, MD, a breast surgeon and associate professor of surgery at the university, was the first to use the technology during surgery in February 2014.

"We're in the early stages of this technology, and more development and testing will be done, but we're certainly encouraged by the potential benefits to patients," she said in a university news release.

Dr. Margenthaler said that 20% to 25% of breast cancer patients who have lumps removed require a second operation because of current technology's inability to spot all cancer cells.

"Our hope is that this new technology will reduce or ideally eliminate the need for a second surgery," Dr. Margenthaler said.

Better IV Solution

During surgery, an intravenous (IV) saline solution is critical for maintaining blood pressure and hydration, but a study of 264 pancreatic cancer surgery patients found that giving less fluid with more salt led to 25% fewer complications.

Why: The saltier IV draws out excess fluid that can build up in the lungs and extremities, improving the blood flow necessary for healing.

If you're having any type of surgery requiring an IV: Ask your doctor about using a saltier solution.

Harish Lavu, MD, associate professor of surgery, Thomas Jefferson University, Philadelphia.

The technology includes custom video technology, a head-mounted display and a chemical that attaches to cancer cells and makes them glow when viewed with the glasses. The glasses can detect tumors as small as 1 millimeter in diameter (the thickness of about 10 sheets of paper), according to the study, published in the *Journal of Biomedical Optics*.

Dr. Achilefu has filed a patent for the technology. The research was funded by the U.S. National Cancer Institute.

The American Cancer Society has more about cancer surgery at *cancer.org*.

Get Checked for Diabetes While Getting Your Teeth Cleaned?

New York University, news release.

The dentist's office may be a good place to screen people for diabetes, a recent study suggests.

About eight million of the 29 million Americans living with diabetes are undiagnosed, the researchers noted.

"In light of findings from the study, the dental visit could be a useful opportunity to conduct diabetes screening among at-risk, undiagnosed patients—an important first step in identifying those who need further testing to determine their diabetes status," wrote principal investigator Shiela Strauss. She is an associate professor of nursing and codirector of the Statistics and Data Management Core for New York University's Colleges of Nursing and Dentistry.

The NYU study of 408 dental patients found that blood collected from the mouth during dental procedures was 99% as accurate for hemoglobin A1c (HbA1c) testing as finger-prick blood samples.

Testing HbA1c is recommended by the American Diabetes Association for diagnosing diabetes and for monitoring blood sugar levels among those with diabetes.

The study was published in the *American Journal of Public Health*.

While diabetes screening at dental visits can help all people at risk for the disease, those aged 45 and older would likely get the greatest benefit, the researchers said.

Dental screening for diabetes is still in development. Individuals should consult with their primary care physicians to test for prediabetes and diabetes.

The American Academy of Family Physicians has more about diabetes at *familydoctor.org*.

Why You Should Question Getting a CT Scan or MRI for a Headache

Research letter titled "Headaches and Neuroimaging: High Utilization Costs Despite Guidelines," published in *JAMA Internal Medicine*.

Did you know that 97% to 99% of CT scans for headache turn up normal? This is why medical societies such as the American Academy of Family Physicians, the American Academy of Neurology and the American Headache Society have, for a long time, recommended against routine use of CT and MRI scans for headaches and emphasized the value of neurologic exams instead. Their

guidelines were drafted and put under doctors' noses back in the year 2000. Yet that use of CT and MRI for headache—despite their ineffectiveness, cost and (in the case of CT scans) radiation—has substantially increased instead over time.

Who's to blame?

GOING OVERBOARD

Imaging tests for headaches here in the US cost $1 billion each year. If they were helpful and necessary, the money would be well-spent, but the only patients who may need a CT scan or MRI if headache is the main complaint are folks whose neurological examination—a physical exam preferably done by a neurologist—detects warning signs of a tumor or blood clot, for example, that an imaging test could confirm. What has been happening, though, is that doctors are increasingly sending patients who complain of easily diagnosed tension headaches and migraines for CT scans and MRIs.

This costly habit was uncovered in a study that spurred a call for doctors to know and stick to the guidelines. The researchers used information on outpatient care from a special database called the National Hospital Ambulatory Medical Care Survey to identify headache diagnoses and use of CT or MRI. The analysis showed that the rate of CT and MRI use to investigate headache and migraine tripled from 5% to 15% between 1995 and 2010, suggesting ongoing and worsening overuse of imaging technology.

REASONS FOR OVERUSE

Further research is needed to sort out why CT scans and MRIs appear to be overused in people complaining of headache or migraine. In certain instances, it may be because the doctor is sincerely trying to get to the root of the problem. In others, it is because the doctor is concerned that if a health emergency occurs later, a patient's lawyer will cry negligence if a CT or MRI was not done. In other instances, it may be because the doctor has a financial interest in having imaging done...and, in others, it may be because a patient bugged his or her doctor so much that the doctor simply capitulated against his better professional judgment.

WHEN IMAGING IS WARRANTED

If a thorough neurological exam, which looks at reflexes, coordination and motor strength (gripping, walking on heels), among other signs of neuromuscular health, is abnormal and your headache can't be diagnosed based on your symptoms, an imaging test might be needed, according to the year 2000 guidelines. Headaches that might be worrisome and require a look-see from imaging, according to the American Headache Society (*americanheadachesociety. org/*) and American College of Radiology, are those that are either very different from headaches you normally have (if you are headache-prone) or those that come on very suddenly and severely, including those that come after exertion. In addition, a headache that comes with a constellation of symptoms that include fever, seizures, vomiting, loss of coordination or a change in vision, speech and alertness is a cause for immediate medical attention that will likely include a CT or MRI scan.

But if you are simply prone to headaches, before asking your doctor to order an imaging study—or blindly agreeing to his recommendation to have one done—you might want to check out the patient resources page of the American Headache Society or ask your doctor for a referral to a headache-management specialist, a type of neurologist who can provide counseling about headache as well as both drug and nondrug strategies for headache and migraine relief.

Marijuana: A Safer Solution to Chronic Pain Relief?

Study titled "Medical Cannabis Laws and Opioid Analgesic Overdose Mortality in the United States, 1999-2010," published in *JAMA Internal Medicine.*

Don't kid yourself—if you use an opioid-based pain drug, such as OxyContin, Percocet, Vicodin or Dilaudid, it could kill you. Thousands of people who use opioids for pain control die from overdose each

New Hope for Paralysis

Electrical stimulation of the spinal cord recently allowed four adults with paraplegia to voluntarily move previously paralyzed muscles. The finding may allow researchers to develop new treatments for individuals who have this type of paralysis.

National Institute of Biomedical Imaging and Bioengineering.

year—and the number is increasing. In fact, opioid-overdose deaths have quadrupled within 10 years, according to the Centers for Disease Control and Prevention, and three out of four of these deaths involve prescription pain medications, not street drugs. Most of the people who die—60%—aren't using the drugs illegally either. They have legitimate prescriptions. This is a huge problem.

Enter medical marijuana. A recent study has revealed some very interesting facts about medical marijuana and relief of chronic pain and patient safety. Meanwhile medical marijuana is becoming legal in more and more states. *Here's why you should be thinking about it if you or a loved one suffers from chronic pain…*

MAKING THE CONNECTION

A team of investigators from the University of Pennsylvania decided to take a look at the incidence of opioid-related deaths in states that have legalized medical marijuana. They reasoned that since pain control is a major reason why people use medical marijuana, states that have legalized or decriminalized the herb might have lower rates of opioid-related deaths.

To test its theory, the team analyzed medical marijuana laws and 10 years' of death certificates from the entire United States. The research team discovered that, in states that allowed medical marijuana, the overall average annual death rate from opioid overdose was almost 25% lower than it was in states where medical marijuana remained illegal.

Keep in mind that, whatever you might think of marijuana as a recreational drug, we are not talking about recreational use here—we are talking about marijuana as an alternative to potentially dangerous and addictive drugs that often lose effectiveness with long-term use and, thus, lead people with chronic pain to up their dosages to get the same effect.

Now, it's true that the University of Pennsylvania study doesn't show the degree to which the decline in opioid death rates in states with legal medical marijuana is due to patients switching from opioids to marijuana. More research is needed on that issue. And the study is not a carte blanche invitation for everyone with chronic pain to start using marijuana. Marijuana is not an across-the-board solution for everyone with intractable pain. But the study does provide yet more scientific evidence in support of marijuana as a medical treatment. At minimum, it suggests that rather than being a so-called "gateway drug" to opiate use, as we were told years ago, marijuana can be a lifesaving alternative to opiates.

Doctors Regrow Large Areas of Muscle Lost in Injured Soldiers

Stephen Badylak, DVM, PhD, MD, surgical professor, University of Pittsburgh, and deputy director, McGowan Institute for Regenerative Medicine.
Peter Rubin, MD, F.A.C.S., chair, department of plastic surgery, University of Pittsburgh.
David Lowenberg, MD, orthopedic surgeon, Stanford School of Medicine, California.
Nick Clark, Youngwood, Pennsylvania.
Science Translational Medicine news briefing.

Doctors now can grow back large amounts of muscle lost to a traumatic injury, using tissue drawn from pigs as a "homing beacon" to coax the body's own stem cells into repairing the wound.

Five patients with huge wounds in their leg muscles—including three injured during military service in Iraq and Afghanistan—experienced substantial regrowth following treatment with the pig tissue and intense physical therapy, a recent study reported.

Three of the five patients had at least a 25% improvement in function following the treat-

Playtime for Stem Cells

The silicone that gives the molding toy Silly Putty its "stretch" forms a pliable surface that could make it easier to transform cells into stem cells, which may help treat spinal cord injuries, Alzheimer's disease and more.

University of Michigan.

ment, and all five reported improved quality of life, the researchers noted.

The findings were published in an April 2014 issue of *Science Translational Medicine*.

Trauma caused by a car crash or an explosive device can cause irreparable damage to a person's muscles if too much muscle mass is torn away, said lead author Stephen Badylak, DVM, PhD, MD, a surgical professor at the University of Pittsburgh and deputy director of the McGowan Institute for Regenerative Medicine.

"When you lose so much muscle that the gap is too large for the normal restorative processes to occur, the end result is typically filling that gap with scar tissue," Dr. Badylak said in a journal news briefing. The scar tissue causes a loss of function in that muscle, he said, potentially disabling the patient.

RESEARCH DETAILS

Dr. Badylak's team hit upon the idea of using an "extracellular matrix" drawn from pig tissue to promote regrowth of muscle. Extracellular matrix is a component of body tissue that functions outside of the body's cells. Made mostly of collagen, the extracellular matrix provides structural and biochemical support to surrounding cells.

Such materials already are used in hernia repair and breast reconstruction, to provide structural support and protection for surgical sites, said study co-author Peter Rubin, MD, FACS, chair of the department of plastic surgery at the University of Pittsburgh.

But researchers discovered that the implanted pig tissue promotes healing by releasing biochemicals called peptides into nearby human tissues.

"These peptides that are released serve as a homing device for the body's own stem cells," Dr. Badylak said. Stem cells located in nearby human tissues are drawn to the site of the wound, where they begin replacing the lost muscle.

After testing the process on mice, doctors started a clinical trial involving five men aged 27 to 37. All had lost 58% to 90% of muscle in one of their legs.

The men underwent surgery that cut away all the scar tissue from the wound location, and then surgeons implanted the extracellular matrix into the wound.

The patients all started aggressive rehabilitation within two days of the surgery, Dr. Badylak said. This was done to provide the stem cells guidance in the repair of muscle.

"When those cells get there, they depend upon local environmental cues to say, 'OK, now that I'm here, what do you want me to do?' One of the most important cues are the mechanical forces that are asked of the site," he said.

The goal was to improve their ability to perform day-to-day tasks such as walking up stairs, getting out of a chair and raising a leg to a sitting position.

SUCCESS STORY

One of the patients, Nick Clark, lost massive amounts of muscle and nerve tissue from his left leg in a 2005 skiing accident. He had terrible balance in his left leg, he said, and sometimes relied on canes or ankle braces to stabilize his stride.

Clark underwent the experimental surgery in 2012. "The second day I was in the hospital, they had me walking up and down the halls of the hospital," he said in the news briefing. "It was pretty tough. It was painful. But it was worth it."

He now can balance on his left leg for several minutes at a time, and has more strength pushing off with his left foot.

"My balance is still not 100%, but it's improved quite a bit," said Clark, 34, of Youngwood, Pennsylvania. "Now I can almost keep pace with a normal person walking, maybe 90%. Before the surgery, I had about half the pace of a normal walk."

EXPERT COMMENT

The procedure represents an important medical advance, according to a trauma expert who was not involved in the study.

"I think it will set a new treatment paradigm in people with significant muscle injury, which we in the trauma world see quite frequently," said David Lowenberg, MD, an orthopedic surgeon at Stanford School of Medicine. "They took something that's a huge problem and found a way to fix it relatively inexpensively, and it's not technically difficult to do."

Dr. Lowenberg helped train military doctors to deal with such large wounds as part of a distinguished scholars program, and saw firsthand the physical trauma caused by war. "The number of large muscle defects in our wounded warriors is real," he said.

The cost of the procedure could decline even more in coming years. "There are new ways to manufacture these scaffolds that are even more cost-efficient and you won't have to depend on the animals to process from," Dr. Lowenberg said.

WHAT HAPPENS NEXT

For now, study author Dr. Badylak said, the research serves as "a demonstration of the true movement of bench-top basic science through preclinical animal work to treatment at the bedside."

He said the next step is to train surgical and physical therapy teams at other leading institutions on the process. "That way we can show this is an approach that can work," Dr. Badylak said.

Once the procedure is proven effective, Dr. Badylak believes it could be used by any surgical hospital as a low-cost way to heal wounds that were previously thought irreparable.

"The approach we've taken is intended to be the type of approach that can be utilized anywhere that good surgery is available," he said.

info The U.S. National Institutes of Health has more about stem cells at *http://stem cells.nih.gov/info/basics/Pages/Default.aspx,*

U.S. Seniors' Health Poorest, Global Survey Shows

Steffie Woolhandler, MD, professor, CUNY School of Public Health, Hunter College, New York City, and co-founder, Physicians for a National Health Program

David Blumenthal, MD, president, and Robin Osborn, vice president and director, International Program in Health Policy and Practice Innovations, both Common-wealth Fund.

Health Affairs, online

Seniors in America have more chronic health problems and take more medications than seniors in 10 other industrialized countries do, according to a recent global survey.

The United States also stood out among the 11 nations surveyed by The Commonwealth Fund for having more seniors struggling to get and afford the health care they need.

Eighty-seven percent of US adults who are 65 and older suffer from at least one chronic illness, and 68% have at least two illnesses, which were the highest rates found, the survey showed. Also, 53% of older Americans take at least four medications, another record high, and 21% spend at least $2,000 in yearly out-of-pocket health care costs, which was second only to Switzerland.

STUDY DETAILS

For the survey, the researchers collected responses from more than 15,000 older adults in Australia, Canada, France, Germany, the Netherlands, New Zealand, Norway, Sweden, Switzerland, the United Kingdom and the United States.

Almost all of the other countries have some form of universal health insurance, and American seniors have Medicare, but Osborn said striking differences emerged in the survey.

Although the U.S. senior group was the youngest of all the countries in the report, *they were also among the sickest:* 25% of older Americans saw at least four doctors in the past year, second only to Germany at 39%.

In addition, more Americans (19%) said they skipped essential health care because they could not afford it, and 11% said they had trouble paying their medical bills. In France, only 3% of seniors said they skipped health care because of cost, and in Norway only 1% said they had trouble paying medical bills.

In terms of out-of-pocket costs, only the Swiss spent more than Americans. In the United States, 21% spent $2,000 or more a year, compared with 22% in Switzerland and 2% in the United Kingdom. In France, on the other hand, virtually no one spent out-of-pocket costs.

Only 57% of U.S. seniors said they were able to see their doctor the same or the next day when they were sick, compared with 83% in France and New Zealand, and 81% in Germany.

Americans use of emergency rooms was one of the highest, at 39%. Thirty-five percent of these visits were for conditions their doctors could have dealt with had they been available, the researchers found.

When a specialist was needed, 86% of U.S. seniors and 82% of seniors in Switzerland were able to see one within four weeks—the highest rates in the survey. Seniors in Canada (46%), Norway (46%) and Sweden (50%) were the least likely to get appointments that quickly.

U.S. seniors, like seniors in the other countries, appear to suffer from poorly coordinated care or gaps in communication between doctors: 35% of U.S. seniors reported having such problems, as did 41% in Germany and 37% in Norway. In France, only 7% said they had these problems. But, the survey showed, American seniors also had better doctor/patient relationships than seniors in many other countries.

Medication Smarts

Drugs That Work Against Each Other

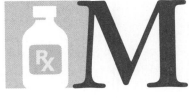

Most people who have a chronic health problem such as osteo-arthritis, high blood pressure or diabetes are accustomed to taking medication to help control their symptoms.

But if you have more than one chronic condition—and take medication for each of them—you could be setting yourself up for other problems.

The risk that often goes undetected: Taking medication prescribed for one disease may actually worsen another health problem. This situation, known as "therapeutic competition," has received surprisingly little attention from the medical profession.

ARE YOU AT RISK?

Therapeutic competition can occur at any time in a person's life. But the risk increases with age—the older we get, the more likely we are to have chronic medical conditions and use more medications. Because our bodies metabolize medication less efficiently as we age, we're also more likely to develop side effects that can worsen other health problems.

Modern medicine has not done very much to help the situation. For one thing, polypharmacy—the use of multiple medications—has become more common than ever before.

For people with more than one chronic medical condition, frequent conflicts occur if you have…

HIGH BLOOD PRESSURE

If you also have chronic obstructive pulmonary disease (COPD), drugs that you take to ease your breathing, such as the beta-adrener-

David Lee, PharmD, PhD, assistant professor in the College of Pharmacy at Oregon State University in Portland. Dr. Lee is also a coauthor of a recent paper on therapeutic competition that was published in the journal *PLOS ONE*.

gicagonist *albuterol* (Proventil) or a corticosteroid, may raise your blood pressure.

If you are also being treated for depression, an antidepressant such as *venlafaxine* (Effexor) or *duloxetine* (Cymbalta) could push your blood pressure higher. COX-2 inhibitors such as *celecoxib* (Celebrex), commonly used for osteoarthritis, also may increase blood pressure.

DIABETES

Corticosteroids taken for COPD can raise blood sugar levels, worsening diabetes. If you have an enlarged prostate and take an alphablocker such as *tamsulosin* (Flomax) or a betablocker such as *atenolol* (Tenormin) for high blood pressure, the drug can mask symptoms of low blood sugar, such as shakiness.

COPD

If you also have high blood pressure or angina and take a non-selective beta-blocker such as *propranolol* (Inderal), the drug could worsen lung symptoms.

HEART DISEASE

COPD drugs, including albuterol…tricyclic antidepressants such as *imipramine* (Tofranil), taken for depression…and COX-2 inhibitors for osteoarthritis also can make heart disease worse.

ATRIAL FIBRILLATION

Osteoporosis drugs, including bisphosphonates such as *alendronate* (Fosamax)…and Alzheimer's drugs, including cholinesterase inhibitors such as *donepezil* (Aricept), may worsen atrial fibrillation.

OSTEOPOROSIS

Corticosteroids used to treat COPD often lead to significant bone loss. Glitazones taken for diabetes and proton pump inhibitors such as *omeprazole* (Prilosec), commonly prescribed for gastroesophageal reflux disease (GERD), can accelerate bone loss.

GERD OR PEPTIC ULCERS

Warfarin (Coumadin) or *clopidogrel* (Plavix), often prescribed for atrial fibrillation or heart disease, as well as nonsteroidal anti-inflammatory drugs (NSAIDs), can cause bleeding that worsens GERD and ulcers. Bisphosphonates taken for osteoporosis may aggravate esophageal damage that commonly occurs with GERD and ulcers.

HOW TO PROTECT YOURSELF

If you have more than one chronic condition and take two or more medications to treat them, it is crucial that you watch for signs of therapeutic competition, such as new symptoms that are unexplained or begin soon after a new medication is started. Any new health condition actually may be an adverse effect of medication.

Important steps to avoid therapeutic competition…

•**Try to cut back on the drugs you take.** The less medication you're on, the less likely one of your drugs will adversely affect another condition. Ask your doctor whether it's advisable to reduce the overall number of prescriptions you take. A drug you have been taking for years may no longer be necessary. You may also be able to make lifestyle changes—such as getting more exercise—that will allow you to cut back on blood pressure or diabetes medication.

•**Get the right medication.** If it seems that a drug is worsening another condition, ask your doctor about less harmful alternatives. Some medications are more selective—that is, their effects on the body are more focused on the target illness, making unintended consequences for other conditions less of a danger.

Example: Nonselective beta-blockers, such as propranolol, often worsen COPD symptoms, but medications with more selective action, such as *metoprolol* (Lopressor), are usually just as effective for the heart problem they're prescribed for without adversely affecting your lungs.

GET A YEARLY MEDICATION CHECK

If you suffer from multiple ailments, you need to tell all your doctors about the medications you take. Also, talk to your pharmacist each time you pick up a new prescription to make sure your drugs aren't working against each other.

To ensure that no drug-related problems develop: Once a year, have a pharmacist (ask one at your drugstore) review all your medications. This service includes a discussion of side effects, interactions and alternatives. For many people, Medicare Part D and some private health plans will pay for this service. If not, it usually costs less than $100.

A Shocking Side Effect of Everyday Drugs

Jack E. Fincham, PhD, RPh, professor of pharmacy administration at Presbyterian College School of Pharmacy in Clinton, South Carolina. He serves as a panel member of the FDA Nonprescription Drugs Advisory Committee.

You wouldn't be surprised if a narcotic painkiller made you feel a little sleepy or you developed an upset stomach after taking an aspirin-like painkiller for a few days.

What most people don't know—and their doctors don't talk about—is that popular prescription and over-the-counter (OTC) drugs can affect your body and your mind.

A hidden risk: Let's say that you start taking a new drug. Weeks or even months later, you begin to feel depressed or suffer some other psychiatric symptom. You might assume that something's wrong with you when, in fact, the drug could be to blame. Common offenders you need to know about—psychiatric side effects can occur with any dose, but the greater the drug amount, the greater the risk…

PAINKILLERS

Naproxen (Aleve, Naprosyn and others). It's one of the most popular pain relievers because it's less likely to cause stomach upset than other nonsteroidal anti-inflammatory drugs (NSAIDs), such as aspirin or *ibuprofen* (Motrin). But it's more likely than other OTC painkillers to cause depression.

How it hurts: The exact mechanism isn't clear, but naproxen affects the central nervous system in ways that other NSAIDs do not. Some people who take naproxen every day—for chronic arthritis, for example—have reported drowsiness, reduced concentration and/or depression.

My advice: Be aware of your mood when using naproxen. Even though this drug is less likely to cause stomach upset than other NSAIDs, you should watch for signs of depression while taking naproxen. If depression develops, ask your doctor for advice.

BLOOD PRESSURE DRUGS

Beta-blockers, such as *propranolol* (Inderal) and *sotalol* (Betapace), work by blocking the effects of epinephrine (also known as adrenaline), thus slowing the heart rate.

How they hurt: Damping down the heart's action can cause fatigue and depression. Because these drugs affect many different body systems, including the brain, they've also been linked to mania and other mood problems in some people.

My advice: Beta-blockers are typically used to treat serious conditions such as high blood pressure and cardiac arrhythmias, so never stop taking this medication without consulting your physician. You may be able to switch to a different drug (such as a calcium channel blocker) for high blood pressure.

If you must take a beta-blocker, use nondrug approaches to improve your energy levels and mood. Be sure to exercise regularly, rely on positive thinking and get enough sunlight, which the body uses to produce vitamin D (low levels have been linked to depression).

COLD REMEDIES

Guaifenesin. This is one of the most common ingredients in OTC decongestants and cold remedies, such as Robitussin and Mucinex. As an expectorant, guaifenesin thins mucus, making it easier to cough it up.

How it hurts: Guaifenesin has wide-ranging effects on the central nervous system. In some people, these changes can lead to fatigue and/or depression. When guaifenesin is combined with other ingredients such as *pseudoephedrine* (a common decongestant), side effects can also include anxiety.

My advice: For most people, drinking water helps to thin mucus about as well as a pharmaceutical expectorant does. When you're stuffed up, drink a few more glasses of water—or tea or juice—than you usually consume during an average day.

ALLERGY DRUGS

Nonsedating antihistamines. Don't believe the labels—so-called "nonsedating" allergy drugs may have less noticeable side effects than older antihistamines (such as Benadryl), but they are sedating.

Some people with seasonal or year-round allergies who use drugs such as *loratadine* (Claritin) or *cetirizine* (Zyrtec) complain about drowsiness—and depression.

How they hurt: All antihistamines have anticholinergic effects (caused by blocking a neurotransmitter in the central nervous system). While some people have no side effects, others notice that they're agitated and/or confused. For some people, these antihistamines also may lead to depression or concentration problems.

My advice: Since unwanted sedation is the most common side effect, take antihistamines at bedtime. Pollen counts and allergy symptoms tend to be worse in the morning, so taking an antihistamine at night will also help you feel better when you wake up.

Worth a try: Break the tablets in half (assuming that the medication isn't timed-release). Many people get the same allergy relief with fewer side effects from a lower dose.

HEARTBURN MEDICATIONS

H2 blockers. Some patients who take these heartburn drugs, including *cimetidine* (Tagamet) and *ranitidine* (Zantac), have reported suffering from depression, confusion and even hallucinations. These and other side effects usually occur in older adults, who tend to accumulate higher drug levels in the body.

How they hurt: Ironically, the psychiatric side effects of H2 blockers are probably related to lower stomach acidity—the effect that these drugs provide to fight heartburn. Too much stomach acid (or a weak esophageal muscle that allows acid reflux) is obviously a problem, but reduced acid may have its own risks. For example, people who take these drugs every day tend to absorb smaller amounts of folate and other nutrients—an effect that can lead to mood problems.

My advice: Most people can reduce—or even eliminate—heartburn without the daily use of potent drugs. Simple approaches that work include not eating within a few hours of bedtime...and avoiding "trigger" foods such as chocolate or alcohol. If you need more relief, you may be able to get by with the occasional OTC antacid, such as Mylanta or Maalox.

How to Supercharge Your Medications

Thomas Kruzel, ND, a naturopathic physician at the Rockwood Natural Medicine Clinic in Scottsdale, Arizona. Dr. Kruzel is author of *The Homeopathic Emergency Guide. RockwoodNaturalMedicine.com*

When you get a new prescription, most doctors don't talk about dietary supplements. If a conversation does take place, it probably focuses on the potentially dangerous interactions that can occur when people take a prescription medication and a supplement.*

The other side of the story: While some supplements can cause dangerous interactions with certain drugs, the reverse is also true—certain supplements can actually boost the effectiveness of a prescription drug and/or reduce its side effects. In some cases, this beneficial effect may allow you to take a lower dose of the drug...or even discontinue it at some point.

DRUG-BOOSTING SUPPLEMENTS

If you are interested in using a supplement as part of a medication regimen, always discuss this with your doctor. Medical supervision is necessary to ensure that you are using the combination safely.

Medication-supplement pairings that often work well...

•**Diabetes medication and alpha-lipoic acid.** Alpha-lipoic acid is an endogenous (made

*To see if a drug you have been prescribed may interact with a supplement you are taking, ask your doctor. You can also go to *nlm.nih.gov/medlineplus*, and click on "Drugs & Supplements."

in the body) antioxidant that helps transform blood sugar (glucose) into energy. It is found in foods such as red meat and liver, though it is difficult to get enough from food to work effectively with your medication for type 2 diabetes.

When taken in the larger doses that are found in supplements, alpha-lipoic acid lowers blood sugar and may reduce pain, itching and other symptoms caused by diabetes-related nerve damage (neuropathy). For diabetic neuropathy, I typically recommend 400 mg to 500 mg of alpha-lipoic acid, twice daily. For general antioxidant benefit, 100 mg to 300 mg daily is usually sufficient.

If you're taking a diabetes medication that lowers blood sugar, such as *metformin* (Glucophage) or *glyburide* (DiaBeta), the addition of alpha-lipoic acid may allow you to use a smaller drug dose. If your glucose levels are stabilized through diet and regular exercise (without medication), you may want to take alpha-lipoic acid indefinitely.

Caution: Taking too much alpha-lipoic acid with a diabetes drug could lead to excessively low blood sugar, which can cause anxiety, sweating, shakiness and/or confusion. Alpha-lipoic acid also may interact with chemotherapy drugs and thyroid medication such as *levothyroxine* (Synthroid). Talk to your doctor before taking alpha-lipoic acid with any prescription medication.

• **Cholesterol medication and CoQ10.** Co-enzyme Q10 (CoQ10) is a critical component of the energy-producing mitochondria of the cells in your body. It is found in foods such as meat and fish. CoQ10 levels decline as we grow older. Cholesterol-lowering statin drugs also deplete CoQ10.

Food generally does not provide a therapeutic amount of CoQ10. When taken in supplement form, CoQ10 (100 mg to 200 mg daily) helps prevent the muscle pain that can occur as a side effect of statin medication. Research shows that CoQ10 itself has a mild cholesterol-lowering effect and may reduce the risk for cardiovascular disease.

Caution: CoQ10 may increase bleeding risk when taken with aspirin, *warfarin* (Coumadin)

and other blood thinners. Talk to your doctor before taking CoQ10 with any prescription medication.

• **Antidepressant medication and vitamin B-12.** Vitamin B-12 is required for red blood cell formation and neurological function. This vitamin is naturally present in animal foods, such as clams, beef liver, red meat and eggs.

It's well-known that vitamin B-12 levels decline with age—largely due to a loss of the stomach acid that is needed to absorb this vitamin. Strict vegetarians also tend to have low levels of B-12.

In a recent study, patients with a vitamin B-12 deficiency who took an injectable form of the vitamin—1,000 micrograms (mcg) weekly for six weeks—while also taking an oral antidepressant reported a significantly greater reduction in depression symptoms than those taking the oral medication alone.

Oral vitamin B-12 supplements (100 mcg daily for adults under age 50) or sublingual (under-the-tongue) tablets (1,000 mcg daily for adults over age 50) can be used to help make antidepressants more effective. No adverse effects have been linked to excess vitamin B-12 intake from food or supplements in healthy adults. However, when higher doses than those described above are used (to treat a severe B-12 deficiency or anemia, for example), the treatment should be supervised by a doctor.

• **Blood pressure medication and magnesium.** Magnesium is an extremely versatile mineral. It promotes the health of your heart and blood vessels and regulates the effects of calcium and other important nutrients in the body. Healthy adults can usually get plenty of magnesium from nuts, green vegetables and whole grains.

However, in order to get enough magnesium to help lower blood pressure, people with hypertension usually need a supplement (400 mg to 500 mg, twice daily). Magnesium citrate is the most absorbable form of the mineral.

Many blood pressure drugs relax and dilate the arteries, which allows blood to circulate with less force. Combining magnesium with a blood pressure–lowering medication can result in even lower blood pressure, which may allow you to take a reduced dose of the drug. When adding magnesium to a blood pressure medication regimen, check your blood pressure daily at home until your doctor says it's stable.

Caution: Taking too much magnesium with a blood pressure drug may lead to low blood pressure. Symptoms include fatigue and light-headedness. Magnesium supplements can also cause diarrhea, so you may need a lower dose.

Is Your Medication Dose Wrong for You?

Heather Whitley, PharmD, an associate professor in the Auburn University Harrison School of Pharmacy in Auburn, Alabama. She is also associate affiliate professor at The Institute for Rural Health Research at The University of Alabama, Tuscaloosa.

I f you are a man and take a sleeping pill in the middle of the night, you may fall asleep quickly and wake up feeling refreshed. If you're a woman and take the same pill, you may fall asleep just as fast but find that you are slogging through the morning with a drug-powered hangover.

Just a fluke? Absolutely not.

An under-recognized problem: While scientists have long suspected that men and women don't respond in the same ways to certain drugs, a growing body of research shows that these differences are more significant than previously thought.

Why this matters: You may be taking a drug—or be prescribed one in the future—in a dose that's not right for you…or in a class that is not the most effective for your condition. What you need to know…

HOW GENDER SLIPPED UNDER THE RADAR

Since 1992, when the sedative *zolpidem* (Ambien) was first introduced in the US, the recommended maximum dose for men and women has been the same—10 mg.

A startling finding: Recently, evidence came to light that women who took the same dose of zolpidem as men had blood levels that were 45% higher. The "standard" dose, in other words, was essentially an overdose for women.

Meanwhile, zolpidem has also been implicated in cases of so-called "sleep driving," in which people who have taken the drug drive their cars while not fully awake.

Now the FDA has stepped in and cut the recommended dose of zolpidem for women in half, to 5 mg. The daily dose for the extended-release version is up to 12.5 mg for men and 6.25 mg for women.

But it's not just sleeping pills that affect men and women differently. Entire classes of medications—such as beta-blockers, opioid painkillers and heart medications—have sex-specific effects.

WHY HAVEN'T WE HEARD MORE ABOUT THIS?

Until the early 1990s, women of childbearing age were excluded from most drug-based research. The majority of drugs were tested only in men. Based on these results, doctors assumed that any research that cleared a medication as being safe and effective for men would also apply to women—but they didn't really know.

Today, medications are routinely tested in roughly equal numbers of men and women—but there are still hundreds, maybe thousands, of drugs on the market whose outcomes have never been analyzed based on gender. What's more, data do not always separate outcomes based on age, ethnicity and other factors. So the recommended dose may not be the optimal amount for certain people.

WHICH DRUGS ARE SUSPECT?

You'd expect that a small woman would require a lower dose of medication than a large man. But size is only one difference.

Because women have a higher percentage of body fat, on average, drugs that are lipophilic—that is, accumulate in fatty tissue—cause longer-lasting effects in women than in men. On top of that, women tend to metabolize (break down) some medications more slowly than men, so women can be more likely to accumulate higher-than-expected concentrations of those drugs in their bodies.

A woman's digestive process is also generally slower than a man's, which means that women may have to wait for a longer time after meals in order to take some medications "on an empty stomach."

Trust your gut: If you start taking a new medication and your instincts tell you that something's wrong, pay attention. You may need a different drug or dose.

The research on sex-based drug effects is still in the early stages. There are probably hundreds, if not thousands, of drugs that affect men and women differently.

Among the drugs that women should use with caution...

SEDATIVES

Benzodiazepine sedatives, such as *diazepam* (Valium), accumulate in fat and have longer-lasting effects in women. Women may find themselves feeling drowsy the next day...less alert than usual...and having slower reaction times. (Zolpidem, the medication discussed earlier, has similar effects.)

My advice: If you are a woman taking one of these medications for anxiety, back spasms or any other condition, ask your physician, "Could I take a lower dose because I'm a woman?"

BLOOD PRESSURE DRUGS

Beta-blockers, such as *metoprolol* (Lopressor), *atenolol* (Tenormin) and *propranolol* (Inderal), have stronger effects on women. For example, women who take them tend to have a greater drop in blood pressure and heart rate than men, particularly during exercise.

My advice: All patients should be started on the lowest possible dose, then gradually adjusted (titrated) every few weeks until the desired effects are achieved.

Let your doctor know if you're experiencing dizziness, fatigue or other symptoms—this could signal that you're taking a dose that's too high for you.

Calcium channel blockers, including *amlodipine* (Norvasc) and *felodipine* (Plendil), are among the most commonly used drugs for high blood pressure. One potential side effect of these drugs is edema (fluid accumulation in the body)—and women tend to experience more of this edema than men.

My advice: Rather than taking a diuretic to manage edema, women (and men) who have this side effect might do better without a calcium channel blocker at all.

They can frequently switch to an ACE inhibitor such as *lisinopril* (Zestril), which also provides blood pressure–lowering effects—and does not cause edema. Alternatively, adding an ACE inhibitor to the calcium channel blocker can reverse edema.

PAINKILLERS

Opiate analgesics, such as morphine, *oxycodone* (OxyContin) and *hydromorphone* (Dilaudid), have a greater analgesic effect in women.

In fact, women usually get pain relief from a 30% to 40% lower dose than that required for men. Women who do not take the lower dose are also more likely than men to experience side effects, including unwanted sedation.

My advice: Tell your doctor that you want the lowest effective dose. It can always be increased if you need more relief.

HEART MEDICATION

Low-dose aspirin is routinely recommended to prevent heart attacks and/or strokes. This benefit has been shown to occur in both men and women who have already had a heart attack or stroke but is less clear-cut in those who have not. Clinical studies have found that low-dose aspirin helps prevent stroke in healthy women ages 55 to 79 and heart attack in healthy men ages 45 to 79. Preventive low-dose aspirin may be especially beneficial for men and women with cardiovascular risk factors, such as high blood pressure, high cholesterol, diabetes, family history or smoking.

My advice: Men and women should discuss with their doctors whether they need low-dose (81-mg) aspirin to prevent a heart attack or stroke, especially since even small doses of aspirin increase the risk for gastric bleeding. Unlike some other drugs in which side effects are amplified for women, low-dose aspirin is less likely to cause gastric bleeding in women than in men.

Getting the Most from Drug Ads

Charles B. Inlander, a consumer advocate and health-care consultant based in Fogelsville, Pennsylvania. He was the founding president of the nonprofit People's Medical Society, a consumer advocacy organization credited with key improvements in the quality of US health care, and is author or coauthor of more than 20 consumer-health books.

I'm a big fan of drug ads. Even though plenty of people despise these lengthy interruptions in their favorite TV programming, a lot can be gained from these ads if you know what to look for.

Prior to 1997, when the FDA eased its rules to allow direct-to-consumer (DTC) prescription drug advertising, pharmaceutical companies promoted their prescription drugs almost exclusively to health-care professionals. Consumers knew very little, if anything, about the medication choices that were available to them. And studies reported that the average doctor prescribed the same 10 drugs to about 90% of their patients.

Before the law changed, a friend of mine saw various doctors for his severe summer allergies, and each prescribed drugs that made him extremely drowsy. When DTC advertising started, my friend saw a TV ad for the allergy drug Claritin. What struck him was that it promised to not make him drowsy, and he needed to take only one pill every 24 hours. He asked his allergist about it, and the doctor agreed he should try it. The drug worked perfectly. Later, his doctor said he hadn't thought of Claritin.

How to watch drug ads...

•**Don't fall for the hype.** Most drug ads feature attractive actors and engaging music. Don't let that distract you. Listen for what condition the drug treats...what makes it different and/or better than a product you now use (if any)...and use the information to have a discussion with your doctor about the best course of treatment for your problem.

•**Don't let the ad scare you.** The FDA requires that prescription drug ads disclose the most common and dangerous side effects of an advertised drug—this is not, by the way, required for advertised over-the-counter (OTC) drugs. Remember, most drug side effects are rare. Because all drugs have potentially serious side effects, including all OTC products such as aspirin, always talk to your doctor about this before starting any new medication.

•**Use the ad to find a cheaper alternative.** Advertised drugs are usually either the newest or the most expensive medications in their categories. Big-name prescription drugs such as *Zocor* (for cholesterol) and *Xanax* (for anxiety) are now available in generic form—at a fraction of the original cost.

My advice: Ask your doctor if there is a less expensive, yet effective alternative to the advertised drug. There usually is!

What's Really in That Generic Drug?

Jack E. Fincham, PhD, RPh, professor of pharmacy administration at Presbyterian College School of Pharmacy in Clinton, South Carolina.

Generics cost 80% less, on average, than brand-name drugs. They contain the same active ingredients and supposedly do the same job. What's not to like? A lot, it turns out. In June 2014, two large manufacturers of the generic version of the heart drug Toprol-XL issued a recall because the drug wasn't dissolving properly—a problem that was identified when patients taking the drug started complaining of chest pain and other heart symptoms.

This isn't an isolated incident. Generic drugs may be similar to their brand-name counterparts, but they are not identical. *What you need to know about generic drugs...*

DOUBTS ABOUT QUALITY

For years, major medical groups such as the American Heart Association (AHA) have expressed concerns that generics may cause more side effects than brand-name drugs—and the AHA as well as many other such groups advise always getting a doctor's approval before using a generic drug.

Generics account for about 80% of all prescriptions in the US and save Americans billions of dollars a year, but some experts worry that patients, in some cases, are trading quality for economy—and may be taking serious risks.

Sobering statistics: A survey of more than 500 doctors found that nearly 50% worried about the overall quality of generics...and more than 25% said that they would hesitate to prescribe these drugs for themselves or their families.

THE FACE-OFF

Key differences between generic and brand-name drugs...

•**Bioequivalence.** You would think that the amount of a drug that's absorbed by the body would be the same in generic and brand-name versions. This isn't always the case.

According to FDA guidelines, generics are required to reach maximum blood concentrations that are between 80% and 125% of the levels achieved by brand-name drugs. Suppose that you switch to a generic that delivers medication at the low end of the range. You may find your symptoms aren't as well-controlled as they used to be. If the drug is at the high end, you'll be more likely to have side effects.

•**Timed-release.** Medications that release their active ingredients slowly are among the trickiest to copy. Even when the active ingredient is the same in two versions of the same drug, how it is released in the body might be different.

•**Fillers.** The active ingredients in generic and brand-name drugs are the same, but the extra ingredients—such as binding agents, preservatives and pill coatings—may be different. These ingredients are supposed to be inert. But recent research suggests that they may affect how drugs dissolve or how they're absorbed by the body.

•**Testing.** The same investigational drug studies that are needed for FDA approval of brand-name drugs are not required for all generic drugs. For example, the FDA requires only a very small number of people (sometimes just 20) for its bioequivalence studies.

HOW TO PROTECT YOURSELF

There's no reason to swear off generic drugs. The cost savings can be tremendous, and most generics provide the same benefits—with no greater risk for side effects—as brand-names. But you have to choose them carefully. *My advice...*

•**Be wary of timed-release medications.** Also called extended-release, they are used for conditions such as pain, depression and asthma that require long-term control...or for convenience. They're usually designated with abbreviations such as ER (extended release), LA (long acting) or LTR (long-term release).

Problems with the timed-released components are more of an issue with generics than with brand-name drugs. This doesn't mean you should avoid generics. What matters is the predictability of the timed-release drug. If your symptoms are well-controlled by a generic version, stick with the same drug—preferably one that's made by the same manufacturer (see below). You're more likely to have problems when you first switch from a brand-name drug to a generic substitute.

•**Take exactly the same drug.** Pharmacies use generic products from multiple manufacturers. Different drug companies use different manufacturing techniques as well as different ingredients. Even if you think you're taking the same drug, there may be subtle variations in such areas as effectiveness and side effects each time the prescription is filled. You can avoid these variations by making sure that your prescription comes from the same company.

What to do: Check the prescription bottle for the manufacturer of the drug you take. If it's not there, your pharmacist can tell you. Also, ask him/her if it's possible to use a single company for each refill.

This is crucial if the drug has a narrow therapeutic index (NTI)—a fine line between an effective dose and a toxic dose.

Examples: Some blood-thinning drugs (such as *warfarin*)...drugs used for seizures (such as *phenytoin*)...and antipsychotic drugs (such as *lithium*).

•**Track results.** Be suspicious if a drug that you've been taking for months or years suddenly seems less effective or seems to be causing new side effects. It's possible that your condition has changed—or you could be receiving a drug made by a different manufacturer.

Important: If you start using a new pharmacy, let the pharmacist know the manufacturers of all your medications. Also, ask your doctor to give you copies of all your test results. Track your numbers—for cholesterol and blood sugar, for example. If you notice a change, tell your doctor right away. It's possible that you just need a dosing adjustment. It's also possible that a generic isn't the best choice for you.

•**Switch drugs.** If you're not getting the best results from a new generic medication, don't assume that you need a different drug. You might simply need to switch to the brand-name version.

What to do: Ask your doctor to prescribe the brand-name drug for a few months. If you notice an improvement in your symptoms and test results, it might be worth sticking with it even if it costs more. Or if you are not happy with the results of your generic but would rather avoid the high cost of a brand-name, ask your pharmacist to recommend another generic.

Can Medical Marijuana Ease What Ails You?

Gregory T. Carter, MD, rehabilitation-medicine specialist and medical director, St. Luke's Rehabilitation Institute, Spokane, Washington. Dr. Carter has written two textbooks on the medicinal uses of cannabis and coauthored more than 200 peer-reviewed journal articles.

Would you use cannabis (marijuana) if your doctor recommended it for, say, nerve pain or to help control muscle spasms? Twenty-three states, plus the District of Columbia, have now legalized it for such medical uses.*

But do the benefits of medical marijuana truly outweigh the risks? Who should consider trying it—and what's the best way to use it safely? Here, answers to some common questions...

•**What conditions is marijuana most likely to help?** Several—but because research has been impeded by political considerations, the level of evidence varies for each condition.

Beginning nearly 30 years ago, the prescription drug *dronabinol* (Marinol) was approved by the FDA for treating appetite loss in AIDS patients. It's a synthetic version of one of the active compounds in cannabis.

Since then, cannabis has been shown to relieve nausea in cancer patients. Unlike the synthetic version, it's not a single agent. It contains 80 to 100 different medicinally active compounds known as cannabinoids.

Recent lab and animal studies suggest that cannabis can be an effective treatment for cancer itself. The active compounds have been shown to limit tumor invasiveness and the activation of chemical signals that stimulate growth in some types of cancers.

Patients who have nerve pain often get more relief with cannabis than with other prescription medications, such as *gabapentin* (Neurontin). Cannabis also has been used successfully to treat muscle spasms, seizures and other neurological conditions such as multiple sclerosis. And it seems to be effective at controlling the tics and behavior problems caused by diseases such as Tourette's syndrome. Some people also use it for fibromyalgia and glaucoma.

•**If my doctor prescribes cannabis, what type should I buy?** Cannabis dispensaries (in states where medical uses are permitted) typically sell many different strains, which affect users in different ways. The best medical strains have a high concentration of cannabidiol (CBD) and cannabinol (CBN), with relatively small amounts of tetrahydrocannabinol (THC), the compound responsible for most of the intoxicating effects.

Bear in mind that even in states that have legalized it, insurance does not cover the cost of medical marijuana, which ranges from $200 to $500 an ounce.

•**Is it better to smoke medical marijuana or eat it?** Neither. It's unlikely that the small amount of smoke from medical doses increases

---

*Medical marijuana has been legalized in Alaska, Arizona, California, Colorado, Connecticut, District of Columbia, Delaware, Hawaii, Illinois, Maine, Maryland, Massachusetts, Michigan, Minnesota, Montana, Nevada, New Hampshire, New Jersey, New Mexico, New York, Oregon, Rhode Island, Vermont and Washington. Seven states—Alabama, Florida, Iowa, Mississippi, Tennessee, Utah and Wisconsin—allow medical marijuana for specific conditions, such as epilepsy.

the risk for emphysema or other lung diseases, but the smoke does contain carcinogens. Why take chances? Edible forms of cannabis—such as baked goods, shakes and candies—are effective, but it's difficult to control your intake. The absorption rate will depend on what's already in your stomach, and it can take up to two hours to feel the effects.

The best way is to use a vaporizer. The medicinal compounds vaporize at a much lower temperature than is required for combustion (smoking). The inhaled vapor gives the same rapid onset as smoking—you'll feel the effects within a few minutes. Vaporized cannabis is safer than inhaled smoke. Vaporizers are sold online and at dispensaries for around $100 to as much as $400.

You can also buy sublingual tinctures at dispensaries. You put a few drops under your tongue. You'll feel the effects almost as quickly as from smoking. This form of medical marijuana can be just as effective as other forms, but concentrations are not standardized, so it can be a bit harder to provide the correct dose.

•**What is the right dose?** Everyone reacts differently to cannabis, and some strains are more potent than others. If your doctor prescribes cannabis, don't leave the office without detailed instructions—how much to use…how often…and what to expect.

Marijuana also interacts with certain medications you may be taking, such as sedatives, including the tranquilizer *lorazepam* (Ativan) and the sleep drug *zolpidem* (Ambien), so be sure to also discuss all medications you take.

•**What are the risks?** Your motor skills and reaction times will be diminished, particularly within the first few hours. You don't want to drive, operate power tools or engage in other tasks that require serious concentration while the drug is active in your body, which varies widely depending on the person and the strain of cannabis but is typically four to six hours.

•**What about addiction?** Few people who use cannabis for medical purposes will become dependent, develop cravings or go on to abuse other drugs. But the potential for addiction is obviously a concern, just as it is with alcohol and some types of medication. If you have a history of alcoholism or other forms of addic-

tion, talk to your doctor about this before using cannabis.

The US government still classifies cannabis as a Schedule 1 drug—that is, a substance with no medical benefits and a high potential for abuse. Although federal law prohibits the use of medical marijuana, doctors now prescribe it in states where it has been legalized by the state legislatures.

Antibiotic Caution

Martin J. Blaser, MD, director of the Human Microbiome Program in the departments of medicine and microbiology at New York University School of Medicine, New York City. He is author of *Missing Microbes: How the Overuse of Antibiotics Is Fueling Our Modern Plagues*.

Antibiotics are effective at killing bacteria and stopping infections. But they're not very discriminating. Each dose kills many different organisms, including ones that you may need to stay healthy.

In the US, doctors routinely prescribe antibiotics for infections that usually are caused by viruses (which aren't affected by the drugs) or for conditions that usually get better with no treatment.

Antibiotics can be lifesaving drugs. I don't advise people to never take them. But doctors need to prescribe antibiotics more judiciously. *Important…*

•**Don't insist on antibiotics just because you (or your child) has an ear, sinus or upper-respiratory infection.** The vast majority of these infections are caused by viruses. Even when bacteria are to blame, the infections usually clear up on their own. Ask your doctor if he/she is sure that an infection needs to be treated.

•**Ask for a narrow-spectrum drug.** Doctors often prescribe high-powered, broad-spectrum antibiotics (such as the Z-Pak) because they knock out many common infections. But the broad-spectrum drugs also kill more innocent organisms.

•**When possible, it's better to take a narrow-spectrum antibiotic (such as penicil-**

lin) that's less likely to kill beneficial organisms. It's not a perfect solution, because all antibiotics kill multiple strains of bacteria. But "targeted" drugs may be somewhat less likely to cause long-term problems than broad-spectrum antibiotics.

Expired Drugs Are Still Good

Sharon Horesh Bergquist, MD, a physician with the Emory Clinic in Atlanta. She is assistant professor of medicine at Emory University, Atlanta. *EmoryHealthCare.org*

Do not throw away prescription and over-the-counter drugs just because they are past their expiration dates. These dates are not when the drugs will go bad—they are merely the dates beyond which the drugmakers no longer guarantee full potency. While there is a lot of variability among different drugs, drugmakers tend to be overly conservative with these potency guarantees because they don't want to go to the expense of testing drug longevity over longer periods.

A 20-year Food and Drug Administration study found that 88% of the 122 medicines that were properly stored and tested still were perfectly fine a full year after their expiration dates, and the average expiration date could be extended by five-and-a-half years.

Expired drugs do not "spoil" as some expired foods do. There has not been a single confirmed case of an expired medication becoming toxic. The only potential risk from using an expired medication is that the drug might have lost some of its potency. A past-its-use-by-date pain medication might retain only 90% or 95% of its original potency, for example.

But using expired drugs is not worth the risk for lower potency when your life depends on the potency of the medication.

Examples: Replace your EpiPen when it reaches its expiration date if you have a potentially lethal allergy. Replace your nitroglycerine pills when they reach their expiration date if you have them for a serious heart condition.

Store medications in a cool, dry place out of direct sunlight. A bedroom drawer or kitchen cabinet can be a good spot (though not the kitchen cabinet above the stove). Do not store medications in the bathroom, where heat and humidity can reduce their useful life.

Medicine is especially likely to remain effective if it is in tablet or capsule form. Ointments, creams, liquid medications and any medications requiring refrigeration are significantly less likely to remain viable long after their expiration dates.

Dangerous New Painkiller

G. Caleb Alexander, MD, MS, codirector of the Johns Hopkins Center for Drug Safety and Effectiveness, Baltimore. He is a practicing general internist and pharmacoepidemiologist and an ad hoc member of the FDA Drug Safety and Risk Management Advisory Committee. *jhsph.edu/cdse*

The Food and Drug Administration (FDA) recently approved a new painkiller called *Zohydro ER* (hydrocodone extended-release), even though its own expert advisory committee voted 11 to two against it.

Zohydro ER is the first hydrocodone therapy without acetaminophen and thus has a lower risk for liver injury. But Zohydro ER and its fellow "opioid" painkillers are extremely addictive, even compared with other pain medications. Opioids caused more than 16,600 overdose deaths in the US in 2010—that's more than 75% of the total number of deaths from pharmaceutical drugs. In fact, it's more than 43% of all overdose deaths, including those from illegal drugs—and Zohydro ER is even more powerful than most of the previous opioids on the market.

Patients can build up a tolerance to opioids over time, diminishing the drugs' effectiveness. Some patients even develop opioid-induced hyperalgesia, a condition that causes opioids to increase pain rather than reduce it. And opioids can have unpleasant side effects including constipation and drowsiness.

Opioids can be a painkilling option for a short-term problem, such as after the removal of wisdom teeth—and some patients have chronic and debilitating pain, making opioids a reasonable choice. But opioids should be prescribed only as a last resort.

Common Cold Meds May Pose Health Threats

Hartley Atkinson, PhD, managing director, AFT Pharmaceuticals Ltd., Auckland, New Zealand.

Victoria Richards, PhD, associate professor of medical science, School of Medicine, Quinnipiac University, North Haven, Connecticut.

Frank H. Netter, MD, School of Medicine, Quinnipiac University, North Haven, Connecticut.

Houman Danesh, MD, director, Integrative Pain Management, Icahn School of Medicine at Mount Sinai, New York City.

Andrea Fischer, spokeswoman, U.S. Food and Drug Administration.

Jodie Wertheim, spokeswoman, McNeil Consumer Healthcare.

New England Journal of Medicine.

Over-the-counter sinus and pain remedies that combine two common ingredients—*phenylephrine* and *acetaminophen*—might cause serious side effects such as high blood pressure, dizziness and tremors, New Zealand researchers warn.

These side effects occur because acetaminophen (the main ingredient in Tylenol) boosts the effects of phenylephrine, according to a report in a March 2014 issue of the *New England Journal of Medicine.*

Products containing this drug combination include Tylenol Sinus, Sudafed PE Sinus, Benadryl Allergy Plus Sinus and Excedrin Sinus Headache.

"What we found was surprising because it hasn't been studied or reported," said lead researcher Hartley Atkinson, PhD, managing director of AFT Pharmaceuticals, Ltd., in Auckland.

Phenylephrine, which replaced pseudoephedrine in many over-the-counter medications, relieves nasal congestion from colds, allergies and hay fever. *Pseudoephedrine* had become a source for creating the illegal drug methamphetamine, and the U.S. Food and Drug Administration asked manufacturers to voluntarily remove it from their products.

When phenylephrine is combined with acetaminophen, blood levels of phenylephrine rise to four times higher than when the same amount of phenylephrine is used alone, Dr. Atkinson said.

"Basically, if you give the combination, a lot more phenylephrine absorbs into your body

Painkillers Linked to Blood Clots

A meta-analysis of six studies of *venous thromboembolism*—a type of clot that includes deep vein thrombosis and pulmonary embolism—showed an 80% higher clot risk in people who use *naproxen, ibuprofen* and other nonsteroidal anti-inflammatory drugs (NSAIDs) compared with nonusers. For patients known to have increased risk for venous thromboembolism because of genetic factors or extended immobility, *acetaminophen* may be a safer pain reliever. Talk to your doctor.

Patompong Ungprasert, MD, an instructor in the department of rheumatology at Mayo Clinic, Rochester, Minnesota, and leader of an analysis published online in *Rheumatology.*

than what you would be expecting," Dr. Atkinson said.

Side effects can also include insomnia, headache, heart palpitations, anxiety and urine retention.

Dr. Atkinson noted that labels on products containing phenylephrine warn of possible side effects for people with heart disease or prostate problems. These warnings, however, refer only to the dose of phenylephrine approved for that product.

People with these conditions need to know that in actuality the dose might be higher, he said.

Similar increases in phenylephrine levels might occur with drugs that contain vitamin C, which is metabolized in the same way as acetaminophen.

"In a lot of countries, there are drugs that contain acetaminophen, phenylephrine and vitamin C together, which could cause an even greater interaction," Dr. Atkinson said.

HOW THE ADVERSE REACTIONS WERE FOUND

Dr. Atkinson stumbled upon this drug interaction while developing a new drug containing acetaminophen, *ibuprofen* (the main ingredient in Advil) and phenylephrine. Ibuprofen does not cause harmful side effects when combined with phenylephrine, he said.

This drug interaction is a problem regulatory agencies need to consider, Dr. Atkinson said.

EXPERT COMMENT

Another expert agreed the findings are worrisome.

"This article sheds light on a previously unknown reaction of acetaminophen with phenylephrine, which essentially raises the possibility of an overdose with a single dose," said Houman Danesh, MD, director of integrative pain management at the Icahn School of Medicine at Mount Sinai, in New York City.

"Taking medications which contain ibuprofen with phenylephrine may be safer with regards to phenylephrine toxicity," Dr. Danesh said. "However, ibuprofen has increased risks of stomach ulcers, kidney issues and heart issues as well. So, once again, consult with your doctor."

INDUSTRY RESPONSE

The FDA is aware of the problem, but agency spokeswoman Andrea Fischer said it has limited ability to regulate.

"Both phenylephrine and pseudoephedrine are generally recognized as safe and effective and may be marketed without premarket approval by the FDA," Fischer said.

Likewise, it's permissible to combine either nasal decongestant with acetaminophen, she said.

According to McNeil Consumer Healthcare, the Johnson & Johnson subsidiary that makes some of these dual-ingredient remedies, combination acetaminophen-phenylephrine drugs are safe.

"Based upon clinical studies, years of use and post-marketing surveillance, we believe over-the-counter doses of acetaminophen and phenylephrine, when taken together, are considered safe," said Jodie Wertheim, a McNeil spokeswoman.

"When used as directed, over-the-counter medicines containing acetaminophen and phenylephrine are both effective and well-tolerated," she added.

Not everyone is convinced, however.

"Consumers should look at the labels arefully and talk with the pharmacist or with their doctor to understand exactly what they're taking," said Victoria Richards, PhD, an associate professor of medical sciences at the Frank H. Netter MD School of Medicine at Quinnipiac University in North Haven, Connecticut.

info Learn more about phenylephrine from the U.S. National Library of Medicine at *http://www.nlm.nih.gov/medlineplus/druginformation.html.*

Men's Health

The Real Truth About Testosterone

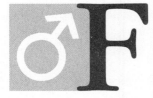

For many men, it's the holy grail: A treatment that promises to beef up their muscles…rev up their sex drive…improve their stamina and concentration…and perhaps even help prevent a heart attack.

So it's no surprise that prescriptions for testosterone shots, gels and patches have nearly quadrupled over the last decade. About 3% of American men over age 40 now use testosterone therapy.

But is it safe? The answer to this crucial question depends on many factors that aren't clearly spelled out in the slick advertising—and, in some cases, even by the doctors who prescribe testosterone therapy.

What every man needs to know about testosterone therapy…

HOW THE RESEARCH STACKS UP

Testosterone is manufactured by the body and plays a key role in a man's health. It helps maintain his bone density…builds his muscles…allows him to produce sperm…and fuels his libido.

A man's testosterone levels start to decline, however, after age 30—usually by about 1% a year. This is not an illness—it's a fact of aging. If a man's testosterone drops farther than normal, though, it can cause fatigue, reduced sex drive, an increase in fat and a decrease in muscle. Some research suggests that low testosterone may also increase a man's odds of having a heart attack, diabetes and other serious health problems.

No wonder so many men are turning to testosterone therapy, which drug companies are now marketing in successful "low T" ads. The problem is, however, that many doctors are growing increasingly concerned that men

Peter J. Burrows, MD, a practicing urologist in Tucson and a clinical assistant professor of urology at The University of Arizona College of Medicine, also in Tucson.

Testosterone Testing Can Be Done Until 2 PM

Current guidelines call for men who suffer from erectile dysfunction to have their testosterone levels tested between 8 am and 11 am, when levels usually are highest.

But: A recent study has found that men over age 45 can be tested up until 2 pm. Only younger men showed a clinically significant decrease earlier in the day and should be tested as close to 7 am as possible.

Study of 2,569 men, ages 26 to 84, by researchers at Southern Illinois University School of Medicine, Springfield, published in *The Journal of Urology*.

whose testosterone levels are simply declining are loading up on the hormone, perhaps to the detriment of their health. Adding to those worries is recent research raising new questions about the safety of testosterone therapy.

Troubling recent finding: In research published in *The Journal of the American Medical Association*, men using testosterone had nearly a one-third increase in the rate of heart attacks and stroke.

Of course, this research doesn't prove that testosterone increases cardiovascular risks. Other studies have shown the opposite—that men with higher testosterone may have fewer heart attacks. So what's going on? It's possible that the underlying low testosterone, rather than the treatment, was the cause of the increased heart attack risk. It's also possible that men who start testosterone feel so much better that they overextend themselves and get more exercise—and sex—than their hearts can handle.

For now, there is no clear explanation for the mixed research findings—that's why it's so important to use caution when considering testosterone therapy.

WHO CAN BENEFIT?

Even with these new safety questions, it's widely agreed that men who meet the clinical criteria for low testosterone need hormone replacement—the benefits outweigh the risks. But what about men whose testosterone levels

are waning but do not meet that criteria? That's where it gets more complicated.

Researchers still argue over what testosterone level is "normal." When they test men of different ages, they find levels ranging from the low-300s to as high as 1,000 (expressed in nanograms per deciliter—ng/dL—of blood). The cutoff points between "healthy" and "deficient" are somewhat arbitrary. They're based on averages, not optimal levels.

For now, testosterone replacement is FDA-approved only for men with a clinical deficiency—currently defined as testosterone levels below 300 ng/dL. This condition (hypogonadism) is usually caused by problems in the testicles or the pituitary gland—both play a role in regulating a man's testosterone levels.

PLAY IT SAFE

For a reasoned approach to testosterone therapy, here's my advice…

• **Don't automatically blame testosterone.** The drop in testosterone in older men isn't caused only by their age. It can be due to chronic diseases, such as high blood pressure and kidney disease. Painkillers can cause it, too. (About three-quarters of men who take long-acting opioids, such as extended-release *oxycodone*, develop very low testosterone.) Stress is also a factor.

Bottom line: Consider using testosterone only after other health problems have been addressed—and corrected.

Obesity and a sedentary lifestyle are common causes of low testosterone. Overweight men who exercise and lose weight can increase testosterone naturally by up to 25%—in some cases preventing the need for hormone replacement.

• **Take the test.** If your doctor has ruled out any physical ailment that may be causing symptoms, get your testosterone level tested (both total and free levels). Low testosterone is easily diagnosed with a blood test. Have the test early in the day, when testosterone levels tend to be highest. If your level is low, ask your doctor to repeat the test on another day, since levels can vary.

• **Get your heart checked out.** If your testosterone level is low, don't start replacement therapy without getting your heart checked out with a stress test, complete blood count (CBC) and tests for cholesterol and high blood pressure. Any cardiac condition that shows up on these tests must be resolved before beginning testosterone therapy.

Even though the research is not yet definitive, there are enough studies linking testosterone use to heart attack and other cardiovascular problems—especially in men with risk factors for heart disease, including smoking and obesity—that it's not worth taking a chance on this.

•**Use the right dose.** Since a man's optimal testosterone level is still not clearly defined, I advise a conservative approach. When choosing a dose, I try to get patients' blood levels within the upper one-fourth of the range generally recommended by endocrinologists—say, about 750 ng/dL—but no higher.

Different forms of supplemental testosterone are equally effective. Injections are the cheapest, but they must be repeated every 10 to 14 days. Most men learn how to administer the shots themselves.

Patches are another option, although some men don't like them, since they can trigger a rash. Testosterone gels and creams are the easiest to use, but they're expensive—and the medication can transfer to other people through skin-to-skin contact. They're usually applied to the shoulders or upper arms.

Testosterone-Suppression Therapy for Prostate Cancer

Testosterone-suppression therapy does not help early-stage prostate cancer. The treatment, called primary androgen deprivation therapy (ADT), does not extend these patients' lives, and it has significant side effects, including impotence, diabetes and bone loss. Primary ADT is appropriate only for men with very aggressive prostate cancer as shown by a PSA greater than 50 or a PSA score that doubles in less than 12 months.

Grace L. Lu-Yao, PhD, MPH, a cancer epidemiologist at Rutgers Cancer Institute of New Jersey and professor of medicine, Robert Wood Johnson Medical School, New Brunswick, New Jersey. She led a study published in *JAMA Internal Medicine*.

•**Go for checkups.** For anyone on testosterone therapy, it's crucial to get regular checkups. I advise men to get their testosterone levels checked at three months, then every six months. After that, if they're doing well, they can come in once a year for testing of lipid levels and liver function (testosterone can affect both). I also order tests every six months to monitor a man's red blood cell (RBC) counts—testosterone increases RBC levels, which can boost his risk for blood clots.

Other tests you'll need: A prostate specific antigen (PSA) test to check for prostate cancer every six months. Testosterone replacement doesn't cause prostate cancer, but it can cause tumors that are already present to grow more rapidly. Men with untreated prostate cancer should not take testosterone. However, testosterone can be given to those who have been successfully treated for prostate cancer. Studies show it does not trigger cancer recurrence.

In general, men who have low testosterone will feel better within a month after starting testosterone therapy. Optimal testosterone levels should help with weight loss and can boost natural production of the hormone—so many men find that they no longer need treatment.

5 Things That Can Ruin a Man's Sex Life

Steven Lamm, MD, medical director of the Preston Robert Tisch Center for Men's Health at New York University Langone Medical Center. He is coauthor of *The Hardness Factor: How to Achieve Your Best Health and Sexual Fitness at Any Age. DrStevenLamm.com*

An erection is a manly miracle—a complex, coordinated effort of brain, blood vessels, nerves, muscles and hormones that increases blood flow to the penis sixfold. But because so much has to go right for a man to have an erection, there's also a lot that can go wrong.

The problem is called erectile dysfunction (ED)—the inability to get or sustain an erection hard enough to have enjoyable and satisfying sex. And it's a very common problem. Nearly

Medication May Blunt Love

Sexual dysfunction is a well-known side effect of long-term antidepressant use, but a recent study shows that these drugs may actually stifle feelings of love and attachment toward partners, especially among men. The effect was stronger for men taking selective serotonin reuptake inhibitors (SSRIs), such as *paroxetine* (Paxil) and *escitalopram* (Lexapro), than for those taking tricyclic antidepressants, such as *clomipramine* (Anafranil).

Donatella Marazziti, MD, professor of psychiatry, University of Pisa, Italy.

one in five men have ED, including 44% of men ages 60 to 69 and 70% of men 70 and older.

A prescription ED drug such as *sildenafil* (Viagra), *vardenafil* (Levitra) or *tadalafil* (Cialis) can help. But this pharmaceutical solution isn't necessarily the best solution, because ED drugs don't address the underlying causes of ED—some of which can kill you.

What most men don't realize: An erection is the best barometer of a man's overall health—particularly the health of his circulatory system. The easier it is to achieve erections, the healthier the man. By identifying and correcting the factors that might be undermining erections, a man not only can restore his sex life—he might save his life.

Here, five factors that can ruin a man's sex life and what to do about them…

HEART DISEASE

An artery leads directly to the penis and subdivides into three more arteries, supplying the robust flow of blood on which an erection depends. If those arteries are narrowed or blocked, it's likely that there's a problem with all your arteries—including the arteries supplying blood to your heart.

Troubling recent finding: A decade-long study published in *Journal of Sexual Medicine* shows that men over age 50 with ED are 2.5 times more likely to develop heart disease, and men under age 50 are 58% more likely. And a study of men with ED who were already diagnosed with heart disease shows that they are twice as likely to have a heart attack and 90% more likely to die of heart disease, compared with men who have heart disease but not ED.

What to do: Eat a Mediterranean diet, emphasizing vegetables, fruits, whole grains, beans, fish and healthy fats (in olive oil, avocado and nuts). It's a diet proven to prevent and treat heart disease—and several studies from Italy show that a Mediterranean diet also can prevent and cure ED.

Other conditions that increase the risk for ED: Type 2 diabetes, obesity, gout and sleep apnea—and studies show that these conditions also are helped with a Mediterranean diet.

Important: If you have ED, make an appointment with your doctor, tell him/her about your problem and ask for a complete workup to check for cardiovascular disease.

ALCOHOL

Alcohol is a central nervous system depressant, and despite what many people think, it dampens sexual arousal—and that's particularly true for older men.

What to do: Limit yourself to no more than one to two drinks per day. (A drink is one 12-ounce beer, a four-ounce glass of wine, 1.5 ounces of 80-proof spirits or one ounce of 100-proof spirits.)

What not to do: Washing down fried foods with beer (or any alcohol) is a double whammy. Eating fried food immediately spikes the level of blood fats such as triglycerides, impeding blood flow to the penis for several hours.

MEDICATIONS

ED can be a side effect of taking one or more prescription medicines. The most common offenders are drugs to treat high blood pressure, heart ailments, depression and allergies.

Telltale sign: You start a new medication, and you suddenly notice that you're having erectile difficulties.

What to do: Talk to your doctor about using a different medication to treat your health problem. For example, one class of antidepressants (selective serotonin reuptake inhibitors, or SSRIs) often leads to libido issues and ejaculation problems contributing to ED, but the antidepressant *bupropion* (Wellbutrin) rarely does.

LACK OF EXERCISE

Regular exercise lowers your heart rate and blood pressure and helps clear life-threatening plaque from arteries—all of which translates into preventing or reversing ED.

Important recent finding: A recent study in *Journal of Sexual Medicine* found that men who have risk factors for heart disease were 50% more likely to suffer from ED if they did not exercise regularly. Another study shows that exercise can improve ED even in men who are already taking a drug for ED.

What to do: Walk! It is a proven way to prevent and treat ED. When researchers from Duke University studied men with an average age of 62, they found that those who walked briskly for 30 minutes, four days a week, were 66% less likely to have ED.

STRESS

Too much stress can undermine erections by slowing the production of hormones (including testosterone, the master male hormone) and by impeding blood flow to the penis.

What to do: The best way to reduce stress is to spend at least 20 to 30 minutes a day doing something you personally enjoy—whether it's watching your favorite comedian on Netflix, participating in a hobby such as woodworking or going for a walk with your dog.

When Sex Is Over Too Quickly

Steven Lamm, MD, medical director of the Preston Robert Tisch Center for Men's Health at New York University Langone Medical Center. He is coauthor of The *Hardness Factor: How to Achieve Your Best Health and Sexual Fitness at Any Age. DrStevenLamm.com*

When it comes to men's sex lives, we hear a lot about erectile dysfunction (ED). But another condition—premature ejaculation (PE)—affects even more men.

Recent research: While PE has traditionally been considered a man's problem, a recent study found that it can also distress his sex partner—almost one-quarter of women reported that the issue had led to a relationship breakup, largely because the men were so focused on their own sexual performance that they neglected their partners.

WHAT'S NORMAL?

Studies show that most men ejaculate after about five minutes of sexual intercourse.

When it's a problem: Even though most men occasionally finish more quickly than they would like—after a long period of abstinence, for example, or from the excitement of being with a new partner—it's called premature ejaculation only under certain circumstances. This includes when the man usually ejaculates within one minute of penetration (or before penetration occurs)…the man is unable to delay even when he tries…and/or he is frustrated by the inability to last longer and it causes distress.

As long as men and their partners are satisfied with their sex lives, there's nothing to worry about. But, because of PE, many men struggle with a sense of failure and inadequacy.

GET CHECKED

Few men will admit to sexual problems, even to their doctors…and doctors often don't ask. But if you have PE and are bothered by it, tell your doctor. PE can always be treated. Some men just need help coping with anxiety. Others have

Happy Statin Side Effect

Statins can boost sexual performance in men with erectile dysfunction (ED) who are taking the drugs to reduce cholesterol. Erectile function scores were 24% better in men taking statin medications than in men not using them. Statins may improve erectile function by helping blood vessels dilate properly and boosting blood flow to the penis.

Analysis of 11 clinical trials involving a total of 647 people by researchers at Robert Wood Johnson Medical School, Rutgers University, New Brunswick, New Jersey, published in *Journal of Sexual Medicine*.

unrealistic expectations. Some men have a lifelong problem with PE, while others develop it later in life. PE can also be caused by medical issues, including a hormone imbalance (such as hyperthyroidism), infection/inflammation of the prostate gland, genetic factors or even ED. (With ED, men fear losing the erection and ejaculate prematurely.)

Also: Some men as they age may have delayed ejaculations. They may be unable to ejaculate during intercourse or for several hours or days afterward. Side effects from medication, especially for depression, can increase time between ejaculations as well.

WHAT HELPS

If your doctor has ruled out any physical causes for PE, there are simple steps you can take that may improve or reverse PE. *You may want to try these strategies before considering medication...*

•**Wear a condom.** Even if you don't need condoms for contraception or disease prevention, they reduce sensation for some men who are hypersensitive and can help you last longer.

•**Pause and squeeze.** This form of behavioral training can help men recognize the feelings of impending ejaculation before it's too late to stop. It doesn't work for all men, but it's worth a try.

What to do: During sex (or masturbation), stop the stimulating movements before you're ready to ejaculate. Squeeze the top of the penis where the head meets the shaft to stop the urge to ejaculate. Keep squeezing for several seconds.

Wait about 30 seconds, then resume the activity—and stop-squeeze again when you feel you're getting close. Keep doing it until you're ready to finish. Your partner can also do it as part of foreplay. With practice, you can develop the "habit" of lasting longer.

•**Try a topical anesthetic.** You can apply over-the-counter numbing sprays or creams (such as Promescent) to the penis. They have topical anesthetics that reduce sensation and delay ejaculation.

Don't overdo it when using these products. Reducing sensation can make it more difficult to sustain an erection. Also, some of the numbing

agent can be transferred to your partner, which reduces her sensations. But a topical anesthetic does work for some men.

•**Try different positions.** Some sexual positions are more stimulating than others. In general, the man-on-top position produces the most friction and stimulation. You might last longer with other positions—say, with the woman on top. In this position, you can use your hands and pelvis to guide her body into angles and movements that are less stimulating to the most sensitive parts of your penis.

•**Psychotherapy may also help improve sexual skills,** increase self-confidence and improve self-esteem—all of which can ease PE.

MEDICATIONS THAT HELP

Some men can learn to delay ejaculation with the behavioral and sexual techniques mentioned earlier, but it may take time and practice. The reality is, many men find medication to be more effective. Your urologist or internist can help you decide which is best for you.

•**Antidepressants.** The selective serotonin reuptake inhibitor (SSRI) antidepressants, such as *sertraline* (Zoloft) and *paroxetine* (Paxil), aren't FDA-approved for PE, but doctors often prescribe them "off-label" for this condition.

These drugs' sexual side effects, including reduced libido and delayed ejaculation, can help men with PE. Studies have shown that men who take these drugs can last anywhere from about four to eight times longer.

The doses prescribed for PE are lower than those used for depression, so other side effects

---

Kegel Exercises for Men

Kegel exercises are not just for women. Pelvic floor exercise can help treat incontinence and sexual dysfunction in men. Pelvic muscles, like all muscles, weaken with age. To strengthen them, men should tighten the muscles used to cut off the flow of urine midstream. Hold the contraction for a few seconds, then release. Repeat the exercise 10 to 15 times for each set.

Andrew L. Siegel, MD, urologist, Bergen Urological Associates, Hackensack, New Jersey, and author of a paper about Kegel exercises for men, published in *Urology*.

(such as mouth dryness and sometimes nausea) are usually minor and tend to disappear within a few weeks.

•**PDE-5 inhibitors,** such as *sildenafil* (Viagra) and *tadalafil* (Cialis), do more than help with erections. They also appear to help men with PE. These medications increase levels of nitric oxide, a blood gas that dilates blood vessels and increases blood flow to the penis. At high levels, nitric oxide inhibits ejaculation. A man with a firmer, more reliable erection also tends to be more confident and less likely to rush through sex.

Some men find that taking both a PDE-5 inhibitor and an SSRI antidepressant works best. One study found that men who used both medications increased their intercourse time to more than three minutes from less than one minute. However, PDE-5 inhibitors can cause headaches, nausea and other side effects and should not be taken with medications that contain nitrates, alpha-blockers or *cimetidine* (Tagamet).

The Truth About Sexual-Enhancement Herbs for Men

Laurie Steelsmith, ND, LAc, licensed naturopathic physician and acupuncturist in private practice in Honolulu. Dr. Steelsmith is coauthor, with her husband Alex Steelsmith, of *Great Sex, Naturally: Every Woman's Guide to Enhancing Her Sexuality Through the Secrets of Natural Medicine. DrLaurieSteelsmith.com*

Herbal supplements might seem like a good idea if you are a man who is having "trouble" in the bedroom. They're easy to buy—locally or online—and you don't have to discuss this embarrassing problem with your doctor.

Or maybe you think these natural products are safer than Viagra or other pharmaceuticals and may, in fact, have health benefits that go beyond improving your sex life.

But…some of the most common herbs for male sexual enhancement have been bashed by the medical establishment—yohimbe, maca, horny goat weed and even ginkgo biloba.

Alcohol Lowers Sperm Count

Alcohol lowers sperm count. The more alcohol younger men drink, the lower their sperm count. Men who consumed 40 or more drinks a week had sperm concentrations 33% lower than men who consumed five drinks a week.

Study of more than 1,200 men, ages 18 to 28, led by researchers at University of Southern Denmark, Odense, published in BMJ Open.

How much weight should you give that news? First, let's examine what's being said about male sexual-enhancement herbs. Then let naturopathic sex-health and Traditional Chinese Medicine expert Laurie Steelsmith, ND, LAc, reveal the real dos, don'ts and dangers of these herbs.

THE DANGER OF SEXY SUPPLEMENTS

A recent article by a team of British and Italian researchers said that the business of selling herbal supplements for male sexual enhancement—or dysfunction—is a major health hazard. Because these supplements are marketed as "natural," many consumers assume that they are safe. In fact, they can cause serious side effects in some users.

In their exposé, the researchers focused on supplements that contained four herbs commonly used to treat male sexual dysfunction—yohimbe, maca, horny goat weed and ginkgo biloba. In brief, they concluded that all of these herbs were linked to dangerous side effects, including cardiovascular problems, mood swings, anxiety, hallucinations and addictive behavior.

Dr. Steelsmith, however, believes that these researchers have been overly harsh. "They are making herbs, such as ginkgo, out to be radical villains, which they are not," she said, adding that ginkgo and maca have long-term safety records. She also said that horny goat weed is safe when used according to the principles of Traditional Chinese Medicine. But she agreed that the researchers made some good points about yohimbe, which can cause high blood pressure, dangerously low blood pressure, increased heart rate and palpitations, breathing difficulties, headaches and anxiety among other symptoms. "It is a potentially dangerous herb.

Unlike the other herbs discussed, I don't think it should be sold over the counter, but certain formulations of the herb can be used with medical supervision," she said.

PRACTICE
"SAFE SEX SUPPLEMENTS"

Most common sex-enhancement herbs are safe and effective when used correctly, said Dr. Steelsmith, who is coauthor of the book *Great Sex, Naturally*. Rather than self-treating, it is best to consult a naturopathic doctor or similarly trained professional who can properly diagnose your health concern and treat you with specially compounded herbal extracts and extracts from high-quality professional-grade manufacturers. *Here are her expert thoughts on the sex-boosting herbs mentioned in the British-Italian study…*

•**Yohimbe.** Rather than use over-the-counter extracts, always consult a naturopathic doctor if you want to try yohimbe. Dr. Steelsmith reserves such treatment for patients who are in good health but have erectile dysfunction that does not respond to other less potentially toxic remedies. If yohimbe is right for you, a naturopath will treat you with a prescription form of the herb called alpha yohimbine HCl, said Dr. Steelsmith. The naturopath will monitor you while you take yohimbe to make sure that the dosage is optimal and side effects are kept at bay. Men with kidney problems or psychological issues should not take or be treated with this herb.

•**Horny goat weed.** This herb is useful for men who have decreased libido, a slow metabolism and chronically cold hands and feet. In Traditional Chinese Medicine, horny goat weed is never prescribed on its own but rather in combination with herbs that support its ability to boost sexual energy while preventing side effects of overstimulation, said Dr. Steelsmith. Because horny goat weed can act as a stimulant, it is not for you if you suffer from insomnia or anxiety symptoms. Dr. Steelsmith also does not recommend it's use in people who are on blood-thinning medications.

Important: Make sure that the herbal extract prescribed by the naturopath is a standardized extract that contains at least 20% of the active compound icariin.

•**Maca.** This Peruvian herb, traditionally used to increase male sexual potency and endurance, enhances male fertility, said Dr. Steelsmith. It increases sperm production and renders those critters into super-triathlete swimmers (it keeps them strongly mobile, that is). So if a man is ready to start a family, Dr. Steelsmith often prescribes maca. It is generally safe, but be aware that it can increase blood pressure, an issue that you should discuss with the naturopath, especially if you already have high blood pressure.

•**Ginkgo biloba.** Besides boosting memory and cognitive function, ginkgo biloba can boost libido and enhance sexual performance. It is especially useful in both men as well as women who are suffering sexual dysfunction as a side effect of antidepressant medication, said Dr. Steelsmith. A word of caution, though…ginkgo is a natural blood thinner and can interact with blood-thinning drugs as well as other drugs that are broken down by the liver (and most are)—so if you are on a blood thinner or any other type of medication or supplement, ginkgo biloba may not be the right herb for you. This aside, Dr. Steelsmith said that it is safe at the dosages that naturopaths use to treat erectile dysfunction. The product prescribed should be a standardized extract of 24% ginkgo flavone glycosides.

Beside these herbs mentioned in the alarming Brit-Italian study, Dr. Steelsmith treats patients with *Tribulus terrestris*, which acts similarly to DHEA, an essential building block of estrogen and testosterone that can help keep you young and fit. The extract should contain 45% of the active ingredient protodioscin. It is especially

Circumcision for Cancer?

In a recent study, men circumcised after age 35 were 45% less likely to develop prostate cancer than uncircumcised men. The reason is unknown, but the link was most apparent in black men, who have higher rates of the disease than white men.

University of Montreal.

useful in men whose low sex drive is attributed to low testosterone, said Dr. Steelsmith. The herb may support testosterone production. Dr. Steelsmith cautioned that lithium and diabetes drugs can interact with this herb, so anyone taking those medications is not a candidate for use of this herb.

MORE THAN JUST SEX

Before grabbing any herb or drug to fix a sexual-performance problem, it's wise to reflect on the underlying cause of the problem and make the necessary lifestyle changes, said Dr. Steelsmith. Are you stressed or sleep-deprived? Anxious or depressed? Is a physical health condition getting in the way of good sex? Treating the root cause may solve your sexual dysfunction without any other measures.

Viagra Linked to Melanoma Skin Cancer Risk

From study titled "Sildenafil Use and Increased Risk of Incident Melanoma in US Men: A Prospective Cohort Study," published in *JAMA Internal Medicine.*

When the drug *sildenafil* (Viagra) was approved for the treatment of erectile dysfunction (ED) in 1998, the "little blue pill" quickly became the punch line of many a joke on late-night television. It also became big business, with billions of dollars in sales per year.

Melanoma, the deadly form of skin cancer, has big numbers, too. It's the eighth most common cancer diagnosis…and it kills nearly 10,000 people in the US each year.

What do Viagra and similar drugs have to do with melanoma, you may wonder? Perhaps quite a lot, according to the latest research. *Here's what men need to know to protect themselves…*

GOOD FOR SEX, BAD FOR SKIN

Researchers used data from the Health Professionals' Follow-up Study that began back in 1986 when nearly 52,000 male health professionals completed a questionnaire on their medical history and lifestyle practices. The men were between 40 and 75 years old at the beginning of the study. Then, every two years thereafter, participants updated their info using additional questionnaires.

In 2000, cancer-free participants were asked whether they had ever been treated for erectile problems and whether they had used sildenafil. (Other ED drugs that work in similar ways were not approved until 2003, so they weren't included in this analysis.) The study also gathered data on the men's known skin cancer risk factors—number of moles, natural hair color, history of blistering sunburns, places of residence (to assess ultraviolet light exposure), family history of melanoma, etc. Of the nearly 26,000 men who completed this questionnaire, 5.3% reported taking sildenafil for ED in the previous few months and 6.3% reported having used it at any time.

Then, tracking the men until 2010, the researchers found that 142 participants developed melanoma and 3,610 developed nonmelanoma skin cancer. *After adjusting for the effects of various known melanoma risk factors, the researchers discovered that…*

• **Use of sildenafil at any time was associated with 92% increased risk for melanoma,** while recent use was associated with an 84% increased risk, compared with men who did not use the drug at all.

• **There was no difference in risk for nonmelanoma skin cancers** (such as squamous cell and basal cell skin cancer) between the men who had used the ED drug and those who had not. Given that certain factors such as sun exposure affect a person's risk for all three main types of skin cancer, the lack of any link between the nonmelanoma skin cancers and ED medication suggests that the drug has some detrimental effect with regard to melanoma specifically.

• **When participants who had diabetes,** high blood pressure or heart disease were excluded (since these conditions can affect sexual function), the association between sildenafil use and melanoma was even more pronounced. Compared with men who never used the ED

Stop Getting Up at Night

• **Big bellies mean more trips to the bathroom.** According to recent research, the health habits of 409 men with moderate or severe lower urinary tract symptoms, such as urgent urination, were studied for two-and-a-half years.

Result: 39% of men with the largest waists (greater than 39.3 inches) urinated more than eight times in a 24-hour period, compared with 27% of men with 35- to 39.3-inch waists. The average man urinates no more than seven times a day.

Theory: Large waist size increases risk for pelvic dysfunction, including frequent urination—and erection and ejaculation difficulties.

Steven Kaplan, MD, professor of urology, Weill Cornell Medical College, New York City.

• **Going too much at night may be a sign of something else.** Frequent trips to the bathroom at night may indicate diabetes or heart failure for both men and women. Try limiting beverages close to bedtime. If that doesn't help, keep a diary for three days, noting all of the times you urinate. If one-third or more of your bathroom trips occur at night, talk to your doctor.

Tiffany Sotelo, MD, assistant professor of urology, George Washington University School of Medicine & Health Sciences, Washington, DC, quoted in *Woman's Day.*

• **Do this once a week for better prostate control.** Men who exercised just one hour a week had a 13% reduction in the need to get up twice or more during the night to urinate, according to a recent study of men with benign prostatic hyperplasia (BPH). More exercise provided even greater benefit.

Why: Exercise helps curb inflammation (a factor in BPH).

Kate Wolin, ScD, associate professor of surgery, Loyola University Chicago Stritch School of Medicine.

drug, recent users had a 2.24 times higher risk for melanoma, while those who had ever used it had a 2.77 times higher risk.

• **No association was found between ED itself and increased melanoma risk…**meaning that the drug, rather than the condition the drug was meant to treat, appeared to be responsible for the link.

WHAT'S THE CONNECTION?

Sildenafil and the other ED drugs approved later on—*tadalafil* (Cialis) and *vardenafil* (Levitra)—work by inhibiting an enzyme called PDE5A. That then leads to other changes that allow smooth muscle relaxation, improved blood flow and, voilà, penile erection. That same enzyme, however, also would normally work against melanoma cell proliferation, especially in the 50% of melanoma tumors that are fueled by a particular genetic mutation. In other words, by taking ED drugs that target PDE5A, men may be opening a chemical pathway that allows melanoma cells to flourish.

This study does not prove that ED drugs cause melanoma…and it was not designed to address questions about medication dosages, cumulative effects of long-term use or the relative risks of the various types of ED drugs. But clearly, men should now be on alert about this risk, and more research is needed—especially considering the fact that melanoma rates are increasing most rapidly in men over age 50…the same group that is most likely to use ED medication.

If you have taken or are considering taking any ED medication: Talk to your doctor about how to weigh the benefits against the potential dangers, including an increased risk for melanoma…discuss the lifestyle changes and alternative treatments that can improve sexual function without drugs…and be especially sure to get regular whole-body skin checkups from your dermatologist.

Male Breast Cancer Is Different

Fatima Cardoso, MD, director of the breast unit at the Champalimaud Cancer Center, Lisbon, Portugal.

Christopher Pezzi, MD, director of surgical oncology, Abington Memorial Hospital, Abington, Pennsylvania.

Courtney Vito, MD, assistant clinical professor of breast and surgical oncology, City of Hope Cancer Center, Duarte, California.

San Antonio Breast Cancer Symposium, presentation.

Men's breast cancer differs in some ways from women's, recent research finds.

One important difference is in the rates of survival. The study found that while survival for men with breast cancer has improved, it hasn't kept pace with the strides made in treating breast cancer in women.

"Although we saw a significant improvement in overall survival for male breast cancer patients over time, the prognosis for men with breast cancer has not been improving as much as for women with the disease," Fatima Cardoso, MD, director of the breast unit at the Champalimaud Cancer Center in Lisbon, Portugal, said in a news release from the American Association for Cancer Research.

"This is largely because male breast cancer is a rare disease—it accounts for just 1% of breast cancers—and we know very little about its biology and how best to treat patients," Dr. Cardoso said.

STUDY DETAILS

In the recent study, Dr. Cardoso and her team followed more than 1,800 men with breast cancer. The men were diagnosed between 1990 and 2010 and they were treated at 23 medical centers in nine countries. The average age of men at diagnosis was almost 69 years old, the study reported.

The researchers found that only 77% of men got endocrine therapy such as *tamoxifen* for their cancer when it was indicated. They also found that even though 56% of the cancers were diagnosed when the tumors were very small, only 4% of the men had breast-conserving surgery. Most had a mastectomy, Dr. Cardoso found.

Most of the men, 92%, had cancer known as estrogen receptor positive, the kind that requires estrogen to grow. In women, 70% of breast cancers are ER-positive.

Far fewer of the men's cancers were of the types known as HER2 and triple negative, which occur in women, the researchers found.

After a follow-up of nearly six years on more than 1,000 men, 63% were still alive, according to the study.

Dr. Cardoso presented the study's findings at the 2014 San Antonio Breast Cancer Symposium. The symposium is a partnership of the University of Texas Health Science Center, the American Association for Cancer Research and Baylor College of Medicine.

Studies presented at medical meetings are generally viewed as preliminary until published in a peer-reviewed medical journal.

EXPERT COMMENT

The study conclusions ring true, said Courtney Vito, MD, assistant clinical professor of breast and surgical oncology at City of Hope Cancer Center in Duarte, California. Vito has conducted similar research and says the recent findings echo many of her findings.

"The problem is, men tend to seek medical attention later than women," she said. "And men don't always get the treatment they need."

Some men notice a symptom, such as a lump, and brush it off, never thinking about the possibility of breast cancer, Dr. Vito said. "Men should take a lump in the breast as seriously as a woman should," she said. Men who notice a change in breast skin, such as redness, or a change in appearance of the nipple, or a discharge, should get it checked out.

"Any man who has breast cancer deserves genetic testing," Dr. Vito added, to see if the cancer is driven by genetic risks.

Christopher Pezzi, MD, director of surgical oncology at Abington Memorial Hospital in Abington, Pennsylvania, recently reported on 13,000 cases of male breast cancer. The recent findings are largely in keeping with his research.

"Overall, we also did find significant differences between breast cancer occurring in men and women. But it is also worth noting that we also found that there was a great deal of similarity and overlap in the disease presentation, and many areas where the tumors presented and behaved in very similar ways," Dr. Pezzi said.

"It is good to see male breast cancer being studied," he said.

info To learn more about breast cancer in men, visit American Cancer Society at *www.cancer.org/cancer/breastcancerinmen/*.

"Watchful Waiting" Not Always the Best

Jennifer R. Rider, ScD, MPH, assistant professor of medicine, Channing Division of Network Medicine, Brigham and Women's Hospital and Harvard Medical School, both in Boston. She is coauthor of a study published in *The New England Journal of Medicine*.

Men under 65 with localized prostate cancer should consider radical prostatectomy rather than "watchful waiting."

Recent finding: Among Swedish men whose cancers were found through digital rectal exams (DREs) before age 65, 18% treated with surgery had died from the cancer after an average of 13 years…compared with 34% who had died in the watchful-waiting group.

"Killer Stress" Is Real

Rebecca Shannonhouse, editor, *Bottom Line/Health*, Boardroom Inc., 281 Tresser Blvd., Stamford, Connecticut 06901.

Plenty of people I know complain of "killer stress." But that's just hyperbole, right? Actually, no, according to a recent study. When researchers looked at health data on 1,293 men, they found that 64.3% of those who reported the most everyday stress had died by the end of the 21-year study. Those who had less daily stress had a much lower death rate (28.7%).

"There are lots of ways that stress can harm you," explains Carolyn Aldwin, PhD, director of the Center for Healthy Aging at Oregon State University in Corvallis and lead author of the study. Persistently high levels of stress hormones have been linked to heart disease, diabetes and even cancer. It's no surprise that people who are stressed also tend to smoke more and drink more.

No one can avoid stress. The key is to control how you react—which is probably more important than the stress itself, recent research has shown. *What to do…*

•**Plan for stress.** You can often avoid stress just by predicting it and working around it. What's better—being blindsided when there are tense moments at a family reunion or bracing yourself beforehand for a little stress? Do you go insane when you're stuck in rush-hour traffic? Leave earlier or later.

•**Don't glamorize stress.** Some people think that living with lots of stress is heroic. Don't believe it. Setting aside at least 10 to 15 minutes a day for stress-reducing strategies—such as slow, deep breathing, meditation and yoga—could actually extend your life!

Osteoporosis and Men

Tamara D. Rozental, MD, associate professor of orthopedic surgery, Harvard Medical School, Boston.

Up to one in four men over age 50 will break a bone due to osteoporosis.

Problem: A recent analysis that looked at 439 patients' medical records found that men are less likely than women to be screened for osteoporosis and far less likely to be treated for the condition after a fracture.

Why it matters: Treating the fracture but not the underlying cause puts patients at risk for future breaks.

Playing the Field May Lower Prostate Cancer Risk

University of Montreal, news release.
Marie-Elise Parent, PhD, adjunct professor, department of social and preventive medicine, University of Montreal.

Having sex with more than 20 women might have some risks for men, but a recent study suggests it could also have an unexpected health benefit.

STUDY FINDINGS

Canadian researchers report that such promiscuity lowers the risk of prostate cancer by 28%. The same did not hold true if a man had sex with a similar amount of men, however.

In fact, having that many male partners doubled the chances of prostate cancer, the study found.

Quantity seemed key: If a man had only one male sexual partner, prostate cancer risk was no greater than if a man never had any male sexual partners, the study found.

Apparently, it is the frequency of ejaculations that may explain the difference between one female partner and many, the study authors said.

"It is possible that having many female sexual partners results in a higher frequency of ejaculations, whose protective effect against prostate cancer has been previously observed in [other] cohort studies," said lead researcher Marie-Elise Parent, PhD, of the University of Montreal.

In this study of more than 3,000 men, those who had more than 20 female partners were also 19% less likely to get a more aggressive type of prostate cancer. But having more than 20 male partners upped the chances of a less aggressive prostate cancer fivefold, the researchers found.

They theorize that any benefit to men from having multiple partners may be offset when having sex with men because of the possibility of more exposure to sexually transmitted diseases, and the potential of the prostate being harmed by anal sex.

The researchers also reported that having a relative with prostate cancer doubled the chances of a man getting the disease himself.

The findings were published in the journal *Cancer Epidemiology*.

info For more information on prostate cancer, visit the American Cancer Society web site at *www.cancer.org/cancer/prostatecancer*.

Hot Flashes in Men?

Aging men with declining hormone levels can experience the same symptoms as menopausal women—weight gain, lower sexual desire and hot flashes, which are called night sweats when they happen during sleep. Hot flashes are much less common in men than in women, though, since hormone levels usually decline more gradually in men.

An overlooked cause of hot flashes in both sexes is sleep apnea, a condition in which the airway partially collapses during sleep, causing breathing to pause. It can trigger heart palpitations, severe sweating and frequent awakenings.

Men (and women) can get some relief by using cooling gel pillows (such as the Chillow) and avoiding any food, caffeine or alcohol within four hours of bedtime. Talk to your doctor about hormone replacement therapy for both sexes. You should also see a sleep specialist, who can test for sleep apnea.

Steven Y. Park, MD, sleep medicine physician in New York City and author of *Sleep, Interrupted. DoctorStevenPark.com*

Do You Pee in Your Pants After You Pee? There's a Cure for That

Geo Espinosa, ND, LAc, CNS, naturopathic physician, director of integrative urology, New York University Langone Medical Center, New York City.

Have you heard of post-micturition dribble? The term might not be familiar, but the sight of it probably is—a wet spot

---

New Prostate Cancer Test

The Prostate Health Index (PHI), a new blood test, is three times more accurate than the prostate-specific antigen (PSA) test. Because the protein that is measured by the PSA test can be elevated due to prostate cancer—or prostate inflammation or enlargement—this test often leads to unnecessary biopsies.

Now: The PHI test, which analyzes three different protein markers, was found to be more accurate and reduced the need for unnecessary biopsies by 31%.

William J. Catalona, MD, director, Clinical Prostate Cancer Program, Robert H. Lurie Comprehensive Cancer Center of Northwestern University, Chicago.

---

smack on the front of a man's pants. It happens when the last few drops of urine leak out after a gent thinks he's done using the bathroom. It can happen to women, too.

But you can fix it.

The first thing to know is that post-micturition dribble—which we will refer to as urinary dribble here—is not a sign of a dangerous health problem. It sure is annoying and embarrassing, though...a major cause of stress, not at all surprisingly.

How many people have urinary dribble is not exactly clear, but it's not rare. A Finnish study, for example, asked people about it and found that 6% of adults between the ages of 18 and 79 have it—more men than women. In an American study, 11.8% of men and 8.5% of women between the ages of 30 and 79 said they have it.

According to Geo Espinosa, ND, LAc, the director of integrative urology at New York University's Langone Medical Center, those percentages are probably low...because urinary dribble is the sort of problem that many people, especially men, are too embarrassed to admit having.

PMD is not caused by poor hygiene or problems with the bladder or, for men, the prostate. It differs from stress incontinence (involuntary urination caused by weakness of the pelvic floor muscles) or urge incontinence (urination caused by involuntary contraction of the blad-

der muscles). Although weakened muscle tone does cause urinary dribble in men—and we'll explore the solution for that below—in women, it is not muscle weakness but rather anatomical glitches that are generally responsible for urinary dribble.

WHY WOMEN DRIBBLE AFTER THEY PEE

Urinary dribble is occasionally found in women who have anatomic abnormalities that prevent complete emptying of the bladder. *Abnormalities include...*

•**A tiny pouch, called a diverticulum, on the wall of the urethra (the tube that carries urine out of the body).** Urine can become temporarily trapped in this pouch, only to trickle out later. Most women adapt to having a diverticulum and wear a pad to catch moisture. Another option is to have the diverticulum surgically removed.

•**An abnormal opening** between either the vagina and bladder or vagina and ureter (a tube that connects the kidney to the bladder) through which urine can leak. This kind of abnormality is corrected by surgically sealing off the opening.

WHY MEN DRIBBLE

For men, gravity and muscle weakness are responsible for urinary dribble. The male urethra doesn't run in a straight downhill line. It has a little dip in the middle of it, creating a pool where urine can collect. Normally, a muscle called the bulbocavernosus that fits around the urethra will automatically squeeze to force the urine out, but this muscle can lose its tone, especially in men older than 50. Instead, movement and gravity will cause the last few drops of urine that pool up in the dip of the urethra to involuntarily spill out of the body at an unpredictable time, leading to those embarrassing wet spots.

STRENGTH TRAINING FOR MEN WITH URINARY DRIBBLE

The problem is correctable. "Like any other muscle, the bulbocavernosus will be strengthened only by working it out," said Dr. Espinosa. The muscle is part of the pelvic floor, the area between the scrotum and the anus. To work the pelvic floor muscles, sit or lie down. Then tighten your muscles as if you were trying to hold in your urine (and trying not to pass gas). Don't hold your breath or squeeze muscles in your abdomen or buttocks, as some men tend to do, because the extra effort will make focus on the pelvic floor muscles more challenging.

Hold those muscles tight for 10 seconds and then relax for 10 seconds. Repeat this exercise six to 10 times for one set, and complete two or three sets each day. You may have guessed it—this is the male version of the Kegel exercise, an exercise that many women do to strengthen their pelvic floors.

In his practice, Dr. Espinosa recommends a biofeedback session or two for a man to most effectively learn how to work his pelvic floor muscles. Here's how it works. Band-Aid–like stick-on sensors are placed around the pelvic area, and a small rectal sensor is inserted a little way into the anus. Sensors are also placed on the abdomen. How does all that go over with patients—especially the rectal sensor? Dr. Espinosa says that his patients don't mind. The sensors are small and do not cause discomfort. All together, they help the biofeedback therapist see which pelvic muscles are being used. The therapist can then guide the patient to contract only the muscles that need strengthening to prevent urinary dribble.

Urinary dribble is cured within three months in about 60% of Dr. Espinosa's male patients. The remaining 40% achieve partial cure and adapt to living with some dribble, although a few may need surgery to correct the problem. The key to cure, he emphasized, is to be very regular and disciplined about doing the exercises.

And as a big bonus, Dr. Espinosa added, exercising the bulbocavernosus muscle can help sexual performance, because that same muscle also helps create and maintain erections. You get a two-for-one!

Better Prostate Cancer Treatment

Emmanuel Antonarakis, MD, assistant professor of oncology, Johns Hopkins Sidney Kimmel Comprehensive Cancer Center, Baltimore.

Men whose prostate tumors contain an abnormal protein called AR-V7 are less likely to respond to two widely used prostate cancer drugs, *enzalutamide* (Xtandi) and *abiraterone* (Zytiga), a recent study has found.

Possible explanation: AR-V7 lacks a molecule that is targeted by these drugs.

If you have metastatic prostate cancer: Ask your doctor about a blood test for AR-V7. If you test positive, ask your doctor to recommend other chemotherapy or immunotherapy drugs or radiotherapy.

Better Biopsies

Jesse Le, MD, resident physician in the department of urology at UCLA's David Geffen School of Medicine, California.
Samir Taneja, MD, director of the division of urologic oncology at NYU Langone Medical Center, New York City.

Prostate cancer patients should not rely on a conventional biopsy when deciding between surgery and active surveillance.

Reason: A conventional "blind" biopsy may fail to reveal the true extent of the cancer.

Better: A targeted biopsy, which fuses an MRI with a 3-D ultrasound to more accurately determine the grade of the cancer and help doctors decide whether treatment or surveillance makes the most sense.

Three US centers are experienced in MRI-targeted biopsies—Smilow Comprehensive Prostate Cancer Center at NYU Langone Medical Center, New York City…National Institutes of Health in Bethesda, Maryland…and UCLA Medical Center in Los Angeles. Or check local academic medical centers—some recently have started programs.

Cell Phones Can Harm Sperm

Analysis of 10 studies by researchers in the biosciences department at University of Exeter, UK, published in *Environment International*.

Cell phones may harm male fertility. In a recent analysis of 10 studies, the sperm of men who carried cell phones in their front pants pockets were 8% less able to move toward an egg than the sperm of men who did not carry the phones. Cell phones emit radio-frequency electromagnetic radiation that may negatively impact sperm quality.

Prostate Cancer Link

Stephen J. Freedland, MD, associate professor of surgery, Duke University School of Medicine, Durham, North Carolina.

Prostate cancer is linked to high triglycerides. For every 10 points a man's triglyceride level rises above a baseline of 150 mg/dL after prostate removal, his risk for cancer recurrence increases by about 3%, according to a 15-year study.

Possible reason: High lipid levels may fuel tumor growth.

If you've had prostate surgery: Ask your doctor about statins, diet, exercise and other therapies to keep your triglycerides down.

Natural Cures

Pinch Here...Poke There...17 Natural Remedies You Always Have with You

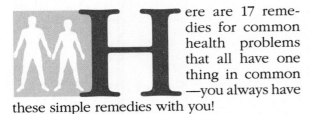

Here are 17 remedies for common health problems that all have one thing in common —you always have these simple remedies with you!

•**Dry mouth.** When it's important for you to seem calm and sound confident, don't let your dry mouth get in the way. Gently chew on your tongue. Within about 30 seconds, you will manufacture all the saliva you need to end this uncomfortable condition. If people notice, they will just think that you're chewing gum or sucking a candy.

•**Burned fingertips.** If you get a minor burn on your fingertips, simply hold your earlobe— it's an acupressure point. Place your thumb on the back of the lobe and the burned fingertips on the front of the lobe. Stay that way for one minute. It works like magic to relieve the pain.

•**Hiccups.** *Here are two remedies...*

•Pretend that your finger is a mustache. Place it under your nose, and press in hard for 30 seconds. *That should do it, but if not...*

•Take a deep breath. Without letting any air out, swallow. Breathe in a little bit more, then swallow. Keep inhaling and swallowing until you absolutely can't inhale or swallow anymore. Then, in a controlled way, slowly exhale.

•**Motion sickness.** Pull out and pinch the skin in the middle of your inner wrist, about one inch from your palm. Keep pulling and pinching, alternating wrists, until you feel better. It shouldn't take too long.

•**Leg cramps.** The second you get a cramp in your leg, "acupinch" it away. Use your thumb

---

Joan Wilen and Lydia Wilen are health investigators based in New York City who have spent decades collecting "cures from the cupboard." Their most recent book is *Bottom Line's Treasury of Home Remedies and Natural Cures.* They are authors of the free e-letter *Household Magic Daily Tips. BottomLinePersonal.com/household-magic.com* and your index finger to pinch your philtrum—the skin between your nose and upper lip. Pinch it for about 20 seconds until the pain and the cramp disappear.

•**Stomachache.** This remedy came to us from an Asian massage therapist. If you are having stomach discomfort, massage the acupressure points at the sides of your knees, just below the kneecaps. This will relieve your stomachache.

•**Warts.** First thing each morning, dab some of your own spittle on the wart (but do not lick the wart). "First thing" means before you brush your teeth. We don't know why it works—it just does.

•**Hemorrhoids.** Edgar Cayce, who is often called the father of holistic medicine, recommended this exercise for the treatment of hemorrhoids…

•Stand with your feet about six inches apart, hands at sides.

•Then raise your hands up to the ceiling, and if balance isn't a problem for you, gradually rise up on your toes at the same time.

•Bend forward, and bring your hands as close to the floor as you can get them.

•Go back to the first position, and do it again.

Perform this exercise for two or three minutes twice every day, one hour after breakfast and one hour after dinner, until your hemorrhoids are relieved.

•**Choking cough.** When you're not actually choking on something but you just are coughing as though you are, raise your hands as high as you can and the choking cough will stop.

•**Tension headache.** Tense all the muscles in your face, neck, jaw, scalp and shoulders. Hold that tension for at least 30 seconds. Then, suddenly, relax completely, letting go of all the tension, and your headache along with it.

•**Gas.** Try this yoga pose called the wind-relieving pose. Lie on your back with your legs and arms extended. As you exhale, draw both knees to your chest. Clasp your hands around them. While holding only your right knee with both hands, release your left leg and extend it along the floor. Hold this pose for one minute. Draw your left knee back in toward your chest, and clasp your hands around both knees again. Then while holding only your left knee, release your right leg and extend it along the floor. Hold this pose for up to a minute. Finally, draw both knees to your chest. Then with an exhalation, release and extend both legs.

•**Fatigue.** If you are having a hard time staying awake or paying attention, here are five energizing strategies. *Try the one that is doable in your situation…*

•Chinese theory is that "tiredness" collects on the insides of your elbows and the backs of your knees. Wake up your body by slap-slap-slapping those areas.

•Run in place for about two minutes.

•Energy lines directly connected to internal organs and body functions run through your earlobes. Use your thumbs and index fingers to rub your earlobes for about 15 seconds. This should wake up your entire nervous system.

•This visualization exercise will help you overcome drowsiness. Sit back, close your eyes, and let all the air out of your lungs. Imagine a bright blue-white energizing light entering and filling your entire body as you inhale slowly through your nostrils. Then open your eyes. You will feel refreshed.

•Boost your energy by belting out a few bars of a favorite cheerful song. Inhale deeply as you sing to bring more energizing oxygen into your lungs and increase circulation in your body.

4 Spices That Could Save Your Life

Bill Gottlieb, CHC, editor of *Healing Spices: How to Use 50 Everyday and Exotic Spices to Boost Health and Beat Disease*, founder and president of Good For You Health Coaching, and author of 14 health books and natural healing books. *BillGottliebHealth.com*

Certain spices have been touted as good for our health. For example, cinnamon helps regulate blood sugar…ginger eases indigestion…and garlic can lower high blood pressure.

What most people don't realize: Several other commonly used spices are just as healthful (if not more so). *Here are four "secret" super-spices with healing powers...*

BLACK PEPPER

Black pepper is rich in *piperine*, the pungent compound that triggers a sneeze when it hits the nerve endings inside your nose. Hundreds of studies show that piperine also triggers healing—energizing and protecting nearly every organ and system in your body. *Two standout benefits...*

●**Cancer.** Cellular and animal research demonstrates that piperine fights cancer. In a test of 55 natural compounds, piperine scored number one in killing triple-negative breast cancer, the most virulent type. In another study, it killed aggressive HER2 breast cancer cells—and even stopped the deadly HER2 gene from activating. Other research shows that piperine can slow, stop or kill prostate, colorectal, lung, cervical, liver and stomach cancers. Piperine also slows angiogenesis, the growth of new blood vessels that feed tumors. It even enhances the effectiveness of radiation and chemotherapy.

●**Arthritis and gout.** Piperine is anti-inflammatory—and studies show that it can stop destructive inflammation in cartilage cells (loss of cartilage is the cause of osteoarthritis) and reduce inflammation associated with gout. It also reverses the symptoms of arthritis in lab animals.

How to use: For the highest level of piperine, buy whole black peppercorns and grind as needed. (Green and white peppercorns are not as rich in piperine, and once the peppercorn is ground, piperine begins to decrease.) Add freshly ground black pepper liberally and often—in cooking and at the table. Try to add freshly ground pepper at the end of cooking because the benefits break down the longer the spice is heated.

Also helpful: Studies show that just smelling black pepper (in the form of black pepper oil) can cut nicotine cravings in smokers and strengthen "postural stability" in older people (thereby helping to prevent falls). Put a drop of oil on a tissue, and inhale for two minutes, two to three times a day. Black pepper oil is available at Amazon.com and other online retailers.

OREGANO

Two major components of oregano—*thymol* and *carvacrol*—have been proven to have healing powers...

●**Heart disease and stroke.** In a study published in *Journal of International Medical Research*, people with high LDL (bad) cholesterol were divided into two groups—one group ingested oregano extract with every meal and one group didn't. Three months later, the oregano group had greater decreases in LDL, lower levels of C-reactive protein (a biomarker of artery-damaging inflammation) and greater increases in arterial blood flow.

In other studies, researchers found that oregano is more powerful than any other spice in stopping the oxidation of LDL—the breakdown of cholesterol by unstable molecules called free radicals that drives the formation of arterial plaque. Oregano also stops the activation of cytokines, components of the immune system that attack oxidized cholesterol, sparking the inflammation that worsens heart disease.

●**Infections.** Oregano is antimicrobial. It can kill the parasite giardia more effectively than *tinidazole*, a prescription antiparasitic drug. It decimates *Candida albicans*, a yeast that can multiply in the intestinal tract and trigger a range of health problems, such as arthritis and depression. And it can neutralize *Staphylococcus aureus*, a common hospital-acquired infection.

How to use: You can buy oregano fresh or dried. I recommend using the dried form because it concentrates the therapeutic compounds. It often is used in salad dressings, marinades, chili and in Italian and Greek dishes. For optimum benefits, try to use at least one teaspoon of dried oregano daily.

Also helpful: During the winter, consider using oregano oil in supplement form to prevent colds and flu. Follow the directions on the label.

BASIL

Basil is a traditional medicine in Ayurveda, the more than 5,000-year-old natural healing system from India, where it's used to treat diabetes, digestive disorders, skin problems and infections. The variety native to India is holy basil, and there are at least 30 more varieties worldwide. All of them contain basil's four main healing components—the antioxidants orientin and vicenin and the volatile oils eugenol and apigenin—that can help regulate blood sugar.

•**Type 2 diabetes.** In one study, people with type 2 diabetes who included more basil in their diets saw an average drop of 21 mg/dL in fasting blood sugar and a 15.8 mg/dL drop in postmeal blood sugar. In a similar, smaller study, three people with type 2 diabetes had remarkable decreases in fasting blood sugar levels when they added basil to their diets three times a day for five weeks—from 250 to 110 mg/dL, from 200 to 80 mg/dL, and from 230 to 90 mg/dL (99.9 mg/dL and lower is normal...100 to 125.9 mg/dL is prediabetes...126 mg/dL and higher is diabetes).

How to use: Dried basil has a larger concentration of the health-giving volatile oils than fresh. I recommend one-quarter to one-half teaspoon daily. Use dried basil in full-flavored sauces. Fresh basil still is rich in health-giving compounds. An easy way to enjoy fresh basil is to toss a handful of leaves into your favorite hot pasta and dress with extra-virgin olive oil.

SAGE

The botanical name for sage—*Salvia officinalis*—comes from the Latin *salvare*, meaning "to save" or "to cure." *And sage lives up to its name...*

•**Memory problems.** One hour after people took a supplement of sage oil, they had better memory, more focused attention and more alertness, reported researchers in *Journal of Psychopharmacology.* In another study, people who smelled sage had a stronger memory and were in a better mood.

•**Anxiety.** In a study published in *Neuropsychopharmacology,* people who took a supplement of dried sage leaf were less anxious and felt calmer and more content than when they took a placebo.

Why it works: Sage may block the action of cholinesterase, an enzyme that destroys acetylcholine, a brain chemical that plays a role in memory, attention and alertness. Sage also might improve the functioning of cholinergic receptors on brain cells that receive acetylcholine.

How to use sage: Because of its robust flavor, sage is best used in hearty dishes such as pot roast, meat loaf and stuffing. It also goes well with squash, sweet potatoes and apples.

However: The amounts that improve mental and emotional functioning aren't easy to get with diet, so you may want to take a sage leaf supplement. I often recommend the herbal extract from Herb Pharm because it's made from the whole leaf that has been grown organically. Follow the directions on the label.

What a Top Naturopath Has in His Own Medicine Cabinet

Mark Stengler, NMD, a naturopathic medical doctor and founder of Stengler Center for Integrative Medicine, Encinitas, California. He is coauthor of The Natural Physician's Healing Therapies. *MarkStengler.com*

Sometimes you need powerful, fast-acting medications. But prescription and over-the-counter drugs can present serious risks. It's estimated that more than two million adverse drug reactions occur in the US every year and are responsible for more than 100,000 deaths annually.

I strongly recommend and use natural remedies. They contain lower doses of chemically active agents. They're less likely than drugs to cause dangerous side effects. And they often work just as well, sometimes better. All are available at health-food stores and online.

Important: Always check with your doctor before taking any new medication or supplement.

LESS JOINT PAIN

Aspirin and related painkillers often irritate the stomach and increase the risk for ulcers. Natural analgesics are much gentler and just as effective.

Boswellia, a tree found in India, Africa and the Middle East, has a milky resin that inhibits the body's production of inflammatory molecules. A study that looked at patients with osteo-arthritis of the knee found that boswellia extract relieved pain and stiffness as effectively as the drug *valdecoxib* (Bextra), which has been withdrawn from the market because of side effects. A small percentage of boswellia users experience digestive upset. If that happens, reduce the amount. If you don't start to feel better within 48 hours, stop taking it. If you are taking it for chronic pain, give it two weeks.

Dose: 750 milligrams (mg), two to three times daily during flare-ups.

Curcumin is the active ingredient found in the spice turmeric. In a study, rheumatoid arthritis patients reported that it helped relieve morning pain and stiffness.

Caution: Taking curcumin with blood thinners can increase the risk for bleeding.

Dose: 500 mg, three times daily. You can take it every day to keep pain and inflammation down or just take it during flare-ups.

LESS STRESS AND ANXIETY

Chamomile tea is a gentle relaxant that has traditionally been used as a "nerve tonic." Other herbs have similar effects. *One of my favorites...*

Passionflower. Despite the name, passionflower is more relaxing than arousing. It increases brain levels of *gamma-aminobutyric acid* (GABA), a neurotransmitter that dampens activity in the part of the brain that controls emotions, making you feel more relaxed. In one study, participants drank either passionflower tea or a placebo tea before going to bed. Those who drank passionflower tea slept better and were more likely to wake up feeling refreshed and alert.

How to use it: Steep one teaspoon of dried passionflower in three ounces of just-boiled water. Drink it two to three times daily when you're stressed. Or take passionflower capsules or tinctures, following the label directions.

MIGRAINE RELIEF

There are many drugs for treating migraines, but they're rife with side effects—and may increase the risk for liver damage or even a heart attack.

Butterbur, a member of the daisy family, is an effective alternative. It contains two potent anti-inflammatory compounds, petasin and isopetasin, which may help blood vessels in the brain dilate and contract more normally. A study published in *Neurology* found that people who used butterbur had a 48% reduction in the frequency of migraines. You also can use butterbur to reduce migraine intensity.

Dose: For prevention, take 50 mg of Petadolex (a butterbur extract) three times daily, with meals, for one month. Then reduce the dose to twice daily. For treating a migraine, take 50 mg three times daily until the migraine is gone.

EASE MUSCLE SORENESS

For an aching back or sore arms, apply an ice pack or a heating pad...or alternate cold and warmth. *Also helpful...*

Arnica is a plant in the daisy family that reduces muscle soreness and swelling. It also helps bruises heal more quickly.

A recent study from the Australian Institute of Sport in Canberra, Australia, published in *European Journal of Sport Science*, found that the topical application of arnica reduced the level of achiness for up to three days after a vigorous workout. The participants included men who ran in five bouts of eight-minute bursts on a treadmill, followed by two minutes of walking on a flat surface. They applied arnica gel or a placebo gel every four hours.

How to use it: Apply a small amount of cream or tincture to the sore areas. Repeat every hour as necessary. Don't apply if the skin is broken.

Helpful: If a large area is sore, you can take arnica orally instead. Take two pellets of a 30C potency three times daily for one to two days.

REDUCE HEARTBURN

I advise patients to start with natural approaches, including sleeping on their left side (sleeping on the right side makes heartburn worse)...avoiding "trigger" foods, such as onions and chocolate...and maintaining a healthy weight (excess weight makes stomach acid more likely to enter the esophagus and cause heartburn). *Also helpful...*

Melatonin, a supplement that is often used for insomnia, also is effective for heartburn. A study published in *Journal of Pharmacology* found that melatonin reduces the amount of acid produced in the stomach without blocking it altogether. This is important because you need stomach acid for good digestion—you just don't want too much of it.

Dose: 3 mg to 6 mg, taken daily at bedtime.

INFLUENZA FIGHTERS

A healthy immune system is the best way to protect against flu. *Starting at the beginning of flu season (typically early October), take...*

Influenzinum, a homeopathic remedy that I've recommended for more than 15 years. The makers of influenzinum reformulate it annually based on the flu viruses that are expected to predominate that year.

Dose: Three pellets (of a 9C potency) dissolved under the tongue, once a week for six weeks.

N-acetylcysteine (NAC), an antioxidant, reduces both the chance that you will get the flu and the severity of symptoms if you do get sick. An Italian study found that only 25% of older people who were injected with flu virus after taking NAC for six months experienced flu symptoms, versus 79% who took a placebo.

Dose: 1,000 mg daily in tablet form for prevention during the flu months (typically October through April). If you get the flu, increase the dose to 4,000 mg daily until you recover.

Also helpful: 2,000 international units (IU) of vitamin D daily. During the peak flu months, increase the dose to 5,000 IU.

COLD RELIEF

Don't waste your money on often ineffective over-the-counter cold medicines. *Instead...*

Pelargonium sidoides, a South African plant, has been tested in more than 20 clinical studies. It relieves congestion, sore throat and other cold symptoms. It is available in syrups, lozenges, capsules and tablets. Follow the dosing instructions on the label.

Restore Your Health and Life with DHEA

Andrew Rubman, ND, medical director, Southbury Clinic for Traditional Medicines, Southbury, Connecticut. SouthburyClinic.com.

Some folks think that the key to the "fountain of youth" is to hold onto their sex hormones for as long as they possibly can—even through artificial means. And when you think of hormone replacement, estrogen and testosterone are probably the two hormones that come to mind. But there is another hormone, available as an over-the-counter dietary supplement, that's increasingly getting attention as more evidence emerges of its wide array of possible health benefits. It won't turn you into a 22-year-old live wire, but it has been known to help relieve depression, slow osteoporosis and improve sex, and when used properly, it may protect you from heart disease, too.

A LIFESAVER

The hormone is dehydroepiandrosterone (DHEA). It's actually an essential building block of estrogen and testosterone and the most abundant steroid hormone in the body—at least when you're young. Bloodstream levels peak at around age 20 and then steadily decline. Sadly, by age 60, your DHEA levels are typically down to 5% to 15% of what they were in your 20s. This loss has got to be tied in with the aging process—at least some researchers think so. Experimental studies have shown that DHEA boosts the body's production of estrogen and testosterone and may have an anti-inflammatory effect on blood vessels. This means that DHEA could help prevent cardiovascular disease.

Despite the promising research on the effect of DHEA on blood vessels, the consensus in mainstream medicine has been that, while DHEA might be a mood-booster and help you get your groove on, it probably does not have a strong effect on heart health. But a Swedish study of 2,416 men ages 69 to 81—the largest study yet to be done—suggests otherwise.

The five-year study kept track of participants' DHEA levels and incidents of coronary heart disease (the cause of heart attack) or stroke. Although no association between DHEA levels and stroke was found, the lower a man's blood level of DHEA, the higher his risk of coronary heart disease. In fact, low DHEA levels were associated with an 82% increased risk of coronary heart disease.

Whether DHEA supplements would help prevent heart disease has yet to be formally studied, but it seems reasonable given these findings.

WISE USE FOR IMPROVED HEALTH

Some doctors, such as Andrew L. Rubman, ND, *Daily Health News* contributing medical editor and a naturopathic physician in Southbury, Connecticut, strongly believe that DHEA supplementation is an important key to restoring health. He often prescribes oral drops, which are faster-acting and much better absorbed than tablets. Only about 5% of the DHEA in tablets will survive after being broken down in the stomach, but DHEA in oral drops passes directly into the bloodstream through the lining of the mouth, explained Dr. Rubman, who prepares his own formulation of the DHEA for his patients.

Although DHEA is available over the counter, it should be taken only under the care of a naturopathic physician who is knowledgeable about proper use of DHEA, said Dr. Rubman. Such a doctor can guide you to the best, purest product (not all brands are accurate and honest about what the supplement actually contains or how much of the active ingredient is actually in it), instruct you about appropriate dosage and monitor your use to protect you from side effects. *Yes, side effects—DHEA use does come with precautions...*

HANDLE WITH CARE

Like all medications, pharma-based and natural, DHEA supplementation has its dangers, especially at high doses or if done for longer than three months without proper monitoring. That's because, in raising testosterone and estrogen levels, supplemental DHEA can potentially increase the risk of hormone-sensitive cancers, such as breast, ovarian and prostate cancer, as well as colorectal cancer.

Besides these risks, women can experience side effects such as loss of head hair, facial hair growth and a deepening of the voice. Possible side effects for men include breast enlargement, shrunken testicles, reduced sperm production and erectile dysfunction. And both men and women can experience oily skin, acne, high blood pressure, insomnia and fatigue. Dr. Rubman stressed that, when considering DHEA therapy, query doctors to make sure they are very experienced with it. Interpretation of DHEA-monitoring tests requires specialty training. Naturopathic doctors may be more up on it than mainstream doctors, but don't assume. Be sure to ask about their experience anyway. You can find a naturopathic doctor in your area through the American Association of Naturopathic Physicians.

Hypnosis: 6 Medical Problems It's Been Proven to Help

Marc I. Oster, PsyD, a psychologist and professor of clinical psychology at the Illinois School of Professional Psychology at Argosy University in Schaumburg, Illinois. *MarcOster.Homestead.com*

Don't confuse medical hypnosis with the flamboyant stage shows that feature a swinging watch, a performer in a glittery jacket and volunteers from the audience, all quacking like ducks.

Hypnosis-enhanced therapy is a legitimate treatment for various medical problems—and unlike many treatments, it is noninvasive and totally safe.

Here's what hypnosis really helps...

IRRITABLE BOWEL SYNDROME

IBS is a mysterious, often debilitating condition that causes cramps and intermittent episodes of diarrhea, pain and constipation. Medications to treat it aren't very effective.

Several well-designed studies of hypnotherapy for IBS have shown that IBS patients who were treated with hypnosis had "substantial, long-term improvement" of gastrointestinal symptoms, along with less anxiety and depression. It's possible that hypnosis alters how the central nervous system responds to intestinal signals. It also diverts people's attention from their intestinal sensations and causes them to perceive less discomfort.

PAIN RELIEF

Hypnosis doesn't necessarily reduce pain, but it does alter how people react to it. Studies have shown, for example, that hypnotized dental patients have a higher pain threshold. They also have less anxiety, which reduces sensitivity to pain.

One study, which looked at patients with burn injuries, used virtual-reality technology to induce hypnosis. Patients wore a fiber-optic helmet that immersed them in a make-believe environment. As they descended into a snowy, three-dimensional canyon, an audiotape with a clinician's voice prepared them for what they would experience during the treatment of the burn.

Result: They had a decrease in both pain and anxiety—and their need for potent pain-killers was reduced by half.

HELP QUITTING SMOKING

About 65% to 70% of smokers who are treated with medical hypnosis quit successfully, according to research. That's much better than the quit rate from going cold turkey (about 20%) or using stop-smoking drugs including nicotine therapy (35% to 40%).

Hypnosis isn't a miracle cure for smoking or other addictions. Anyone who takes the time to schedule appointments with a therapist already is highly motivated. The success rate would be lower for those who remain on the fence about quitting. That said, hypnosis still is more effective than standard treatments.

BETTER CANCER CARE

The radiation therapy that's used to treat some cancers often causes fatigue as a side effect. Researchers at Mount Sinai Hospital, New York City, found that cancer patients who underwent hypnosis during a common kind of counseling called cognitive-behavioral therapy experienced less fatigue than participants in a control group.

The study, published in *Journal of Clinical Oncology*, showed that after six months, the average patient treated with hypnosis had less fatigue than 95% of those who weren't hypnotized.

LESS SURGICAL PAIN

Another study of cancer patients found that those who had a single, 15-minute hypnosis session prior to their surgery required less sedation and experienced less nausea, pain and fatigue than those in a nonhypnosis group.

Mount Sinai researchers analyzed 20 studies on hypnosis and surgery, and they found that in 89% of cases, hypnotized surgical patients had less pain, used less pain medication and recovered faster.

CHRONIC FATIGUE

A six-month study at Beth Israel Deaconess Medical Center, Boston, showed that 73% of participants who had chronic fatigue syndrome reported increased energy, more restful periods of sleep and better concentration at work. This is far better than the national average of 23% of people who improve with other types of therapy.

HOW YOU CAN TRY HYPNOSIS

Because of its long association with parlor tricks, hypnosis still is a subject of confusion.

A few facts: You don't go into a trance during hypnosis…you are more in control of yourself than usual, not less…and you won't do anything that you don't want to do.

A specially trained therapist will use guided imagery to focus and direct your imagination. It is the same technique sometimes used during meditation.

Example: While you relax, the therapist will encourage you to breathe slowly and deeply…to imagine a soothing scene (such as walking in the woods)…and to keep your mind focused on just that one thing. This is known as the induction phase. Your brain activity slows, but you still are focused and alert.

At this point, medical hypnosis diverges from traditional meditation. While you are in a relaxed state, the therapist will guide your thinking toward particular issues.

Suppose that you have arthritis and that your arm always hurts. The therapist might describe a scene in which you're walking to a lake…submerging yourself in icy water…and feeling your arm go pleasantly numb. The positive effects can last for minutes to hours to forever.

Research has shown that people who are mentally and physically relaxed are more receptive to taking in new ideas and feeling in new ways.

To find a hypnotist who can help you, look for a licensed health-care professional who offers hypnosis as only one part of his/her practice. Someone who only does hypnosis may not have the understanding of health-care issues to properly diagnose and treat you. The website for the Societies of Hypnosis (*societiesofhypnosis.com*) has referral pages that can help you find an expert in your area.

Expect to complete between four and 10 sessions. The cost per session is about the same as you would pay for other types of counseling.

Example: Depending on where you live, you might pay about $150 for a session with a psychologist. You will pay less if you see a social worker, nurse or mental-health counselor.

Most insurance companies do not cover hypnosis per se, but they may cover therapy that includes hypnosis. Medicare covers "hypnotherapy" for certain conditions.

Natural Cures for Psoriasis

April Abernethy, ND, a naturopathic physician and interim chief scientific and medical officer at the National Psoriasis Foundation in Portland, Oregon. She is also a member of the board of directors at International Dermatology Outcome Measures, an organization working to establish common measurements of treatment effectiveness and outcomes.

Living day in and day out with psoriasis—known for its silvery scales and itchy, painful red patches (plaques) on the skin—is hard enough for the more than 7.5 million Americans who have the disease.

But researchers are now finding that people with psoriasis also may be more likely to develop other inflammation-based conditions such as diabetes and cardiovascular disease. People with psoriasis should be screened for these conditions and talk to their doctors about ways to reduce other risk factors they may have for these diseases.

Problem: Even though drugs, such as *apremilast* (Otezla) and *adalimumab* (Humira), that inhibit parts of the immune system involved in psoriasis are now available, any therapy that suppresses immunity can increase the risk for infections, gastrointestinal upset and other conditions.

Solution: There's mounting evidence that natural therapies can be used to reduce overall inflammation and help support the immune system. These drug-free approaches can improve the effectiveness of psoriasis medication and sometimes even eliminate the need for it (with your doctor's approval). First, try the dietary approaches in this article—they should result in improvements that increase over time. Supplements also can be used.

PUTTING YOUR DIET TO WORK

Eating the right foods (and using supplements when needed) can increase your ability to fight psoriasis on a systemic level by reducing inflammation and helping regulate your immune system—two key factors linked to psoriasis. *My advice…*

•**Go for anti-inflammatory foods.** Americans eat lots of processed foods—most of which promote inflammation in the body. Meanwhile, whole, nutrient-packed foods such as fresh fruits and vegetables help attack the inflammatory process that is increased in psoriasis.

Good choices: Beets, blueberries, kale or other leafy greens, salmon, garbanzo beans, quinoa, lentils, nuts and ginger. For other food choices, go to *Psoriasis.org*, and search "anti-inflammatory diet."

•**Get more vitamin D.** People with psoriasis, like many Americans, are often deficient in vitamin D, which is known to help regulate immune function and inhibit inflammation. That's why it's important to consume foods that contain vitamin D, such as oysters, shrimp, salmon, sardines and any fortified milk. Vitamin D supplements also may be needed. If you have psoriasis, ask your doctor for a blood test to check your vitamin D level.

•**Spice things up.** Turmeric, which gives mustard its bright yellow color and curry its distinctive flavor, contains the medicinal compound curcumin.

A study published in the journal *BioFactors* showed that turmeric helps healthy, new skin cells form more quickly. If you don't like curry or mustard (you would need to eat 1 g to 3 g a day to get the therapeutic effect), you can try turmeric in supplement form—400 mg to 600 mg two to three times a day.

Talk to your doctor first if you take antacids, diabetes drugs or blood thinners, since turmeric may interfere with these medications—and if you have a history of gallstones (turmeric may cause stomach upset in these people).

•**Load up on omega-3s.** Get lots of anti-inflammatory omega-3 fatty acids.

Daily amounts needed to fight psoriasis: Seven ounces of salmon…a small avocado…or two tablespoons of ground flaxseed (store in the refrigerator to prevent spoilage). If you don't like fish and other omega-3–rich foods, consider taking 2 g to 3 g daily of a fish oil supplement. Choose one that has more EPA than DHA, and check with your doctor first if you take a blood thinner or diabetes medication—fish oil could interact with them.

A 2014 study published in the *Journal of the American Academy of Dermatology* found that among many common supplements taken by people with psoriasis, fish oil—which may reduce tumor necrosis factor-alpha (TNF-alpha), a protein associated with systemic inflammation—demonstrated the greatest benefit.

FOR CRACKED SKIN AND PLAQUES

Among the more troubling symptoms of psoriasis are dry, cracked skin (that may even bleed) and the red, scaly, itchy plaques that can develop on the elbows, scalp, torso and other areas.

What works best…

•**Oregon grape root.** When used topically, this powerful, little-known antibacterial herb (also called Mahonia) helps reduce skin irritation and topical infections common to people with psoriasis.

A research review published in the *British Journal of Dermatology* showed that Oregon grape root reduced the development of red, raised psoriasis plaques and healed psoriasis-related cracked skin.

Oregon grape root is found in tincture form at health-food stores, and you can add two or three drops to your favorite skin cream. The herb also can be found in over-the-counter creams containing 10% Mahonia, which has been shown to help control mild-to-moderate psoriasis plaques.

FOR ITCHING AND FLAKING

Soaking in the high concentration of mineral salts found in the Dead Sea in Israel is a centuries-old remedy for the itching and flaking associated with psoriasis.

What helps: Adding one-quarter to one-half cup of Dead Sea (or Epsom) salts to a warm (not hot) bath has been shown to ease itching skin and remove dead, flaking skin cells. Dead Sea salts have a higher concentration of minerals than Epsom salts and are available online and at health-food stores and spas.

A substantial body of research, including a study published in the *Journal of Dermatological Treatment*, has shown that psoriasis patients who regularly take such baths report significant improvements in itch and irritation levels within three weeks.

For even greater benefits: Mix the salts with colloidal oatmeal, such as Aveeno. Take these baths two to three times a week.

Natural Cures for Bad Breath

Mark Stengler, NMD, a naturopathic medical doctor and founder of Stengler Center for Integrative Medicine, Encinitas, California. He is coauthor of The Natural Physician's Healing Therapies. MarkStengler.com

Persistent bad breath can indicate gum disease, a sinus infection or digestion problems…or it can be a sign of excessive toxins in the body. Bad breath that doesn't clear up with natural remedies should be evaluated by a doctor.

Solutions: One teaspoon of chlorophyll taken orally after meals. It's a traditional breath freshener that helps neutralize strong odors and remove toxins from the body. Supplements that contain chlorella, alfalfa and spirulina have similar effects.

Also helpful: A probiotic powder supplement that contains at least four billion organisms per dose. Mix it in water, swish it around your mouth and then swallow it. The beneficial organisms can prevent the buildup of odor-causing mouth bacteria. Taking probiotics also promotes the growth of beneficial intestinal bacteria that improve digestion and help improve breath—as well as reduce body odors.

Do You Have a Gallstone? How to Avoid Surgery

Sarah Brewer, MD, MSc, a general practitioner, registered nutritionist and registered nutritional therapist with a private practice in Guernsey, Channel Islands. Dr. Brewer is also author of *Overcoming Gallstones: Nutritional, Medical and Surgical Approaches.*

You probably don't give much thought to your gallbladder—that four-inch, pear-shaped sac tucked beneath your liver. When it's working properly, it stores a liquid (bile) that plays an important role in digesting dietary fats.

But for more than 25 million Americans, this organ harbors one or sometimes even hundreds of gallstones. These hard deposits of cholesterol, calcium and/or other substances can be as small as grains of sand or as large as golf balls.

The good news is that gallstones usually cause no symptoms or only a single "attack" marked by abdominal cramps that may be accompanied by nausea or vomiting.

What to watch out for: Because the gallbladder can be removed relatively easily via minimally invasive laparoscopic surgery, some doctors recommend removal for patients who would do just as well with nonsurgical approaches.

A SAFER APPROACH

Even though gallbladder removal (using laparoscopy or the traditional "open" approach) can be necessary or even lifesaving in some cases, it's wise to consider whether you can avoid surgery. Not having a gallbladder can lead to such problems as poor digestion of dietary fats.

If your gallstones are "silent" (they have not caused you discomfort but were detected during an imaging test for another condition), or you've had just a single painful episode, your best bet is usually to wait it out—if the symptoms get worse, you *might* need surgery.

More often, you can stop gallstones from growing (or forming in the first place) with the following simple steps...

•**Lose weight—and lose it slowly.** People who are overweight or obese are far more likely to develop gallstones than those who are lean. They are also more likely to have one or more painful episodes.

In people who are overweight, bile (the digestive fluid that's stored in the gallbladder) tends to contain more cholesterol—the main constituent in about 70% of gallstones. Weight loss is among the most effective ways to prevent gallstones, but only if you lose weight at a reasonable pace—for example, no more than two pounds a week.

Here's why: Studies have shown that faster weight loss can trigger an increase in stone formation and/or symptoms because the gallbladder doesn't empty completely on diets that cut too many calories (for example, less than 1,500 calories daily for men and less than 1,200 calories daily for women). Stored bile becomes "stagnant" and is more likely to form stones.

•**Cut fat—but not too much.** Doctors used to recommend low-fat diets for weight loss. It makes sense to eat less fat because a diet that's high in cholesterol and saturated fat can increase stone formation—especially if you're not getting much fiber, which acts like a sponge to mop up fats.

But not getting enough fat has the same effect as consuming too few calories—it allows bile to "sit" in the gallbladder. That's why I recommend a Mediterranean-type diet that contains healthful fats (such as olive oil, fatty fish and nuts) along with plenty of fruit and vegetables.

Also helpful: Supplements that contain milk thistle and/or globe artichoke.* Follow label directions. These supplements stimulate bile production and reduce the concentration of cholesterol and other stone-causing substances.

•**Get more omega-3 fatty acids.** Omega-3s, found in fatty, cold-water fish, reduce the amount of cholesterol in bile—by up to 25%, according to research.

Important: Eat fish. You'll get all the omega-3s that you need from two to four weekly servings of fish. Good choices include salmon, kippers, sardines and mackerel. Compared with fish consumption, the evidence is not as strong for taking fish oil supplements to reduce gallstone risk.

•**Eat high-fiber foods.** A Harvard study analyzing long-term fiber intakes of nearly 70,000 women found that every 5 g increase in daily fiber reduced the need for gallbladder surgery by an average of about 10%. Eat at least five daily servings of high-fiber foods.

Good options: Beans (such as kidney and soybeans)…whole grains (such as oats)…and fresh vegetables (such as dark greens).

•**Load up on vitamin C.** Research has shown that women who consume the most vitamin C–rich foods are less likely to have gallstones or gallstone-related symptoms than those who get the least of these foods. Women

*If you take a prescription drug or have a chronic medical condition, check with a doctor or pharmacist before trying supplements. People with a history of hormone-related cancer, such as prostate or breast cancer, should not take milk thistle. Those with a ragweed allergy should not take milk thistle or artichoke supplements.

When You Do Need Gallbladder Surgery

Gallstones rarely cause problems when they stay put. They usually cause symptoms, such as fever, abdominal pain, nausea or vomiting, when they migrate into other areas, such as the small ducts that lead to the intestine. Most people need surgery to remove the gallbladder only if their symptoms are frequent (two or more episodes) or unusually painful…if they develop cholecystitis, an infection/inflammation that occurs when a stone blocks the cystic duct…or if a stone lodges in the duct leading to the pancreas. In these cases, surgery is advisable because the risk for complications, such as jaundice and chronic cholecystitis and pancreatitis, is high. Whether it's minimally invasive (laparoscopic) or "open," surgery to remove the gallbladder carries a risk for infection or the accidental severing of the bile duct. If surgery is advised, look for a surgeon who has significant experience performing this operation.

who got even more vitamin C from supplements were 34% less likely to have problems than women who didn't take a supplement. Vitamin C is also believed to reduce gallstone risk in men.

My advice: In addition to consuming vitamin C–rich foods (such as citrus fruits and berries), take 500 mg of vitamin C four times daily (to maintain steady blood levels and maximize absorption). The "ester-C" form of vitamin C is nonacidic and easier for the body to absorb—and less likely to cause diarrhea at the doses recommended here.

•**Get extra magnesium.** Many Americans don't get enough of this important mineral. Low magnesium has been linked to elevated LDL "bad" cholesterol, high blood pressure—and a higher risk for gallstones. A large study that followed more than 42,000 men for 16 years found that those with the highest magnesium intakes (more than 409 mg daily) were 33% less likely to develop gallstone disease than those with the lowest levels (less than 288 mg daily).

My advice: Regularly consume magnesium-rich foods, such as beans, nuts, brewer's yeast, salmon, leafy greens and dark chocolate. If you are not sure that you're getting enough, take 150 mg to 300 mg daily of a magnesium citrate supplement, which is the most readily absorbed.

•**Enjoy a little coffee.** One study linked two to three cups of coffee a day to a 20% lower risk of developing gallstones. Decaf coffee, caffeinated tea or soft drinks did not have this protective effect—perhaps because of their lower amounts of caffeine, a compound that increases the flow of bile.

New Constipation Cure

Applying self-pressure to the perineum (area between the anus and genitals) significantly reduced constipation for 72% of adults in a recent study. Patients also used traditional methods, such as increased fiber intake and stool softeners, but those who added this form of daily acupressure saw the most improvement.

How it works: Applying moderate pressure to the perineum for even a few seconds when you feel the urge to defecate can break up stools and relax the anal sphincter muscles.

Ryan Abbott, MD, visiting assistant professor of medicine, David Geffen School of Medicine, University of California, Los Angeles.

Fight Thyroid Disease Naturally

Jamison Starbuck, ND, a naturopathic physician in family practice and a guest lecturer at the University of Montana, both in Missoula. She is past president of the American Association of Naturopathic Physicians and a contributing editor to The Alternative Advisor: The Complete Guide to Natural Therapies and Alternative Treatments.

Hypothyroidism is one of those conditions that often hovers just beneath the radar. You feel lousy, then get used to dragging yourself around and may not even think it's important enough to tell your doctor about it. Of course there's a simple blood test for hypothyroidism (underactive thyroid), and treatment—a daily synthetic thyroid replacement hormone pill, or *levothyroxine*—is fairly straightforward. But in my opinion, thyroid replacement hormone alone usually doesn't take care of the problem, because it helps patients feel better—but not great. That's not good enough!

Here's what most people don't realize: A major cause of hypothyroidism is an autoimmune condition known as Hashimoto's thyroiditis (in some cases, hypothyroidism is due to other causes such as thyroid surgery or thyroid cancer). As an autoimmune disease, Hashimoto's throws the immune system out of whack so that it goes on the attack, for unknown rea-

sons, against the thyroid gland. This means that you've got a bigger problem than an empty gas tank—your whole body needs some tuning up. *If your doctor has told you that you have Hashimoto's, talk to him/her about adding the following natural approaches to your standard thyroid replacement regimen…*

1. Avoid food allergens. Food allergies are linked to autoimmune disease. Gluten and wheat allergies are particularly common in people with thyroid disease. To find out if you have food allergies (believe it or not, many people who have food allergies aren't aware of it), ask your doctor for an IgG blood test. If it's positive, avoiding the foods you're allergic to will increase your vitality and nicely augment your hormone replacement therapy.

2. Try supplements and tweak your diet. Low iodine, zinc and selenium can reduce thyroid hormone production—a bad situation when you already have low thyroid levels. That's why I prescribe low-dose supplements—300 micrograms (mcg) of iodine…30 mg of zinc… and 100 mcg of selenium daily—for my patients with Hashimoto's. (Before trying these supplements, be sure to check with your doctor—especially if you have any other chronic health condition or take medication.) Also, avoid "goitrogens"—foods that suppress thyroid function by interfering with the absorption of iodine, which plays such a key role in keeping this gland healthy. Goitrogens include raw kale and broccoli and soy (in any form). Cooked green veggies are OK—heat deactivates the goitrogenic substances.

3. Get some natural sunlight. When our eyes are exposed to sunlight, it fuels the pineal gland in the brain to produce thyroid hormone. To get this thyroid benefit, take your sunglasses off for at least 30 minutes a day when you're outdoors. (If you have an eye disease, such as glaucoma, this is not advisable.)

4. Do aerobic exercise for 20 minutes, four times a week. Moderate exercise increases thyroid hormone production and boosts the immune system by improving circulation, enhancing cardiac function and relieving stress.

5. Improve circulation to your thyroid gland. Hashimoto's often impairs blood circulation to the thyroid gland. To promote better blood flow, you can try yoga or simply do a "shoulder stand" for a few minutes every day—raise your hips and legs above your head while you lie on your back. (Don't do this if you have glaucoma, high blood pressure or neck problems.)

Is This Parkinson's Disease Cure on Your Spice Rack?

Kalipada Pahan, PhD, professor of neurological sciences, Floyd A. Davis Professor of Neurology, Rush University Medical Center, Chicago. His study appeared in the *Journal of Neuroimmune Pharmacology.*

The Bible makes several references to it. The ancient Egyptians used it to preserve their mummies. The ancient Greeks and Romans used it to help them digest their feasts of lamb and wine. We know it's great for diabetes and glycemic control.

And now we find out that this substance fights Parkinson's disease. What is it?

"Cinnamon," said Kalipada Pahan, PhD, professor of neurologic sciences at the Rush University Medical Center in Chicago. "Besides being a commonly used spice, cinnamon has a long history as a medicine. Medieval physicians used it to treat arthritis, coughing, hoarseness and sore throats. In fact, it was once so valuable, wars were fought over it."

Dr. Pahan has shown that cinnamon can prevent symptoms of Parkinson's disease that include tremors, slow, jerky movement, stiffness and loss of balance. Or at least he's shown that cinnamon has this effect in mice acting as experimental models of Parkinson's disease.

Mouse studies often translate to humans when further research is done—so, given how devastating Parkinson's disease can be...and how familiar and safe cinnamon is...these cinnamon studies merit our attention right now. As Dr. Pahan put it, "If these results are repeatable in Parkinson's disease patients, it would repre-

sent a remarkable advance in the treatment of this neurodegenerative disease."

The first thing to know is that we are not talking about just any kind of cinnamon, but a specific, authentic kind.

Two types of cinnamon are sold in the United States—Chinese cinnamon (sometimes sold as Saigon cinnamon) and Ceylon cinnamon. Chinese cinnamon, or cassia, is the more common, less expensive type of cinnamon and is what you generally find in supermarkets. You know it—the usual cinnamon powder or that hard, aromatic curl of wood that you plunk into hot apple cider or cocoa. But this is not really "true" cinnamon and does not have its health benefits. Ceylon cinnamon is true cinnamon, and its sticks are softer and flakier than those of Chinese cinnamon. The powder is also lighter and sweeter smelling. There is virtually no way of knowing whether the powdered cinnamon you buy is true cinnamon or cassia or a mix unless it is specifically marked. Ceylon cinnamon is what Dr. Pahan is referring to when he talks about the spice. So even just for general health, keep that in mind the next time you head out to the grocery store to replenish your spice rack—you may need to go to a higher-end market or even order online to get Ceylon cinnamon.

HOW DOES IT WORK?

As you may know, cinnamon is loaded with antioxidants. It may be therapeutic in Parkinson's disease because its antioxidant effects counteract nitric oxide, a free radical that attacks proteins essential to supporting adequate levels of dopamine. Dopamine is the chemical in our brains that not only makes us feel happy and motivated but also controls many of our muscle and limb movements.

It's known that the amount of proteins like DJ-1 and Parkin decrease in the brains of patients with Parkinson's disease. "We have found that these proteins also decrease in the brains of mice with Parkinson's disease because of nitric oxide production," said Dr. Pahan. He found that after the mice ate ground cinnamon, their livers turned the cinnamon into an element, or metabolite, that cinnamon breaks down into during digestion, called sodium benzoate. Once the sodium benzoate got to the brain, it decreased the production of nitric oxide, which stopped the loss of Parkin and DJ-1, protected brain cells and allowed the mice to move around more normally, with steadier legs and less need for rest and downtime. According to Dr. Pahan, it's possible that cinnamon could also prevent or lessen the symptoms of other diseases, such as types of palsy and Lewy body dementia, which are also caused by dopamine dysfunction.

HOW TO USE CINNAMON

Dr. Pahan's findings are potentially great news for people with Parkinson's disease and those who worry that they carry the potential for it in their genes. As it stands, Parkinson's disease patients must rely on drugs, such as *levodopa*, to replace dopamine, but these drugs neither cure nor change the course of the disease. They only provide temporary relief. Over time, symptoms become increasingly harder to control, and the drugs often have a wide range of serious side effects.

"Cinnamon, however, and its metabolite sodium benzoate, could potentially be among the safest approaches to stop the progression of Parkinson's disease once it's diagnosed," said Dr. Pahan.

You've probably heard of sodium benzoate. It's a common food preservative found in salad dressings, juices, condiments and cosmetics. The National Institutes of Health's National Center for Complementary and Alternative Medicine has concluded that sodium benzoate and true cinnamon are safe and that true cinnamon is safe even in large amounts—but this is not true for cassia (Chinese cinnamon) because it contains coumarin, which, besides being a blood thinner, can damage the liver.

Unless you're allergic to cinnamon, Dr. Pahan suggests taking one teaspoon a day. But don't attempt to just swallow a teaspoon of dry cinnamon powder "straight-up"! It will make you gag and could cause you to cough and inhale the powder into your lungs, which is dangerous. Instead, mix cinnamon into food or drink.

You can bet there's much more research coming on cinnamon and Parkinson's—meanwhile, generous helpings of this richly antioxidant spice could be well worth trying.

Relief for Vets

More than 200,000 US troops who fought in the Persian Gulf War developed fatigue and other symptoms of Gulf War Illness.

Recent study: 80% of those who took 100 mg of coenzyme Q10 for three-and-a-half months reported improvement.

Neural Computation

How to Get Rid of Funky Fungus

Jamison Starbuck, ND, a naturopathic physician in family practice and a guest lecturer at the University of Montana, both in Missoula. She is past president of the American Association of Naturopathic Physicians and a contributing editor to *The Alternative Advisor: The Complete Guide to Natural Therapies and Alternative Treatments.*

No doubt about it, fungus is funky. Among the most widespread external fungal infections in humans are "athlete's foot" and "jock itch." There's also "yeast," the layman's term for the fungal infection–causing organism known as candida. You can be pretty sure that you have a fungal infection if you notice a few key signs—an area of scaling, peeling skin that may itch, burn, even crack and be very sore… or nails that are discolored (usually yellow or white), brittle, thick, cracked and crusty.

Conventional medical providers prescribe topical or oral antifungals such as *clotrimazole* (Lotrimin), *fluconazole* (Difulcan) or *griseofulvin* (Grifulvin V). These drugs can reduce the problem, and I sometimes prescribe them myself when the infection is severe. However, unless you strengthen your resistance to fungal intrusion, your problem will likely return when you stop the medication and you're exposed to fungi again. *For better results…*

●**Load up on probiotics.** Fungi—like bacteria—are found in and on our bodies at all times, but they cause problems only when their populations get out of control due to such factors as diet. Having lots of healthful bacteria throughout your body will take up much of the cellular space and nutrition the fungi need. That's why I often prescribe the healthful bacteria in probiotics—sometimes up to 30 billion colony-forming units (CFUs) of acidophilus and bifidus per day—for fungal infections. This dose is safe for most adults, though some people can get a loose stool or diarrhea. If this occurs, reduce or discontinue the probiotic.

•**Eliminate all simple sugars.** Forgive me, sugar lovers, but giving up simple sugars for at least 14 days will help reduce the fungi in your body. This means no candy, cookies, desserts, bread, muffins, bagels, pastries or any sort of alcohol. Fungi feed on simple sugars and refined carbohydrates. To help starve out the excess fungi in your system, keep these items out of your diet for two weeks (eat them only sparingly thereafter).

•**Use vinegar and sunlight.** Fungi, which usually thrive in dark, moist areas of our bodies, don't do well in an acidic environment. If you have a topical infection, swab it with a solution of white vinegar and water three times a day. Start with a 50/50 vinegar-water solution, and increase the vinegar strength until it stings. If your fungal rash is cracked, sore or bleeding, topical vinegar can be painful, so avoid it. If possible, also expose your rash to direct sunlight for about 10 minutes, twice daily. These approaches are cheaper than drugstore antifungals and often more effective.

When a fungal infection affects your nails: Fungi often hide beneath the nail (in the nail bed), where it is almost impossible to apply medicine. For this reason, I often prescribe liquid ketoconazole, in addition to the recommendations above, and advise patients to apply it at the edges and as far underneath the nail as is possible. Toenails need to be treated on a daily basis for six months...fingernails require at least three months of treatment.

Pain

Conquer Pain Safely

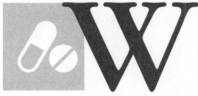

What's the first thing you do when you're hurting? If you are like most people in pain, you reach for aspirin, *ibuprofen* (Advil, Motrin), *naproxen* (Aleve) or a similar non-steroidal anti-inflammatory drug (NSAID). Each day, more than 30 million Americans take these popular medications. Another roughly seven million take a different class of painkiller, *acetaminophen* (Tylenol) each day.

The risks most people don't think about: Even though NSAIDs are as common in most American homes as Band-Aids and multivitamins, few people realize that these medications often cause stomach and intestinal bleeding that leads to up to 20,000 deaths every year in the US. And while previous studies have suggested that these drugs also threaten heart health, an important new meta-analysis found that the risks are more significant than once thought. In fact, ibuprofen and other NSAIDs—taken in doses that many people consider normal—increased the risk for "major vascular events," including heart attacks, by about one-third.

SAFER PAIN RELIEF

The good news is, it's still fine to take an NSAID for arthritis, a headache or other types of short-term pain up to two or three times a week. It is also safe, with your doctor's approval, to take a daily low-dose aspirin (81 mg) to prevent heart attacks and stroke.

What not to do: It is never a good idea to depend on these drugs to relieve chronic pain. As a doctor who specializes in treating arthritis pain, I rarely recommend these medications for long-term use because there are safer analgesics that are just as effective.

Vijay Vad, MD, a sports medicine physician and researcher specializing in minimally invasive arthritis therapies at the Hospital for Special Surgery in New York City. He is author of *Stop Pain: Inflammation Relief for an Active Life.* *VijayVad.com*

My favorite alternatives to oral NSAIDs (ask your doctor which might work best for your pain)…

ANALGESIC CREAMS

You've probably seen over-the-counter pain-relieving creams, such as Zostrix and Capzasin. These products contain capsaicin, which causes a mild burning sensation and appears to reduce substance P, a neurotransmitter that sends pain signals to the brain. Capsaicin products work well for some people suffering from osteoarthritis or rheumatoid arthritis, back pain, shingles and diabetic nerve pain (neuropathy). *Many people, however, get better results from…*

•**Voltaren Gel.** In the heart study mentioned earlier, oral *diclofenac* (Voltaren) was one of the riskiest NSAIDs. But a topical version, Voltaren Gel, which is available by prescription, is less likely to cause side effects, even though it's just as effective as the tablets. Voltaren Gel is good for pain in one joint, but if your pain is in several joints, supplements will offer more relief.

How it's used: Apply the gel (up to four times a day) to the area that's hurting—for example, your knee or wrist.

Helpful: Apply it after a bath or shower, when your skin is soft. More of the active ingredient will pass through the skin and into the painful area. Voltaren Gel should not be combined with an oral NSAID.

PAIN-FIGHTING SUPPLEMENTS

If you need even more pain relief, consider taking one or more of the following supplements. Start with the first one, and if pain has not decreased after eight weeks, add the second, then wait another eight weeks before adding the third, if necessary.

Important: Be sure to check first with your doctor if you take blood thinners or other medications because they could interact.

•**Curcumin.** There's been a lot of research on the anti-inflammatory and painkilling effects of curcumin (the compound that gives the curry spice turmeric its yellow color). One study found that it reduced pain and improved knee function about as well as ibuprofen.

Typical dose: 1,000 mg, twice daily.

•**Fish oil.** A huge amount of data shows that the omega-3 fatty acids in fish oil have analgesic and anti-inflammatory effects.

Scientific evidence: One study found that 60% of patients with neck, back and joint pain who took fish oil improved so much that they were able to stop taking NSAIDs or other medications.

Typical dose: 2,000 mg daily.

•**Boswellia.** Boswellia (or frankincense) is an herbal medicine that reduces both pain and inflammation. It's effective for all types of joint pain, including osteoarthritis and rheumatoid arthritis.

Scientific evidence: In one study, patients with knee arthritis took boswellia or a placebo for two months, then switched to the opposite treatment for another two months.

Results: The people taking boswellia had less pain and more knee mobility than those taking placebos.

Typical dose: 300 mg to 400 mg, three times daily.

HOW TO USE TYLENOL FOR PAIN

If you prefer an oral medication over the options listed above, ask your doctor about switching from NSAIDs to acetaminophen (Tylenol). It's not an anti-inflammatory, but it's an effective pain reliever that doesn't cause stomach upset or bleeding—or trigger an increase in cardiovascular risks. I've found that people who limit the dosage of acetaminophen are unlikely to have side effects.

Caution: Taking too much of this drug can lead to liver damage, particularly if it's used by someone who consumes a lot of alcohol or has underlying liver disease, such as hepatitis.

My recommendation: No more than 2,000 mg daily of acetaminophen (this dosage is lower than the limits listed on the label).

Important: In calculating your total daily dose, be sure to factor in all sources of acetaminophen. More than 600 prescription and over-the-counter drugs, including cold and flu medications and allergy drugs, contain the active ingredient acetaminophen. For a partial list of medications that contain acetaminophen, go to *KnowYourDose.org/common-medications*.

To be safe: Get a liver function test (usually covered by insurance) every six months if you regularly take acetaminophen.

The Chronic Pain-Depression Connection

Gary Kaplan, DO, founder and medical director of the Kaplan Center for Integrative Medicine in McLean, Virginia. He is also clinical associate professor of family medicine at Georgetown University School of Medicine in Washington, DC, and author of *Total Recovery: Solving the Mystery of Chronic Pain and Depression.* KaplanClinic.com

Anyone who lives with unexplained chronic pain knows that it can be depressing. In fact, of the more than 47 million American adults who suffer from chronic pain—often with no identifiable cause—at least two-thirds also have depression.

It's no coincidence, according to Gary Kaplan, DO, a pain expert who believes that the two disorders may be an important symptom of the same underlying condition—inflammation in specific cells of the brain. *Here he supplies advice for people who are suffering from unexplained chronic pain…*

1. Create a time line of life and health. On one sheet of paper, write down the major traumas of your life—physical and emotional—along with the dates (or approximate dates) they happened. On another sheet, write down the dates your pain, depression or illnesses began. By comparing the two, you should be able to see a correlation between them.

2. Consider psychotherapy. If you recognize a pattern in your time line, some of your pain could be due to unresolved feelings about the traumas. Unresolved guilt, shame, resentment and anger inflame neurons in the central nervous system. But resolving these issues can reduce or reverse inflammation.

MRIs of patients who have post-traumatic stress disorder (PTSD) have shown that with cognitive behavioral therapy or eye movement desensiti-

zation and reprocessing—in which certain eye movements and discussion of the trauma are combined—neuron function can return to normal.

3. Avoid NSAIDs. Occasional use of non-steroidal anti-inflammatory drugs (NSAIDs), such as Aleve or Motrin, is fine, but frequent use (three or more times a week) can, over time, lead to chronic intestinal inflammation, which can spread to other organs, including the brain.

4. Ask about medication. I sometimes prescribe low-dose (1.25 mg to 4.5 mg) *naltrexone* (a medication that is used to treat addiction), which can return microglia to a noninflammatory state. Other drugs that may help include *minocycline*, an antibiotic, or an angiotensin receptor blocker, a medication that relaxes blood vessels. If you have chronic pain, ask your doctor about these.

EXTINGUISH YOUR INFLAMMATION CYCLE

Certain lifestyle factors can promote pain-causing inflammation. *What helps…*

•**Test your diet.** For six weeks, avoid all foods with wheat, soy, milk and milk products (foods that often trigger allergies or sensitivities that promote inflammation). Eat only fresh fruits, vegetables, brown rice, fish, chicken and eggs—these foods, in general, are the least likely to cause inflammation.

After six weeks, add back one category of food—such as dairy—per week. Note whether these foods have a negative effect on your energy, mood or level of pain. If so, eliminate that food from your diet entirely.

•**Try meditation.** Research shows that meditation builds new neuronal tissue and helps create a natural resilience to future trauma. Your meditation doesn't have to be a formal program—you can start by simply sitting quietly in a room for 20 minutes each day, allowing your body to gradually relax while you focus on your breathing. Aerobic exercise and adequate sleep also help control inflammation.

Is Your Head Where It Should Be?

Steven Weiniger, DC, member, postgraduate faculty, Logan University, Chesterfield, Missouri, and managing partner, *BodyZone.com*, a national online health information resource and referral directory for posture-exercise professionals. A past delegate to the White House Conference on Aging, he lectures widely on posture and exercise and is author of *Stand Taller, Live Longer: An Anti-Aging Strategy*.

Are you part of the poor-posture epidemic? It's estimated that two out of every three American adults now have forward head posture (FHP), an increasingly common condition in which the head juts out past the shoulders, placing excessive stress on the neck and back.

FHP can be caused by such simple things as texting, driving or even the type of glasses you wear, but it can trigger a surprisingly wide variety of troubling health conditions—from neck, back and shoulder pain…to headaches, digestive issues, breathing difficulties and even arthritis.

Good news: FHP can often be corrected with simple exercises and lifestyle changes.

WHAT CAUSES FHP

A main culprit of FHP is frequent computer use—people tend to lean forward in an effort to see their computer screens. Texting is another common cause, as most people hunch over their smart phones.

Other triggers include: Bucket seats in cars—they encourage an unnatural bend in the body…reading or watching TV while on an exercise machine at the gym—straining to see the page or screen forces the head out of alignment…bifocals—these glasses force you to tilt your head backward and stick your chin out in order to see through the lower portion of the lenses…carrying a heavy backpack—the load causes your head to protrude forward…and the natural process of aging—as the neck muscles weaken, the head drifts forward.

Startling fact: Every inch that your head moves forward past your spine adds 10 pounds of pressure to the neck and back, which often leads to muscle and joint pain and headaches. A forward-hanging head also compresses the rib cage, compromising the lungs' ability to expand by as much as 30% and slowing down digestion. What's more, over time, FHP can cause the spine to stiffen, limiting range of motion and contributing to osteoarthritis.

Recent study: When more than 800 adults over age 65 were followed for about five years, those who began leaning forward at an earlier age were 3.5 times more likely to require assistance bathing, dressing, eating and getting in and out of chairs than those who started leaning forward later.

EASY TO SELF-DIAGNOSE

A simple photo is often all you need to determine whether you have FHP. Put on some gym clothes and stand as you normally would in a straight but not stiff position. Then have a spouse or friend snap a full-length photo of you from the side. Look at the photo—the middle of your ear should be lined up with your shoulder, hipbone and ankle. If your head is forward, the alignment of your body is off. Save the photo as a baseline, and have a photo taken monthly to monitor your progress once you begin using the strategies below.

HOW TO HELP YOURSELF

•**Become more aware of your head position.** Lying down on the floor, flat on your back, take a moment to notice where your gaze naturally falls—if you have FHP, you will likely be looking slightly back and away from your feet (those who have healthy posture will be looking straight up at the ceiling).

To recognize the proper head position: While still lying on your back, gently lift your head just off the floor and tuck in your chin to give yourself a slight double chin. Then, keeping your chin tucked, put your head back down. If you're looking straight up at the ceiling, your head is now in the proper "level-head" position.

Take five slow breaths here, then relax on the floor for two to three minutes to let your head align with your torso and pelvis. Do this two to three times a day to help retrain your body. If you have discomfort in your low back, put a small pillow under your knees.

•**Perform chin tucks every day.** Initially, do these exercises on the floor. Lying down in the level-head position, take a deep breath in…while exhaling, press your chin into a tuck. Release and repeat for five cycles, two to three times a day.

If the stretch in the back of your neck feels too intense or you can't keep your head level, try propping your head up on an inch-thick book wrapped in a thin towel. (Use a book you don't want, since you're going to be removing pages.) After doing this exercise a few times a day for three or four days, remove about an eighth of the pages. Repeat for a few more days and remove another small section of pages, continuing this cycle until the book is empty and your head is flat on the ground.

As chin tucks become easier, you don't have to do them lying down and can do them regularly throughout the day—at your computer or even walking down the street.

●**Make other changes to your daily routine.** The average American logs about 11 hours of screen time per day—including time spent on computers, using smart phones and watching TV. At work and at home, make sure your computer screen is at eye level. If you use a laptop, use a laptop stand and purchase a separate keyboard. When using a smart phone for texting or e-mail, try to hold it at eye level. When wearing bifocals for reading, adjust the glasses on your nose rather than changing your head position. These strategies will help keep your ears in line with your shoulders and may even help prevent wrinkles caused by squinting.

And before driving, be sure the seat is not tilted excessively backward—this forces you to hold your head at an angle that contributes to FHP.

●**Use a cervical pillow for sleeping.** Cervical pillows improve spinal alignment by cradling the head and supporting the neck, usually with an indentation or cutout in the middle of the pillow. You may need to try several pillows before finding the one that's most comfortable for you. I like the cervical pillows by Therapeutica (*TherapeuticaInc.com*) and Tempur-Pedic (*TempurPedic.com*) and the Chiroflow Water Pillow (*Chiroflow.com*).

If after two to four weeks of trying these strategies you're still experiencing health problems related to FHP, be sure to see a chiropractor or physical therapist.

Noninvasive Devices May Help Migraines

U.S. Food and Drug Administration, news release.

Two recent prescription devices approved by the U.S. Food and Drug Administration (FDA) may provide some relief for people with migraine headaches who don't tolerate migraine medications well, according to a recent study.

One device—the Cefaly—is designed to prevent migraines, while the other device—the Cerena—is meant to be used when migraines first start, according to an FDA news release.

"Patients have been looking for alternative migraine treatments. Because these devices aren't ingested or metabolized like drug therapies, they don't necessarily have the same types of side effects," Michael Hoffmann, a biomedical engineer with the FDA, said in the news release.

Migraines involve severe pulsing or throbbing pain in one part of the head. These intense headaches can also cause people to develop nausea and vomiting as well as sensitivity to light and sound. About one-third of people with migraines experience an aura, or visual effects such as flashing lights, dots or a blind spot, which marks the onset of the headache, said the FDA.

Migraines can last as long as 72 hours if left untreated. These headaches affect 37 million people in the United States. Although anyone—even children—can get migraines, women are affected more often than men, the FDA reported.

"There are many drugs to reduce migraine pain and symptoms," said Eric Bastings, MD, a neurologist with the FDA, in the news release. "Although these drugs are quite effective, they are not for everyone. Some can make you tired, drowsy or dizzy. Some can affect your thinking. And some migraine drugs can cause birth defects; so pregnant women can't use them," he said.

The Cerena Transcranial Magnetic Stimulator can be used as soon as patients feel a migraine coming on. It's held against the back of the head. After pressing a button, a very short magnetic pulse stimulates the area of the brain that processes visual information, the FDA said.

The Cefaly transcutaneous electrical nerve stimulation device is also FDA-approved as a preventative treatment for migraine. Patients can use this device daily before a migraine develops. This portable, battery-powered device involves an electrode patch that is placed on patients' foreheads. The patch is connected to a headband. The device sets off an electrical current to stimulate a large nerve in the head that has been linked to migraines, the agency said.

"It's a set-time therapy—running for 20 minutes and stopping automatically," Dr. Hoffmann noted.

Reported side effects for both devices were minor and resolved quickly, including:

- **Skin irritation**
- **Discomfort**
- **Sleepiness**
- **Dizziness**
- **Pain at site of application**

The FDA researchers noted the safety and effectiveness of the Cerena and Cefaly have not been evaluated in use by children, pregnant women and those with pacemakers.

info The U.S. National Institute of Neurological Disorders and Stroke provides more information on migraine pain at *http://www.ninds. nih.gov/disorders/migraine/migraine.htm*.

Take Control of Tension Headaches

Yacov Ezra, MD, assistant head of neurology at Soroka University Medical Center and a lecturer at Ben-Gurion University, both in Be'er Sheva, Israel.

Taking a painkiller now and then may not be a problem if you have occasional tension headaches. But it's a different story if you frequently get that steady ache on both sides of your head—you probably know the feeling…it's a little like your head is being squeezed in a vise! With regular use, nonsteroidal anti-inflammatory drugs (NSAIDs) such as *ibuprofen* (Motrin) can lead to stomach problems and other side effects, while *acetaminophen* (Tylenol) can put the health of your liver at risk.

There is also the trap of getting "rebound" headaches—a common complication when a frequent headache sufferer overuses medication to fight the constant pain.

A missing link: In the quest to quell the pain of tension-type headaches, one crucial point often gets overlooked—up to 88% of these headaches are believed to be caused by stress. On top of that, nearly half of people suffering from chronic tension-type headaches also have depression or anxiety disorders, which painkillers don't treat.

Many doctors prescribe *amitriptyline* (Elavil), a tricyclic antidepressant, to boost mood and help regulate pain signals. This drug helps some people with tension-type headaches, but it, like other medication, has its share of bothersome side effects—dizziness, drowsiness and dry mouth, to name just a few. What's the answer?

RESEARCH UNCOVERS A BETTER SOLUTION

To test how tension-type headache sufferers would respond to a drug versus a nondrug approach, researchers gave 98 people with frequent or chronic tension-type headaches the choice of using amitriptyline or trying "hypnotic-relaxation therapy"—a technique that induces a deeply relaxed, focused state.

The results, published in the journal *Headache*, showed that the headache sufferers, who met with therapists to learn hypnotic relaxation, not only preferred this technique over the medication but also found it far more effective because it works as both a treatment and preventive. Specifically, after up to a year of follow-up, 74% of patients in the hypnotic-relaxation group had a 50% reduction in headache frequency, compared with 58% of patients in the amitriptyline group.

Even though this study did not include painkillers such as NSAIDs, researchers believe that hypnotic relaxation offers benefits over those medications, too. For example, with hypnotic relaxation, headache sufferers are not putting themselves at risk for the rebound headaches that so often occur with frequent use of painkilling medication.

So what does this research mean for the average sufferer of tension-type headaches? Anyone can use hypnotic relaxation. People with tension headaches who try the technique are usually surprised by the simplicity of it. In fact, it takes just a few minutes to learn the progressive muscle relaxation and focused breathing exercises underlying the technique. *How to begin…**

●**Find a quiet,** private space that's distraction free. Turn off your cell phone.

●**Get comfortable on a chair or couch (sitting or lying down).**

●**Close your eyes and empty your mind of thoughts (as much as possible).** When intrusive thoughts return, simply acknowledge them and allow them to "drift away."

●**Breathe slowly and deeply,** visualizing tension leaving your body with each exhale. Imagine vitality entering your body with each inhale.

●**Progressively relax your body's major muscle groups,** beginning with your toes and then moving through the calves, thighs, hips, stomach, hands, arms, shoulders, neck, face and head. Stay in this relaxed state for a number of minutes, noticing the rising and falling of your chest. Now, imagine that you are at the top of a flight of 10 steps. Tell yourself that you are going to walk down the steps and count backward from 10 as you picture yourself descending each step. Feel yourself becoming more relaxed with each step.

How to create a hypnotic trance: Your next task is to self-induce a hypnotic trance using what is known as a "safe-place technique."

What to do: With your eyes closed and while breathing deeply, mentally take yourself to a place that feels calm and safe. This could be a quiet forest, a sunny beach or a serene mountaintop. What do you see, smell, hear and taste? How do you feel in this place? Engage all your senses. After a few minutes, begin repeating suggestions to yourself that reinforce a sense of well-being and lack of pain in your head.

These suggestions may include statements such as: The muscles in my head and neck are completely relaxed…my head is completely pain-free. The entire relaxation session

*If you have difficulty with this technique, consult a trained hypnotherapist who is also a medical doctor or psychologist.

Botox for Head Pain

Botox injections help more than just chronic migraines. They can help frequent episodic migraines, TMJ-related headaches and cluster, cervicogenic and post-traumatic headaches. In his experience, approximately 70% of patients treated with Botox for headache pain see significant improvement.

Alexander Mauskop, MD, director of the New York Headache Center and CEO of Migralex, Inc., both in New York City.

takes only about 10 minutes. Ideally, headache sufferers should use hypnotic relaxation three times daily to guard against stressors that trigger tension-type headaches…it can also be used as soon as a headache starts to develop so the sufferer can quickly gain control over the pain. If pain medication is still needed, hypnotic relaxation will likely allow for a reduced dose.

What to Take for a Tension Headache—No Drugs Needed

Trupti Gokani, MD, board-certified neurologist and director of the Zira Mind & Body Center in Glenview, Illinois. Her special interests include alternative approaches to headache management and women's issues. *ZiraMind AndBody.com*

What can you take when a tension headache grabs hold? Integrative neurologist Trupti Gokani, MD, director of the North Shore Headache Clinic in Highland Park, Illinois, suggested trying any or all of the following options. Products are available at health-food stores and/or online. *Consider taking…*

●**A few bites of food or a big drink of water.** If hunger or dehydration is triggering your headache, the pain may disappear once you assuage your body's basic needs. Just about any healthful food will do…but stay away from known headache triggers such as processed meats, aged cheeses, red wine and anything with monosodium glutamate, Dr. Gokani said.

•**Butterbur supplements.** Though various supplements may prevent headaches when taken regularly, butterbur works best to help halt a headache you already have. This anti-inflammatory herb should be taken as soon as you feel the pain coming on. Try the brand Petadolex (*Petadolex.com*), which contains a purified form of butterbur free from liver-damaging pyrrolizidine alkaloids.

Caution: Do not use butterbur if you are pregnant or have liver disease.

•**Some whiffs of an aromatherapy remedy.** Finding the right scent may require some experimentation, Dr. Gokani said, because an aroma that soothes pain for one person can irritate another.

Options to try: Essential oil of lavender… basil…or clary sage.

To use: Sprinkle three drops of the desired essential oil onto a tissue or handkerchief and take a sniff every few minutes…or sprinkle three drops onto a hot or cold compress and apply to your forehead until the pain lets up.

•**Ask yourself why you have this headache.** A tension headache usually has an underlying trigger.

Consider: Do you need a break from your computer screen? Are you working in a poorly lit room? Might a short walk or a chat with a friend help relieve whatever stress you're under? Once you identify the root problem and take action to rectify it, your pain should ease up.

Neck Pain Relief…at Last

Pierre Côté, DC, PhD, associate professor, Faculty of Health Sciences, and director, Centre for the Study of Disability Prevention and Rehabilitation, University of Ontario Institute of Technology (UOIT), Oshawa.

Most of us will suffer from neck pain at some point in our lives—it's the fourth-leading cause of chronic disability in the US. It's no wonder that we call an aggravating, unrelenting person or situation "a pain in the neck."

GETTING A GRIP ON NECK PAIN

Until now, no one really knew for sure what specific types of exercises worked best for neck pain. Now a recent study from Canada has answered this important question. The right treatment can reduce pain so that a person can return to his/her normal activities faster. Don't be too impatient about mild neck pain. It will usually get better within a week, so give that much time to allow the pain and stiffness to subside before running off to a doctor for treatment.

RELIEF FOR NEW, MILD NECK PAIN

Gentle stretching and range-of-motion exercises, done all by yourself in the privacy of your home, help keep your neck muscles toned and limber and are usually enough to bounce back from mild neck pain caused by muscle strain from, for example, spending too much time in front of your computer or whiplash from a minor car accident. If that sounds simple, it is, but the fact is that many people do the opposite when they have any kind of neck pain—they try to not move their necks…often wearing a protective neck collar or brace. Bad choice!

Instead, try doing five to 10 repetitions of these simple movements three to four times daily (the sequence doesn't matter, but do them slowly)…

•**Act as if you are saying "no" by slowly rotating your head from right to left and back again,** making sure to turn your head as far as it will comfortably go to enhance range of motion.

•**Act as if you are saying "yes" by nodding your head up and down,** gently stretching your head up as if to view the ceiling and flexing it down as if to look at the floor to work on range of motion.

•**Act as if you are saying "maybe" by tipping your head from side to side, moving each ear toward that side's shoulder.**

Also, keep active in general, but avoid any activities or movements that aggravate the neck pain. Remember, you want a good stretch, not a strain.

RELIEF FOR LONG-TERM, PERSISTENT PAIN

What happens when nagging neck pain doesn't go away in a week or so and your doctor has no real solution? You don't have to just grin and bear it. Ongoing neck pain can be eased with a combination of range-of-motion exercises (described above) and flexibility and strengthening exercises or routines, particularly qigong and Iyengar yoga.

Home-based range-of-motion exercises are not any less effective than expensive supervised intensive rehabilitative neck-strengthening exercises. So why not consider making a simple set of range-of-motion neck exercises part of your daily routine…and have some fun? Learn something new and kick your health and well-being up a big notch by trying a class in qigong or Iyengar yoga.

FOR SEVERE NECK PAIN

Severe neck pain and stiffness that's really bad and lasting might be the sign of a number of other conditions, such as cervical dystonia or a pinched nerve (often accompanied by a shooting pain down the arm). To find out exactly what's wrong and what the remedy is, it is best to consult a medical doctor, physiotherapist or chiropractor who can make a diagnosis, refer you to a specialist and set up a treatment plan.

Fibromyalgia: New Research Helps Unravel the Mystery

Anne Louise Oaklander, MD, PhD, an associate professor of neurology at Harvard Medical School and director of a diagnostic and research laboratory at Massachusetts General Hospital that studies neurological causes of chronic pain and itch, both in Boston.

For the roughly five million American adults with fibromyalgia, the muscle soreness, body aches and telltale painful "tender points" on the shoulders, neck, back, hips, arms and legs are all too familiar.

Even though the American College of Rheumatology has recognized fibromyalgia as an illness since 1990, most doctors have been uneasy about diagnosing it because there has been no way to test for the condition. X-rays and blood tests can rule out other conditions, such as rheumatoid arthritis, but fibromyalgia has been a diagnosis based on symptoms alone. The recent research findings may change that.

What important recent studies have uncovered: According to several studies published in 2013, one conducted by researchers at Massachusetts General Hospital, nearly half of people with fibromyalgia have evidence of a disease called small-fiber polyneuropathy (SFPN).

A form of peripheral neuropathy, SFPN involves damage to specific nerve cells that can trigger pain and the digestive problems that often accompany fibromyalgia.

How was this discovery made? Skin biopsies were the key tests that uncovered abnormalities in the nerve cells of 40% of SFPN sufferers who were tested.

Meanwhile, researchers at Albany Medical College found another interesting piece of the puzzle—excessive nerve fibers lining the blood vessels within the skin of people with fibromyalgia. Since these fibers control the flow of blood, oxygen and nutrients to muscles during exercise, this abnormality might explain the deep muscle pain of fibromyalgia.

These recent findings do not mean that the name has been changed—fibromyalgia (fibro, the Latin term for fibrous tissue…and the Greek words myo, meaning muscle…and algia, meaning pain) perfectly describes the condition's primary symptoms of chronic, widespread muscle pain.

Even though the discoveries described above don't apply to all fibromyalgia patients, they give researchers some clues to follow toward cracking the disease's formidable mystery.

NEW HOPE FOR BETTER TREATMENTS

Scientists may be intrigued by this new evidence, but what does it mean for people who suffer from fibromyalgia? The most immediate—and significant—implication has to do with testing. Fibromyalgia symptoms can vary widely, so the diagnosis can be challenging even for experienced rheumatologists.

Now that fibromyalgia has been linked to SFPN, people with fibromyalgia symptoms may want to ask their doctors about testing for SFPN. A skin biopsy from the lower leg is currently the best way to diagnose SFPN. The sample can be mailed to an accredited lab—for example, at

Massachusetts General Hospital—for analysis. It is usually covered by insurance.

In the meantime, the following medications (in addition to the nondrug approaches described) can help relieve symptoms of fibromyalgia...

•**FDA-approved medications.** *Pregabalin* (Lyrica), an *anticonvulsant*...and *duloxetine* (Cymbalta) and *milnacipran HCI* (Savella), both serotonin and norepinephrine reuptake inhibitors (SNRIs), have been shown to reduce pain and improve function for some people with fibromyalgia. Researchers do not know exactly why these drugs work, but some data suggest that they affect pain signaling in the brain and spinal cord.

•**Nortriptyline (Pamelor).** An older tricyclic antidepressant that has also been proven effective for chronic pain relief, nortriptyline is not specifically FDA-approved for fibromyalgia. But it and several other off-label medications, including the *anticonvulsant gabapentin* (Neurontin)—available cheaply as generic drugs—have strong data supporting their use for fibromyalgia.

NONDRUG APPROACHES...

Medication isn't the only treatment for fibromyalgia symptoms. *Other good options...*

•**Exercise.** Don't think this is just another plug for exercise. The research showing exercise's effect on fibromyalgia pain is very strong. Whether it's walking, strength training or stretching, exercise improves emotional well-being and lessens muscle wasting, an unfortunate consequence of avoiding exercise due to pain.

•**Vitamin D.** This inexpensive vitamin supplement has just begun to prove its mettle for some people with fibromyalgia. A study published in January 2014 in the journal *PAIN* indicates that vitamin D supplements may reduce chronic pain linked to fibromyalgia for those whose blood tests show a low level of the nutrient. The optimal vitamin D dose depends on the level of deficiency.

Joint Pain: Is It Arthritis?

Harris H. McIlwain, MD, a pain specialist who is board-certified in internal medicine, rheumatology and geriatric medicine. With a private practice in Tampa, Florida, Dr. McIlwain is author of 28 books on topics including arthritis, osteoporosis, back pain and fibromyalgia.

That stabbing, aching pain in your joints may mean that you just have a touch of garden-variety osteoarthritis. Or so you tell yourself.

What most people don't realize: When osteoarthritis wears down the cartilage covering the ends of your bones, it can lead to bony growths known as osteophytes, an often undetected source of severe joint pain.

Commonly known as bone spurs, these smooth or pointed growths on normal bone tissue also can form in response to stress on a joint—as may occur from repetitive motion activities, such as running or typing. Regardless of the trigger, bone spurs can rub against other bones, ligaments, tendons or nerves and are marked by painful inflammation.

Why this matters: It's important to distinguish bone spurs from run-of-the-mill arthritis so that you can take the necessary steps to stay ahead of potentially debilitating joint inflammation. If not dealt with in the right way (and at the right time), bone spurs often require powerful additional treatment to control the pain, and this treatment can have bad side effects. You want to deal with bone spurs early.

What you need to know to determine whether you have bone spurs—and the therapies that help most...

MORE THAN ARTHRITIS

How do you tell whether your joint pain is partly or completely due to bone spurs?

Clues to watch for: Osteoarthritis pain tends to come and go gradually—like the general stiffness that affects a large area of your body, such as your lower back, in the morning but eases by afternoon.

A bone spur, on the other hand, may cause chronic localized pain that's bad enough to make you not want to move your back, neck, hip, finger or some other joint that may be affected. You may have bone spurs in more than one place, but one spur could cause more pain, depending on its location and the amount of physical activity in that area.

The more sudden and severe the pain, the more likely that a bone spur is the culprit. Numbness, tenderness and weakness may also occur. If a parent or sibling has suffered from bone spurs, you're at increased risk, too—research suggests there is a genetic component.

HOT SPOTS FOR BONE SPURS

Any joint can develop a bone spur, but here are the most common locations and how the pain and other symptoms may vary in each part of your body...

•**Knees.** Bone spurs in the knee—a common location for those that occur with osteoarthritis—often resemble a pointy bird's beak on X-rays. The resulting discomfort is typically a blend of arthritis and bone spur pain—both sore and sharp.

•**Feet and/or heels.** Acute pain that occurs with every step—the kind that makes you want to avoid walking—can signal bone spurs in the feet and/or heels (often called "heel spurs"). Corns and calluses may also build up over heels or toes as the body tries to protect the area by providing added padding. Therefore, if you have pain along with corns and/or calluses, ask your doctor to check for a bone spur.

•**Hips.** Arthritis in the hips generally produces a deep aching and stiffness that occurs when you stand or walk. Bone spurs at the side of the hip—where the bony prominence can sometimes be felt—trigger pain when the hip is flexed, such as when riding a bike.

•**Hands and/or shoulders.** Jabbing pain (rather than a dull throb) is the telltale sign.

•**Neck and/or spine.** Bone spurs at these locations usually do not cause pain unless accompanied by arthritis, but they can pinch the spinal cord and irritate surrounding nerves.

GETTING DIAGNOSED

If you have one or more bone spurs, the usual arthritis treatments—including nonsteroidal anti-inflammatory drugs (NSAIDs), such as *ibuprofen* (Motrin) and *naproxen* (Aleve)...stretching...and warm heat—often don't make a dent in your joint pain.

Because bone spurs usually are not large enough to feel externally, an X-ray is the easiest way to diagnose them. In certain areas, such as the neck, more advanced imaging tests, such as MRI or CT scans, may be needed to diagnose them.

My advice: If your joint pain doesn't respond to the therapies described earlier and you suspect that you may have bone spurs, you don't need a definitive diagnosis provided by an X-ray. Ask your physician whether you may have bone spurs, and get his/her OK to promptly try the approaches below. If you don't start treatment quickly, the serious pain that bone spurs typically cause may limit your use of the joint, progressively weakening muscles surrounding it and creating an even worse problem.

FINDING THE BEST TREATMENT

Among the best therapies for joint pain due to bone spurs...

•**Alternate heating pads and ice packs in 20-minute intervals.** Use ice first to ease acute pain, then moist heat to penetrate inflamed areas. Do this twice a day.

•**Get acupuncture.** Acupuncture has been shown to reduce pain and improve functional mobility. Your acupuncturist will tailor a treatment plan for your bone spur.

•**Eat inflammation-fighting foods.** Processed foods promote inflammation, while certain whole foods, such as salmon, nuts, beets, leafy greens, olive oil and berries, fight it. Include as many of these foods in your daily diet as possible.

•**Use targeted supplements.** These include fish oil, turmeric and ginger. There is strong research showing that these supplements help fight painful inflammation.

My advice: You can take one or all of these supplements, depending on the intensity of your pain. Daily dosages are up to 3 g of fish oil...three 400-mg to 600-mg tablets or capsules of turmeric...and two 500-mg to 1,000-mg capsules of ginger, taken with food. It usually takes about two months for turmeric to work.

Caution: Talk to your doctor before using any of these supplements if you take any type of medication (especially a blood thinner) or have a chronic medical condition.

•**Try ultrasound therapy.** Ultrasound uses sound waves that can penetrate more than two inches into the body to reach the painful area. Often used for shoulder or heel pain caused by bone spurs, it can be administered by a medical doctor or physical therapist.

Caveat: The pain relief provided by ultrasound may be long-lasting but sometimes lasts only a few weeks.

WHEN TO CONSIDER SURGERY

One of the biggest misconceptions about bone spurs is that they need to be removed surgically. The truth is, when strategies such as those described in this article are used, the inflammation may lessen after a period of weeks or months even though the spur does not go away.

In determining the need for surgery, location of the bone spurs is the key factor. For example, bone spurs located in the neck can press on nerves or even the esophagus, which can interfere with swallowing.

Generally, however, the risks associated with surgery, such as infection, outweigh the benefits for most bone spurs. If you have tried the regimen described above for bone spurs for about a year but still have not gotten adequate pain relief, then ask your primary care doctor for a referral to an orthopedic surgeon.

Shingles: You Could Have It and Not Even Know It

Anne Louise Oaklander, MD, PhD, director of a diagnostic and research laboratory at Massachusetts General Hospital that studies neurological causes of chronic pain and itch and associate professor of neurology at Harvard Medical School, both in Boston.

Many people think that shingles is just a rash, so they wait for it to go away like poison ivy and sunburn do. That's a big mistake. If you suspect that you may have shingles, take action right away—it's a neurological emergency.

The rash that we see on the skin, which develops on half the body only, usually in a band around the torso or above and around the eye, is just the tip of the iceberg.* The center of the infection is deep inside the body, within sensory nerve cells close to the spinal cord or brain. In some cases, the infection can spread into the spinal cord or brain to cause myelitis or encephalitis, stroke or spinal-cord injury.

A recent study published in the journal *Neurology* found that the risk of having a stroke years later was up to 74% higher in people who had been diagnosed with shingles before age 40. The virus also can cause vision loss or hearing or balance problems.

But the most common complication of shingles is post-herpetic neuralgia (PHN), where pain persists after the rash heals. The pain can be intense—some people compare it to childbirth or passing a kidney stone. It gradually improves, but that can take months or years, and sometimes it never goes away. The nerve damage that causes pain also can lead to intense itching, known as post-herpetic itch. Although both are treatable, the medications often have side effects that make them unpleasant to use.

The best way to avoid getting shingles (and its complications): Get vaccinated. For people age 60 and older, the onetime vaccination reduces the risk of getting shingles by half and reduces the chance of the persistent pain of PHN

*To view photos of the shingles rash, go to *shinglesin fo.com.*

by two-thirds. It is even more effective in adults ages 50 to 60, reducing shingles risk by 70%.

Even so, a sobering recent study shows that less than 7% of adults who are eligible for the shingles vaccine have received it—even though it has no major side effects.

Why are so few people getting vaccinated? One reason is that there are widespread misconceptions about who should get this vaccine. Everyone in the US has been exposed to chicken pox by his/her adult years and is at risk for shingles. However, many people think only adults in their 70s and 80s, who tend to be at greatest risk for the illness, should receive the vaccine.

The truth is, the shingles vaccine is important for people who are younger than that, but there's not a consensus even among government agencies. The CDC recommends it for adults who are age 60 and older, while the FDA has approved it for people age 50 and older. Ask your physician for his recommendation.**

Contrary to popular opinion, even children, college students and adults in their 30s and 40s can develop shingles, although far less often than older adults. Impaired immunity—not only from aging but also from immune-suppressing drugs or chronic diseases such as HIV, cancer or rheumatoid arthritis—is the main shingles risk factor. But young people who don't have these conditions can still develop the illness.

To give yourself—and loved ones—the best chances of avoiding shingles, here are additional misconceptions you should know about the condition…

MISCONCEPTION #1: You can't develop shingles more than once. Having shingles boosts your immunity and offers some protection against a rapid recurrence. But that "booster effect" can wane, and you can have a second attack. Furthermore, people with impaired immunity may not experience this effect and can have recurrent or prolonged episodes. So even if you've had shingles, talk to your doctor about vaccination.

MISCONCEPTION #2: The pain will end in a few weeks. Everyone with shingles

**Because the shingles vaccine contains a live virus, it is not recommended for people undergoing radiation or chemotherapy…those with some cancers…or patients with HIV or other conditions that affect the immune system.

breathes a sigh of relief when the painful rash is gone—usually within two to four weeks. But in some cases, the problem continues. The older you are, the longer the pain can continue. Sometimes, it never completely subsides.

MISCONCEPTION #3: There's no harm in taking a wait-and-see approach. Shingles symptoms can start days or a week before the rash appears. You may notice pain or itching in a band on one side of your body before the rash appears. If pain occurs on the chest, some patients worry that they could be having a heart attack. Even without the rash, a one-sided area or band of pain or itching is highly suspicious for shingles, particularly in older or immunosuppressed patients.

Savvy doctors will consider starting treatment with antiviral medications even during this early "prodrome" stage, when these drugs may abort an attack.

Even when started after the rash appears, antivirals significantly reduce the severity of the rash, its pain and also the risk for PHN and other complications. So if your regular doctor can't see you immediately when you first notice symptoms, go to an urgent-care center or an emergency room.

If the doctor orders a blood test to identify shingles, ask to start antiviral medications immediately. These medications, specifically *acyclovir* (Zovirax), *famciclovir* (Famvir) or *valacyclovir* (Valtrex), can reduce the risk for PHN.

Important: Quick treatment is particularly important if the rash occurs anywhere near the eye. See an ophthalmologist immediately. Most people do not realize that shingles can cause corneal ulcers, glaucoma and even blindness.

In addition to antiviral drugs, you'll probably be given steroid eyedrops to reduce inflammation and possibly a short-term course of oral steroids. Steroids can impair immunity, so don't take them unless you've already started an antiviral drug.

MISCONCEPTION #4: There's not much you can do for the painful rash. Even though antiviral medication is the main treatment, low doses of *nortriptyline* (Pamelor, Aventyl) can reduce pain. The drug also improves sleep and reduces the risk for PHN by about 50%.

Although originally marketed to treat depression, *nortriptyline* and other tricyclic anti-depressants are unsurpassed in their ability to treat neuropathic or nerve-injury pain such as that caused by shingles. Inexpensive generics are available, and one dose lasts more than 24 hours. But they must be taken for a few weeks to fully kick in, and they can have side effects, such as dizziness and weight gain, so discuss these drugs with your doctor.

AN EXPERIMENTAL SHINGLES TREATMENT

Transcranial magnetic stimulation, a noninvasive procedure that uses magnets to trigger firing of certain neurons in the brain, appears to relieve post-herpetic neuralgia (PHN) in some patients who suffer pain three months or longer after their shingles rash has healed.

This approach is still in the experimental stages, but has been approved by the U.S. Food and Drug Administration to treat migraines and treatment-resistant major depressive disorder. Clinical trials are often available. Visit Clinical Trials.gov for a possible trial near you. (Search "transcranial magnetic stimulation and PHN")

The Secret Muscles That Can Cause Chronic Pain

Jo Ann Staugaard-Jones, MA, an advanced Pilates and Hatha yoga instructor based in Andover, New Jersey. She is a former professor of kinesiology, exercise science and dance at County College of Morris in Randolph, New Jersey, and author of *The Anatomy of Exercise & Movement* and *The Vital Psoas Muscle. Move-Live.com*

Most people have heard plenty about the core—that band of muscles in the abdomen, low back, hips and pelvis. But what if there were some far less well-known muscles that could be causing all your trouble? Say hello to the psoas (pronounced SO-as) muscles! Ignoring these crucial muscles can lead to low-back pain and poor posture.

What you need to know…

WHERE ARE THEY?

Located deep within the center of the body, the psoas major muscles are the only muscles that connect the upper and lower extremities of your body. As a pair of muscles on both the right and left sides, they run from the lower spine, past the front of the pelvis, through either side of the groin and attach to the inside of the femurs (thighbones).

So what exactly do these muscles do? The psoas muscles help with the transfer of weight when you're walking or running. When you extend your leg back, for example, the psoas on that side lengthens…when you lift your knee, it contracts. The psoas muscles also act as stabilizers of the lower spine, the pelvis and the legs, aiding body alignment and posture.

What goes wrong: If the psoas muscles are shortened for long periods of time—as occurs when sitting, for example—they can tighten on one or both sides. If the psoas on one side of the body is tighter than the other (from leaning to one side while sitting, for instance), it can also torque the spine, affecting your posture and gait. An imbalance on one or both sides can lead to inflammation and pain while walking.

Unlike toned abs, you can't see the psoas muscles. Because you can't touch your psoas muscles either, it can be difficult to tell if they're the cause of your back pain and poor posture.

There are some clues, however, that may indicate that these muscles are tight or weak—for example, you may also feel discomfort in the hip sockets, the glutes or even the sacroiliac joints, which are in the back of the pelvis. The pain can be in one spot or travel throughout the path of the muscle.

KEEPING YOUR PSOAS MUSCLES IN SHAPE

The first step to keeping the psoas muscles in top shape is to stand up. Instead of sitting for long periods of time, get up and move around at least every hour. *To help prevent or relieve psoas-related pain, also do these three exercises every other day (as with any exercise program, check with your doctor first)…*

Exercise #1: **Lunge.** Also known as the "runner's stretch," the lunge strengthens and stretches the psoas and thigh muscles.

What to do: Stand with your left foot forward and right leg back (about three to four feet apart). Bend your front knee until it's directly

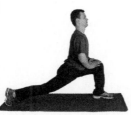

over your toes, at about a 90-degree angle. Slide your right leg straight back until it is almost parallel to the floor. Keep your feet facing forward, and don't let your front knee extend beyond your toes. Your spine should be straight, and you can rest your hands on the floor or the front of one thigh. Hold for up to 30 seconds, then repeat on the other side.

Exercise #2: **Teaser or Boat pose**. This position, used in both Pilates and yoga, works the psoas muscles and several other core muscles.

What to do: Sit on the floor with your legs extended out in front. While keeping your

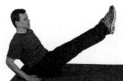

hands on the floor behind your hips, lean back slightly and balance just behind your "sits" bones (beneath your buttocks). Then gently raise one leg and then the other as high as possible, so that your body is in a "V" position. Hold for 10 seconds while keeping your chest lifted and your torso long. If you're able, extend your arms forward for added challenge. Repeat three times, or hold longer.

Exercise #3: **Windmill.** This exercise strengthens and stretches the psoas muscles and oblique (side abdominal) muscles.

What to do: While standing with your arms extended out to each side and your knees slightly bent, lean forward and touch your left hand to your right ankle as you extend your right arm upward and look up toward the ceil-

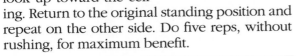

ing. Return to the original standing position and repeat on the other side. Do five reps, without rushing, for maximum benefit.

End Your Back Pain... for Good

Patrick A. Roth, MD, FACS, chairman of the department of neurosurgery and director of the neurosurgical residency training program at Hackensack University Medical Center in Hackensack, New Jersey. He is also the founder of the North Jersey Brain & Spine Center in Oradell, New Jersey, and the author of *The End of Back Pain*.

You're lucky if you haven't suffered a backache recently. It's common...make that very common.

In any three-month period, 25% of adults will suffer at least one day of back pain. Over the course of a lifetime, about 85% of us will experience back pain at some point.

My story: As a spinal surgeon and a former back pain sufferer, I've examined this malady from all angles. What I have discovered is that contrary to our culture of "pop a pill" or "go under the knife," the best course of action starts with discovering your "hidden" core.

FINDING YOUR HIDDEN CORE

If I told you that you needed to strengthen your core, you might assume that means doing crunches to work on your abdominal muscles, or abs. While washboard abs are the most visible and easily trained part of your core, they are only part of a larger muscle group that makes up the core.

In fact, strengthening your abs without also working on your hidden core can make back pain worse. That's because unbalanced core muscles cause an unstable spine.

The muscles you don't see: Your core is a group of muscles that encircles your midsection—front, sides and back. And most of the muscles lie deep inside your body—hidden from view. Taken together, these muscles form an internal brace around your spine, holding it erect, protecting it from damage. In order to reduce or limit back pain, you need to strengthen all your core muscles equally.

THE HIDDEN CORE WORKOUT

The workout I've developed targets all the inner muscles that make up your body's natural support system. Don't worry—even if you're not in great shape, you can start by doing the exercises at your own pace. However, do each of the exercises below so that you'll strengthen all the muscles equally to keep your spine in balance.

Here's the drill: Perform the exercises three times a week...and focus on maintaining proper form. Even if your back is aching, do the exercises if you can—they often give some immediate relief and help prevent future flare-ups.

Give it time: It may take three to four weeks before you notice significant pain reduction.

Important: These exercises can be safely done by most people, but check with your doctor first. See your doctor right away if you have back pain and severe leg pain (a sign of sciatica) or you have a history of cancer (back pain could be a sign that cancer has spread).

EXERCISE 1: Front plank. This exercise focuses on the muscles at the front of the core—the rectus abdominis (the abs) and the transverse abdominis—and the obliques, which are on the sides of the core.

What to do: Start by lying on your stomach on a carpet or mat. Place your hands on the floor at about the level of your ears, with your elbows bent and close to your sides.

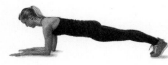

Slowly lift your body off the floor using just your forearms and rising up on your toes. Your elbows and hands should remain on the floor. Keep your back straight by contracting your front abdominal muscles. (If you cannot lift your body as described, try supporting your lower body from your knees rather than your toes.)

Breathe normally...and hold the position for 10 seconds. As you are able, increase the amount of time you hold the position. A minute is a good goal for most people.

EXERCISE 2: Side plank. This strengthens the sides of your core—the internal and external obliques.

What to do: Start by lying on the floor on your right side, with your feet together. Prop yourself up on your right elbow, with your right hand and forearm flat on the ground and your forearm perpen-

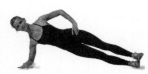

dicular to your body. Put your left hand on your left hip. Contract your abdominal muscles, and raise your hips off the floor until your back is straight.

Breathe normally, and hold the raised position for 10 seconds. As you are able, increase the amount of time you hold the position to 60 seconds. Repeat on your left side.

EXERCISE 3: Birddog. This exercise strengthens the back muscles that support your spine, including the multifidus muscles and the erector spinae muscles.

What to do: Start on your hands and knees, with your wrists below your shoulders (hands facing forward) and your knees below your hips. Stabilize your spine by tightening your abdominal muscles.

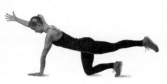

Simultaneously extend your right arm straight forward and your left leg straight back until both are parallel to the ground. Remember to keep your back and neck straight, without sagging or arching.

Hold this position for two seconds, then return to the starting position. Repeat, using the other arm and leg. Do the cycle five times. As you are able, increase the amount of time you hold the position each time for up to 10 seconds.

START RUNNING

If you have back pain, you've likely been advised to do only low-impact aerobic exercises and avoid running. I disagree. After years of examining runners, I noticed that their disks (and spines) tend to be healthier than those of nonrunners. Unexpected, right? But it makes sense.

All weight-bearing exercises stimulate bone cells so that the bones themselves become stronger. Similarly, disks also improve with high-impact exercise—the cells that make up the gel of a disk proliferate, retaining more water and becoming "fuller," which cushions the bones of the spine, reducing pain.

If you want to try running (and it doesn't cause you knee or hip pain), start slowly. Walk for one mile—and three times during that walk, run for 20 to 30 seconds. Thereafter, double the number of times you run until you're running more than walking. Try to work up to at least 30 minutes, three times a week.

---

30 Handy Aids for Achy Hands

Jim Miller, an advocate for older Americans, writes "Savvy Senior," a weekly information column syndicated in more than 400 newspapers nationwide. Based in Norman, Oklahoma, he also offers a free senior news service at *SavvySenior.org.*

People typically don't think about how much they use their hands until their hands get stiff and painful.

Arthritis, carpal tunnel syndrome and other conditions can make performing everyday tasks such as turning a doorknob, fastening a button, brushing your teeth, preparing a meal or using a computer mouse difficult and painful. There are various assistive devices and other products to help ease the burden of having achy hands. *Here are some of the best ones...*

KITCHEN AIDS

•**Dexter DuoGlide** knives have soft, textured handles and curved blades that let you chop foods using a rocking motion with less hand strain. Available in six models—paring knife, utility knife, bread slicer, all-purpose knife, cook's knife and chef's knife. From $22.50 to $64.85. *Dexter1818.com*

•**Anolon 14-Inch French Skillet** ($59.99) and **Circulon 6-Quart Covered Chef Pan** ($79.99) both have a large, ergonomically designed handle and a second helper handle on each pan that makes them easier to lift and move around when cooking, cleaning or serving. *PotsAndPans.com*

•**West Bend Electric Can Opener** is a hands-free can opener that starts and stops automatically once you lock the can in place. A built-in magnet keeps the lid from falling in the food once open. $45.99. *WestBend.com*

•**Zim Jar Opener** has a V-shaped grip that holds the lid still as you use both hands to twist open a jar or bottle. Available in wall-mounted ($18.88) and under-counter-mounted ($16.99)

versions, these openers require installation. *Amazon.com*

Alternative: Hamilton Beach Open Ease Automatic Jar Opener is a small, battery-operated device that opens twist-lids from one to four inches in diameter at the push of a button. $10.99. *Amazon.com*

•**Good Grips Eating Utensils** (fork, small spoon, teaspoon, tablespoon, soup spoon and rocker knife) are stainless steel with large, soft 1 ⅜-inch, nonslip grips that are easy to grasp. The fork and spoons also have a special twist built into the metal shaft that allows them to be bent to any angle for either left- or right-handed use, which helps people with limited hand-to-mouth reach. $10.95 per utensil. *NCMedical.com*

•**OXO Good Grips** makes easy-to-grip cooking and baking utensils with large, soft handles. They range from spatulas and whisks to pizza wheels and ice cream scoops. Large-handled utensils spread your fingers so that they don't close completely around the tool, which reduces hand stress and makes the utensils more comfortable to grasp. Typically from $5 to $13 per item. *OXO.com*

HOUSEHOLD HELPERS

Lever faucet handles. If you have twist-handle kitchen or bathroom faucets, check the brand and then see if lever-styled replacement handles are available through the manufacturer's website or through a home-improvement store. Lever handles provide greater leverage for easier turning.

Example: Danco Decorative Lever Handle, $16.89 each at The Home Depot. If lever-style replacement handles are not available, replace your faucets with lever-handle faucets.

The following items can be found at *Maddak. com...*

•**Doorknob extenders fit over standard doorknobs,** converting them into easy-to-turn door levers. $21.70 for a package of two.

•**Key turners attach to a key.** Each turner has two finger holes in the handle to improve grip and leverage. $7.76.

•**Big lamp switch is a large,** three-spoked knob adapter that provides better leverage for turning a lamp switch. $10.12.

PERSONAL CARE

Simplehuman triple wall-mount pump holds liquid soap, shampoo and conditioner and has a T-bar lever at the base of each container that you pull for one-handed dispensing. $70. *Simplehuman.com*

Simplehuman sensor pump is a touch-free liquid-hand-soap dispenser that sits by the kitchen or bathroom sink. Place your hand under the spout to dispense the soap automatically. $40. *Simplehuman.com*

Touch N Brush. The Hands-Free Toothpaste Dispenser can hold any size tube of toothpaste and attaches to the bathroom mirror or the wall with suction cups. Just touch the pump arm with your toothbrush head to get a strip of toothpaste without squeezing the tube. $9.20. *Amazon.com*

Oral-B and Sonicare electric toothbrushes with handles that are easier to hold and are wider than standard manual brushes. Prices for the Oral-B toothbrushes run between $39.99 and $169.99 (*OralB.com*). Sonicare toothbrushes cost between $39.95 and $189.95 (*Sonicare.com*).

Cheaper alternative: Foam tubing can be cut down to size and fit onto your toothbrush handle to create a large, soft handgrip. This also can be used on eating utensils, pens and pencils. Available in ¼-inch, ⅜-inch and 1⅛-inch widths, this tubing is slip-resistant and does not absorb water. $14. *Maddak.com*

Philips Sonicare AirFloss cleans between your teeth by shooting microbursts of air and water droplets, eliminating the need for string floss. $89.95. *Bestbuycom*

EASIER DRESSING

Button Hook Zipper Pull is a rubber-grip hand tool with a four-inch-long wire-hook buttoning aid at one end for fastening and unfastening buttons and a brass hook at the other end for pulling zipper tabs. $11.99. *EasyComforts.com*

Zipper pulls are three-inch-long polypropylene pulls that attach to zipper tabs, making them easier to grasp. $4.99 for a set of 12 in assorted colors. *EasyComforts.com*

Lock Laces are elastic shoelaces that convert lace-ups into slip-ons. To ensure a good fit, they include a spring-activated locking device that can tighten and loosen the shoelaces. Available in a variety of colors for $7.99 or $9.99 per pair. *LockLaces.com*

EASIER DRIVING

These are available at Amazon.com…

Car key turner (around $6) is a curved, five-inch-long plastic handle that attaches to the key to provide leverage.

Kinsman gas cap removal tool ($22.89) works like a wrench and fits most gas caps.

Steering Wheel Cover ($10 to $15) fits over the steering wheel to make the wheel larger in size and easier to grip. There are numerous options, including heated versions.

READING, WRITING AND COMPUTING

For book readers, electronic e-readers are ideal because they're lightweight and easier to hold than regular books and don't require traditional page turning. But if you like paper publications, there are bookholders such as…

Levo Book Holder Floor Stand ($169) and **Corner Table Clamp Book Holder** ($99) that hold hardcovers, paperbacks, magazines and cookbooks in any position. Levo also offers holders for e-readers and tablet computers that cost between $99.99 and $229.99. *Levostore.com*

The Pencil Grip is a small rubber grip that fits on pencils and pens to make holding easier and reduce hand fatigue. $1.79. *ThePencilGrip.com*

Pen Again is a Y-shaped pen that cradles your index finger to relieve hand stress when writing. $4.99. *PenAgain.com*

3M Ergonomic Mouse has a vertical-grip handle design that keeps your arm in a more

---

Back Pain Is Not Affected by Weather

Researchers found no connection between study participants' pain and changes in temperature, humidity or precipitation. (These findings apply only to musculoskeletal pain caused by tissue damage, sprains, falls and overuse—not arthritis.)

Study of 993 cases of sudden back pain by researchers at George Institute for Global Health, University of Sydney, Australia, published in *Arthritis Care & Research*.

neutral position to reduce wrist and hand stress when using a computer. $59.73 *Amazon.com*

Contour RollerMouse sits directly in front of the computer keyboard, giving you the ability to control the cursor with your fingertips, eliminating the reaching and gripping of a traditional mouse. $199.95 to $265. *RollerMouse.com*

Natural Osteoarthritis Relief

Harris H. McIlwain, MD, a pain specialist in private practice in Tampa, and coauthor of Diet for a Pain-Free Life. *IPainFreeDiet.com*

Eating foods that have been shown to lower inflammation may help relieve your pain, so make sure your diet includes plenty of these—broccoli, red grapes, tea (black or green), pineapple, blueberries, strawberries, spinach, plums, cabbage, brussels sprouts and salmon. Supplements that may help ease osteoarthritis pain include sulforaphane, bromelain, ginger, turmeric and curcumin. Check with your doctor first—these supplements and some of the foods above may interact with certain medications, including blood thinners. Follow directions on the supplement label. Also helpful are regular—twice daily for five to 10 minutes—soaks in a warm bath or whirlpool.

Knee Pain While Using Stairs May Be First Sign of Arthritis

Philip Conaghan, MB, BS, PhD, professor of musculoskeletal medicine, University of Leeds, England. University of Leeds, news release.

Having knee pain while using the stairs may be an early sign of arthritis, a recent study suggests.

BACKGROUND

"At present, we have little concept of 'early' osteoarthritis and often only see people when

Arthritis and Your Kidney

People with rheumatoid arthritis have a 25% risk of developing chronic kidney disease, compared with a 20% risk for people who don't have the chronic inflammatory disorder. Factors that contribute to the higher risk in rheumatoid arthritis patients include the severe inflammation that is characteristic of the first year of rheumatoid arthritis and the use of corticosteroids. High blood pressure, obesity and high cholesterol also are linked to chronic kidney disease.

Study by researchers at Mayo Clinic, Rochester, Minnesota, published in *American Journal of Kidney Diseases*.

they have significant, longstanding pain and loss of function," said research leader Philip Conaghan, MB, BS, PhD, a professor of musculoskeletal medicine at the University of Leeds in England.

"This research is vital to understanding early symptoms of knee osteoarthritis," he said.

NEW STUDY

The study included more than 4,600 people who were at high risk for arthritis. Researchers followed the volunteers for up to seven years.

Using stairs was the first weight-bearing activity in which people with early knee arthritis noticed pain. They later developed pain while walking, standing, lying or sitting, and finally, while resting in bed.

"Knowing this will help us intervene earlier, perhaps leading to more effective ways of treating this very painful condition," Dr. Conaghan explained.

The study was published in the journal *Arthritis Care & Research*.

info The U.S. National Institute of Arthritis and Musculoskeletal and Skin Diseases has more about osteoarthritis at *www.niams.nih.gov.* Search "osteoarthritis."

You Need Exercise—Not a Knee Replacement

Mitchell Yass, DPT, founder and director of PT2 Physical Therapy and Personal Training. He is author of *Overpower Pain: The Strength-Training Program that Stops Pain without Drugs or Surgery. MitchellYass.com*

Did you know that knee-replacement surgery is virtually epidemic in this country? The number has doubled over the past decade. And among Medicare beneficiaries, the number of knee replacements has increased by more than 160%. One recent research paper reported that four million Americans now have knee implants—including half a million who had to have their knee replacement redone at least once. What explains all the extra knee replacements?

Is it possible that a lot of unnecessary operations are being done?

KNEE-REPLACEMENT RAMPAGE

A recent study showed that just about one-third of all knee replacements are inappropriate. The patients had relatively low levels of pain that could have been managed in other ways, and/or their knee X-rays showed little evidence of substantial arthritic changes. Many patients who were inappropriately given knee replacements were under age 55, and for them, considering that the life expectancy of the artificial joint is 15 to 20 years, another—and then perhaps another—arduous replacement operation will be needed.

Why are so many people so willingly getting an operation that is expensive, can take a year for full recovery and is certainly not without serious risks, including deadly blood clots? Most patients—and their doctors—jump to the conclusion that they need a knee replacement because of pain due to arthritis, but pain is not a reason for knee replacement or necessarily a sign of knee arthritis.

Studies that have looked at pain in relation to arthritic changes have shown that only about 15% of people with X-ray evidence of knee arthritis actually have knee pain. One study even showed that sham surgery relieved knee pain caused by

Injections Beat Pills for Arthritis

For treating knee osteoarthritis, injections are generally more effective than pills, says Raveendhara Bannuru, MD, PhD. Injections of hyaluronic acid or cortisone usually relieve pain better than any oral medicine, including *acetaminophen* (Tylenol) and non-steroidal anti-inflammatory drugs (NSAIDs) such as *celecoxib* (Celebrex).

But: The long-term safety and efficacy of injected corticosteroids is uncertain, and injected hyaluronic acid is expensive.

Best: Nondrug treatments such as exercise and physical therapy should be tried first.

Raveendhara Bannuru, MD, PhD, is director of Center for Treatment Comparison and Integrative Analysis and researcher at Center for Arthritis and Rheumatic Diseases, both at Tufts Medical Center, Boston. He led an analysis of 137 randomized trials involving more than 33,000 patients, published in *Annals of Internal Medicine.*

osteoarthritis just as well as real surgery. Clearly the relationship between osteoarthritis and knee pain cannot be directly correlated.

THE REAL CAUSE OF KNEE PAIN

Most people who suffer knee pain experience the pain around the kneecap. The pain is caused by an imbalance in the strength of the quadriceps muscles on the front of the thigh and the hamstring muscle on the back of it. The quadriceps naturally get a lot more use from walking and everyday activity and naturally tend to be much stronger than the hamstrings. When the hamstring muscles are weaker than the quads, the quads shorten. This increases tension on the kneecap. Instead of painlessly gliding along with the joint, the kneecap presses against the joint...painfully.

THE REAL SOLUTION

If you have knee pain, try the exercises on the next page to improve and balance your leg muscles and avoid the type of knee symptoms that have convinced too many people—and their doctors—that they need knee-replacement surgery. (Check with your doctor first—but there is seldom a good medical reason not to try exercises before going to surgery.) How many reps should you do? Do each exercise 10 times, take a one-minute break, then repeat two more sets. How frequently? Two or three times a week.

•**Loosen the Quads.** Stand near a wall for support. If your left knee is the most bothersome, turn your right side to the wall and rest your right hand against it. Then, reach back with your left hand to grip your left foot or ankle. Gently pull the foot toward the buttocks until you feel a stretch in the front of your thigh. Hold for about 20 to 30 seconds. Repeat on the other side whether or not you have problems with the other knee to keep all the muscles in balance.

•**Strengthen the Hamstrings.** Practice the straight leg dead lift. To do this, stand with your legs hip width apart, hands at hip level either holding hand weights or grasping a pole (such a broomstick) horizontally in front of you. Bend forward from your hips, keeping your legs straight (without "locking" your knees) and letting your hands (holding weights or a pole) run down your thighs until you begin to feel a pull at the back of the thighs. Then immediately return to the start position. Do three sets of 10 repetitions.

•**Strengthen the Calves.** Mitchell Yass, DPT, founder and director of PT2 Physical Therapy and Personal Training says that in his experience, strengthening the calves can help offset excessive tightening of the quads and can strengthen the hamstrings. To do this exercise, stand facing a wall, counter or sturdy chair and place both hands on it to keep your balance. Rise up onto the balls of the feet (lifting your heels)…then, gently lower your heels to the ground. Once you feel that you can keep your balance when doing this exercise, you can hold dumbbells, which will create more muscle resistance and help strengthen the calves even more.

By the third week of doing these exercises, you should notice a significant improvement. But even if you are completely rid of pain, you ought to keep up your exercise routine to keep the pain from returning.

Fast Help for Achilles Tendinitis

Johanna S. Youner, DPM, podiatric surgeon in private practice in New York City. *HealthyFeetNY.com*

Achilles tendinitis, a painful inflammation of the tendon that runs from the lower calf to the heel, typically takes about two to three months to heal. Avoiding high-impact activities such as running will prevent further tissue damage. You can still stay active by doing low-impact exercise, such as walking, swimming and cycling.

"Contrast" baths increase blood flow to the area and help speed healing.

What to do: Once a day, immerse the sore area in warm water (use a bathtub or large basin) for five minutes, then cool water for five minutes. Repeat two or three times, ending with cool water. You can also do this with heating pads and ice packs. (People with diabetes should check first with their doctors, since their feet may be very sensitive to temperature changes.)

Supplements also can help heal a painful Achilles tendon. I recommend choosing one from each of the following categories: Vitamin C, glucosamine or chondroitin sulfate to help build ligaments…fish oil, boswellia extract, devil's claw or quercetin to decrease inflammation…and the enzymes pancreatin, papain,

Knee Surgery Could Lead to Arthritis

Recent study: All 31 knees operated on to repair tears of the meniscus (cartilage that stabilizes the knee joint) developed arthritis within one year, compared with 59% of the 165 knees that didn't have surgery. Talk to your doctor about whether surgery is really necessary and whether physical therapy, including targeted muscle exercises, is a better option for you.

Frank Roemer, MD, associate professor of radiology, Boston University School of Medicine and University of Erlangen–Nuremburg, Germany. His study was presented at a meeting of the Radiological Society of North America.

bromelain or trypsin to relieve pain. Check with your doctor, since they could interact with medications. Follow label directions.

Fix Your Feet for Under $75

Johanna S. Youner, DPM, a podiatric surgeon in private practice and attending physician at New York–Presbyterian/Lower Manhattan Hospital, both in New York City. *HealthyFeetNY.com*

Aching feet can be more than an annoyance. If you don't take proper care of your feet, it can throw off the alignment of your body, leading to knee, hip and back problems. Calluses can crack and turn into nasty infections. Athlete's foot can lead to thickened, painful toenails that make it difficult to even walk.

Good news: For less than $75, you can choose a handful of excellent over-the-counter (OTC) products that will relieve foot pain and keep your toenails and the skin on your feet healthy—without seeing a doctor.

Caution: If your foot pain is daily or doesn't improve with the products mentioned in this article, see a podiatrist for advice.

FOR BETTER SUPPORT

Even though shoes generally protect your feet from the surface you're walking on and from the weather, they don't always provide much support.

Fortunately, well-made, foam-padded insoles that go inside your shoes work like shock absorbers, alleviating pressure and stress on the foot. Insoles help restore balance, increase stability and reduce pain—not just in your feet but also in your knees, hips and back.

Important: If an insole does not feel comfortable in the shoe, then it's not right for you—these are not devices that are "broken in." *Before you buy expensive, custom-fit orthotics, consider trying these OTC insoles…*

•**Superfeet insoles are available in a variety of styles for men's and women's shoes.** For example, Superfeet Delux Dress-fit ($29.95,

Bursitis vs. Arthritis

The difference between these two painful conditions is the location of the inflammation.

Bursitis is caused by inflammation of the bursa (a small, fluid-filled protective sac between bones and soft tissue), which can occur when the area is injured by overuse. Bursitis symptoms include swelling, stiffness and pain.

Arthritis has similar symptoms, but the inflammation is caused by the degeneration of a joint. The treatment initially is the same—rest, ice packs and nonsteroidal anti-inflammatory drugs (NSAIDs) for pain.

If your symptoms have not subsided in a few days, see your doctor, who can offer other treatments, such as corticosteroid injections.

Sabrina Strickland, MD, associate professor of orthopaedic surgery, Weill Cornell Medical College, New York City.

Zappos.com) are slim enough to slip inside any women's shoe, but they work best in flats or shoes with heels up to one-and-a-half inches. The insole's structured cup under the heel adds shock absorption, and the support in the arch helps stabilize the foot. Superfeet Premium Blue insoles ($44.95, *Zappos.com*), available for men and women, are designed for cleated athletic footwear and most types of casual and dress shoes.

•**Powerstep ProTech Full Length Orthotics** ($30 to $40, *Amazon.com*), also available for men and women, are especially helpful for pain in your arch or heel due, for example, to plantar fasciitis. If you have this condition, which causes inflammation of the tissue along the bottom of the feet, you'll likely benefit a lot by using these insoles.

Important: Insoles can be transferred from shoe to shoe (depending on the size of each one) but should be replaced yearly or more often if they no longer relieve pain.

TO FIGHT DRY SKIN AND CALLUSES

Dry skin can be a year-round problem for your feet. Also, corns (painful, bumpy thickenings that form on the skin) can develop on the tops and/or sides of your toes where they rub against your shoe.

Calluses (areas of dry, hard and thickened skin) can crack, especially when they are on the heel. If the cracks deepen, they can hurt, bleed and become infected.

To prevent dry skin and calluses on your feet, you need a moisturizing cream that contains a keratolytic (descaling) agent to strip away the layers of dead skin so the moisturizer can do its work. *To restore your feet's skin, try one of the following products with keratolytic agents…*

•**Gehwol Med Callus Cream** ($16.99 for 2.6 ounces, *Amazon.com*).

•**Kerasal One Step Exfoliating Moisturizer Foot Therapy** ($10.79 for one ounce, *CVS.com*).

Apply the cream after your shower, when the skin is softened a bit. Twelve to 24 hours later, rub the area gently with a pumice sponge, which is less damaging to use than a pumice stone. Be very gentle if you have cracks in your feet, especially if you've lost some of the feeling in your feet (due to neuropathy, for example). If you're using one of the moisturizing products and it stops working, switch to the other.

FOR FUNGAL INFECTIONS

These common infections—often due to athlete's foot, which can be contracted by walking barefoot in a public shower, for example—cause thickened, disfigured toenails that sometimes curl inward.

You'll need a doctor's prescription for antifungal cream, such as Ertaczo or Naftin…or maybe even oral medication, such as *terbinafine* (Lamisil). *To speed the recovery process and help prevent recurrences, try this nail cream…*

•**Kerasal's Fungal Nail Renewal Treatment** ($27.49 for 0.33 ounce, *CVS.com*) contains acids and other ingredients that soften the nail, reduce its thickness and improve its appearance, usually within two weeks of nightly use.

Sleep Solutions

Foods That Help...Foods That Harm Your Sleep

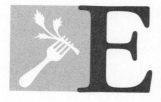

Even though most people would rather avoid taking sleeping pills, insomnia can be so unnerving that many sufferers will do almost anything to get some sleep.

But now there's even more to worry about than the pills' possible side effects, such as headache, nausea and diarrhea.

Startling recent research: In a study of more than 34,000 men and women, regular use of prescription sleeping pills was linked to a more than fourfold increase in death and a 35% increased cancer risk over a two-and-a-half-year period.

Fortunately, there is a safer and better way to get a good night's sleep—it can be as simple as eating the right foods at the right time.

SLEEP-PROMOTING FOODS

Certain foods contain compounds that interact with your body's natural chemistry to trigger the sleep process or to help maintain it. *Include in your meals...*

•**Tryptophan.** Found in turkey, this essential amino acid is widely believed to be responsible for the sleep-inducing spell that overcomes people after feasting on the big bird at Thanksgiving. The postprandial drowsiness is, in fact, more likely due to carbohydrate-rich foods served with the meal. However, a diet that includes plenty of tryptophan-rich foods will help you feel less anxious and more relaxed, which can help promote sleep.

Bonnie Taub-Dix, RDN, CDN, a registered dietitian and director and owner of BTD Nutrition Consultants, LLC, on Long Island and in New York City. She is author of *Read It Before You Eat It. BetterThanDieting.com*

Michael Breus, PhD, Scottsdale, Arizona–based clinical psychologist who is board-certified in clinical sleep disorders. He is a coauthor, with Debra F. Bruce, PhD, of *The Sleep Doctor's Diet Plan: Lose Weight Through Better Sleep. TheSleepDoctor.com*

Tryptophan acts as a building block for the sleep hormone melatonin and the calming neurotransmitter serotonin.

Surprisingly, chicken and beef have about the same amount of tryptophan as turkey. Other sources include most animal protein and dairy products, such as milk and yogurt. Dates, peanuts and tofu also are good sources. What foods contain the most tryptophan per gram? Spinach, shellfish and egg whites.

•**Complex carbohydrates.** When you eat complex carbohydrates, the body releases insulin, which not only metabolizes sugar but also removes amino acids that compete with tryptophan. This process allows more sleep-promoting serotonin and melatonin to enter the brain.

Complex carbohydrates include whole-grain bread, whole-grain pasta, beans, peas and brown rice.

HERBS AND SPICES

Though scientists are not sure why, the spices garlic, nutmeg and turmeric have been shown to promote sleep—and so have the herbs dill, parsley and sage.

Consider cooking with these spices and herbs whenever you can. Drinking herbal tea with nutmeg a few hours before bedtime is also a good sleep promoter.

VITAMINS AND MINERALS

The vitamins and minerals essential to getting restful sleep every night include…

•**B vitamins, such as B-3 (niacin), B-6, B-12 and folic acid, which regulate the body's use of tryptophan and other types of amino acids.**

Vitamin B–rich foods include: Broccoli, potatoes and whole grains.

•**Vitamin D acts as a sleep-promoting hormone in the body.** The body produces vitamin D in response to exposure to sunlight. Getting 15 minutes of sunlight a day is important for adequate vitamin D—and for sleep.

Foods that contain vitamin D include: Herring, salmon, tuna and vitamin D–fortified milk and cereals.

•**Calcium,** which aids the brain in using tryptophan to produce serotonin.

Calcium-rich foods include: Dairy products, leafy green vegetables and salmon and sardines canned with their soft bones.

•**Magnesium,** which calms nerves and relaxes muscles to help promote quality sleep.

Magnesium-rich foods include: Avocados, bananas, halibut, pineapple, almonds and tofu.

•**Zinc.** A deficiency of zinc is associated with insomnia, so it helps to include foods with an abundance of this mineral in your diet.

Zinc-rich foods include: Calf's liver, oysters and other shellfish, wheat germ and pumpkin seeds.

My advice: Most people can get an adequate amount of these sleep-regulating vitamins and minerals by eating a balanced diet of whole, nonprocessed foods. Taking a multivitamin/mineral supplement that has these vitamins and minerals also helps ensure that you are getting enough of the nutrients.

BEST BEDTIME SNACKS

It is best to stop eating three to four hours before bed so that the sleep process does not have to compete with the digestion process. However, if you had only a small dinner or ate early, don't go to bed hungry. This elevates levels of the stress hormone cortisol, which will keep you awake.

The best bedtime snack has a small amount of protein plus some complex carbohydrates. It should have no more than 200 calories and be eaten at least one hour before bed so digestion doesn't interfere with sleep.

Good bedtime snacks: Yogurt with banana slices, almonds and granola…a small helping of warm oatmeal with milk and banana slices…or, my personal favorite, a slice of cheesecake (this tasty treat's carbs do the trick for me—just make sure it's a small slice!).

•**Warm milk.** It's not a myth—warm milk at bedtime really will help you get to sleep. It settles the stomach, and the ritual of drinking it can help you calm down and fall asleep more easily.

•**Cherry juice.** A study published in *Journal of Medicinal Food* found that people who drank eight ounces of tart cherry juice in the morning and eight at night for two weeks had about 17 minutes less awake time during the night than when they drank a non-cherry juice. Tart cherries are high in melatonin, a hormone that regulates the body's sleep-wake cycles. The brand used in the study was Cheribundi.

Helpful: Tart cherry juice has 140 calories in eight ounces, so you may want to cut back on calories elsewhere.

FOODS THAT SABOTAGE SLEEP

You know that an evening coffee can leave you tossing and turning in the wee hours. *But other foods hurt sleep, too....*

•**Premium ice cream.** Brace yourself for a restless night if you indulge in Häagen-Dazs or Ben & Jerry's late at night. The richness of these wonderful treats comes mainly from fat—16 to 17 grams of fat in half a cup of vanilla and who eats just half a cup?

Your body digests fat more slowly than it digests proteins or carbohydrates. When you eat a high-fat food within an hour or two of bedtime, your digestion will still be "active" when you lie down—and that can disturb sleep.

Also, the combination of stomach acid, stomach contractions and a horizontal position increases the risk for reflux, the upsurge of digestive juices into the esophagus that causes heartburn—which can disturb sleep.

•**Chocolate.** Some types of chocolate can jolt you awake almost as much as a cup of coffee. Dark chocolate, in particular, has shocking amounts of caffeine.

Example: Half a bar of Dagoba Eclipse Extra Dark has 41 milligrams of caffeine, close to what you'd get in a shot of mild espresso.

Chocolate also contains theobromine, another stimulant, which is never a good choice near bedtime.

•**Beans.** Beans are one of the healthiest foods. But a helping or two of beans—or broccoli, cauliflower, cabbage or other gas-producing foods—close to bedtime can make your night, well, a little noisier than usual. No one sleeps well when suffering from gas pains. You can reduce the "backtalk" by drinking a mug of chamomile or peppermint tea at bedtime. They're carminative herbs that aid digestion and help prevent gas.

•**Spicy foods.** Spicy foods temporarily speed up your metabolism. They are associated with taking longer to fall asleep and with more time spent awake at night. This may be caused by the capsaicin found in chile peppers, which affect body temperature and disrupt sleep. Also, in some people, spicy foods can lead to sleep-disturbing gas, stomach cramps and heartburn.

Don't make this mistake: Drinking alcohol to help you sleep. Alcohol should be avoided within three hours of bedtime. Drinking it right before going to bed reduces the rapid eye movement (REM) sleep, which is the time your brain organizes and stores memories.

BETTER SLEEP...LOSE WEIGHT

If you're trying to lose weight, you must get a good night's sleep. A recent study published in *Annals of Internal Medicine* found that dieters who spent only five-and-a-half hours sleeping each night lost 55% less fat compared with those who slept for eight-and-a-half hours a night. The dieters who slept less had higher levels of ghrelin, a hormone that promotes hunger.

Gentle Ways to Get Better Sleep

Jamison Starbuck, ND, is naturopathic physician in family practice and a guest lecturer at the University of Montana, both in Missoula. She is past president of the American Association of Naturopathic Physicians and a contributing editor to *The Alternative Advisor: The Complete Guide to Natural Therapies and Alternative Treatments.*

When you're really wrestling with insomnia, it's tempting to go to your doctor and ask for one of the sleep medications we see advertised on TV—Ambien or Lunesta—or an older tranquilizing drug such as Valium. While short-term use of one of these drugs might make sense for a person who feels his/her overall health is being threatened by insomnia, I generally advise against this approach. Sure, these drugs may temporarily allow you to sleep, but they don't cure insomnia. *My advice...*

•**Do some detective work.** Thinking about your own sleep issues and making some written notes can be a big help. When do you typically go to bed? How often do you have insomnia? Do you have trouble falling asleep or wake in the middle of the night? Also, look at when your problem started to determine whether it coincided with any health issues, use of new medications or habits, such as working late hours, that could lead to insomnia.

• **Get your doctor involved.** Discuss your notes with your doctor. Chronic pain, hormonal changes (including those related to hyperthyroidism and menopause) and serious illness, such as cancer and heart or lung disease, can cause insomnia. If any of these conditions is to blame, getting proper treatment may well take care of the insomnia, too.

After you've consulted your doctor, try these gentle methods…*

• **Avoid high-protein dinners.** Protein is often hard to digest. Eating a lot at dinner can lead to gastrointestinal distress that may result in insomnia. Instead, eat foods that are easy to digest (such as soup and salad) for dinner, and have larger, protein-rich meals midday.

Also helpful: Take a 2,000-mg omega-3 supplement with your evening meal. When taken before bedtime, these healthful fats can have a calming effect on the brain, promoting sleep.

• **Try Calms Forté.** This homeopathic preparation is effective and extremely safe.

Typical dose: One tablet under the tongue at bedtime and whenever you wake up in the middle of the night (up to six tablets per 24-hour period). Calms Forté, made by Hylands, is available at natural groceries and pharmacies.

• **Add skullcap.** If the steps above don't give you relief, you may want to also try this potent herb to relax the "busy brain" experience that often keeps people awake. I recommend using skullcap in tincture form—30 to 60 drops (one-sixteenth to one-eighth teaspoon) in a cup of chamomile or spearmint tea at bedtime.

Note: Skullcap can make some people too sleepy. If you are sensitive to medication, try just 10 drops of skullcap at bedtime—or simply drink chamomile or mint tea as a sedative.

*Check with your doctor before trying supplements, especially if you take medication and/or have a chronic medical condition.

Better Bedtime Reading

Adult volunteers who used electronic readers or tablets, such as iPads, for four hours before bedtime had a harder time falling asleep…got less rapid eye movement (REM) sleep…and felt less alert and rested the next morning than when they spent the same amount of time reading a printed book.

Why: Tablets emit blue light directly into the reader's eyes, which can suppress the sleep hormone melatonin and disrupt the circadian clock.

Anne-Marie Chang, PhD, associate neuroscientist, Division of Sleep and Circadian Disorders, Brigham and Women's Hospital, Boston.

• **Use melatonin with care.** If you'd rather try this popular sleep aid, do so thoughtfully. Melatonin is a hormone. Taking too much can trigger irritability. Melatonin supplements may also raise women's estrogen levels, increasing overall inflammation in the body. I recommend taking no more than 3 mg of melatonin in a 24-hour period and often start my patients on a daily dose of only 1 mg. Take melatonin 30 minutes before bedtime.

To Get to Sleep Fast, Do These 6 Easy Yoga Moves

Loren Fishman, MD, assistant clinical professor of rehabilitation and regenerative medicine, Columbia Medical School, New York City, medical director, Manhattan Physical Medicine and Rehabilitation, and author of several books on yoga for health, including *Healing Yoga: Proven Postures to Treat Twenty Common Ailments—from Backache to Bone Loss, Shoulder Pain to Bunions, and More.*

Losing a good night's sleep is a bummer, isn't it? You walk around in a groggy fog the next day and run the risk of getting snippy with coworkers, friends and loved ones because sleep deprivation has made you grumpy. So many factors in modern daily life can make it tough for us to fall asleep, stay asleep and rest peacefully.

Yoga is a powerful tool to relieve stress and help your body relax and prepare for sleep. By stretching muscles, yoga poses trigger mechanisms in the body that send powerful relaxing signals to the brain. When performed daily, yoga can make us into better sleepers.

Do the following yoga routine nightly at bedtime. Poses can even be done while in bed. Otherwise, do them on a cushioned surface on the floor. A plush blanket or towel will do if you don't have carpeting or a yoga mat.

•**Seated forward bend.** This will give a great stretch to your legs and back muscles. To prepare for the forward bend, sit with your legs straight in front of you. First, stretch one leg and then the other by extending from the hip through the heel to elongate the leg. Then relax your legs and stretch your arms straight upward to

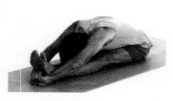

feel your torso and back extend long and lean. Now you are ready to bend forward from the hips and reach out with your hands to grasp your ankles or feet (or as far down your legs as you comfortably can—you should be stretching, but not straining). Let gentle, deep breaths help you relax into the stretch. Hold this pose for one to three minutes.

•**Revolved abdomen pose.** This pose massages the abdominal organs, gives a nice

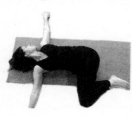

stretch to the lower back and muscles across the rib cage and opens the chest so you can breathe more deeply. To do it, lie on your back, bend your knees to your chest and stretch your arms out to your sides. With bent knees pressed together, inhale. Then, while exhaling, twist from your hips to lower your legs to the right while turning your face to the left. Again, give yourself a nice stretch, but do not strain or force yourself to go deeper into the pose than you comfortably can. Hold the pose for five breaths, then bring your knees and head back to center. Repeat the pose on the opposite side by dropping

your knees to the left while turning your head to the right. Hold the pose for five breaths.

•**Reclining big toe pose.** This is a leg lift that gives a good stretch to the muscles all down the back of the leg. Unless you are very limber, you will need a prop to help you get the most stretch. The prop can be a long belt, scarf, cord or necktie that you can brace against the arch or ball of your foot and use as a lever to stretch your leg until your foot faces the ceiling. To do this

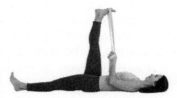

posture, lie on your back, take a deep breath, and, while gently exhaling, bend your right knee to your chest and loop the prop around the arch or ball of the right foot, holding the ends of the prop in both hands. Inhale while straightening your knee so that your right heel is turned toward the ceiling. Guide the prop to comfortably increase the stretch. Hold this pose for a minute or two and then repeat with the other leg.

•**Child's pose.** This restorative yoga pose helps get more blood flowing in the head and can be so deeply relaxing that when you roll out of it, you may just nod off to

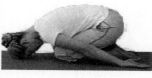

sleep like a baby. Begin by kneeling so that you are sitting on your heels, and take a nice, deep, relaxing breath. Bend forward while exhaling and place your forehead on the floor (or on your bed if that's where you are doing the exercise). Place your arms at your sides so that the hands, palms turned up, are near your feet. As you breathe, especially focus on relaxing your back and shoulders. Hold this pose for five to seven long, slow deep breaths.

•**"Stop-action" breathing.** This is an easy and deeply relaxing breathing technique that strengthens the respiratory system. While lying down on your back in bed, exhale completely through the nose. Then inhale a little bit of air— just enough for a count of two or three seconds. Hold that little bit of breath for two or three seconds and, without exhaling, take another two or three seconds of breath, hold, and keep on taking those little sips of air, inhaling and pausing, until your lungs are full as if you've just taken only one big breath instead of a series of small ones. Hold for a second or two. Then slowly exhale in the same manner, exhaling a little bit for two or three seconds, pausing with breath held for two or three seconds and continuing like this until you've completely exhaled air from the lungs. Do four or five rounds of this breathing technique, taking a normal breath between each round of the stop-action breaths.

•**Corpse pose.** If you're not in your bed yet, it's time to crawl into it and get into this pose—you're going to be asleep soon! Lie on your back with your legs stretched out and your arms comfortably at your sides, palms turned up. Slowly inhale and exhale through the nose, feeling your abdomen expand and contract. While you do so, start mentally scanning your body, beginning at your toes and working your way up to the top of your head, assessing whether you are holding tension anywhere. Mentally release muscular tension as you go, allowing your body, inch by inch, to comfortably sink into the surface it is lying on. You may fall asleep in the process or you might simply hold the pose for five breaths and then slowly transition into your favorite sleeping posture to fall asleep.

New Treatments for Sleep Apnea

David Rapoport, MD, professor of medicine and director of the Sleep Disorders Center, New York University Medical Center, New York City.

People who have obstructive sleep apnea stop breathing for very short intervals during the night, disrupting sleep and increasing the risk for diabetes, heart attack and stroke. In addition to conventional treatments such as continuous positive airway pressure (CPAP) machines and oral mouthpieces that advance the jaw, newer treatments include Provent Sleep Apnea Therapy (*ProventTherapy.com*), which is a small disposable patch that fits over each nostril. A central valve produces pressure

FDA OKs Nonsedative Sleeping Pill

Suvorexant (Belsomra), recently approved by the FDA, is the first drug to treat insomnia by altering the action of brain chemicals called orexins, which regulate the sleep-wake cycle. The new drug may be an alternative to sedative-hypnotic sleeping pills, which can be addictive. It is available in 5-mg, 10-mg, 15-mg and 20-mg doses, and the lowest effective dose should be taken within 30 minutes of bedtime.

Caution: People taking suvorexant should avoid driving the next day, since it can impair alertness.

David Rapoport, MD, director, Sleep Medicine Program, New York University School of Medicine, New York City.

in the airway so that it remains open during sleep. The Winx Sleep Therapy System (*Apni cure.com*) uses a soft mouthpiece that is connected to a small vacuum console. The device creates suction to open the throat. For more about sleep apnea, see Chapter 1, "Allergies, Asthma and Respiratory Disorders."

The Sleep Solution for Depression

Donn Posner, PhD,CBSM (Certified in Behavioral Sleep Medicine), director, behavioral sleep medicine program, Sleep Disorders Center, Lifespan Hospitals. He also is coauthor of *Cognitive Behavioral Treatment of Insomnia: A Session-by-Session Guide*.

Do you lie awake night after night, struggling to catch the sleep that eludes you…then feel exhausted and miserable during the day? Don't just suffer stoically—insomnia is serious! It increases the risk for high blood pressure, obesity, diabetes, anxiety and substance abuse. What's more, although insomnia often is considered a sign of depression, recent research reveals that the insomnia can come first and double a person's risk of developing depression.

There's an option that can get you the deep, blissful sleep you need. It's completely safe and drug-free, and because it addresses the underlying causes of insomnia (unlike medication), its benefits persist even long after treatment ends. It's called cognitive behavioral therapy for insomnia (CBT-I), and just a few sessions can go a long way to restore normal sleep patterns. CBT-I has been shown to relieve insomnia for a wide variety of people, including older adults and those who suffer from chronic pain, fibromyalgia, cardiovascular disease, mood disorders and other health problems. It can even help people who have been taking sleeping pills for years.

IS THIS SLEEP SOLUTION FOR YOU?

It's important to know that a few restless nights should not be considered insomnia. True chronic insomnia means difficulty initiating or maintaining sleep, despite adequate opportunity to sleep, that occurs at least three times a week and lasts for at least three months. How long can it take you to fall asleep before it's a problem? Most experts in the field consider 30 minutes of lying awake, either before first falling asleep or after having woken up in the middle of the night, as the cut-off. In addition, insomnia leads to some daytime consequences—for instance, fatigue, memory problems, difficulty concentrating, poor work performance or even anxiety about being unable to fall sleep. Insomnia is not just a nighttime disorder…it's a 24-hour disorder.

If you think that your sleep pattern fits the above description of insomnia, talk to your doctor—a medical problem could be interfering with your slumber, and you may find that sleep comes more easily once that underlying condition is addressed. If your insomnia persists, however, you should strongly consider trying CBT-I.

WHAT TO EXPECT DURING TREATMENT

The first step with CBT-I is for you to find a sleep specialist who offers it. To do this, ask your doctor for a referral to a qualified professional with expertise in CBT-I…or find a practitioner through the National Sleep Foundation (*sleepfoundation.org*) or contact the nearest certified sleep center and say that you're interested in CBT-I.

Once you choose a sleep specialist, you can expect to undergo a thorough evaluation of all areas of functioning to determine all the factors that are contributing to your sleep problems. Genetic makeup, internal rhythm, social life, home life and work life are all evaluated…and you are instructed to keep a sleep diary to help pinpoint problematic patterns. Your therapist also tries to determine whether an emotional issue or even another sleep disorder precipitated your insomnia. When the evaluation is complete, the therapist creates an individualized treatment plan, typically consisting of four to six weekly one-hour sessions.

Then the real work begins. As the name implies, CBT-I involves both behavioral and cognitive elements. *Though therapy is tailored to each patient, a typical protocol includes the following…*

•**Sleep restriction.** You may be instructed to stop napping…stay active in the evening to avoid dozing off in front of the TV…go to bed later than you usually do…and get out of bed at precisely the same time every morning regardless of how well you slept. Your sleep therapist also may restrict the amount of time you spend in bed, for instance, by allowing you only 30 minutes more than your actual sleeping time—so if you usually get just five hours of sleep, you'll be told to spend no more than five and a half hours in bed. Only as your "sleep efficiency" improves do you start going to bed

Sleep Disorder Predicts Brain Disease

According to a recent study, up to 90% of people with rapid-eye-movement sleep behavior disorder (RBD) will develop a brain disease, such as Parkinson's, up to 15 years later. RBD causes people to act out their dreams, often hurting themselves or their bed partners. In healthy brains, the muscles are paralyzed during sleep to prevent this. See your doctor if you or your bed partner experiences these behaviors.

John Peever, PhD, associate professor of cell & systems biology, University of Toronto, Canada.

earlier and staying in bed longer. The idea is for you to be very sleepy at bedtime…which makes it much easier to fall asleep.

•**Stimulus control.** You are cautioned against using your bed at any time of day for anything other than sleeping or sex. That means no lounging on the bed to read, watch TV, talk on the phone or surf the Internet. For times when you do go to bed and do not fall asleep (or fall back to sleep) within 15 to 20 minutes, you are told to get up and go do something in another room, returning to bed only when you feel sleepy again—and repeating this instruction as many times as necessary.

The rationale: When a person habitually struggles to fall asleep, he "works" at what should be a natural process…and he becomes conditioned to associate the bed with anxiety, frustration and effort. In contrast, by getting out of bed whenever he cannot sleep, he gives up that struggle. If he applies this rule consistently, over time the bed becomes a trigger for sleep rather than for wakefulness.

•**Sleep hygiene.** Typically patients are advised to avoid caffeine after noon…and to avoid exercise, alcohol, heavy meals and nicotine within two hours of bedtime. Your sleep therapist also reviews your bedroom environment to make sure it is dark and cool enough to be conducive to sleep. (Many people keep their bedrooms too warm for good sleep.)

•**Anxiety abatement.** The therapist teaches you how to deal with the anxiety you may feel before heading to bed. For instance, you may often think, *I'll be a wreck if I don't get to sleep…or I can't stand lying awake like this!* As you learn to counteract that "catastrophic thinking" with rational thoughts—*I can function OK even if I don't sleep for eight hours…*or *Insomnia is unpleasant but hardly unbearable*—your anxiety lessens and sleep comes more easily. You also may be shown relaxation techniques to practice during the day and at bedtime.

Commitment is key: Too many people try one or two of the techniques for a few nights, and then if they don't immediately start sleeping better, they get frustrated and give up. It takes dedication and commitment to make CBT-I work because you have to rebuild your innate sleep

drive and realign your body's natural rhythms before you'll be able to sleep well. It can take a week or two to start seeing real progress.

Covering the costs: The Affordable Care Act now requires insurance companies to cover behavioral health treatments, but benefits vary depending on the state you live in, your insurance plan and your sleep therapist's professional degree. The price for a course of CBT-I treatment averages about $460 for up to six sessions. It's also worth noting that you may end up saving money in the long run. A recent study showed that older adults with insomnia spent an average of $1,100 more on health care over a six-month period compared with those who did not have insomnia—and that, after completing as few as three sessions of CBT-I, participants' total health-care costs dropped significantly.

So even if you have to pay out of pocket, you may want to consider CBT-I an investment in yourself. Chances are good that it will end up saving you anxiety, aggravation and money… promoting optimal health overall.

How Healing Hands Provide Sleep for Dementia Patients

Michael Reed Gach, PhD, founder of *Acupressure. com*. He is based in Kihei, Hawaii, and is the author of seven books and numerous self-healing CDs on the topic of acupressure and health, including the fully guided CD *Sleep Better.*

If you live with someone who has Alzheimer's disease or another type of dementia, he or she may be keeping you up at night—even keeping you up all night—with restlessness just as a newborn baby would. But the feeling of dealing with an Alzheimer's patient overnight is worlds apart from that of dealing with a beautiful new baby's nighttime fussing. In fact, it can be maddening, exhausting and frustrating for caregivers.

Difficulty falling or staying asleep as well as "sundowning" (becoming agitated in the late afternoon or early evening) are common among people with dementia. Although medication can help calm agitation in a person with dementia, it won't necessarily improve his or her sleep quality. In fact, medication for sleep can make patients drowsy at the wrong times and unsteady on their feet, causing falls. It also can increase confusion and reduce a patient's self-care abilities. But there is a safe, effective nondrug technique that can relieve dementia-related sleep problems—acupressure. And if you are a caregiver, you can easily learn it and do it at home.

Acupressure is based on the same principles as acupuncture—but no needles are used. Acupressure simply involves using the fingers and hands to press certain parts of a person's body. The pressure is applied to meridian points, a highway of human energy flow, explained Michael Reed Gach, PhD, acupressure educator and founder of *Acupressure.com*, an online hub for self-healing. Acupressure can release stress and tension, increase circulation and reduce pain—all of which leads, as you might imagine, to better sleep.

PROVEN TO IMPROVE SLEEP

Acupressure was recently shown, in a scientific study from Turin, Italy, to relieve sleep problems in nursing home residents who had insomnia and either Alzheimer's disease or mild cognitive impairment (a mild form of dementia that may or may not worsen to full-blown dementia). The study included 129 people between the ages of 69 and 96 who received acupressure on a pressure point called HT7 ev-

---

Sleep and Alzheimer's

A long-term study of initially healthy 65-year-olds found that those who slept the least (about five hours or less without waking) tended to have fewer neurons (brain cells) in a part of the brain that controls sleep.

Also: Many in the study who developed Alzheimer's disease were those who had fewer neurons and less sleep.

To protect your brain: Keep neurons healthy with good sleep habits, and seek treatment if you suspect you may have a sleep disorder.

Andrew Lim, MD, assistant professor of neurology, University of Toronto, Canada.

---

ery day for eight weeks. (To find HT7, follow a line on the palm side of the hand from the space between the little finger and ring finger to the crease where the hand and wrist meet.) Residents were much better able to fall asleep and stay asleep and also got more overall hours of sleep when they had acupressure treatment. Plus, the need to use sedative drugs for sleep among these residents decreased.

ACUPRESSURE TECHNIQUES FOR YOU

Although having some formal training in acupressure is ideal, anyone can learn the basics of this hands-on therapy to help another person—including a person with dementia. *Here is some guidance from Dr. Gach to improve sleep…*

When the person with dementia is in bed and ready for sleep, sit beside him or her and…

•**Locate the two main acupressure points for relief of agitation, anxiety and sleep problems.** These are HT7 (the spot on the wrist in line with the space between the little finger and ring finger) and a spot on the forearm, called P6, that's in line with the middle finger but about two inches (three fingers' width) below the wrist.

•**Apply firm, steady pressure to each point, one after the other** (which point is first doesn't matter), using a finger, thumb or, if you have arthritis that makes this uncomfortable, a knuckle. For P6, Dr. Gach suggests clasping the person's forearm so that you press your thumb on the P6 point while pressing your fingertips into the corresponding spot on the other side of the arm.

How much pressure to apply? It should be the kind that "hurts good," similar to the kind of smarting relief you feel from a nice massage of sore muscles. Although it mildly hurts, it also feels good. So when doing acupressure on a person with dementia, you will have to carefully observe and patiently ask the person about his or her comfort level and not go beyond it. (Explaining that this "massage" will help with sleep can be a good strategy, too.)

•**Hold the pressure for two to three minutes on each spot,** and, if possible, encourage the patient to breathe slowly and deeply. "But even if the patient doesn't understand what acupressure is or why you are doing it, it will still have the desired effect," said Dr. Gach. "The body will respond even if the brain doesn't fully comprehend the purpose of it."

Also, although you might think anxiety and aggression are symptoms that might get in the way of giving acupressure to a person with dementia, studies have shown that acupressure and similar hands-on healing techniques, such as massage therapy, are well-tolerated and symptom-relieving solutions for people with dementia. In addition to improving sleep, acupressure relieves anxiety and agitation and decreases aggression and combativeness.

EMPOWER YOURSELF

Of course, you can use these acupressure techniques on anyone, including yourself, to help the body naturally fall asleep and sleep well. But these techniques are particularly empowering for caregivers of people with dementia, who may feel helpless in the face of a disease that can only get worse, said Dr. Gach. "Even if you can't stop the disease or reverse it, you can at least be empowered to help with the symptoms."

Hidden Causes of Daytime Sleepiness

Shelby Harris, PsyD, a psychologist and director of the Behavioral Sleep Medicine Program at the Sleep-Wake Disorders Center at Montefiore Medical Center in New York City. *DrShelbyHarris.com*

Insomnia seems to be the granddaddy of all sleep problems. But what about people who sleep too much or those who constantly feel sleepy even when they get "normal" amounts of sleep?

What's new: Some researchers are now finding that excessive sleepiness is more prevalent than previously thought—perhaps affecting up to 5% of American adults.

The average adult sleeps roughly six to nine hours a night. If you get this amount of sleep or more but still feel sleepy during the day—and/or you remain sleepy after a 20-minute nap or need multiple naps that interfere with your daily activities—a medical condition could be the cause.

Excessive sleep and daytime sleepiness are common symptoms of dozens of health problems, including hormone disorders (such as thyroid disease)...depression...nutritional deficiencies (including low vitamin D or iron levels)...and medication side effects from such drugs as painkillers, antidepressants and antihistamines. That is why people who are concerned about sleeping too much or feeling sleepy during the day should consult their primary care doctors.

However, if you are generally healthy but are still sleeping too much, you could have hypersomnia. With this sleep disorder, a person typically will sleep a full night but will be unrefreshed and sleepy throughout the day.

Possible causes of hypersomnia...

ADVANCED SLEEP PHASE DISORDER (ASPD)

If you go to sleep earlier than most people and wake up hours before you'd like, your body clock probably needs resetting.

Patients with ASPD are typically exhausted and ready to sleep in the early evening (around, say, 7 pm) and wake up at 2 am or 3 am. Even though they sleep the normal six-to-nine hours, their body clocks have advanced by several hours.

Warning signs: Suspect ASPD if you have the above symptoms for more than a week.

Diagnosis: In most cases, a sleep specialist can diagnose ASPD by learning about your sleep schedule (usually from a sleep diary you keep to record your regular sleep patterns).* Actigraphy, in which the patient wears a small sensor on the wrist to help the specialist identify sleep patterns, may also be used. The patient can wear the sensor in his/her own home.

Treatment: You can reset your body clock with bright-light therapy. This involves sitting near a light box (available online and at some pharmacies for about $60 to $200) for one to two hours in the early evening before bedtime. The full-spectrum light mimics sunshine and delays the release of melatonin, a sleep-inducing hormone.

Some individuals can achieve a normal sleep-wake schedule (for example, 10 pm to 6 am)

*To find a sleep specialist near you, consult the American Academy of Sleep Medicine, *SleepEducation.com*.

within a month or less. Others need to use a light box for longer.

Consult your doctor before using a light box. It may not be appropriate if you have certain eye conditions, such as glaucoma or cataracts. Also, work with a sleep specialist who can advise you on the proper time to use the light box. Insurance may not cover the cost of this therapy—check with your insurer.

NARCOLEPSY

This is a neurological disease that interferes with the brain's ability to control sleep-wake cycles. It causes sudden, and irresistible, bouts of daytime sleepiness. For example, patients may nod off in the middle of a conversation or while eating. Patients who don't have such sleep attacks still can be chronically sleepy even if they think they are sleeping at night (with narcolepsy, frequent nighttime awakenings disturb normal sleep).

Warning signs: Narcolepsy is often accompanied by episodes of cataplexy, a sudden loss of muscle tone while awake, which leaves the patient unable to move or speak.

Diagnosis: Patients have an overnight sleep test (polysomnogram) to identify abnormalities. In a second test (multiple sleep latency), a patient takes a series of five naps spaced two hours apart. People with narcolepsy will sleep during most or all of the nap periods…will fall asleep in eight minutes or less…and will enter REM sleep soon after falling asleep.

Treatment: Medications can target the predominant symptoms of narcolepsy.

Examples: *Sodium oxybate* (Xyrem) helps control cataplexy and sleep attacks…*zolpidem* (Ambien) or other sedatives are helpful for those who mainly suffer from disturbed sleep…and *modafinil* (Provigil) is a stimulant that reduces daytime sleepiness and can minimize sleep attacks. Sometimes several drugs are prescribed at the same time. Patients usually need to take them long term, but symptoms tend to subside with treatment.

Lifestyle changes, such as limiting caffeine, scheduling naps and managing stress, are also helpful.

PERIODIC LIMB MOVEMENT DISORDER (PLMD)

If you kick and twitch while you sleep, you'll want to sleep more during the day. Patients with PLMD usually are not aware of their nighttime limb activity (unless someone tells them). The main symptom is daytime sleepiness. The leg jerks cause frequent, brief awakenings and interfere with deep sleep—in patients and their bed partners.

Warning signs: Most people with restless legs syndrome (RLS)—uncomfortable sensations that can be relieved only by moving the legs—also have PLMD. PLMD is also linked to narcolepsy and other sleep disorders.

Diagnosis: An overnight sleep test measures the frequency and severity of leg movements and detects any other sleep disorders.

Treatment: Medications that block abnormal muscle movements and improve sleep. These include *pramipexole* (Mirapex), *clonazepam* (Klonopin) and sometimes a narcotic medication.

SLEEP APNEA

Snoring, snorting or gasping for breath during sleep are some of the widely known symptoms of sleep apnea, but daytime sleepiness is also a red flag for the condition.

Patients with apnea stop breathing for anywhere from just a few seconds to more than a minute—a cycle that interrupts their sleep. Apnea is dangerous because it increases risk for dementia, high blood pressure, heartbeat irregularities and other cardiovascular diseases.

Warning signs: In addition to sleepiness during the day, people with sleep apnea may wake up with a dry mouth and a headache from diminished oxygen.

Sleep and Memories

Do you have an accurate memory? It may depend on how well you slept the night before.

Recent research: People who are sleep-deprived are more likely to develop false memories, a finding that could call into question the reliability of crime eyewitnesses.

Psychological Science

Diagnosis: If you experience chronic daytime sleepiness or your bed partner says that you snore or gasp for breath while sleeping, you may have sleep apnea. (If you sleep alone, you can record yourself at night.) A sleep study is used to confirm the diagnosis—it measures your breathing patterns and blood oxygen levels.

Treatment: A positive airway pressure (PAP) device. Used at home, it supplies a constant stream of air into the nose/mouth while you sleep. PAP can often eliminate the interrupted breathing patterns of sleep apnea and daytime sleepiness. For those who can't tolerate PAP devices, an oral appliance or a small device placed in each nostril can be used as an alternative, but it may not work in all patients. There are surgical treatments for sleep apnea, which are beneficial in about 50% of cases.

Also helpful: Weight loss. Most apnea patients are overweight. In these cases, losing as little as 10% of one's body weight often can help.

Note: Though uncommon, some people have positional sleep apnea (they have it only when sleeping on their backs). If this is the case for you, training yourself to sleep on your side may help (try putting a tennis ball in the pocket of a T-shirt worn backwards). A sleep specialist can tell if your sleep apnea is related to sleep position.

Dangerous Restless Legs

Study of 12,556 male health professionals with RLS led by researchers at Brigham and Women's Hospital and Harvard Medical School, both in Boston, published in *Neurology*.

Restless legs may harm health as much as smoking, excess weight, high blood pressure, history of heart attack, depression, insomnia and increasing age. In restless legs syndrome (RLS), which affects 4% to 14% of the population, uncomfortable sensations in lower limbs produce an urge to move the legs. The symptoms usually are worse at night when lying down or sitting and may lead to sleep deprivation. See your doctor if you have RLS—diagnosing and treating the condition can lead to better sleep and improved overall health.

Don't Use Just Any Old Pillow

William J. Lauretti, DC, an associate professor in the department of chiropractic clinical sciences at the New York Chiropractic College in Seneca Falls, New York, and spokesperson for the American Chiropractic Association in Arlington, Virginia. He is author of numerous journal articles and textbook chapters on neck and back pain.

Do you wake up stiff and achy? Don't be so quick to blame it on your age or arthritis—it just might be due to what you're sleeping on…

Plenty of people agonize about buying a mattress—you can easily spend $1,000 or more, and there are all those features to choose from (such as pillow toppers and coil counts).

The truth is, there's no unbiased research showing that any of these features will reduce pain. The best mattress for you is simply the one that feels best for you.

The features offered in pillows, however, do matter. That's why pillows should never be selected as an afterthought. How to select a pillow based on where you need support and how you sleep…

PILLOWS FOR NECK PAIN

I usually advise people to sleep on their sides because it's a neutral position that's easy on the back, shoulders and knees.* But side-sleeping leaves a large gap between the downward-facing shoulder and the head. A too-thin pillow will allow your head to dip down, which puts a lot of stress on the neck.

Best pillow for side-sleepers: One that's thick enough to fill the space between your ear and the mattress. It will support your neck and head and keep them in line with your spine. A firm foam pillow is ideal because the weight of your head won't compress it very much while you sleep.

Good products: BackJoy SleepSound Pillow, $99.99, *BackJoy.com/sleep*. Or you could try a water pillow so you can customize your

---

*We all have a preferred sleep position, but certain positions are better for various types of pain than others. I have found that patients can adopt a new sleep position if it helps their pain.

pillow height. Chiroflow Premium Water Pillow, $46.17, *Amazon.com*.

Best pillow for back- and stomach-sleepers: A feather pillow. You can shape a feather pillow and make it thicker under the neck for better support and thinner under the head so that it remains flat.

Good product: 700-Fill-Power Sateen White Goose Down Pillow, $199, *LLBean.com*.

If you like the feel of a feather pillow but are allergic, try the Grand Down All Season Down Alternative Standard Pillow Set, $34.40, *Amazon.com*.

Another option for neck pain is a thin conventional pillow with a "neck bone" support pillow placed under the neck.

Good product: Original Bones NeckBone Chiropractic Pillow, $14.99, *Amazon.com*.

You can also try a specialized pillow that is thicker at the ends, with a slight cavity in the middle and built-in neck support. These pillows help keep the head at the right height while supporting the neck. In addition, they provide flexibility for people who like to change from back-sleeping (when they would use the thinner middle part of the pillow) to side-sleeping (when the thicker end would be appropriate).

Good product: Core Products Core 200 Tri-Core Pillow Standard Support, $37.99, *Amazon. com*.

PILLOWS FOR BACK PAIN

For back pain, the usual advice is to sleep on your back on a superfirm mattress. Back-sleeping does give good support, but many people aren't comfortable in this position, and it tends to increase snoring.

I have found that back pain patients tend to do better when they sleep on their sides. It keeps the spine straight and is generally less stressful than stomach- or back-sleeping.

Stomach-sleeping tends to produce a forward curve in the low back, jamming the joints together and causing pain. Back-sleeping can be better, but if the mattress is too soft, it causes a forward curve in the low back. And if the mattress is too firm, it flattens the low back, which can lead to tight muscles.

Insomnia Can Worsen Tinnitus

A survey of 117 people with tinnitus found that the more difficulty they had falling asleep, the more severe their symptoms.

If you have tinnitus: Talk to your doctor about ways to ensure a good night's sleep, which can help ease your symptoms.

Kathleen L. Yaremchuk, MD, chair, department of otolaryngology–head and neck surgery, Henry Ford Hospital, Detroit.

Best pillow pick: When sleeping on your back, use a feather pillow that's "fluffed" to provide more lift under the neck, and flattened out a bit under the head. When sleeping on your side, use a fairly thick and firm foam pillow to support the head and fill the gap between the head and bottom shoulder. See feather pillow and foam pillow recommendations mentioned earlier.

PILLOWS FOR SHOULDER PAIN

It's a challenge to find a comfortable position when you have shoulder arthritis or a history of shoulder injuries. If you sleep on your stomach, you would have to keep your head turned all night, which could make shoulder pain worse. Of course, sleeping on the "bad" shoulder can be painful as well, but lying with the bad side up is also tricky because the shoulder isn't supported by a pillow or the mattress.

Best pillow pick: A large body pillow. While on your side, hug the pillow to your chest and rest your top-side arm (with your painful shoulder) on top of it. It will support the shoulder and keep it from "folding" while you sleep.

Good product: Dreamland Body Pillow, $21.20, *Amazon.com*.

PILLOWS FOR KNEE PAIN

Back-sleeping is ideal when your knees hurt, but as mentioned earlier, few people can comfortably sleep on their backs. And stomach-sleeping is a problem because it overextends the knees. Side-sleeping is less stressful to the knees, but this position can be uncomfortable when the bones of the knees press together.

Best pillow pick: While sleeping on your side, placing a pillow between your knees will prevent them from rubbing against each other and keep your upper hip at a comfortable angle.

Good product: Remedy Contoured Memory Foam Leg Pillow, $17.99, *Walmart.com*.

You can also put a body pillow between your knees.

HELPFUL RESOURCE

For reviews of additional types of pillows, go to *SleepLiketheDead.com/pillow-reviews.html*.

How to Pull an All-Nighter

Eric J. Olson, MD, codirector, Mayo Clinic Center for Sleep Medicine, Rochester, Minnesota, quoted in *The Wall Street Journal*.

If you must stay up all night, coffee or other caffeinated drinks can help, but wait to drink them until the hours between midnight and 7 am, when your body naturally tends to shut down. Keep protein bars around for energy-boosting snacks—avoid high sugar intake, which can cause a sugar crash afterward. Try to be in an active environment—noise and activity make it easier to stay awake. If you are doing something unstimulating, such as driving, it may be best to pull over and take a 20-minute nap to boost performance. The day after an all-nighter, try to take a short nap after lunch and then sleep without interruption that night.

Transform Nightmares into Sweet Dreams

Barry Krakow, MD, sleep medicine specialist, founder and medical director, Maimonides Sleep Arts & Sciences, Ltd., Albuquerque, New Mexico, and author of several books on sleep disorders. *NightmareTreatment.com*

If you are a horror-movie buff, you know who Freddy Krueger is—the character from the iconic slasher movie *A Nightmare on Elm Street*. This murderous villain stalked his victims in their dreams. The movie's director, Wes Craven, is said to have been inspired, in part, by news reports about a group of Cambodian war refugees who suffered nightmares that were so horrific that many refused to sleep. Some even died—likely as a result of the severe sleep deprivation caused by their nightmares.

Although death is an extreme and exceptional, if unproven reaction to a nightmare, frequent nightmares can be a consequence of serious trauma, depression, anxiety disorder, run-of-the-mill stress and even sleep apnea. About one in 12 people are tormented by frequent nightmares. That's a lot of anxious, tired people. If you are one of them, don't think that nothing can be done about the problem. The solution may be much easier—and entertaining—than you think.

HOW TO STOP NIGHTMARES

Imagery rehearsal therapy (IRT), co-developed more than 25 years ago by Barry Krakow, MD, a sleep disorders expert who founded Maimonides Sleep Arts & Sciences, Ltd., in Albuquerque, New Mexico, has been scientifically proven to reduce nightmares and improve sleep quality—and the proof has been in studies of people with posttraumatic stress disorder (PTSD). In fact, the landmark study of IRT, which involved people with PTSD, showed that just three sessions of IRT spread over four weeks reduced nightmare frequency by more than half. The benefits lasted for six months after treatment ended, with follow-up studies showing that relief can last up to two and a half years.

A recent study of patients with PTSD showed that IRT was just as good as drug therapy with *prazosin* (Minipress), the main drug that is now used to reduce nightmare frequency in people with PTSD, such as war veterans. But you do not have to be in extreme psychological distress to benefit from IRT, especially given its simplicity. "IRT is actually very simple to do," said Dr. Krakow. *It involves just three steps…*

•**Choose a recent nightmare.** "The most important caveat is to not select a nightmare that feels like a replay of a traumatic event that happened in real life," Dr. Krakow cautioned. "You can't change the outcome of something that has really already happened." (Although there are forms of IRT that neutralize nightmares of real-

Pill-free Cure for Insomnia

Just before bed, try this acupressure trick. With your thumbs, press the soles of your feet where the heel and the arch meet. Lie on your back (on a carpeted floor is best), and bend your knees, using your right hand on your right foot and left hand on your left. Press as hard as you can for at least two minutes. You should feel the tension leaving your body.

Joan Wilen and Lydia Wilen are authors of Bottom Line's Treasury of Home Remedies & Natural Cures *and* Secret Food Cures.

life traumas, they should be practiced with a therapist, explained Dr. Krakow. Treatment involves exposure therapy whereby the therapist repeatedly guides a patient through recalling the event to change how he or she feels about and remembers it.)

•**Replay the selected nightmare in your thoughts,** but change the story any way you wish. Dr. Krakow notes that instructions about how to change the story are very open-ended. If, for example, your nightmare involves being chased by a bear, replay it in your daytime recall of it to running after butterflies...or imagine the bear wearing a circus costume and becoming a dancing bear at your command. "The concept underlying the practice is that what you picture in your mind while awake can influence what you picture in your mind while asleep," said Dr. Krakow.

•**Rehearse your revised dream.** You do this by playing it again and again in your mind for five to 20 minutes per day during wake time. After a week, choose a different nightmare to rewrite if another bothersome one exists. Although practice makes perfect, some people practice IRT only a few minutes every other day and still achieve large benefits, perhaps be-

cause they begin to feel that they truly can take control of their nightmares, said Dr. Krakow.

In his experience, most people see results within the first two weeks. Nightmares become less frequent, sleep becomes less interrupted and daytime mood is improved. As for whether people begin to actually dream the daytime story used to replace a nightmare, this occurs in less than 10%, said Dr. Krakow.

The largest improvements usually occur between two weeks and two months from the time of starting IRT, he said. Some people practice IRT for up to a year and others need only a few weeks of doing it to resolve their nightmare problem. "We hear about people picking the practice up again if their nightmares return, so IRT becomes a skill that can be applied as needed. Ideally, someone having a nightmare would wake up in the middle of the night, 'rewrite' the dream right then and there, and be able to go right back to sleep," said Dr. Krakow.

NEXT STEPS IF YOU HAVE NIGHTMARES

With the exception of the curious and tragic case of the Cambodian war refugees, who were clearly suffering from severe PTSD, nightmares themselves aren't dangerous, but they can leave you agitated and startled. If you have been having nightmares at least once a week, Dr. Krakow suggests that you have a complete medical evaluation, including a sleep study, to find out whether a health issue—namely sleep apnea—is causing the nightmares. If you learn that you do have sleep apnea, treating it will reduce the commonly associated health risks, such as high blood pressure, heart attack and stroke. Recent research is also showing exciting possibilities that treating sleep apnea reduces or perhaps prevents nightmares. Otherwise, Dr. Krakow's IRT practice tips may be an empowering and creative way to cultivate sweet dreams and get the restful sleep you deserve.

Women's Health

Women, Reduce Stroke Risk with Potassium

Bananas are rich in it, dried fruits such as raisins, prunes and apricots are, too. Potatoes, white beans and tomato sauce are great sources as well. You may have guessed the nutrient—potassium. And what does getting enough potassium do besides help your muscles move and regulate your blood pressure and heartbeat? It's crucial to heart health, especially for postmenopausal women. And a recent study showed that postmenopausal women who consumed more potassium were less likely to have strokes.

In this study, women who consumed the most potassium (at least 3,194 milligrams [mg] per day) were 12% less likely to suffer any type of stroke than women who consumed the least potassium (less than 1,926 mg per day). And they were 16% less likely to suffer an ischemic

stroke, the most common type, caused when a blood clot blocks oxygen and nutrients to the brain. For women who kept their blood pressure and weight in check and knew to bulk up on potassium, protection against ischemic stroke was more than doubled (a 27% to 30% lower risk) compared with women who consumed a minimum of dietary potassium. That is a huge risk reduction.

Incidentally, even the high-range number for potassium intake mentioned above—around 3,200 mg per day—may be considered on the low side. The World Health Organization recommends 3,510 mg...while the US Department of Agriculture (USDA) recommends 4,700 mg a day. But the sad fact is that most postmenopausal women are nowhere near that goal. In the latest study, the average daily intake of potassium among the 90,000-plus participants was

Sylvia Wassertheil-Smoller, PhD, Dorothy and William Manealoff Foundation and Molly Rosen Chair in Social Medicine Emerita, department of epidemiology and population health, Albert Einstein College of Medicine in Brooklyn. Her study was published in *Stroke*.

Diet Drink Caution

Drinking two or more diet sodas or diet fruit drinks a day resulted in a 30% greater risk for heart attack or stroke than rarely or never consuming these diet drinks, an eight-year observational study of nearly 60,000 women (average age 62) has found.

Theory: Diet sodas and diet fruit drinks (as well as the nondiet versions) have been linked to weight gain and metabolic syndrome, which raise risk for heart disease.

Ankur Vyas, MD, cardiovascular diseases fellow, University of Iowa Health Care, Iowa City.

---

only 2,611 mg—that's barely more than half the daily amount that the USDA says we need!

ARE YOU GETTING ENOUGH?

The irony is that potassium is found in nearly all food groups, especially fruits, vegetables, dairy products and fish and seafood. You can make every meal—breakfast, lunch and dinner—potassium-rich. *See for yourself...*

•**Breakfast or Snack Time.** A banana provides 422 mg of potassium. A cup of cantaloupe, 430 mg. Eight ounces of yogurt gives you up to 579 mg. Toss in a cup of strawberries and you get 255 mg more. Prune juice packs 707 mg in a cup (a cup of stewed prunes, 796 mg). And a cup of orange juice will provide 496 mg. Dried apricots or peaches are sweet and tasty sources of potassium, too, delivering between 378 mg and 398 mg per quarter cup.

•**Lunch and Dinner.** A small baked potato, including the skin, has 738 mg of potassium, a medium sweet potato with skin, 542 mg. Tomato products are great sources of potassium... one-half cup of tomato sauce provides 405 mg. All types of beans, especially white beans (595 mg per half-cup) are excellent sources, too. And a cup of cooked spinach packs 840 mg. Fish and seafood are also great. For example, three ounces of yellowfin tuna provides 484 mg of potassium.

That's just a small sampling, but you can see how having a deliciously varied diet of healthful foods can provide all the potassium you need

for heart health and stroke risk reduction. For more information on the potassium content of foods, the University of Massachusetts School of Medicine has an excellent cheat sheet at *www. umassmed.edu/uploadedFiles/SourcesDietary Potassium.pdf.*

DO YOU NEED A SUPPLEMENT?

The benefits of potassium come from dietary intake. Supplements do not seem to have the same beneficial effect, said Sylvia Wassertheil-Smoller, PhD, who participated in the study on potassium and stroke risk in postmenopausal women. Dr. Wassertheil-Smoller is chair of social medicine at Albert Einstein College of Medicine in Brooklyn, New York. She and other experts agree that having too much potassium in the blood can be dangerous to the heart. So do check with your doctor before taking a potassium supplement. If a potassium supplement is recommended to you, your doctor should monitor your blood potassium levels to make sure they do not go higher than what is healthy and normal.

Vitamin D Deficiency Linked to Breast Cancer Death Risk

Study titled "Meta-analysis of Vitamin D Sufficiency for Improving Survival of Patients with Breast Cancer," published in *Anticancer Research.*

Vitamin D is often in the news because most Americans get too little of it...and because deficiencies are associated with increased risk for cardiovascular disease, diabetes, Alzheimer's disease, osteoporosis and many other serious health problems. And now here we go again—because too-low levels of that same vitamin are linked to nearly double the risk of dying from breast cancer, a recent study shows.

Here's what you should know...

POOLING RESULTS TO SETTLE THE SCORE

Many studies have looked at the association between vitamin D levels and the risk of developing breast cancer, but there has been little exploration of the link between vitamin D and the odds of surviving breast cancer. To address that oversight, researchers looked for studies that investigated a link between breast cancer survival and levels of a vitamin D precursor called 25-hydroxyvitamin D, or 25(OH)D for short. The blood test for 25(OH)D is considered the most accurate way to measure how much vitamin D is in a person's body. Five studies met the researchers' criteria, but their results varied. *However, when the researchers pooled the data from these studies and did a statistical analysis, they found that...*

• **Breast cancer patients** with higher levels of 25(OH)D at the time of their diagnoses had a substantially lower risk of dying from their disease during the study periods, which averaged about 10 years.

• **Women with the highest levels,** around 30 nanograms per milliliter (ng/mL), had a 44% lower risk of dying from breast cancer than women with the lowest levels, around 17 ng/mL.

• **There was a strong dose-related response,** meaning that higher vitamin D levels were consistently associated with reduced mortality risk.

WHAT THIS MEANS FOR YOU

It's important to point out that this study does not prove that 25(OH)D actually helps protect against death from breast cancer. It could be the other way around—the more deadly forms of breast cancer might cause vitamin D to become depleted, making 25(OH)D a marker for disease severity. However, the researchers consider this unlikely because no other studies suggest that cancer reduces 25(OH)D levels. Furthermore, the evidence in support of vitamin D's protective mechanism is bolstered by the fact that cancer death rates are lower in areas of the US

Hidden Heart Risk for Women

Women who suffered childhood sexual abuse (not just physical abuse) are more likely to develop atherosclerosis. Doctors should consider it when assessing cardiovascular risks.

Stroke

(and the world) with ample sunlight, the most abundant catalyst for naturally sufficient vitamin D levels.

Don't DIY with D: The average blood level of 25(OH)D for breast cancer patients in the US is 17 ng/mL—which is too low. The researchers stated that blood levels "in all patients with breast cancer should be restored to the normal range [of] 30 to 80 ng/mL." However, it's important for cancer patients—and everyone else who wants to protect his or her health by optimizing vitamin D levels—to not take a do-it-yourself approach. As we've been warning you for several years, too much vitamin D can be dangerous, increasing the risk for blood vessel calcification, heart rhythm abnormalities and kidney damage.

Prudent: Ask a nutrition-oriented doctor to check your 25(OH)D level and, if necessary, to prescribe an appropriate dosage for supplementation.

HPV Vaccine Might Shield Women Against Throat Cancer

Rolando Herrero, MD, PhD, prevention and implementation group, International Agency for Research on Cancer, Lyon, France.

Marc Siegel, MD, associate professor of medicine, NYU Langone Medical Center, New York City.

Elizabeth Poynor, MD, gynecologic oncologist and pelvic surgeon, Lenox Hill Hospital, New York City.

PLoS One, online

Young women who are vaccinated against the human papillomavirus (HPV) not only protect themselves from cervical cancer, but from throat cancer as well, a recent study suggests.

Many of the increasing number of throat cancers, seen mostly in developed countries, are caused by HPV infection and the HPV vaccine might prevent many of these cancers, the researchers say.

"We found the women who had the HPV vaccine had much less infection than the women who hadn't," said lead researcher Rolando Herrero, MD, PhD, International Agency for Research on Cancer in Lyon, France.

"In fact, there was a 90% reduction in the prevalence of HPV infection in the women who received the vaccine compared to the women who had not," he said.

HPV infection is strongly associated with cancer of the oral cavity, Dr. Herrero noted. "We think that it is possible that the prevention of the infection will also lead to the prevention of these cancers," he explained.

The HPV vaccine has enormous benefit, said Dr. Herrero, "because of the cervical cancer prevention and the anal cancer prevention, and it can even prevent infections in their sexual partners."

A 2011 study in the *Journal of Clinical Oncology* showed that in the US, HPV-positive oral cancers increased from 16% of all oral cancers in the 1980s to 70% in the early 2000s.

The Oral Cancer Foundation estimates that close to 45,750 Americans will be diagnosed with oral and throat cancer in 2015, and more than 8,650 people will die from these conditions.

HPV-linked throat cancer recently came to the public's attention when the British newspaper *The Guardian* reported that actor Michael Douglas's recent bout with the disease might have been caused by oral sex.

STUDY DETAILS

For the more recent study, Dr. Herrero's team randomly assigned more than 7,400 women aged 18 to 25 to either receive the HPV vaccine or a vaccine against hepatitis A, as a comparison.

Women in the HPV vaccine group were given Cervarix, one of two vaccines available for HPV prevention. (The other is Gardasil.)

Four years later, the researchers found the HPV vaccine was 93% effective in preventing throat cancer. Among women who received the HPV vaccine, only one patient showed an oral HPV infection, compared with 15 in the hepatitis A vaccine group, the researchers found.

Because HPV is a sexually transmitted infection, the vaccine is most effective when given before someone is sexually active. Eighty percent of people will test positive for HPV infection within five years of becoming sexually active, said Marc Siegel, MD, an associate professor of medicine at NYU Langone Medical Center, in New York City.

That's why the CDC recommends the vaccine for adolescent girls and boys starting at age 11.

Green Veggies Prevent PMS

Three daily servings of cooked green cruciferous vegetables such as kale, broccoli and brussels sprouts cut risk of developing premenstrual syndrome (PMS) by up to 40%, according to a 10-year study of nearly 3,000 women.

Why: Green cruciferous vegetables are high in iron, which is necessary to produce mood-elevating neurotransmitters in the brain.

Patricia Chocano-Bedoya, PhD, visiting scientist, Harvard School of Public Health, Boston.

CONS AND PROS OF THE STUDY

"The study is really preliminary information," said Elizabeth Poynor, MD, a gynecologic oncologist and pelvic surgeon at Lenox Hill Hospital, in New York City. "It will provide a basis to begin to study how the vaccine will help to protect against throat cancer," she noted.

"It's going to take a while to study those who have been vaccinated to determine that they are protected against throat cancer. This is just the beginning," she said.

"It also really highlights that we need to vaccinate young boys," Dr. Poynor added.

The report was published online in the journal *PLoS One*.

info The U.S. National Cancer Institute has more about HPV and cancer at *http://www.cancer.gov/cancertopics/factsheet/Risk/HPV.*

Vitamin D Deficiency Increases Risk for Pregnancy Disorder

Study of 3,703 blood samples from pregnant women by researchers at University of Pittsburgh Graduate School of Public Health, published in *Epidemiology*.

Low vitamin D increases risk for dangerous pregnancy disorder. Pregnant women who had blood levels of vitamin D lower than 50 nanomoles per liter had 40% higher risk for severe preeclampsia, a potentially fatal condition characterized by high blood pressure and excess protein in the urine.

If you are pregnant: Talk to your healthcare provider about whether you need to take additional vitamin D.

Is It Breast Cancer or Not?

Melissa A. Lazar, MD, assistant professor of surgery at Thomas Jefferson University Hospital and a surgeon who specializes in the treatment of benign and malignant breast disease at the Jefferson Breast Care Center, both in Philadelphia.

It's scary to know that something suspicious appeared on what you thought was a routine mammogram. If your doctor recommends a biopsy, you obviously want to hear that everything's normal after all. But what if it's not? The medical language that's used in these reports can make things sound worse than they really are.

Here are common breast findings and what they really mean…

LOBULAR OR DUCTAL HYPERPLASIA

The lobules in the breasts are milk-producing glands. The ducts are passages that milk travels through to get to the nipples. Many women will eventually develop lobular or ductal hyperplasia. It means that there is an overgrowth of cells in one of these areas.

Is it a worrisome finding? Probably not, as long as the cells don't appear atypical (see below). When researchers at the Mayo Clinic looked at almost 9,000 women who had had benign breast biopsies, about one-third had these proliferating cells.

Hyperplasia is not cancer. It typically does not increase a woman's risk of getting breast cancer. I advise women not to worry about it.

ATYPICAL HYPERPLASIA

This is a little different from the situation described above. Atypical hyperplasia (also known as *proliferative changes with atypia*) is not a cancer. However, women who have been diagnosed with this condition do have to take precautions.

As the name suggests, "atypical" cells don't quite resemble normal cells. Atypical hyperplasia increases a woman's lifetime cancer risk, even in the unaffected breast, making the risk four to five times higher than that of the general population. *My advice…*

•**If the cells were discovered during a core needle biopsy (a sampling of tissue taken from the suspicious area),** I usually advise women to have an *excisional biopsy.* It will remove the entire area that contains the abnormal cells.

Editor's note: You might want to obtain a second opinion on the biopsy results given the findings of a recent study (see "Beware: Breast Biopsy Results May Not Be Accurate" on page 346).

•**Premenopausal women with atypical hyperplasia are advised to take the drug tamoxifen for five years.** It will reduce their risk for breast cancer by about two-thirds. Postmenopausal women will get a similar benefit when they take *raloxifene* (Evista) or *exemestane* (Aromasin). Discuss possible side effects of the drugs, such as blood clots and risk for stroke, with your doctor.

•**Screening guidelines from the National Comprehensive Cancer Network** include annual mammograms and a clinical breast exam

High Blood Pressure Could Cause Psoriasis

Women who have had high blood pressure (hypertension) for six years or more have a 27% higher risk for psoriasis. Women whose blood pressure has been controlled with beta-blockers such as *atenolol* or *propranolol* for more than six years have a 40% higher risk for psoriasis than women who never used those drugs.

Unknown: Whether women using beta-blockers would have a lower risk for psoriasis if they switched to another type of medicine. Psoriasis is a chronic immune system disorder that causes red, raised patches on skin.

Study of nearly 78,000 women from 1996 to 2008 led by researchers at Warren Alpert Medical School, Brown University, Providence, published online in *JAMA Dermatology.*

(a manual exam by a doctor) every six to 12 months.

LOBULAR CARCINOMA IN SITU (LCIS)

Don't let the word "carcinoma" throw you. Some doctors prefer the term *lobular neoplasia* because LCIS isn't a cancer—it is a risk factor.

The term "in situ" means that abnormal cells within the breast lobules haven't broken through the lobule wall and migrated into adjoining tissues or into the bloodstream.

Yet there is a risk. Women with LCIS are more likely to eventually develop breast cancer. The risk increases by 1% every year. A woman diagnosed with LCIS in her 40s is about 20% to 25% more likely to get breast cancer within 15 years than a woman who never had it.

Some women feel that any increase in breast cancer risk is unacceptable. They might ask their doctors if they should have a preventive (prophylactic) mastectomy. It's a difficult decision, particularly because the mastectomy would have to be bilateral (removing both breasts). Women with LCIS are just as likely to develop cancer in one breast as the other.

My advice: I don't recommend mastectomy for most women with LCIS, with the possible exception of those with a strong family history of breast cancer or other risk factors.

Better: Watchful waiting. Your doctor can monitor you closely. If a cancer does eventually develop, it can be treated quickly.

Get an annual mammogram...a clinical breast exam twice a year...and possibly take tamoxifen, raloxifene or exemestane. Women with LCIS who take one of these drugs can reduce their breast cancer risk by about 50%.

DUCTAL CARCINOMA IN SITU (DCIS)

Unlike LCIS, DCIS is a cancer. About 60,000 women in the US each year are found to have DCIS. The abnormal cells are confined inside the milk ducts and thus are not considered invasive. But if you're diagnosed with DCIS, you have to get treated. Treatment options include a lumpectomy followed by radiation to kill any cancer cells that were left behind...or, in some cases, a mastectomy (with or without breast reconstruction). Your surgeon might recommend a mastectomy if the DCIS is extensive or multicentric (more than one tumor, often in different areas of the breast). Once the carcinoma is removed, you will need to be followed closely. There always is the risk for a recurrence, which is 5% to 10% following lumpectomy with radiation and 1% to 2% following a mastectomy.

If the DCIS is *estrogen receptor-positive*, taking tamoxifen for five years is recommended to reduce your risk for recurrence and a new breast cancer.

Beware: Breast Biopsy Results May Not Be Accurate

Study led by researchers at University of Washington School of Medicine and Fred Hutchinson Cancer Research Center, both in Seattle, published in *The Journal of the American Medical Association*.

Breast biopsy findings may not be reliable when it comes to subtle abnormalities, according to a new study.

Researchers asked 115 pathologists to examine biopsy slides, then compared their diagnoses with those from a panel of leading experts who had seen the same slides. The panel of experts was made up of internationally recognized pathologists with highly regarded experience in research and continuing medical education on diagnostic breast pathology.

The outside pathologists were very good at diagnosing invasive breast cancer and agreed with the expert panel in about 96% of cases. For benign findings, they agreed with the experts in 87% of cases. When it came to diagnosing DCIS, they agreed with the experts about 84% of the time.

But with atypical ductal hyperplasia, the pathologists were in line with the experts only 48% of the time. They diagnosed atypia in 17% of readings where the experts had not and missed it in 35% of readings.

Do You Really Need a Mammogram?

Russell Harris, MD, MPH, professor of medicine and adjunct professor of epidemiology, University of North Carolina School of Medicine and Gillings School of Global Public Health, Chapel Hill, North Carolina.

While American doctors follow guidelines that screening should be offered at least every two years to women who are 50 to 74 years old, and although we definitely know that risk of breast cancer increases with age, do you really need a mammogram when you hit 70? A Dutch study says no. In fact, it found that breast cancer screening for women age 70 and older may actually cause more harm than good, leading to unnecessary treatment that puts elderly women at even higher risk than they already are for anemia, gastrointestinal problems, fatigue, infection, memory loss, effects of bone loss (osteoporosis) and heart disease. This all boils down to quality of life in your later years.

And statistics bear this out.

If 1,000 women started biennial mammography screening when they were 50 years old and continued for 10 years, one to three breast cancer deaths would be prevented over the next 15 years.

If 1,000 60-year-old women had biennial screenings for 10 years, three or four deaths would be prevented over the next 20 years. For women in their mid-70s, however, their average remaining life expectancy—about 13 more years—is shorter than the 17-year lag time in which a death attributed to breast cancer could be prevented. Suddenly the number of women being helped by screening starts going down, not up.

But maybe you are 72 and expect to live until 102. Fair enough. In that case, breast cancer screening and next steps if breast cancer is detected should be a personal, individualized decision between you and your health-care provider, according to Russell Harris, MD, professor of medicine, University of North Carolina School of Medicine.

APPROACHING BREAST CANCER DETECTION FROM ANOTHER ANGLE

Dr. Harris said he is not suggesting that all breast cancer screening guidelines should completely go out the window and leave women and their doctors high and dry. His wish—and what he expects to happen, based on discussions with his colleagues in the public health field—is that for older women, at least, there will be new, more individualized guidelines that will be conveyed to gynecologists and primary-care physicians over the next few years. *The same broad leeway being proposed for elderly women should be extended to all women, of every age—and these downsides of breast cancer screening are the rationale...*

•**Cumulative radiation exposure.** Although the amount of radiation received per mammogram is minimal, every time you get a mammogram or are otherwise exposed to radiation in the medical setting, it has a cumulative effect on your body.

•**Possible unneeded treatment.** Some breast cancers are so slow-growing that they would not have caused any harm if they had gone undetected.

•**Side effects of treatment.** As we all know—cancer therapy itself is wrought with side effects. Surgery, radiation, chemotherapy and hormone therapy all come with risks that become riskier with age. Radiation to the breast can damage the heart and lead to lung cancer, and hormone therapy raises a woman's risk for serious blood clots and stroke. For some women, the treatment can be just as devastating as the disease it's meant to conquer.

WHY IT'S A PERSONAL DECISION

Each woman—young, old and in between—needs to evaluate the pros and cons of her own screening in relation to her personal health, family history and life situation. The physician's role is to help women make informed, individualized decisions about breast cancer screening—not to automatically pressure them into decisions based on screening statistics.

Part of being informed means recognizing that screening isn't the only way to protect yourself. There are other approaches to prevention that we've de-emphasized at our peril. It's time to stop putting all our eggs in the screening basket. Screening is not our only hope to reduce the scourge of breast cancer. Maintaining a healthy weight, remaining physically active, not smoking, being moderate in our drinking habits and proactively working with a gynecologist and primary-care physician to know and address personal risk factors are important ways for women to protect themselves against cancer, stay all-around healthy and have a great quality of life.

Do You Really Need a Hysterectomy?

Daniel M. Morgan, MD, associate professor, department of obstetrics and gynecology, University of Michigan Medical School, Ann Arbor. His study appeared in the *American Journal of Obstetrics and Gynecology*.

One of every three women will have an operation to remove her uterus before she turns 60 years old. Something is wrong with that statistic. Shedding a uterus should not be a rite of passage, like sporting silver hair or joining AARP. Doctors may tell you that the operation is no biggie, but removing a body part is always a big deal. Hysterectomies involve anesthesia, often an abdominal incision

and, like all surgery, the risk that something will go wrong.

If you've been told that hysterectomy is the best option to clear up a uterine problem such as endometriosis (a painful condition whereby uterine tissue grows outside of the uterus), fibroids (noncancerous growths) or abnormal bleeding—or if you know someone who was advised to have a hysterectomy—hold on. Although there are times when having a hysterectomy is the right move, such as when cancer is a threat, some procedures are unnecessary, according to researchers from University of Michigan. In fact, a lot of women are getting hysterectomies for no good reason at all. What's more, alternative treatments to hysterectomy don't look like they are being tried as often as they should be.

HOLD ON TO YOUR UTERUS

The University of Michigan team looked through the medical records of 52 Michigan hospitals to evaluate how many of the hysterectomies done in the first 10 months of 2013 were actually appropriate. After weeding out women who had medically valid reasons for heading straight to surgery, such as those with cancer or a life-threatening hemorrhage, the researchers ended up with a study population of about 3,400 women. For each of these, the researchers looked for documentation that other medical treatments had been either tried or at least recommended before the woman's hysterectomy. These other treatments included drug or hormone therapy, endometrial ablation (therapeutic removal of cells that line the uterus) and various other uterus-sparing surgical procedures.

The results: About two-thirds of the women considered or tried at least one other treatment before having a hysterectomy, but most still had hysterectomies done for conditions for which uterus-sparing procedures were available. Most alarming is that nearly one in every five women had her uterus surgically removed for no clear reason. This was particularly seen among the younger women—the rate of needless hysterectomies was 38% in women younger than 40 compared with 8% in women older than 50.

Why would a woman have a hysterectomy for seemingly no medically valid reason? The

Testosterone Cream for Women

Does testosterone cream make sex more pleasurable for women?

Testosterone is known as the "male" hormone—but women's bodies produce some, too. A testosterone deficiency in women may lead to lack of interest in sex. Prescription testosterone cream, which is compounded by a pharmacist and applied to the clitoris in small amounts (0.05 mg to 1 mg) daily, can help improve sensation, desire and arousal. It also increases the size of the clitoris (which may be diminished in postmenopausal women), making it more accessible. The treatment may take a month or more to work.

Barbara Bartlik, MD, a sex therapist in private practice and assistant professor, Weill Cornell Medical College, New York City.

researchers only went by what they could find in the patients' medical records and did not interview any of the patients or their physicians. Their educated guess is that many of the younger women were having hysterectomies to correct abnormal bleeding caused by ovulatory dysfunction. But ovulatory dysfunction is usually a hormonal problem and should be first treated with hormones or other medicines—not a scalpel—according to the American Congress of Obstetricians and Gynecologists. So if young women really are getting hysterectomies to solve bleeding problems, many of the doctors recommending and performing the procedures may be out of line. (But another study will need to be done to investigate if this is really so.)

KNOW YOUR OPTIONS

Before agreeing to a hysterectomy, make sure it is the best and most appropriate treatment for what ails you. Make sure that the doctor fully explains your diagnosis, how the problem can be treated, and the risks and benefits of each and every treatment option. Then, with your doctor, make a list of options to try in order of preference so if the most preferred doesn't work, another option or two can be tried before resorting to a hysterectomy.

Pesticides, Plastics and Chemicals Tied to Earlier Menopause in Women

Amber Cooper, MD, assistant professor of obstetrics and gynecology at Washington University School of Medicine in St. Louis.

Spyros Mezitis, MD, endocrinologist, Lenox Hill Hospital, New York City.

Jill Rabin, MD, co-chief, division of ambulatory care, Women's Health Programs-PCAP Services, North Shore-LIJ Health System, New Hyde Park, New York.

Washington University School of Medicine in St. Louis, news release.

Extensive exposure to common chemicals appears to be linked to an earlier start of menopause, a recent study suggests.

Researchers found that menopause typically begins two to four years earlier in women whose bodies have high levels of certain chemicals found in household items, personal care products, plastics and the environment, compared with women with lower levels of the chemicals.

The investigators identified 15 chemicals—nine (now banned) PCBs, three pesticides, two forms of plastics chemicals called phthalates, and the toxin furan—that were significantly associated with an earlier start of menopause and that may have harmful effects on ovarian function.

"Earlier menopause can alter the quality of a woman's life and has profound implications for fertility, health and our society," senior study author Amber Cooper, MD, an assistant professor of obstetrics and gynecology at Washington University School of Medicine in St. Louis, said in a university news release.

"Understanding how the environment affects health is complex," she added. "This study doesn't prove causation, but the associations raise a red flag and support the need for future research."

STUDY DETAILS

In the study, Dr. Cooper's team analyzed blood and urine samples from more than 1,400 menopausal women, averaging 61 years of age, to determine their exposure to 111 mostly man-made chemicals.

According to the U.S. Environmental Protection Agency, PCBs (polychlorinated biphenyls) have been banned in the US since 1979, but can be found in items made before that time. Furans are by-products of industrial combustion, and phthalates are found in plastics, many household items, drugs and personal care products such as lotions, perfumes, makeup, nail polish, liquid soap and hair spray.

Dr. Cooper said the study's findings could have implications for women's health.

"Chemicals linked to earlier menopause may lead to an early decline in ovarian function, and our results suggest we as a society should be concerned," she said.

Along with reducing fertility, a decline in ovarian function can lead to earlier development of heart disease, osteoporosis and other health problems, the researchers said. Prior research has also linked the chemicals with some cancers, early puberty and metabolic syndrome. Metabolic syndrome refers to a group of health conditions occurring together that increase the risk of heart disease, stroke and diabetes.

"Many of these chemical exposures are beyond our control because they are in the soil, water and air," Dr. Cooper said. "But we can educate ourselves about our day-to-day chemical exposures and become more aware of the plastics and other household products we use."

For example, she suggested that people microwave food in glass or paper containers instead of in plastic, and learn more about the ingredients in their cosmetics, personal-care products and food packaging.

Even though many of the chemicals identified in the study are banned in the U.S. because of health risks, they are still produced in other countries and are common in the environment, Dr. Cooper added.

EXPERT COMMENT

Two other experts say the findings reinforce what endocrinologists had long suspected.

"This important study strengthens the thinking that endocrine-disrupting chemicals affect ovarian function," said Spyros Mezitis, MD, an endocrinologist at Lenox Hill Hospital in New York City.

"Prior research has shown an association with metabolic defects and this research becomes an issue to discuss with patients requesting fertility treatment," he said.

Jill Rabin, MD, is co-chief of the division of ambulatory care in Women's Health Programs at North Shore-LIJ Health System in New Hyde Park, New York. She called the study "important," because "earlier menopause can impact on a woman's quality of life (hot flashes, mood and memory changes) and quantity of life (osteoporosis, fractures, heart disease)."

Both experts called for further research to clarify just how and how much exposure to the chemicals listed in the study might impact people's health.

The study was published online in the journal *PLoS One*.

info The U.S. Office on Women's Health has more about menopause at *http://womenshealth.gov/menopause/*.

Nerve Block Injection Helps Reduce Hot Flashes

David R. Walega, MD, associate professor of anesthesiology, Feinberg School of Medicine of Northwestern University, Chicago. His study was published in *Menopause*.

It's like an inner inferno suddenly erupts, leaving you drenched in sweat and red in the face from heat and embarrassment. No wonder women who suffer from menopausal hot flashes—and that includes about 80% of us at some point in our lives—are desperate for relief. The treatment options leave a lot to be desired, however. Hormone therapy helps but has been linked to increased risk for breast cancer and heart disease...oral medications that reduce hot flashes (*gabapentin, clonidine*) can have intolerable side effects...and botanical therapies such as black cohosh and phytoestrogens haven't proved to be very effective.

A real breakthrough: A treatment usually used to control nerve pain or heavy sweating helps reduce hot flashes, too—and the effects of a single treatment last for six months or more, according to a recent study.

A SINGLE SHOT DOES THE TRICK

To understand the study, you need a little physiology lesson. The stellate ganglion is a collection of nerves located in front of the vertebrae at the base of the neck, connecting to the arms and face. These nerves are part of the sympathetic nervous system that activates our fight-or-flight response when we're stressed, so they're not involved with sensation or movement. When a tiny amount of local anesthetic is injected into this bundle of nerves, a procedure called a stellate ganglion block, it temporarily inactivates the nerves. Doctors typically administer the injection to relieve nerve pain in the head, neck, chest or arm…ease angina…or help control very excessive sweating in those same areas.

Some earlier studies suggested that stellate ganglion blocks also reduced vasomotor symptoms (hot flashes, night sweats) in women—so researchers put it to the gold-standard test by doing a randomized, placebo-controlled study. Participants included 40 women who experienced an average of 10 hot flashes daily, with most hot flashes rating as moderate to very severe. (*Side note:* A severe hot flash lasts up to 20 minutes, feels like a "raging furnace" and is accompanied by weakness, headache, extreme perspiration, anxiety and/or panic attacks. A very severe hot flash is a "boiling eruption" that lasts up to 45 minutes and is characterized by rolling perspiration, heart irregularities, dizziness, nausea, cramps and difficulty breathing!)

Early Menopause Can Hurt Your Brain

Menopause at age 40 or younger may hurt your brain. Premature menopause increased the risk for poor verbal memory by 56% and poor visual memory by 39%.

Likely link: Estrogen levels, which affect brain function, decline at menopause. Low-dose hormone therapy may benefit women undergoing premature menopause. Talk to your doctor about the pros and cons.

Joanne Ryan, PhD, a postdoctoral research fellow in neuropsychiatry at Inserm U1061, Montpellier, France, and leader of a study of 4,868 women, published in *BJOG: An International Journal of Obstetrics & Gynaecology.*

Study procedure: Half of the women were randomly assigned to receive the actual stellate ganglion injection. The other half got a placebo. All study participants kept diaries to record the frequency and severity of their hot flashes, starting two weeks before the procedure and continuing for six months after. In addition to this subjective measure, the researchers also arranged for an objective measure of vasomotor symptoms—at the start of the study and again three months later, each participant wore a skin conductance monitor for 24 hours to measure how much she perspired.

Here are the results, based on…

The objective skin tests: Compared to the start of the study, vasomotor symptoms at three months after the procedure were reduced by 21% in the block group…but were not reduced at all in the sham group.

The women's subjective diaries: For the first three months after the procedure, the women's self-reported symptoms were reduced by about the same amount in both groups—despite the fact that the skin tests showed actual reductions only in the block group—suggesting that a strong placebo effect was at work in the sham group. However, that placebo effect seemed to wear off over time. Compared with the start of the study, the frequency of self-reported moderate-to-very-severe hot flashes occurring in the four to six months after the procedure fell by 52% in the block group but by only 4% in the sham group…while the intensity fell by 38% in the block group but only 8% in the sham group.

How does the procedure work? That's not fully understood, but it could be that the block induces changes in blood flow to regions of the brain that regulate body temperature…and/or that it modulates norepinephrine or nerve growth factor, neurotransmitters that seem to change before and during a hot flash.

If you are interested in trying this treatment: Ask your doctor to refer you to an anesthesiologist who is experienced at doing stellate ganglion blocks. You certainly don't want just anybody injecting your neck, given the many critical nerves and blood vessels there—possible risks include seizure, collapsed lung, nerve damage and temporary numbness or weakness from the neck down. However, injuries are very rare when the procedure is done by a well-qualified practitioner. In this study, the only side effects of the treatment were temporary ones that lasted just a few hours—drooping eyelids, eye redness, warmth in the face, hoarseness—which are normal and expected with a stellate ganglion block.

Neroli Oil Soothes Menopausal Symptoms

Study titled "Effects of Inhalation of Essential Oil of Citrus aurantium L. var. amara on Menopausal Symptoms, Stress, and Estrogen in Postmenopausal Women: A Randomized Controlled Trail," published in *Evidence-Based Complementary and Alternative Medicine*.

A re menopausal symptoms—the hot flashes, night sweats, insomnia and moodiness among all else—cramping your style…stressing your relationships…in short, ruining your life? Sure, hormone replacement therapy (HRT) is an option, but maybe its risks, such as blood clots, gallstones, breast cancer and stroke, have nixed that idea for you.

There's another great way that's helping women wind down and recharge. No, it's not another supplement, mind trick or exercise routine. It's aromatherapy using a lusciously exotic scent—neroli oil.

SNIFF TEST

Neroli oil is extracted from the blossoms of the bitter orange tree and is rich in limonene, a compound that has antianxiety and muscle-relaxing effects. Neroli oil vapor, when inhaled, is known to relieve anxiety, stress and depression, reduce high blood pressure and stimulate an underactive libido. Because symptoms such as mood swings and underactive libido are so common in menopause, a group of Korean researchers decided to scientifically test whether neroli oil had an effect on those and other menopausal symptoms.

Here's what they did. The team recruited 63 healthy menopausal women and divided them into three groups. One group received several vials of a 0.1% concentration of neroli essential oil in scentless sweet almond oil…the other, a 0.5% concentration (in scentless sweet almond oil)…and the third group received plain scentless sweet almond oil (a placebo). The women sat in a comfortable position every morning and evening for five days and inhaled the oil vapor for five minutes at each sitting.

Before and after the five-day treatment period, each woman was given special questionnaires that rated and scored their quality of life and levels of stress and sexual desire. Blood pressure and pulse were also checked, and blood tests were done to measure cortisol (a stress hormone) and estrogen levels.

The results: Compared with the placebo group, women inhaling neroli felt better and had fewer hot flashes. After the five days of daily aromatherapy, their quality-of-life scores improved by an average of 28% in the women smelling 0.1% neroli oil and 20% in the women smelling 0.5% neroli oil compared with an average 7% improvement in women smelling the placebo oil.

Sexual desire also got a lift in the women who inhaled neroli oil, most especially if they were inhaling the 0.5% concentration. It improved by an average 113% in women using the higher concentration and 27% in women using the 0.1% concentration. Meanwhile, sexual desire took a 50% dive in women using the placebo oil.

HOW TO BENEFIT FROM NEROLI OIL

Some pure essential oils, such as clove and cinnamon, come with strong precautions because they can irritate the skin or lungs. Neroli oil is much milder. Still, no undiluted essential oil should be daubed on the skin straight out of the bottle—remember, this is concentrated stuff. A few drops should be placed in a scentless "carrier oil," such as sweet almond oil or jojoba oil.

To approximate your own 0.5% concentration of neroli oil, the ratio should be four drops of the essential oil per ounce of carrier oil. (A good aromatherapy oil will come with its own dropper.)

Don't want to fuss with mixing essential oils and carriers? Another simple way to enjoy aromatherapy is to place up to five drops of an essential oil in a pot of hot water and, keeping a safe distance of about a foot away, breathe the steam. Or consider purchasing an aromatherapy diffuser and vaporizer. They come in different styles and have different user directions that come with the packaging. These gadgets either warm an essential oil or mix it with steam to create a scented vapor. They cost anywhere from a few bucks to about $60 and can be easily found in department stores or online through *Amazon.com* and other sellers.

No side effects were seen in the study, so why not take a few minutes a day to stop and smell the neroli to manage The Change?

Severe Hot Flashes During Menopause May Raise Hip Fracture Risk Later

The Endocrine Society, news release.

A recent study suggests a possible link between certain menopause symptoms—moderate to severe hot flashes and night sweats—and higher rates of hip fractures and weaker bones.

Hot flashes are common during menopause, affecting about 60% of women. The hormonal changes during menopause also affect women after menopause, since they then face a higher risk of weakened bones and osteoporosis.

"Our findings suggest women who exhibit moderate or severe menopausal symptoms are more likely to have issues with bone health than their peers," study coauthor Carolyn Crandall, MD, of the David Geffen School of Medicine at the University of California, Los Angeles, said in a news release from the Endocrine Society. "This is the first large cohort study to examine the relationship between menopausal symptoms and bone health in menopausal women."

While the researchers found an association between some menopause symptoms and bone health, they did not prove that hot flashes and night sweats cause hip fractures. Yet, it's common knowledge that menopausal symptoms are caused by changing estrogen levels, and estrogen levels also affect bone density.

Is It Ever Too Late for Estrogen?

It is generally considered safest to begin estrogen therapy within 10 years after menopause, but this is not a rigid rule.

Some women may decide more than 10 years after menopause that they would like to begin estrogen (to curb hot flashes or night sweats, for example), and this calls for personalized decision-making that weighs the benefits versus the risks for the individual patient. Estrogen has been found to raise risk for blood clots, stroke and breast cancer (especially when taken with progestin). Some women who are not candidates for the pill form of estrogen may still be able to take a low-dose skin patch, gel or spray.

JoAnn E. Manson, MD, DrPH, professor of medicine and women's health, Harvard Medical School, Boston.

STUDY DETAILS

The study analyzed the medical records of more than 23,000 US women aged 50 to 79 who were tracked for eight years, on average.

Compared with women with no menopausal symptoms, those with moderate or severe hot flashes were more likely to fracture a hip. Those with moderate to severe menopausal symptoms also had weaker bones in the neck and spine, as revealed by bone density tests.

"More research is needed to illuminate the connection between bone health and menopausal symptoms such as hot flashes," Dr. Crandall said. "Improved understanding would help clinicians advise women on how to better prevent osteoporosis and other bone conditions. Women who have hot flashes and want to protect their bones may benefit from healthy lifestyle habits such as avoiding smoking and excessive alcohol consumption, exercising and getting sufficient calcium and vitamin D."

The study was published in the *Journal of Clinical Endocrinology & Metabolism*.

info For more about menopause, try the U.S. National Institute on Aging at *http://www.nia.nih.gov/health/publication/menopause*.

The Missing Link in Lupus Care

Donald E. Thomas, Jr., MD, an assistant professor of medicine at the Uniformed Services University of the Health Sciences and an instructor of rheumatology at Walter Reed National Military Medical Center, both in Bethesda, Maryland.

Lupus is a stubborn disease that most doctors treat with a variety of medications. If you're lucky, the disease can be controlled with only an antimalarial drug. Other people with lupus need a "cocktail" of powerful medications.

What most people don't realize: To control lupus, medication isn't enough. Everyone with this disease needs to also manage the triggers that cause flare-ups and can lead to life-threatening complications. Avoiding triggers may allow lupus patients to take smaller doses of stronger immunosuppressant drugs (or even eliminate the need for them) and decrease the frequency and severity of lupus flares.

WHAT IS LUPUS?

About one and a half million Americans—mostly women—are affected with the auto-immune disease known as lupus. With this condition, the body produces antibodies, for unknown reasons, that attack the joints, skin, lungs, kidneys and/or other parts of the body.

About half of lupus patients have a mild form that affects only the joints and the skin. Others have a high risk for organ damage. Systemic lupus erythematosus (SLE), the most serious form of the disease, can affect virtually every part of the body, including not only the skin and kidneys but also the heart, brain and blood vessels.

The signs of SLE differ from patient to patient. One person might have a skin rash but no joint pain.

Someone else might have fatigue and pain but no rash. Others show early signs of heart or kidney disease. This variability makes SLE difficult to recognize—and to treat.

THE DANGER OF UV LIGHT

Even though most people with lupus do take the medication that's prescribed for the disease,

Don't Sweat Flashes

Hot flashes? Don't sweat it. That's the conclusion of research involving about 200 menopausal women.

Study details: Women who have the highest levels of "self-compassion"—that is, the ability to go easy on one's self in difficult or embarrassing situations—find hot flashes and night sweats to be less disruptive than do women who are self-critical.

If you suffer from hot flashes: Try gently telling yourself that this will pass, or make a physical gesture such as placing your hand over your heart.

Lydia Brown, MA, doctoral researcher, The University of Melbourne, Australia.

they could benefit even more by carefully managing one of the most powerful lupus triggers—ultraviolet (UV) light.

Exposure to UV radiation—both from sunlight and indoor lighting—hurts everyone with SLE. UV light causes chemical changes in skin cells that trigger an increase in immune activity and inflammation. In about 30% of lupus patients, UV exposure causes a red rash on exposed skin (photosensitive rash). A so-called "butterfly" rash (covering the bridge of the nose and cheeks) also commonly occurs during or after sun exposure. Those who don't get a rash may still experience some organ damage.

Even brief exposures to UV light can be dangerous. For example, with the help of her doctor, a woman who continued having symptoms even though she always applied sunscreen before going outdoors discovered that her symptoms were triggered by the light from a photocopy machine.

Best UV protection measures...

•**Apply sunscreen lotion all day, every day.** Use a water-resistant product with an SPF of 30 or higher—and make sure that it blocks both UVA and UVB radiation. Apply it every few hours.

Good products: Anthelios SX by La Roche-Posay and sunscreen brands that contain Helioplex.

Also helpful: Use Rit Sun Guard laundry treatment for your outer garments. It adds an invisible coating to clothing that blocks more than 96% of the sun's harmful rays. The treatment lasts for up to 20 washings.

•**Use sunscreen even when you're indoors or driving.** The sunlight that comes through windows can trigger symptoms. Driving with the car windows up decreases UV penetration in the car.

•**Change the lightbulbs.** Indoor lighting also emits UV radiation. Halogen lights emit the most UV light, followed by fluorescent, including both tubes and bulbs.

Best choice: UV-free LED lights, widely available at hardware stores and online.

•**Don't use the UV drying units after manicures or pedicures.** Let the nail polish dry on its own. Or use a dryer that contains a fan but no light.

WHAT ALSO HELPS

Avoiding ultraviolet (UV) light isn't the only self-care step to follow if you have systemic lupus erythematosus (SLE). *Three other important recommendations...*

•**Boost your vitamin D.** Most people with SLE don't produce enough of this important nutrient, in part because they avoid the sun. (Vitamin D is produced in the skin following sun exposure.) The optimal blood level for a person with lupus is around 40 ng/mL. If you've been diagnosed with SLE, your doctor probably orders blood tests four times a year. Be sure that he/she checks your vitamin D level each time, then prescribes an appropriate dose of vitamin D supplement, as needed.

•**Get more omega-3s.** Everyone with SLE should eat fish and other foods high in omega-3 fatty acids, such as flaxseed and walnuts. These healthful fats are thought to ease excessive immune activity and reduce inflammation in the body.

Also: Studies suggest that food sources of omega-3s are more effective than supplements for this disease. If you're not a fish lover, you can get more omega-3s by drinking protein shakes spiked with ground walnuts and flaxseed. One tablespoon daily of olive oil also has been found to have anti-inflammatory properties.

•**Ask about DHEA.** The naturally occurring hormone dehydroepiandrosterone (DHEA) is converted in the body into testosterone and estrogen. Many patients with SLE have levels that are lower than normal. Some patients who take DHEA may be able to reduce their doses of steroid medications—and thus reduce side effects, such as weight gain, diabetes, brittle bones, glaucoma and cataracts.

Important: Take DHEA only under a doctor's supervision, since it can raise risk for certain cancers in some people. Over-the-counter products can contain much lower amounts of the active ingredient than what's listed on the label. Ask your doctor to write a prescription, and get it filled at a compounding pharmacy.

Should You Say Good-Bye to Pelvic Exams?

Mario M. Leitao, Jr., MD, gynecologic oncologist and co-director of Robotic Surgery, and Oliver Zivanovic, MD, PhD, gynecologic oncology surgeon and director of Innovative Surgical Technology, Gynecology Service, department of surgery, both at Memorial Sloan Kettering Cancer Center, New York City.

Ladies, in case you haven't heard, you don't have to endure annual pelvic exams anymore. No more poking and prodding with your feet up in stirrups every year. You heard me right! If you're healthy and not pregnant, the American College of Physicians says that annual gynecologic pelvic exams—no matter what your age—don't really do much healthwise and are not needed. In fact, the College says that the harms, including fear, anxiety, embarrassment, pain and discomfort, outweigh the potential benefits.

That's great, but not all doctors agree with this. And, frankly, you should wonder, too. At best, as with proposed changes about mammography screening, it puts the responsibility for well-being back into the hands of women. That's empowering. But to really make the right decision, a woman needs to be well-informed.

Here's what you need to know to make the best decision about when or whether you should get a pelvic exam...

THE CASE AGAINST THE EXAMS

Whether women need annual pelvic exams has been under hot debate since the American College of Physicians said *No, they don't* in its recently updated guidelines. Two gynecologic oncologists—both from the Memorial Sloan Kettering Cancer Center in New York City—although colleagues, have two very different opinions on the matter. Who's right? Hearing both sides may help you come to the right decision for you.

Pelvic exams, in theory, are done to check for skin growths or rashes or signs of infection, inflammation, tumor growth or other abnormalities of the pubic area, vagina, cervix, uterus and ovaries. "But it's all basically done for the sake of tradition. The value of the examination is not based on published scientific evidence," said Mario M. Leitao, Jr., MD, codirector of robotic surgery in the department of gynecology at Sloan Kettering.

Dr. Leitao went on to say that "even in women who are in their 60s and 70s, there's still no advantage to these exams if they have no medical problems." Instead, Dr. Leitao recommends that women follow guidelines recommended by the American Cancer Society and other medical societies dedicated to cancer prevention and detection.

The American College of Physicians guidelines say that instead of a full pelvic exam, women age 21 to 30 should just have a Pap smear to assess gynecologic cancer risk every three years and women age 30 to 65 should either have a Pap smear every three years or a Pap smear plus a test for human papillomavirus (HPV) every five years. (HPV is a very common sexually transmitted virus that causes genital warts and, if left unchecked, can cause cervical cancer.) Women older than 65 no longer need to have Pap smears or HPV tests if they've had a clean bill of health throughout their lives. Otherwise, they should continue to get Pap smears every three years until they're into their 80s.

IN FAVOR OF PELVIC EXAMS

Now, how about the other side of this? Although Oliver Zivanovic, MD, PhD, director of innovative surgical technology in the department of gynecology at Sloan Kettering, agrees with Dr. Leitao about Pap smear screening and HPV testing, he disagrees with him about the American College of Physicians guidelines about annual pelvic exams. "Pelvic exams are very important to helping doctors detect abnormalities. They provide findings that can save a woman's life."

Yet another professional association—The American College of Obstetricians and Gynecologists (ACOG)—also supports regular pelvic exams. Its position is that the traditional pelvic exam described above should be done every year even for healthy women. Besides picking up on possible diseases and other medical problems, the time spent with the doctor during the exam builds a doctor-patient relationship, according to ACOG.

Dr. Leitao agrees that this is a good point, but says an annual gynecologic exam is mainly of value for the woman who uses a gynecologist as a primary care physician because it presents an opportunity for her to discuss medical issues with a professional and make sure she is getting regular health care.

He also points out that pelvic exams aren't free, despite the fact that most insurance plans include them at no out-of-pocket expense to the patient. "These unnecessary exams are costing us billions of dollars a year," said Dr. Leitao (about $2.6 billion annually, according to the American College of Physicians). "They are financial burdens for women without insurance. For those with insurance or who are on Medicare or Medicaid, the costs put a burden on the health-care system, which impacts the overall cost of health care and impacts the economy." But, in Dr. Zivanovic's view, pelvic exams are an inexpensive way to keep women—as individuals—safe. "A hundred dollars or so a year per woman is worth it to save a human life," he said. Additionally, he believes that a woman should begin annual pelvic exams when she becomes sexually active even if she is younger than 21.

WHERE EXPERTS AGREE

Besides keeping up with cervical cancer screening, Drs. Leitao and Zivanovic, of course, agree that when gynecologic symptoms, such as an unusual discharge, rash or skin growth, appear, a woman should get to her OB/GYN right away. Above all, they agree that the decision to stop or continue annual pelvic exams should not be one-sided but a shared decision between a woman and her doctor after fully discussing her specific medical history and all of the pros and cons of the issue.

Bone Drugs May Protect Against Endometrial Cancer

Sharon Hensley Alford, PhD, department of public health sciences, Henry Ford Health System, Detroit. *Cancer*, news release

Bisphosphonates, which are drugs that treat bone loss, may lower the risk of endometrial cancer, recent research suggests.

The study found that women taking the drugs had about half the risk of endometrial cancer compared with women who don't take the drugs. Endometrial cancer—one of the most common types of cancer in women—affects the lining of the uterus.

Bisphosphonates include medications such as Actonel, Boniva and Fosamax.

STUDY DETAILS

In the study of nearly 30,000 women, researchers examined the medical records of women who took bisphosphonates that contain nitrogen, which have been shown to have the strongest anti-cancer effects. When assessing risk, they accounted for factors such as age, race and smoking status.

The study was published in the journal *Cancer*.

IMPLICATIONS

"Other studies have shown that bisphosphonates may reduce the risk of certain cancers, but we are the first to show that the risk for endometrial cancer may also be reduced," said Sharon

Best Treatment for Varicose Veins

Foam injections and laser therapy are popular alternatives to surgery for treating varicose veins, a common condition in which veins in the legs weaken, swell and become twisted.

Recent finding: In a study of nearly 800 patients, all three procedures were found to be effective and safe, but laser therapy had the highest success rate and fewest complications.

Julie Brittenden, MD, professor of vascular surgery, University of Aberdeen, UK.

Hensley Alford, PhD, a public health researcher from the Henry Ford Health System in Detroit.

"This study suggests that women who need bone-strengthening medications and who have increased risk for endometrial cancer may want to choose the nitrogen form of bisphosphonates because this form may reduce the risk of endometrial cancer," she said.

The study only found a connection between the bone-preserving medications and reduced risk of endometrial cancer. It did not prove cause-and-effect.

info For more about endometrial cancer, visit the American Cancer Society at *www.cancer.org* and search "endometrial cancer."

Drug-Free Bone Builders

Ray Hinish, PharmD, CN, a certified nutritionist and author of *The Osteoporosis Diet: The Natural Approach to Osteoporosis Treatment*. He is owner of The Expert Nutrition Center, Owings Mills, Maryland. *ExpertNutrition.com*

Bone is constantly breaking down and rebuilding, a process called remodeling. If you have osteoporosis or osteopenia (an earlier stage of bone thinning), the rate of breakdown exceeds that of reconstruction.

Result: Porous bones that are brittle and prone to fractures.

A broken bone means pain, tests, repeated doctor visits and maybe even surgery—and that could be just the beginning.

About half of women with osteoporosis (and one in eight men) eventually will have a bone fracture, and many will have more than one.

DRUGS ARE NOT THE SOLUTION

The main class of drugs for treating osteoporosis, the bisphosphonates, have been linked to rare but serious side effects, including severe bone, muscle and joint pain and possibly an increased risk for esophageal cancer (due to inflammation of the esophagus). Other rare side effects include atypical femoral fracture, in which the thighbone cracks, and osteonecrosis of the jaw, in which a section of the jawbone dies and deteriorates.

The risks might be justified if the drugs worked—but often they don't. One study published in *The Journal of the American Medical Association* found that 99.8% of patients who took *alendronate* (Fosamax) did not suffer a subsequent fracture. That sounds impressive, but it turns out that people in the study who took placebos had nearly the same result.

It's estimated that 81 women would have to take alendronate to prevent just one fracture. Put another way, 80 out of 81 patients who take the drug won't benefit at all. *Here are effective, safer treatments…*

CALCIUM-PLUS

Everyone knows that calcium is important for strong bones. But calcium alone isn't enough. Bones are made up of a variety of minerals. You need all of them to increase—or just maintain—bone strength. *Examples…*

•**Magnesium.** Up to 80% of Americans don't get enough magnesium. There is some evidence that people who are low in magnesium are more likely to develop osteoporosis.

My advice: Eat magnesium-rich foods, including dark leafy greens, nuts, fish and whole grains. Because most people don't get enough magnesium from food, I also recommend a daily supplement that contains 500 milligrams (mg).

•**Phosphorus.** It's the second-most-abundant mineral in the body after calcium, and 80% to 90% is found in the bones and teeth.

My advice: Eat phosphorus-rich foods, which include meats, fish, nuts, beans and dairy. Aim for 700 mg of phosphorous a day.

Examples: Salmon (three ounces) has 315 mg…beef (three ounces), 243 mg…yogurt (one cup), 386 mg.

•**Calcium.** You can't have strong bones without calcium—but despite what you've heard, you do not have to consume dairy to get sufficient calcium. Leafy green vegetables—such as kale, spinach and collard greens—are rich in calcium. A four-ounce serving of steamed collard greens or kale has about the same amount of calcium as one cup of milk.

My advice: Since many people don't get enough calcium from their diets, a supplement is helpful. Take 600 mg to 800 mg daily. I recommend any calcium supplement other than calcium carbonate, which is poorly absorbed. Combined with the calcium that you get from foods, it will get you into the recommended daily range of 1,200 mg to 1,500 mg.

Some studies have shown a link between calcium supplements and heart attacks, but a recent study by researchers at Brigham and Women's Hospital found no correlation between calcium supplementation and coronary artery disease, and previous research failed to show a link

Cervical Cancer Is More Common Than Previously Reported

Earlier estimates included women who had had hysterectomies. When they were excluded from the statistics, the actual rate of cervical cancer rose to 18.6 cases per 100,000 women. The US Preventive Services Task Force recommends that women ages 21 to 65 have a Pap smear every three years…and women ages 30 to 65 be tested for HPV every five years.

Anne F. Rositch, PhD, MSPH, is assistant professor in the department of epidemiology and public health at University of Maryland School of Medicine, Baltimore.

when calcium was taken with other supplements such as vitamin D and magnesium.

VITAMIN D

Vitamin D increases the body's ability to absorb calcium from foods and supplements. It also appears to inhibit both the production and activity of osteoclasts, cells that break down bone.

One study found that people who took a daily vitamin-D supplement had a 23% decrease in nonvertebral fractures and a 26% decrease in hip fractures.

Vitamin D is called the "sunshine vitamin" because it is produced in the skin when you're exposed to sun. But most people don't get enough sun to produce adequate amounts.

My advice: Take 2,000 international units (IU) to 4,000 IU of vitamin D daily. And take it with meals for up to 50% better absorption. I recommend the natural D-3 form. It raises blood levels 1.7 times more than the synthetic D-2 form.

LEAFY GREENS

Leafy greens are not only high in calcium, they are rich in vitamin K. Vitamin K works with vitamin D to increase the activity of bone-building osteoblasts.

The Harvard Nurses' Health Study found that women who ate a daily serving of leafy green vegetables, such as spinach, dark green lettuce or kale, were 50% less likely to suffer a fracture than those who had only one serving a week.

My advice: Eat a salad every day. Make side dishes that include spinach, kale or beet greens. Other green vegetables, such as broccoli, cabbage, asparagus and Brussels sprouts, also are high in vitamin K.

ONE PART PROTEIN TO FOUR PARTS VEGETABLES

This ratio seems to be ideal for bone health. You need protein to decrease calcium loss from the body and to increase levels of bone growth factors. But too much protein (particularly from animal sources) increases acidity, which depletes bone minerals.

It's a delicate balancing act. The Framingham Osteoporosis Study found that people who ate the least protein were more likely to have a

Good News for Women

A urine test appears to be nearly as effective as the conventional—and uncomfortable—cervical smear for detecting human papillomavirus (HPV). Testing is critical because HPV is the leading cause of cervical cancer.

TheBMJ.com

bone fracture than those who ate the most. But a Harvard study found that people who ate the most protein (from animal sources) had a higher risk for forearm fractures. (Those who got their protein from soy or other nonmeat sources didn't have the same risk.)

My advice: For every serving of a meat-based protein, consume three to four servings of vegetables to alkalinize your body. An alkaline (low-acid) environment helps prevent bone loss.

EXERCISE WITH WEIGHTS

You need to stress the bones to promote new growth. Lifting weights is the best way to do this, particularly when it's combined with aerobic workouts. A University of Washington study found that women who did both during a 50-to-60-minute session, three times a week, gained 5.2% in spinal mineral density in just nine months.

Don't make it easy. If you can lift a weight more than 10 times, you're not stressing the bones enough. Pick a weight that you can lift only between six and 10 times. You want the last few lifts to be a struggle. When that gets too easy, move up to a heavier weight.

Walking is another good way to build bone. One study found that people who were sedentary lost an average of 7% of bone mass in the spine, while those in a walking program gained 0.5%.

My advice: Wear a weighted vest when you walk. You can build more bone by adding to your body weight. You can buy weighted vests at sporting-goods stores and discount stores such as Target and Walmart. Most are adjustable—you can start with five pounds and work your way up to about 10% of your body weight.

Protect Your Bones from Osteoporosis with Resveratrol

Marie Juul Ornstrup, MD, PhD candidate, department of endocrinology and metabolism, Aarhus University Hospital, Aarhus, Denmark. Her study was published in *Journal of Clinical Endocrinology and Metabolism*.

Strong bones and teeth are not just kid stuff—we especially need ways to promote them as we age because age-related bone loss is no joke. Forget the mere scraped knee if you slip and fall—one false step could mean a broken hip. But a popular supplement, often taken for cardiovascular vigor, can help build strong bones in adults, possibly protecting against osteoporosis.

The supplement is resveratrol, an antioxidant and anti-inflammatory compound famously found in red wine, red grape juice, grapes (it's in the skins) and cacao, peanuts and blueberries.

Because resveratrol has such strong anti-inflammatory properties, Danish researchers reasoned that it might help put the brakes on the inflammation that causes bone weakening. They decided to investigate this in people who have metabolic syndrome, a combination of high blood pressure, high cholesterol and high blood sugar, because their condition puts them at risk for bone weakening. But you don't have to have metabolic syndrome to suffer from systemic inflammation and bone loss...so, anyone who wants to maintain strong bones, pay attention.

The researchers recruited 66 middle-aged men with metabolic syndrome but not osteoporosis and started tracking the effect of resveratrol on bone-forming enzymes and bone density in the men's lower spines. They did this by dividing the participants into three groups. One group received 1,000 milligrams (mg) per day of a natural formulation of resveratrol called transresveratrol (as a 500-mg pill taken twice a day), another group received 150 mg (as a 75-mg pill taken twice a day), and the third group received placebo pills.

The results: It didn't take long for the resveratrol to make its mark. After only four months, the men who took the higher daily dosage of resveratrol had a 16% increase in a bone-forming enzyme called bone alkaline phosphatase, commonly found in children who are going through growth spurts. They also had 3% more bone density than they had at the start of the study. Meanwhile no changes were seen in the placebo group, and minimal changes were seen in the low-dose resveratrol group.

Does this mean that resveratrol can be a natural substitute for osteoporosis drugs, such as Forteo and Fosamax? Probably not—studies show that these drugs have a stronger effect on bone mass than the 3% improvement seen in this study of resveratrol. But who knows? Additional studies of the supplement that look at the impact of different doses over longer time periods may provide more promising information about resveratrol and bone health. In the meantime, resveratrol supplementation might be a smart way to support your body's bone-building potential to protect against bone loss.

GET IT RIGHT

If you are interested in taking a resveratrol supplement, check labels to make sure you are purchasing transresveratrol, since, a synthetic formulation of resveratrol may not deliver the same health benefit as transresveratrol.

Is a Full Bladder Interrupting Your Sleep? You're Not Alone

Amy Hsu, MD, fellow, division of geriatrics, San Francisco VA Medical Center.

Mary Townsend, ScD, associate epidemiologist, Brigham and Women's Hospital, Boston.

Obstetrics & Gynecology

Many women have to get up more than once a night because of a full bladder, a recent study finds.

Researchers found that of over 2,000 women aged 40 and up, one-third said they routinely got up at least twice a night to use the bathroom. Doctors refer to that as nocturia, and it can be a sign that you're drinking too much tea or coffee at night—or a signal of a serious health condition.

"Traditionally, nocturia has been considered a part of other urinary tract disorders," said lead researcher Amy Hsu, MD, a fellow at the San Francisco VA Medical Center.

But in this study, 40% of the women with nocturia reported no other urinary tract symptoms, such as daytime overactive bladder or urine leakage.

That suggests nocturia often cannot be attributed to those conditions, according to Dr. Hsu, who reported the findings in the January 2015 issue of *Obstetrics & Gynecology*.

Mary Townsend, ScD, a researcher at Brigham and Women's Hospital in Boston, said nocturia is increasingly being recognized as a condition unto itself.

"And this study supports that view," said Dr. Townsend, who was not involved in the research.

Dr. Hsu's team found that, not surprisingly, nocturia was more common among relatively older women. For every five-year increase in age, a woman's risk rose by 21%. Nocturia was also more common among women who'd had a hysterectomy, hot flashes or had used vaginal estrogen to treat menopause symptoms.

Bladder problems are common after hysterectomy, and other studies have found a link to nocturia. As for hot flashes, they are notorious for keeping women up at night—which could

Better Fitness Formula for Older Women

The formula 220 minus your age has long been used to set a maximum heart rate. However, this formula was mainly tested on men.

Now: A recent study reveals that while everyone's peak heart rate declines with age, the decline is more gradual in women. If you are a woman over age 70, talk to your doctor about considering a slightly higher target (about five additional beats per minute) to assess your heart health during stress testing and to help set your maximum heart rate for workouts. For men, the current formula still works well. During workouts, your target heart rate is usually 60% to 80% of your maximum heart rate.

Thomas Allison, PhD, MPH, associate professor of medicine, Mayo Clinic, Rochester, Minnesota.

be one reason for the connection to nocturia, according to Dr. Hsu.

On the other hand, relatively few women in the study were actually bothered by their nighttime trips to the bathroom. Only one-quarter said they were at least "moderately" bothered.

SHOULD YOU PAY ATTENTION TO NOCTURIA?

So is nocturia only an issue if it "bothers" you?

"That's a good question," Dr. Hsu said. "If it really doesn't bother you, and you're able to go right back to sleep, then it may not be a problem."

That's especially true, she noted, if you can attribute the nocturia to something benign—like drinking liquids close to bedtime.

However, Dr. Townsend said nocturia can be a symptom of certain health conditions that boost the body's urine production, like diabetes or heart failure. "So, there are still reasons to pay attention to nocturia, even if a woman isn't bothered by it," she said.

Nocturia can also be the result of certain conditions that disrupt sleep, Dr. Townsend said—including sleep apnea and restless legs syndrome.

Hip Replacements Fail More Often in Women

Although the risk of total hip-replacement failure is low, women are 29% more likely than men to need repeat surgery within three years.

Reasons for the failures: Women need prosthetic hips with a smaller-sized femoral head—the rounded ball end of the femur (thighbone)—but a smaller femoral head is more likely to dislocate. Because of differences in anatomy, women's prosthetic hips also are implanted at an angle that is different from men's.

If you need a hip replacement: Ask your surgeon what type of implant you are going to receive. Failure is less common with metal-on-polyethylene or ceramic-on-polyethylene implants than with metal-on-metal implants.

Study of 35,000 people by researchers at Icahn School of Medicine at Mount Sinai, New York City, published in *The Journal of the American Medical Association*.

Weight-Loss Surgery Helps Incontinence

Weight-loss surgery improves urinary incontinence. Of the obese women in a weight-loss program who had urinary incontinence prior to surgery, about two-thirds reported that their incontinence symptoms had improved or disappeared after weight-loss surgery. Other studies have shown that weight loss reduces incontinence because less weight is pressing on the bladder.

Study of 1,565 women by researchers at University of California San Francisco School of Medicine.

encouraged to talk to their health care provider," Dr. Townsend said.

TREATMENT FOR NOCTURIA

Treatment for nocturia might include tackling the underlying cause—such as untreated diabetes—or simple lifestyle changes or pelvic floor physical therapy. And if necessary, Dr. Hsu said, there are medications that can help regulate urine production or calm an overactive bladder.

"I think women should be aware that this condition is common, and not something to be embarrassed about," Dr. Hsu said. "You're not alone."

Two of Hsu's coauthors on the study have received research funding from companies that make drugs for urinary tract disorders.

info The Bladder and Bowel Foundation has more information on nocturia at *http://www.bladderandbowelfoundation.org/bladder/bladder-problems/nocturia.asp*.

Even if nocturia is a woman's only symptom, it can still be significant. "We know that nocturia can lead to lower sleep quality," Dr. Townsend said. "Poor sleep can negatively affect your mood or daytime functioning, including your productivity at work."

And for older women, she noted, getting up at night could lead to a fall and potentially serious injury.

"So women with nocturia—especially those whose symptoms are affecting their mood or ability to function during the day—should be

Index